Sustainable Agriculture Reviews

Volume 49

Series Editor
Eric Lichtfouse
CNRS, IRD, INRAE, Coll France, CEREGE
Aix-Marseille University
Aix-en-Provence, France

Other Publications by Dr. Eric Lichtfouse

Books
Scientific Writing for Impact Factor Journals
https://www.novapublishers.com/catalog/product_info.php?products_id=42242

Environmental Chemistry
http://www.springer.com/978-3-540-22860-8

Sustainable Agriculture
Volume 1: http://www.springer.com/978-90-481-2665-1
Volume 2: http://www.springer.com/978-94-007-0393-3

Book series
Environmental Chemistry for a Sustainable World
http://www.springer.com/series/11480

Sustainable Agriculture Reviews
http://www.springer.com/series/8380

Journal
Environmental Chemistry Letters
http://www.springer.com/10311

Sustainable agriculture is a rapidly growing field aiming at producing food and energy in a sustainable way for humans and their children. Sustainable agriculture is a discipline that addresses current issues such as climate change, increasing food and fuel prices, poor-nation starvation, rich-nation obesity, water pollution, soil erosion, fertility loss, pest control, and biodiversity depletion.

Novel, environmentally-friendly solutions are proposed based on integrated knowledge from sciences as diverse as agronomy, soil science, molecular biology, chemistry, toxicology, ecology, economy, and social sciences. Indeed, sustainable agriculture decipher mechanisms of processes that occur from the molecular level to the farming system to the global level at time scales ranging from seconds to centuries. For that, scientists use the system approach that involves studying components and interactions of a whole system to address scientific, economic and social issues. In that respect, sustainable agriculture is not a classical, narrow science. Instead of solving problems using the classical painkiller approach that treats only negative impacts, sustainable agriculture treats problem sources.

Because most actual society issues are now intertwined, global, and fast-developing, sustainable agriculture will bring solutions to build a safer world. This book series gathers review articles that analyze current agricultural issues and knowledge, then propose alternative solutions. It will therefore help all scientists, decision-makers, professors, farmers and politicians who wish to build a safe agriculture, energy and food system for future generations.

More information about this series at http://www.springer.com/series/8380

Harsh Panwar • Chetan Sharma • Eric Lichtfouse
Editors

Sustainable Agriculture Reviews 49

Mitigation of Antimicrobial Resistance Vol 2. Natural and Synthetic Approaches

Springer

Editors
Harsh Panwar
Department of Dairy Microbiology
Guru Angad Dev Veterinary and Animal Sciences University
Ludhiana, India

Chetan Sharma
Alpine Biomedicals Pvt. Ltd.
Ambala, India

Eric Lichtfouse
Aix-Marseille University, CNRS, IRD, INRAE, Coll France, CEREGE
Aix-en-Provence, France

ISSN 2210-4410 ISSN 2210-4429 (electronic)
Sustainable Agriculture Reviews
ISBN 978-3-030-58258-6 ISBN 978-3-030-58259-3 (eBook)
https://doi.org/10.1007/978-3-030-58259-3

This Springer imprint is published by the registered company Springer Nature Switzerland AG
The registered company address is: Gewerbestrasse 11, 6330 Cham, Switzerland

Preface

> Widespread use of antibiotics promotes the spread of antibiotic resistance. Smart use of antibiotics is the key to controlling its spread.
>
> A. P. J. Abdul Kalam

Antibiotics have drastically improved the health and life expectancy of humans, yet the abrupt increase of antibiotic usage for animals, agriculture and healthcare has induced antimicrobial resistance. Antimicrobial resistance is a global issue challenging the existence of human beings because the number of antimicrobial drugs is very limited. Antimicrobial resistance is leading to resurgence of deadly infectious diseases. The golden era of antibiotics is nearly over due to the emergence of multidrug-resistant bacteria, and as more antibiotics are rendered ineffective. Focus should therefore be shifted toward alternative therapies for treating infections. Here, recent advances in biotechnology, genetic engineering, and synthetic chemistry have opened up new avenues toward the search for advanced therapies. Alternative options do not replace antibiotics but increase the efficacy of antibiotics with alternative techniques and approaches. This book is our second volume on the mitigation of antimicrobial resistance, focusing on natural and synthetic approaches. Chapters present emerging strategies to combat antimicrobial resistance.

Chapter 1 by Valsamatzi-Panagiotou et al. presents an overview of different strategies for prevention and containment of antimicrobial resistance including guidelines of antibiotic stewardship. This chapter also discusses risk factors, mechanisms behind resistance development, and spread. Chapter 2 by Elshaghabee and Rokana describes the potential of probiotics, prebiotics, and synbiotics for the management of antimicrobial resistance. These dietary approaches are often used as prophylactic, yet they can also reduce or even replace the use of antibiotics in some cases. Indeed, co-administration of probiotics and synbiotics with antibiotics can dilute the selective pressure of antibiotics and, in turn, minimize drug resistance.

Chapter 3 by Ng et al. focuses on the potency of various plant-derived antibacterial compounds with focus on flavonoids, phenolic acids, peptides, essential oils, and honey. Those compounds appear both as alternatives to conventional antibiotics and as candidates for combination therapy. Further, Chap. 4 by Varijakzhan et al. details the antimicrobial activity of plant essential oils, which are effective against various pathogens. This chapter discusses the effect of essential oils on the genomes and proteomes of treated microorganisms. To minimize environmental toxicity, research is focusing on low molecular weight polymers with antimicrobial properties and on their applications. On this line, Chap. 5 by Grigoras summarizes the synthesis of quaternary ammonium compounds based on natural and synthetic polymers such as cellulose, chitosan, dextran, pullulan, starch, cashew gum, polylactide, polyamidoamine, polyurethane, polysiloxane, and polymethacrylate. These quaternary ammonium-containing polymers specifically interfere with the metabolism of a wide range of bacteria and fungi.

Chapter 6 by Mishra et al. presents nanomaterials as promising antimicrobials against multidrug-resistant pathogens. The antimicrobial efficacy of nanomaterials can be enhanced along with reduced cytotoxicity, which is explained by their small size, easy penetration to the target cell, and biocompatibility nature. The synthesis, mode of action, and delivery of metallic and nonmetallic nanoparticles are presented. Chapter 7 by Weeks et al. discusses antimicrobial peptides as the next-generation of antimicrobial drugs, with focus on synthesis, classification, properties, antimicrobial efficacy, and clinical applications. Pathogenic microorganisms need iron. In Chap. 8 Holbein et al. use iron chelators (Fig. 1) such as siderophores to restrict iron availability and thus starve pathogens.

Chapter 9 by Premaratne et al. explains that phages can replace or supplement antibiotics in agriculture to control pathogens. Chapter 10 by Jansen et al. focuses on vaccines to fight antimicrobial resistance. Several licensed vaccines for bacteria and virus have already reduced antibiotic consumption and resistance by promoting herd immunity, thereby protecting even segments in population that have not been or cannot be vaccinated.

This book is written by highly qualified scientists working on antimicrobial resistance. The editors are grateful to all the contributors for their enthusiasm and cooperation during the book compilation, review, and revision process. We also

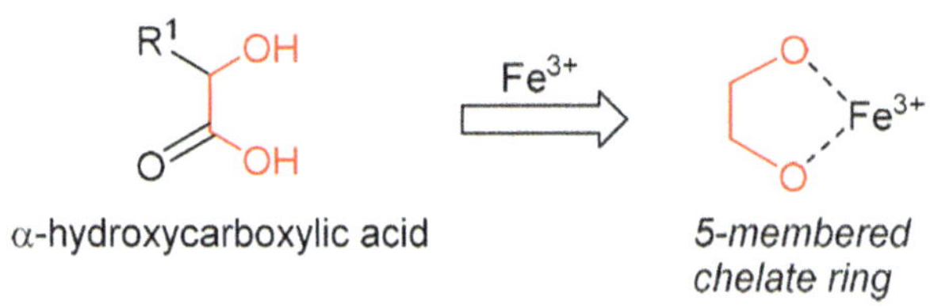

Fig. 1 A siderophore group (left) is able to chelate iron and, in turn, restricts the availability of iron to microbial pathogens. (From Chap. 8 by Holbein et al.)

thank our reviewers for their constructive advice. We also extend our thanks to the Springer Nature team for their cooperation right from acceptance of proposal to the production of this book. This book is aimed at scientists, researchers, and other professionals and is an invaluable and timely review on current research on strategies to abate antimicrobial resistance and is an essential acquisition for anyone involved in this area of biology.

Ludhiana, India Harsh Panwar

Ambala, India Chetan Sharma

Aix-en-Provence, France Eric Lichtfouse

Contents

About the Editors

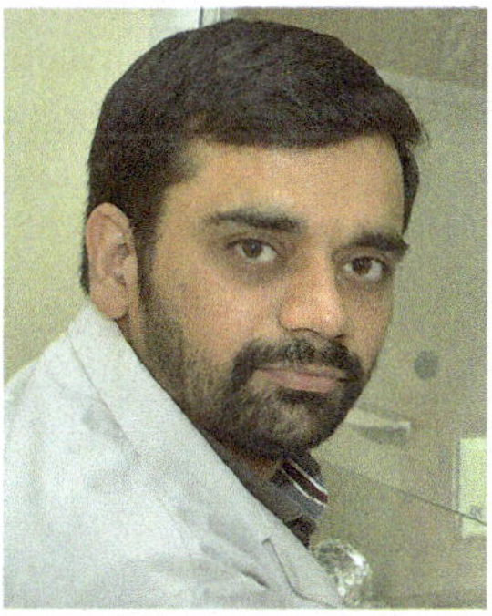

Harsh Panwar is currently Assistant Professor in Dairy Microbiology at Guru Angad Dev Veterinary and Animal Sciences University, India. His research interests include antimicrobial resistance and its mitigation in dairy and food. Dr. Panwar has published more than 40 articles in high-impact journals. He has been awarded Young Scientist Award 2019 by the Association of Microbiologists of India; Indo-Australian Career Boosting Gold Fellowship 2018–19 by Department of Biotechnology, Government of India; Best Teacher 2019 and Best Researcher 2018 Award by Guru Anagd Dev Veterinary and Animal Sciences University; DST Inspire Fellowship by Department of Science and Technology, Government of India; Commonwealth Scholarship by Commonwealth Scholarship Commission, UK; and University Gold Medal by Kurukshetra University Kurukshetra.

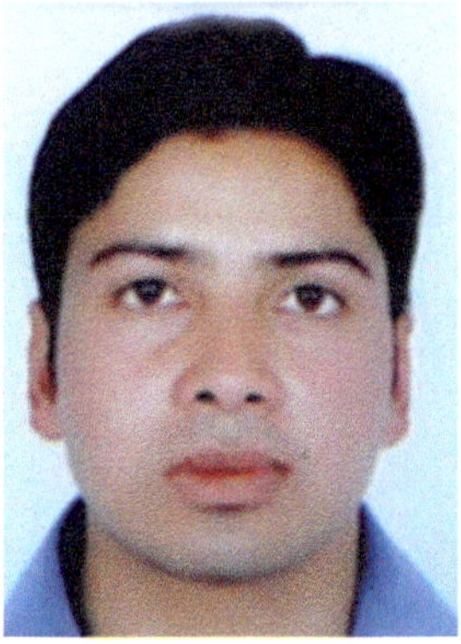

Chetan Sharma is working as a Research Advisor at Alpine Biomedicals Pvt. Ltd. Haryana, India. He has completed his M.Sc. and Ph.D. in Microbiology from Department of Microbiology, Kurukshetra University, Kurukshetra. He has published several research papers of international repute and serves as a reviewer for different journals. He has also edited and published one book by Nova Science Publishers, USA and two books from Springer Nature. His present research interest covers isolation of bioactive compounds from natural sources (plants), medical microbiology, antimicrobial resistance and probiotics.

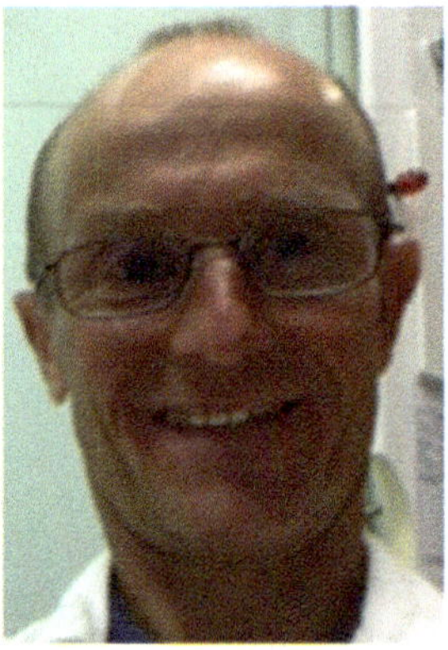

Eric Lichtfouse is Professor at the University of Aix-Marseille University, France, and at Xi'an Jioatong University, China, and Chief Editor of Environmental Chemistry Letters. He has invented carbon-13 dating and discovered temporal pool of individual substances in environmental media. He is teaching scientific writing and environmental chemistry. He has published the book Scientific Writing for Impact Factors. He has awards in analytical chemistry and editing. He is also XTerra Vice-Champion.

Contributors

Riaz Akseer Division of Health Sciences, Abu Dhabi Women's College, Higher Colleges of Technology, Abu Dhabi, United Arab Emirates

Ammar Algburi Health Promoting Naturals Laboratory, School of Environmental and Biological Sciences, Rutgers State University, New Brunswick, NJ, USA

Department of Biotechnology, Science College, Diyala University, Baqubah, Iraq

Maryam Sultan Alhosani Division of Health Sciences, Abu Dhabi Women's College, Higher Colleges of Technology, Abu Dhabi, United Arab Emirates

David S. Allan Chelation Partners Inc., The Labs at Innovacorp, Life Sciences Research Institute, Halifax, NS, Canada

Annaliesa S. Anderson Pfizer Vaccine Research and Development, Pearl River, NY, USA

M. Trisha C. Ang Chelation Partners Inc., The Labs at Innovacorp, Life Sciences Research Institute, Halifax, NS, Canada

Craig Billington Institute of Environmental Science and Research, Christchurch, New Zealand

Tsun-Thai Chai Department of Chemical Science, Faculty of Science, Universiti Tunku Abdul Rahman, Jalan Universiti, Kampar, Malaysia

Wangxue Chen Human Health Therapeutics Research Center, National Research Council Canada, Ottawa, ON, Canada

Michael Chikindas Health Promoting Naturals Laboratory, School of Environmental and Biological Sciences, Rutgers State University, New Brunswick, NJ, USA

Don State Technical University, Rostov-on-Don, Russia

Nalini Chinivasagam Queensland Department of Agriculture and Fisheries, Brisbane, Australia

Chou Min Chong Aquatic Animal Health and Therapeutics Laboratory, Institute of Bioscience, Universiti Putra Malaysia, Serdang, Selangor, Malaysia

Kah-Yaw Ee Department of Agricultural and Food Science, Faculty of Science, Universiti Tunku Abdul Rahman, Jalan Universiti, Kampar, Malaysia

Fouad M. F. Elshaghabee Department of Dairy Science, Faculty of Agriculture, Cairo University, Giza, Egypt

Anca Giorgiana Grigoras "Petru Poni" Institute of Macromolecular Chemistry, Iasi, Romania

William C. Gruber Pfizer Vaccine Research and Development, Pearl River, NY, USA

Bruce E. Holbein Chelation Partners Inc., The Labs at Innovacorp, Life Sciences Research Institute, Halifax, NS, Canada

Department of Microbiology and Immunology, Dalhousie University, Halifax, NS, Canada

Kathrin U. Jansen Pfizer Vaccine Research and Development, Pearl River, NY, USA

Kok Song Lai Division of Health Sciences, Abu Dhabi Women's College, Higher Colleges of Technology, Abu Dhabi, United Arab Emirates

Christian Lehmann Department of Microbiology and Immunology, Dalhousie University, Halifax, NS, Canada

Department of Anesthesia, Pain Management and Perioperative Medicine, Dalhousie University, Halifax, NS, Canada

Swee Hua Erin Lim Perdana University – Royal College of Surgeons in Ireland, Serdang, Selangor, Malaysia

Division of Health Sciences, Abu Dhabi Women's College, Higher Colleges of Technology, Abu Dhabi, United Arab Emirates

Mitali Mishra School of Biological Sciences, National Institute of Science Education and Research – Bhubaneswar, Jatni, Odisha, India

Homi Bhabha National Institute, Anushakti Nagar, Mumbai, Maharashtra, India

Harapriya Mohapatra School of Biological Sciences, National Institute of Science Education and Research – Bhubaneswar, Jatni, Odisha, India,

Homi Bhabha National Institute, Anushakti Nagar, Mumbai, Maharashtra, India

Wen-Jie Ng Department of Allied Health Sciences, Faculty of Science, Universiti Tunku Abdul Rahman, Jalan Universiti, Kampar, Malaysia

Shashank Patole School of Biological Sciences, National Institute of Science Education and Research – Bhubaneswar, Jatni, Odisha, India

Homi Bhabha National Institute, Anushakti Nagar, Mumbai, Maharashtra, India

Robert Penchovsky Department of Genetics, Faculty of Biology, Sofia University "St. Kliment Ohridski", Sofia, Bulgaria

Katya B. Popova Department of Genetics, Faculty of Biology, Sofia University "St. Kliment Ohridski", Sofia, Bulgaria

Aruni Premaratne Institute of Environmental Science and Research, Christchurch, New Zealand

Namita Rokana College of Dairy Science and Technology, Guru Angad Dev Veterinary and Animal Sciences University, Ludhiana, Punjab, India

Chong-Seng Shit Department of Biological Science, Faculty of Science, Universiti Tunku Abdul Rahman, Jalan Universiti, Kampar, Malaysia

Raphael Simon Pfizer Vaccine Research and Development, Pearl River, NY, USA

Warren Thomas Perdana University – Royal College of Surgeons in Ireland, Serdang, Selangor, Malaysia

Aikaterini Valsamatzi-Panagiotou Department of Genetics, Faculty of Biology, Sofia University "St. Kliment Ohridski", Sofia, Bulgaria

Disha Varijakzhan Aquatic Animal Health and Therapeutics Laboratory, Institute of Bioscience, Universiti Putra Malaysia, Serdang, Selangor, Malaysia

Perdana University – Royal College of Surgeons in Ireland, Serdang, Selangor, Malaysia

Ran Wang Jiangsu Academy of Agricultural Sciences, Nanjing, China

James Wassil Pfizer Patient and Health Impact, Collegeville, PA, USA

Present Address: Vaxcyte, Foster City, CA, USA

Richard Weeks Health Promoting Naturals Laboratory, School of Environmental and Biological Sciences, Rutgers State University, New Brunswick, NJ, USA

Shun-Kai Yang Division of Health Sciences, Abu Dhabi Women's College, Higher Colleges of Technology, Abu Dhabi, United Arab Emirates

Hui Zhang Jiangsu Academy of Agricultural Sciences, Nanjing, China

Chapter 1
Strategies for Prevention and Containment of Antimicrobial Resistance

Aikaterini Valsamatzi-Panagiotou, Katya B. Popova, and Robert Penchovsky

Abstract The World Health Organization believes that there were about 480,000 cases of multi drug resistant tuberculosis in 2014 only. In addition, extensively drug resistant tuberculosis was identified in 105 countries during the same year. The methicillin resistant *Staphylococcus aureus* is a widespread cause of severe infections in health facilities and the community worldwide. In this book chapter, we discuss all important strategies for the prevention and containment of antimicrobial resistance, which is a growing problem for healthcare systems around the world. Here we discuss the risk factors and mechanisms of development and ways of spreading of antimicrobial resistance. We focus our attention on various strategies for the prevention of the emergence of antimicrobial resistance *via* the reduction of selective pressure on the pathogenic bacteria.

The risk factors for the development of antibacterial drug resistance are well understood and they have to be mitigated worldwide. The chapter also presents different strategies for containment of widespread infection with antibacterial drug resistant bacteria, including internationally recognized guidelines of antibiotic stewardship. The presented broad scientific area of prevention of antimicrobial resistance would be of interest to both researchers and physicians working or interested in these fields. In addition, we discuss some novel approaches that can be employed to develop new antibiotics against extensively drug resistant microbes. For instance, antisense oligonucleotide technology offers some advantages for antibacterial drug development including fast and comprehensive procedures for drug design.

Keywords Development of antibacterial resistance · Spread of antibacterial resistance · Strategies for prevention of antibacterial resistance · Containment of antibacterial resistance · Antibiotic stewardship

---

A. Valsamatzi-Panagiotou · K. B. Popova · R. Penchovsky (✉)
Department of Genetics, Faculty of Biology, Sofia University "St. Kliment Ohridski", Sofia, Bulgaria

H. Panwar et al. (eds.), *Sustainable Agriculture Reviews 49*, Sustainable Agriculture Reviews 49, https://doi.org/10.1007/978-3-030-58259-3_1

1.1 Introduction

The development of antimicrobial resistance is a worldwide threat that is related to the ability of microorganisms to grow in the presence of an antibiotic(s) that previously inhibited their growth (Allcock et al. 2017; Jampilek 2018). The emergence of antimicrobial resistance is not a new phenomenon although over the last few decades it has accelerated by the overuse along with the misuse of antibiotics in both humans and animals (Fig. 1.1). Antimicrobial resistance can be found not only in hospital units but also at the community level. Due to the ability of bacteria to travel, the crisis worsens because antimicrobial resistance genes are spread among many human pathogenic bacteria. Thus, antimicrobial resistance development constitutes a global issue. The inadequate or lack of methods of prevention and containment also contribute to the emergence of antimicrobial resistance.

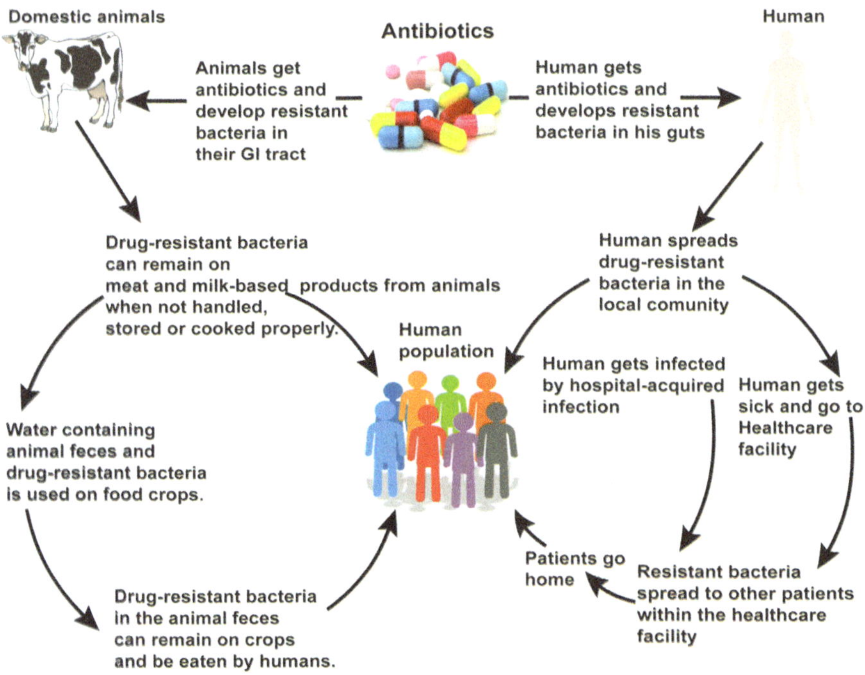

Fig. 1.1 Various ways of the spread of antibiotic resistance in the general human population. According to some studies, previous exposure to antibiotics has a chronicle relation to the development of antimicrobial resistance. For instance, it is reported that individuals who had direct exposure to an antibiotic in the last months seem to have an increased probability to carry a resistant organism (Aiello and Larson 2003). However, exposure to antibiotics sometimes may be involuntary. This is due to the fact that there is extensive use of antibiotics in agriculture, aquaculture, and food animals thus, antibiotics end up in humans through the food chain which may have a significant effect on antimicrobial resistance development (Levy 2014; McEwen and Fedorka-Cray 2002)

In the twenty-first century, antimicrobial resistance is considered to be one of the most serious global public health threats. It should be mentioned that some diseases which were previously thought to be controlled or even eradicated with the use of various antibiotics have returned and they even show resistance to the previously successful therapies. Antimicrobials are very important category of drugs and their use played a crucial role in the decrease of infectious diseases. Especially, at the beginning of the 1900s, their use improved spectacularly patient care. Presently they are considered one of the most successful categories of existing drugs. Indeed, they constitute the primary anti infective drugs that can be administered in intensive care unit patients with known or suspected multi drug resistant bacteria. Nevertheless, the development of multi drug resistance complicates the treatment of infections due to the emergence and spread of organisms that are resistant to antimicrobials. Moreover, multi drug resistance often leads to treatment failures, long term hospitalizations, alternation of the microbiome, and higher severity of infections. Therefore, it contributes to economic and health losses worldwide because more expensive therapies are used to fight resistance and there is an increase in morbidity and mortality rates (Allcock et al. 2017; Bassetti et al. 2017; Fishman 2006; Levy and Marshall 2004; Okeke et al. 2005; Septimus 2018).

In comparison to the past, the number of newly approved antibiotics has decreased dramatically. This highlights the vital need to preserve the antibiotics which already exist for the next generations (Garau et al. 2014). It is also of great importance to focus on strategies for the prevention and containment of bacterial infections. The misuse of antibiotics is related to antimicrobial resistance and multi drug resistance development. Therefore, a reduction in antibiotic use will be followed by a decrease in the emergence of antimicrobial resistance.

Concerted actions are needed to prevent the emergence of new resistant strains and the spread of those which already exist (Okeke et al. 2005). In an effort to strengthen national plans and to promote international collaboration with the main purpose of the containment of antimicrobial resistance and multi drug resistant human pathogenic bacteria, the World Health Organization (WHO) created the resolution WHA67.25 called 'Combating antimicrobial resistance including antibiotic resistance (Mendelson and Matsoso 2014). An integrated model was developed, which comprises three intertwined programs and it is called antimicrobial, infection prevention, and diagnostic (Hughes and Andersson) stewardship model. The model focuses on the creation of a personalized management plan, which aims in the improvement of patient's health and the decrease in the emergence of antimicrobial resistance and multidrug resistant bacterial strains. Actually, national and international collaboration is required to achieve the holistic management of antimicrobial resistance. Eventually, a combination of various strategies and methods should be implemented in a multidisciplinary approach to tackle the emergence of antimicrobial resistance and multi drug resistance (Dik et al. 2016).

1.2 Risk Factors for the Development of Antibacterial Drug Resistance

The antimicrobial resistance is known from the discovery of the first antibiotics and is considered to be a Darwinian response of bacteria to selective pressure provoked by an antibacterial agent (Mendelson and Matsoso 2014; Penchovsky and Traykovska 2015). The exposure to antibiotics, as well as the ingestion of food treated with antibiotics, are closely associated with selective pressure. Antimicrobial resistance is related to antibiotic consumption on a global scale and it is mostly observed in countries where antibiotic use has increased such as the USA and southern countries of Europe, where antimicrobial resistance is considerably higher in comparison with countries with lower consumption of antibiotics in northern Europe (Garau et al. 2014). Some factors which contribute to the spread of pathogenic organisms worldwide are the aging of the population globally, the urbanization, traveling of the population, and climate changes (Bloom et al. 2017).

Antibiotics are one of the most used and, at the same time, the most successful categories of drugs that have managed to decrease infectious diseases and render possible some complex interventions in medicine such as advanced surgery and organ transplantation (Allcock et al. 2017; Wright 2011). Their discovery led to the eradication of many infectious diseases, which were previously thought to be fatal, and there was a conviction among many physicians that these infections will never appear again. This was a miscalculation because the antimicrobial resistance and multi drug resistance impede many established antibacterial therapies (Jansen et al. 2006).

The rapid development of antimicrobial resistance and multi drug resistance constitutes a very alarming issue for human health because it leads to huge health and economic losses worldwide (Okeke et al. 2005; Tagliabue and Rappuoli 2018). The treatment of infections with multi drug resistant bacteria may be delayed due to the time needed to confirm the resistance pattern. The worst scenario is the treatment failure, which leads to an increment in the transmission potential of infections due to the ability of the resistant organism to survive in the host. This also leads to alteration of microbial ecology and as a result, more severe infections with multi drug resistant organisms appear. The change in susceptibility of microbial flora due to the use of hygienic and cleaning regimens should also be mentioned as a contributing factor for antimicrobial resistance development (Aiello and Larson 2003).

Some other risk factors which are pointed as a reason for the development of antimicrobial resistance and multi drug resistance, are the overuse of antibiotics in agriculture, in aquaculture, and in the food industry. Especially, it is reported that annually millions of kilograms of antimicrobials were used for prophylaxis around the world (Levy and Marshall 2004). Sub-therapeutic doses of antibiotics were used as growth promoters in the European Union (EU) until 2006, however, their use still continues both in America and Asia. The use of medically important antibiotics in food animals in the United States is almost 80% (Fig. 1.1), according to an extensive study of researchers from the Center for Disease Dynamics, Economics & Policy

(USA), Princeton Environmental Institute, Princeton University (USA); Institute of Integrative Biology, ETH Zurich (Switzerland); the Université Libre de Bruxelles (Belgium); and the Food and Agriculture Organization of the United Nations (Italy) (Van Boeckel et al. 2017). Meanwhile, the estimated quantity of used antibiotics in China for 2013 in animals was 78,200 tons. The World Health Organization alarms that such unrestrained quantity will lead to the rise of the antibiotic use globally until 2030 and would hinder the efforts toward conserving the efficacy of the current antibiotics. The analysis report for the global progress of antimicrobial resistance for 2017 showed that "*only 64 countries (41.6%) have limited the use of critically important antimicrobials (human and animal) for growth promotion in agriculture*" (World Health Organization 2018; Allcock et al. 2017).

The exponential rise in the income of people living in developing countries renders access to health care facilities easier as compared to the past and leads to an increase in the use of antibiotics. The existence of counterfeit drugs is another problem that plagues developing countries. These drugs might have expired, contain a different dose of the active substance or may have different pharmacokinetics and pharmacodynamics in comparison with the drugs available in developed countries (Selgelid 2007). Some other factors which seem to contribute to the development of antimicrobial resistance globally are the use of a narrow repertoire and poor quality of antimicrobials (Okeke et al. 2005). The abuse of antibiotics plays an important role in antimicrobial resistance development. Some patients do not manage to comply with the instructions of the physician about the duration and the dose of the treatment. Thus, they fail to complete their treatment plan. Another scenario, which is very common, is the use of the leftovers of the pills as self-medication without visiting or taking advice from a physician. This may also promote the development of resistance (Selgelid 2007). It is believed that the increased rate of immunocompromised patients is another fact that is associated with antimicrobial resistance development (Aiello and Larson 2003).

Guidelines for proper antibiotic use in hospital patients, as well as outpatients exist; although sometimes they are not followed properly. This may be attributed to the fact that physicians are afraid of surgical site infections, which leads to the prescription of antibiotics for prophylaxis. At the same time, the lack of diagnostic tools in primary health care may lead to the prescription of antibiotics as empiric therapy. Due to the diagnostic uncertainty, physicians prescribe antibiotics based on the anamnesis of the symptoms, clinical symptoms, and characteristics of the patient. This may finally prove to be wrong due to the lack of confirmation of a bacterial pathogen with a microbiological examination which means that a viral infection sometimes may be mistreated with antimicrobials as it was a bacterial one (Garau et al. 2014).

However, even if the diagnostic tools are available in health care units, the time which is required to confirm the pathogen in combination with patients' demand to be treated as soon as possible may lead to the improper prescription of antibiotics. Another problem is the physician's fear of litigation in cases where they do not prescribe an antibiotic, which might help. Especially, in cases when there is a debate if an antibiotic may slightly or even not at all improve the condition of the patient.

In such circumstances, physicians should think the risk-benefit optimization not only for the individual itself but for the society as a whole. Dilemmas like this are a matter of concern in both hospitals and community settings. It must be pointed out that the improper management of such cases is associated with the development of antimicrobial resistance due to antibiotic misuse. The advertisements of pharmaceutical companies of the newest, most expensive and profitable drugs, which target both physicians and patients create a great problem and seems to contribute to antimicrobial resistance emergence due to the increased demand and pressure of patients who force their physicians to be treated with specific drugs as a result of advertising (Selgelid 2007).

Some basic reasons, which contribute to the dissemination of antimicrobial resistant organisms in healthcare units, are inadequate infection control, shortfalls in hygiene and sanitation along with the lack of proper education and surveillance programs. Bacteria can acquire resistance through the horizontal transfer of genes for resistant traits between them. This is achieved through the help of some genetic elements as bacteriophages, plasmids, transposons, and others. However, antimicrobial resistance may also be intrinsic, which is a result of natural evolutionary processes. Finally, clinical antimicrobial resistance may occur due to therapeutic failure, which may be attributed to the pharmacokinetics of some drugs or interactions among drugs. Acquired antimicrobial resistance is considered the most serious in comparison to inherited and clinical resistance (Hayes and Wolf 1990; Jampilek 2018; Munita and Arias 2016; Okeke et al. 2005; Tenover 2006).

1.3 Ways of the Spread of Antibiotic Resistance

There are many ways by which an individual can be colonized with antimicrobial resistant bacteria (Fig. 1.1). One way is through person-to-person transmission and another way is through direct exposure to an antibiotic through selective pressure. Crowded environments and health care facilities as child care centers are some of the most favorable environments for person-to-person transmission of antibiotic resistant organisms. More specifically in child care centers, the use of broad spectrum antibiotics against resistant organisms or recurrent infections is blamed for antimicrobial resistance development. *Streptococcus pneumoniae* and methicillin resistant *Staphylococcus aureus* (MRSA) are common in child care centers. Especially, it is reported that MRSA has been isolated from children hospitalized in child care centers who did not have any contact with MRSA in a health care center and did not have carriers at home. Penicillin resistant *pneumococci* have also been isolated from some military populations (Fairchok et al. 1996; Hudspeth et al. 2001; Murphy et al. 1996).

In household settings, the use of antibiotics from one family member may lead to antimicrobial resistance in other members of the family. Nonetheless, with the use of methods as cleaning and disinfection, the spreading of antimicrobial resistance microorganisms may be inhibited. Microorganisms are capable to cause cross-contamination if they survive in a home environment. This indicates the great need for the implementation of more researches within the home environment about the sources and routes for transmission of antimicrobial resistance organisms (Aiello and Larson 2003; Kagan et al. 2002; Rydberg and Cederberg 1986).

It is believed that some cleaning and hygienic products may also cause pressure on organisms to develop resistance. The mechanism of action of antibiotics involves some specific targets within the bacterial cell while the mechanism of action of cleaning and hygienic products was thought to involve multiple targets. Cleaning and hygienic products act by degradation and inhibition of the bacteria (White and McDermott 2001). Indeed, alcohols which are used for many years do not have a specific target. However, it was proven that another substance called triclosan, which was used widely in hygienic and cleaning products, acts like some antibiotics by inhibiting the bacterial fatty acid biosynthetic pathway (Chuanchuen et al. 2001; McMurry et al. 1998). Actually, at first, triclosan was discovered and used as an herbicide. Because of its antimicrobial properties, especially in combination with some antiviral and antifungal properties, it started to be used in personal hygienic products, as an ingredient in surgical scrubs, in hand soaps afterward. Unfortunately, it was proved that triclosan inhibits bacteria by having a specific bacterial target. Researches have shown that the use of triclosan is associated with cross-resistance development to clinically relevant antibiotics (Chuanchuen et al. 2001, 2002; Levy 2000, 2001, 2002, Perencevich et al. 2001).

1.4 Major Mechanisms of Development of Antibacterial Drug Resistance

The understanding of the mechanisms of development of antimicrobial resistance has been a subject of great concern. It is believed that the existence of huge bacterial populations and the increment in mutation rates contribute to the rapid evolution of antimicrobial resistance. It is of great importance to know the mechanisms of drug action to understand the sophisticated mechanisms through which bacteria develop antimicrobial resistance (Blair et al. 2015; Hayes and Wolf 1990; Hermsen et al. 2012; Jampilek 2018; Munita and Arias 2016). We should bear in mind that antimicrobial resistance may complicate the treatment of any infection no matter its severity (Kaku et al. 2014; Thampi et al. 2015).

Multiple biochemical routes are used in the classification of the mechanisms of antimicrobial resistance. There are four main mechanisms by which antimicrobial resistance can develop: (i) Modification of the antibiotic molecule that involves inactivation or destruction of the drug. This is achieved with the help of some specific enzymes which are produced by bacteria; (ii) Decrease of antibiotic penetration or efflux. If there is a decrease in the permeability of the membrane, antibiotics will render unable to cross this barrier. In the case of the efflux pumps, there is either overexpression of a pump due to a mutation or a drug is extracted out of the cell

Table 1.1 Mechanisms of drug resistance against antibiotics

Classes of antibiotic	Antibiotics	Mechanisms(s) of resistance
Aminoglycosides	Gentamicin, Streptomycin, Spectinomycin	Phosphorylation, acetylation, nucleotidylation, efflux, altered target
Cationic Peptides	Colistin	Altered target, efflux
Glycopeptides	Vancomycin, Teicoplanin	Reprogramming peptidoglycan biosynthesis
Lipopeptides	Daptomycin	Altered target
Lincosamides	Clindamycin	Nucleotidylation, efflux, altered target
Macrolides	Erythromycin, Azithromycin	Hydrolysis, glycosylation, phosphorylation, efflux, altered target
Oxazolidinones	Linezolid	Efflux, altered target
Pyrimidines	Trimethoprim	Efflux, altered target
Phenicols	Chloramphenicol	Acetylation, efflux, altered target
β-lactams	Penicillins, Cephalosporins, Penems, Monobactams	Hydrolysis, efflux, altered target
Quinolones	Ciprofloxacin	Acetylation, efflux, altered target
Rifamycins	Rifampin	ADP-ribosylation, efflux, altered target
Streptogramins	Synercid	Carbon-Oxygen lyase, acetylation, efflux, altered target
Sulfonamides	Sulfamethoxazole	Efflux, altered target
Tetracyclines	Minocycline, Tigecycline	Monooxygenation, efflux, altered target

through some specific processes; (iii) Changes in the target site. It can be either protected or modified through mutations, enzymatic alterations, complete replacement, or bypass; and (iv) Resistance to global cell adaptations (Blair et al. 2015; Hayes and Wolf 1990; Kaku et al. 2014; Munita and Arias 2016; Piddock 2006; Wright 2011) (Table 1.1).

1.5 Strategies for Prevention of Antibacterial Drug Resistance and Reduction of Selective Pressure

1.5.1 Reduction of Selective Pressure

Several studies mention that selective pressure constitutes a vital reason for the development of antimicrobial resistance. The main cause is considered to be the overuse along with the misuse of antibiotics in daily life. The main mechanism of selective pressure concerns the contact of a bacterial population with an antibiotic which leads to the eradication of susceptible organisms. At the same time, the resistant organisms persist and are able to transmit their resistance coding genes either by vertical gene transfer or through horizontal gene transfer (Essack 2006; WHO 2001a). The first process is a natural evolutionary step that occurs when a parent cell transmits its DNA to the daughter cells. When a mutation for antibiotic resistance occurs, the resistant genes are transferred to their offspring by the process of replication. However, the horizontal transfer of resistant genes occurs between donor bacteria and recipient cells, which are not their offspring.

This is achieved by three mechanisms: transformation, transduction, and conjugation. Transformation is a process in which dead bacteria release exogenous DNA often and it is introduced into other bacteria. Meanwhile, transduction occurs when bacterial viruses, called bacteriophages, infect bacterial DNA. If the phage has incorporated resistance genes from the previous bacterium into its genome, it can transfer those genes into the newly infected bacterium. Unlike the previous two mechanisms, the conjugation requires direct cell-to-cell contact. It often involves a single-stranded plasmid DNA that is transferred from the donor cell through a bridge. Once the plasmid has passed to the recipient, both cells synthesize complementary strands and restore their plasmids (Griffiths et al. 2000).

Undoubtedly the environment plays an important role in the type and frequency of the antimicrobial resistance emergence (Singh et al. 1992). It is believed that sooner or later the use of any antibiotic will induce resistant bacteria. Actually, even nowadays, specific antimicrobial resistance is a growing problem of concern in healthcare worldwide. Therefore, due to the close correlation of antibiotic use to selective pressure, we should apply techniques that will manage to reduce antibiotic use internationally to affect selective pressure. Antibiotic policies should be applied to achieve their rational use. To make this possible, the creation of treatment algorithms and guidelines is necessary. It is suggested that if a bacterium, which is responsible for the infection, has been identified through microbiological procedures and if it is indicated, the type of antibiotics, are the narrow-spectrum antibiotics should be used at the beginning of the treatment. The route of application of an antibiotic, the optimal dose that will minimize selective pressure and the duration of the treatment is also very important. Every treatment plan must be adjusted to the characteristics of the patient. The physician should take into consideration the type and the site of infection, pharmacokinetics and pharmacodynamics, drug interactions, adverse drug reactions and the specific anatomical site where the concentration of the drug is higher (Essack 2006; Medeiros 1997; Pena et al. 1997).

The use of educational interventions both in developing and in developed countries is recommended in an effort to reduce selective pressure. Those interventions should focus on changing the prescribing behavior of physicians and promoting prescription requirement demands. If they fail to do this, they must be strengthened. There is a great need for continuing educational programs adjusted to medical students, resident doctors, doctors, pharmacists, pharmacy attendants, itinerant drug sellers, and other healthcare specialists. Focus group discussions and seminars are also very useful. Their main aim should be to inform physicians about the latest news on the field of antibiotics and to give them instructions for proper use because in their absence physicians will receive information mostly from pharmaceutical companies.

Actually, the information from pharmaceutical companies does not always keep up with rational drug use and the guidelines. The main reason is that the incentives of companies usually focus on economic profits. Some studies after the application of educational programs in developing countries reported that there was an improvement in diagnostic quality and a decrease in the pressure that physicians faced from patients to prescribe antibiotics. At the same time, it is thought that the unjustified prescription of antibiotics decreased due to the physician's extensive and continuing knowledge around the subject of antimicrobial resistance. Some other positive findings were the decrease of polypharmacy along with the cost savings due to a decrease in unnecessary antibiotic use (Adams et al. 2003; Bexell et al. 1996; Chuc et al. 2002; Gutierrez et al. 1994; Okeke et al. 2005; Ross-Degnan et al. 1996; Santoso et al. 1996).

The existence of an infectious disease consultant along with national standard treatment guidelines is of great importance in the health care units and it contributes to more efficient patient management and a decrease in the prescription of non-essential drugs. Nonetheless, better results are expected if educational programs are applied in combination with the interventions mentioned above. The first model list of essential drugs was established by the World Health Organization in 1977 when 120 countries followed the steps of the World Health Organization by the implementation of national essential drug lists. The last revision and update of the World Health Organization model list of essential medicines came in April 2019 at the meeting of the 22nd World Health Organization Expert Committee on the Selection and Use of Essential Medicines.

The main purpose of the creation of the first list was to promote the rational use of antibiotics and reassure the existence of an adequate number of antibiotics, which will be able to cover the needs of every country. Another aim was to increase the awareness of other countries to implement national drug lists, a goal that was achieved successfully. These lists should be continually revised according to the current news adjusted to the condition of every country (Ball et al. 2002; Bennadi 2013; Erbay et al. 2003; Kubin 2002; Laing et al. 2001; Okeke et al. 2005; Saez-Llorens et al. 2000; WHO 2002, 2015).

In a Nigerian teaching hospital, it was observed that although a national drug list existed, there were no educational programs for the physicians. So any decrease in prescriptions was not observed. This example highlights the importance of continuing educational interventions for both healthcare specialists and drug sellers. Moreover, the proper education of consumers is also crucial to understand the importance of their compliance in the physician's instructions for antibiotic use. In detail, the instructions about the duration and the dose of the treatment should be clear and followed strictly. There are many examples in which patients stop the antibiotics without completing the treatment plan that the physician suggested or self-administer drugs to themselves, friends, and family members from previous uncompleted courses that may have expired without consulting any physician. This is the so-called "self-medication". It is a common phenomenon nowadays. It may be attributed to some factors as inaccessibility of healthcare facilities and poverty in developing countries. Although it is also observed in high-income families and in patients with high education who have better access to healthcare facilities.

Patients must avoid self-medication because it seems to play an important role in antimicrobial resistance development. This highlights the importance of patient interventions including education and proper information from the healthcare workers, organizations, and governments. Interventions like these will also contribute to positive results in patient's adherence to medications. Except for the measures mentioned above, the existence of Pharmacy and Therapeutic Committees (PTCs) is recommended in hospital units in developed countries. Their presence seems to have a positive effect not only in monitoring but also in promoting the proper use of antibiotics. The financial capability of the patient to afford some or all the necessary medications prescribed should not be neglected. If a patient cannot afford the drugs, which the physician prescribed, this may lead to the use of unsuitable drugs, underdosing and drug counterfeiting. To avoid such circumstances, antimicrobials should be more available in certain situations. Indeed, there is a great need for national enforcement through legislation (Bavestrello et al. 2002; Harbarth et al. 2003; le Grand et al. 1999; Mabadeje et al. 1991; Okeke et al. 2005; Okeke and Lamikanra 2003; Parimi et al. 2002; Perez et al. 2003; Wayland 2004).

The implementation of some strategies, which focus on the proper antimicrobial use, can potentially lead to a reduction in the emergence of resistance *de novo*. It is widely known that there are a variety of mechanisms, which lead to the development of antimicrobial resistance. Before the beginning of the treatment, it is necessary to ensure that the antibiotics are of high quality. The appropriate dose of a drug along with the optimization of the distribution should be taken into consideration. There is evidence that the selection of antibiotic resistant mutants is related to the dose and the duration of the treatment. Different methods can be applied to avoid the development of antimicrobial resistance. Some of the methods which are reported are combination therapies, antimicrobial bacterial pairing, antimicrobial cycling, and the banning of monotherapy of partner drugs when they should be used in combination therapy (Drlica 2003; Okeke et al. 2005; Phillips-Howard et al. 2003).

It is proved that the consideration of pharmacokinetics and pharmacodynamics properties of the antibiotics are not only crucial in the areas of antibacterial efficacy but also are of vital importance for the prevention of antimicrobial resistance development. The usage of incorrect drug doses with a low resistance barrier promotes the development of antimicrobial resistance. The adaptation of dosing strategies based on the principles of pharmacokinetics and pharmacodynamics is also recommended by the Surviving Sepsis Campaign's (SSC) guidelines. There is a close relationship between dose and antimicrobial resistance development. Single and high antibiotic doses seem to prevent resistance in comparison with multiple low doses. However, more extent research is needed to find out that is the optimal dose that will be capable to treat the bacterial infection and reduce antimicrobial resistance development. The choice of the optimal drug dose is crucial for the outcome especially in intensive care units. There are some parameters for the assessment of the drug dose as Minimum inhibitory concentration (MIC) and Mutation prevention concentration (MPC) which were used in some studies based on dose related prevention of antibiotic resistance development. Apart from the dose of antibiotics, the site of infection, the pathogenic bacteria, and the duration of the treatment course are also important. Especially in self limiting infections, short therapies with antimicrobials are recommended (Barker 1999; Cui et al. 2006; de With et al. 2016; DeRyke et al. 2006; Geli et al. 2012; Markou et al. 2008; Olofsson and Cars 2007; Owens and Shorr 2009; Rhodes et al. 2017; Septimus 2018; Soothill et al. 2013; Zhu et al. 2012).

In recent years, the human microbiota which acts as a barrier against colonization has been researched intensively. Basically, its physiological mechanism of action is to protect the organism from colonization of pathogenic microorganisms and from the overgrowth of the microorganisms which are normally present in the human body – the so called "colonization resistance". There is a widespread belief that the use of antibiotics exerts a negative effect on microbiota and this may have detrimental consequences on human health. The exact mechanism by which antibiotics manage to affect microbiota is either by causing resistance or by damaging the "colonization resistance" which is protective for the organism. Actually, the damage of microbiota depends on its spectrum and some other parameters concerning drug distribution and excretion, the route of administration, the degree of absorption, and the route of elimination of the drug.

The antibiotics should be selected carefully before the start of the treatment in order to figure out if they exert harmful effects on the microbiota. The use of antibiotics, which do not disturb the microbiota, reduces the risk of resistance development, and spread. With the entrance of an antimicrobial drug in the organism, different concentrations gets distributed in different tissues and organs throughout the body. It is very important to choose the optimal route of administration of an antibiotic either oral or parenteral and to be aware of the way how antibiotic is excreted either in bile or through the kidneys in order to achieve the maximum effect. The presence of microbiota in a body site plays an important role in resistance development. In the sites where microbiota is found, the number of bacteria is usually large so if the concentration of an antimicrobial that is prescribed is low this may be related to the development of resistance (Guillemot et al. 1998; Gullberg et al. 2011; Rashid et al. 2012; Soothill et al. 2013; Zhao and Drlica 2001).

In everyday clinical practice, the use of combination therapy is very common. Especially, in the treatment of tuberculosis, multi drug regimens are used in order to prevent bacterial resistance development. Because antimicrobial resistance develops very easy, combination therapy is also used in the treatment of leprosy, human immunodeficiency virus (HIV) and cancer. The synergistic activity that some antibiotics exert when they are used in combination is another reason that renders this therapy important. A common example is bacterial endocarditis in which penicillin and gentamicin are the drugs combined and used successfully for treatment. It should be mentioned that in critically ill patients with unknown pathogens, there is a suspicion for septicemia, and therefore, broad spectrum therapy is needed to target as many as possible species of bacteria, which may be responsible for the condition. That is why in these cases several antimicrobials are used.

Another advantage of the combination therapy is its ability to target resistant bacteria. Augmentin is a combination of amoxicillin and clavulanic acid. Clavulanic acid is a beta-lactamase inhibitor while amoxicillin alone does not have the capability to act against beta-lactamase producing bacteria. In case of use of amoxicillin and augmentin against *Staphylococcus aureus* in patients diagnosed with non-bullous impetigo, *S. aureus* was resistant to amoxicillin and sensitive to the combination therapy with augmentin. Therefore, the use of augmentin broadens the spectrum of action. It seems that combination therapies can enhance the action of old antibiotics. Their application may also decrease the duration of the treatment and this depends on the abilities of the agents, which are added in the treatment course. For example, in *Mycobacterium tuberculosis* infections, the duration of the treatment was shortened after the addition of anti dormancy agents as pyrazinamide and rifampicin. However, before the choice of the treatment with a combination therapy we should bear in mind that there is a risk with the use of this method to create multi drug resistant organisms (Boyd and Nailor 2011; Fox et al. 1954; Mitchison 1954, 1998; Soothill et al. 2013; Traugott et al. 2011).

Another method that can be used for the prevention of antimicrobial resistance development is bacterial-antimicrobial pairing. The bacterial load of different infected sites is measured and the possibility to develop resistance against certain antimicrobials is estimated. If the risk of antimicrobial resistance development is high then the use of some antibiotics should be avoided (Soothill et al. 2013; Williams and Sefton 1999). Since the 1980s, antimicrobial cycling, which is the scheduled rotation of one class of antibiotics with one or more different classes with a similar spectrum of activity was thought to be a promising strategy for reducing antimicrobial resistance in hospitals. The idea is based on the removal of selective pressure for a predetermined period of time by the withdrawal of an antibiotic that is intensively used for the treatment of certain infections and its replacement with another one with similar action. The highest is the rate of the prescription of an antibiotic, the more likely it is to develop antimicrobial resistance. Unfortunately, this method has been the subject of short-term limited investigations and in many of the studies, there was not a complete cessation of the withdrawn agent. In one such trial of antibiotic cycling in United Kingdom, the sulfonamide use was restricted nationally for a period of time, however, no reduction in sulfonamide resistant *Escherichia coli* was observed.

Another study concerned the treatment of Gram negative infections in a surgical intensive care unit. The monthly rotation between different antibiotics led to an improvement in the antimicrobial susceptibility profile of Gram negative organisms in the surgical intensive care unit in comparison with the medical care unit. The efficacy of antimicrobial cycling was documented in 2005 by a review which included both clinical trials and mathematical modeling studies. Due to the poor quality of the majority of the efficacy of the existed clinical trials along with the small number of adequately designed trials the conclusion was that there is not enough evidence in order to consider antimicrobial cycling as a strategy that should be implemented routinely in hospitals in the effort to prevent antimicrobial resistance development (Bennett et al. 2007; Brown and Nathwani 2005; Enne et al. 2001; Okeke et al. 2005).

1.5.2 Diagnostic and Infection Prevention Stewardship

In critically ill patients, any delay in the diagnosis of infection may be associated with an increase in hospital mortality. Thus, in this category of patients, the proper and accurate diagnosis is of vital importance (Ferrer et al. 2014). In the case of infectious diseases, the early microbiological diagnosis in combination with medical knowledge and judgment are very important and contribute to the improvement of the disease outcome. Except for the fact that the diagnosis plays an important role in the optimal therapy, it also helps in the control of infectious diseases and in the prevention of their spread. A laboratory examination is extremely helpful when it is done timely because it provides the physician with information about the presence of an infection, the pathogen that is responsible for the infection and the susceptibility of the pathogen (Dik et al. 2016).

All microbiological examinations must be done before the therapy with an antibiotic starts in order to be more accurate. Proper collection of the specimens is crucial because if the collection is done improperly, this may lead to misdiagnosis. For example, for blood cultures, which are used to diagnose bacteremia, 20–30 ml of blood is needed for adults and the amount of blood, which is needed in children, depends on their age and weight. Two bottles are used (one aerobic and one anaerobic) and before the procedure starts the region from where the blood is taken should be disinfected properly. This aims to decrease the probability of contamination. It was reported that 25% of all positive blood cultures were contaminated. The Infectious Diseases Society of America (IDSA) recommends the use of urine tests only if urinary symptoms exist with an exception in pregnant women and patients who undergo an invasive urinary procedure. This recommendation is because if a urinary test is ordered without the presence of any symptom and the collection of the specimen is done improperly this will lead to overdiagnosis and therefore overtreatment, which accelerates antimicrobial resistance development (Pallin et al. 2014; Septimus 2018; Weinstein 2003).

The choice of the right diagnostic test is of vital importance. The results of the tests are provided within hours, if it is a viral infection or within a day or two, if it is a fungal or bacterial infection. The need for more rapid tests is uncontested. Some new point of care assays may reduce the time needed for diagnosis. Their application may render possible the early differential diagnosis of infectious from non-infectious diseases. It is recommended that the physicians should use an individual plan adjusted on the patient for the management of infectious diseases, which is called a personalized infection management plan.

Although innovative methods as Next generation sequencing (NGS) and Matrix assisted laser desorption/ionization time-of-flight (MALDI-TOF) are promising not only for clinical microbiology but also for antimicrobial resistance prevention, the conventional culture based diagnostics are still used and are considered very effective. The conventional culture based diagnostics include blood, urine, sputum and other cultures in combination with susceptibility tests. Bacterial cultures are important tools because they are both useful and cheap and some isolates can be stored and typed with no other mean. However, the main problem is that the turnaround time of these tests is too long for the early diagnosis of infection. Another problem is that the diagnostic care facilities which provide these tests most of the time are located far away from an individual's primary health care center. A solution would be to make the diagnostic tools available in all primary health care centers to be more easily accessible for the population.

It is reported that the use of procalcitonin (PCT) as a biomarker is helpful in the differentiation of a bacterial from a viral infection, because it is expressed only in response to bacterial infections. Therefore, if it is a viral infection, the procalcitonin level will be low and the use of antibiotics, as treatment, will be avoided. Undoubtedly, there is a great need for the application of more rapid diagnostic tests, based on molecular technologies. Their implementation will help in early and optimal decisions about the management of the available resources and the beginning of the treatment with antibiotics. Although, this type of diagnostics is more expensive in comparison with the conventional methods. Studies about the cost-effectiveness should be done before their massive implementation (Dik et al. 2016; Schuetz et al. 2011; Septimus 2018).

The creation of databases in every microbiological laboratory, which will include all the daily microbiological examinations and the results, will be very useful. It will help with clinical and epidemiological surveillance reports (WHO 2001b). There is a connection between the programs of antimicrobial stewardship, diagnostic stewardship (Hudspeth et al. 2001) and infection prevention stewardship. A pyramid was made and it shows that as serious the condition of a patient is, the more experienced specialists and multi disciplinary team are needed for the disease management. Especially, in specific infectious diseases where the condition of the patient is changing continually and varies over time, the availability of an experienced team is necessary (Dik et al. 2016).

Unfortunately, bacterial cultures, susceptibility tests, and the other tests, which are mentioned above that are common in developed countries, are uncommon or are unreliable in many developing countries. Due to the lack of these tests, most of the times the diagnosis is made based on the clinical signs and symptoms of the patients. Sometimes physicians use even chemotherapy as a diagnostic tool, which means that the confirmation of the diagnosis is made from the recession of the symptoms after the course of the treatment. Another phenomenon that is observed in developing countries is the irrational empirical antimicrobial prescription based on geographically and temporally inconsistent data. All these highlights the great need for systemic surveillance programs internationally. The information that will be collected will help in the modification of empirical antimicrobial prescription and in order to estimate the global burden due to antimicrobial resistance.

At the same time, the design of interventions that will be capable to monitor and control antimicrobial resistance is also important. If data are collected properly, this will help to record treatment failures or associate treatments with outcomes with the help of the International Classification of Diseases 11th Revision (ICD-11) passively or by recruiting sentinel sites actively. In order to gather the collection of surveillance data, quality assured laboratories, and organized health care units are required which most of the time are absent in developing countries. The World Health Organization created the WHONET shareware software, which aims to present surveillance data uniformly and analyze the results of susceptibility tests. This is done to track the local along with the global resistance trends, which are very helpful for the proper use of antibiotics and the management of the infections and diseases globally (Ande et al. 2004; Lim and Cheong 1992; Mutanda et al. 1989; O'Brien and Stelling 1996; Okeke et al. 1999, 2005; Shapiro et al. 2001; Woolhouse et al. 2016).

1.6 Strategies for Containment of Widespread Infection with Antibacterial Drug Resistant Bacteria

1.6.1 Infection Prevention Stewardship

It is important to employ methods, which will reduce the need for antibiotics, as antimicrobial resistance development is associated with their extensive use in the community, hospitals, veterinary medicine, agriculture, and aquaculture. There are variety of ways, which can be applied in order to prevent the spread of infections worldwide. Good hygienic practices and proper food preparation should be followed both in health care units and in the community. Especially, in the community, it is reported that hand hygiene can affect the appearance of diarrhea, acute respiratory tract infections and community acquired infections. Barrier precautions should be used from health care workers in hospital units and the existence of consultants in combination with hospital guidelines for infections and antimicrobial use are of great importance (Allcock et al. 2017; Dik et al. 2016; Okeke et al. 2005). Patients with potentially dangerous resistant bacteria must be isolated in special units or rooms and patient-specific consultations are also recommended. It is reported that in the countries where methods like isolation in special units or in single rooms of hospitalized patients who are colonized with methicillin resistant *Staphylococcus aureus* (MRSA) has led to a decrease in the rate of infections with MRSA. However, in order to have more spectacular results, other measures should be applied in combination with the isolation of the patients (Dik et al. 2016; Levy and Marshall 2004).

Herein lies a paradox, in developed countries hygienic products and health infrastructure are available both in communities and in hospital facilities. Nonetheless, illnesses remain a problem of concern. The mechanism of action of cleaning and hygienic products, which are used, should be tested carefully. The main reason is that the use of antibacterial ingredients as triclosan seems to be associated with cross resistance to relevant antibiotics. The American Medical Association suggests that the use of the hygienic products whose mechanism of antibiotic resistance have been characterized should be stopped. Yet, more studies should be done on this subject. However, no changes are suggested for individual use of cleaning and hygienic products. Only in those products where the mechanism for the potential transfer of resistance is unknown, their use should be limited. Indeed, if a family member is ill, immunocompromised or has a postoperative wound, the use of hygienic products is recommended. In the developed world, there is a strong association between hygiene and better quality of health; while in the developing world there is evidence that hygienic practices contribute to the decrease of infections. Therefore, it is quite difficult to persuade individuals to avoid the use of all types of antibacterial products (Aiello and Larson 2002; Tan et al. 2002; and Council on Scientific Affairs 2002).

It is widely known that over last several decades, the life expectancy of the population has prolonged and at the same time, living conditions are improved. This can be attributed to the existence of better hygienic conditions, antibiotics, and vaccines, which are very important in the control of infections. However, one of these three pillars, the antibiotics tends to weaken due to the presence of many multi drug resistant bacterial strains. This may have a devastating effect on human health. That is the reason why attention should be given in preventive measures as vaccination in order to decrease antibiotic use and thus decrease the antimicrobial resistance development. Vaccines are a very useful tool for physicians in order to prevent bacterial and viral infections. Furthermore, vaccination decreases the demand for therapeutic treatments by preventing the start of an infection and the health consequences of vaccine-preventable infectious diseases. This leads to a decrease in mortality rate and at the same time reduce the health care costs (Tagliabue and Rappuoli 2018). Especially, there is a greater need for vaccination in immunocompromised patients who are at higher risk to suffer from various bacterial infections. Pneumococcal vaccination is recommended for patients with chronic obstructive pulmonary disease, and for elderly and younger patients who have concomitant diseases (Garau et al. 2014; Okeke et al. 2005).

The discovery of every new antibiotic sooner or later is followed by the development of antimicrobial resistance in contrast with vaccines where resistance development is an extremely rare phenomenon (O'Neil 2016). Therefore, vaccines can be used as prophylaxis for longer periods and for the entire population while antibiotics are used therapeutically only after an infection is manifested. The way by which vaccines act is by inducing a protective immune response against multiple antigenic targets. With the vaccination, the selection has lower opportunities to act in comparison to the use of antibiotics. In contrast with antibiotics, which can be used immediately, vaccines need some time from a week to several months to exert fully their protective properties but they induce a memory that can last for years. It should be pointed out that with the use of vaccines, infections as polio, diphtheria, *Haemophilus influenza*, Meningococcus A and C and several strains of *Pneumococcus* were eliminated and smallpox was eradicated. However, the refusal of many parents to have their children vaccinated led to the reemergence of smallpox in many developing countries such as France and others.

The discovery of new vaccines was benefited from new technologies, while there is a decline in the discovery of new classes of antibiotics. The World Health Organization has documented a list with the priority pathogens which includes twelve families of bacteria that threaten the public health and highlights the importance of vaccines. A report "Tackling drug-resistant infections globally" that includes the main reasons and methods to reduce antimicrobial resistance and a section for vaccines was published in 2016 by a group of experts (O'Neil 2016; Tagliabue and Rappuoli 2018).

Every year since 2004, 'Palio meetings' are organized. The meeting takes place in Siena, Italy, close to an event, the horse race of "Palio di Siena". For that, the meetings are called the "Palio meetings". That is a forum in which the most important issues for vaccines are discussed worldwide. The last meeting was held in July 2017 in Wavre, Belgium and its title was "Prioritizing vaccines to fight antimicrobial resistance". The main purpose of the meeting was to find ways to make vaccines one of the primary tools used to tackle antimicrobial resistance and increase public confidence in vaccination. They concluded that to achieve this purpose, evidence based cases are needed which will support the fact that vaccines are very important for prophylaxis and their use is associated with the prevention of antimicrobial resistance development. Indeed, it should not be neglected that the use of vaccines aims at protection from illness as well as, the long side effects that an illness may cause to an individual. During the last decade new vaccines are developed, thanks to the introduction of new technology, the so-called "reverse vaccinology 2.0" (Barocchi et al. 2016; Black et al. 2015; Black and Rappuoli 2010; Bloom et al. 2017; Rappuoli et al. 2009; Saul and Rappuoli 2009; Tagliabue and Rappuoli 2018).

There are reports which show that antibiotic use in livestock is related to antimicrobial resistance development in humans and animals and due to this correlation Denmark has restricted the use of antibiotics in pigs. It is believed that if primary and secondary infections are controlled there will be no need for antibiotic use (Kruse et al. 2019). The only measure which is available and capable to prevent infectious diseases and most viral infections in animals is the vaccination. The rapid development of antimicrobial resistance against antibiotic and anthelmintic drugs necessitates the use of vaccines instead of chemotherapy. The benefit of vaccines use is double and concerns both animals and humans. With their use animals are protected from infections and therefore, this protects humans from zoonotic infections (Pastoret and Jones 2004).

Thus, to achieve better control of antimicrobial resistance development mass vaccination campaigns should be organized for both humans and animals to manage the maximum coverage of the populations. More research should be done on vaccines especially they should focus on pathogens that are blamed for multi drug resistance infections. The pathogens which are of great concern based on the prioritized classification of the US are *E. coli,* which already developed resistance to 3rd generation cephalosporins and fluoroquinolones; *K. pneumoniae,* which developed resistance to 3rd generation cephalosporins and carbapenems; MRSA; *S. pneumoniae* which developed resistance to penicillin; Non-Typhoidal *Salmonella* (NTS) and *Shigella* which developed resistance to fluoroquinolones; and *Neisseria gonorrhoeae* which has reduced susceptibility to 3rd generation cephalosporins (Whitehouse 2014).

Another route of spread of resistant bacteria and resistant genes between humans is the food chain. Actually, the food acts as a vector. Soil, water, animal and human fecal material are some sources where resistant bacteria may be found. The theory that there is a connection between antibiotic use in agriculture and the development of antimicrobial resistance is supported by numerous scientific studies (Carattoli 2008; Depoorter et al. 2012; Mayrhofer et al. 2006; Silbergeld et al. 2008; Srinivasan et al. 2008; Stine et al. 2007; Zirakzadeh and Patel 2005). The use of antibiotics is not limited only in agriculture but also in animal production. This is an explanation about the presence of *Salmonella* Typhimurium strains in some humans after the consumption of poultry and pork meat. Therefore, it seems that both agriculture and aquaculture may constitute sources of transfer of resistant bacteria (Verraes et al. 2013).

Animal as well as plant products may be contaminated with resistant bacteria if they are washed with water contaminated with human or animal feces or sewage discharges. Seafood is particularly prompt to bacterial contamination. We should bear in mind that food can be contaminated by the environment after food processing or through the presence of other contaminated food when they are stored or handled together. The first way of contamination is called "post-contamination" while the second one is called "cross-contamination". During the procedure of food processing, some microorganisms are added for technical reasons as starter cultures, probiotics, preventing pathogenic microorganisms to develop. The purpose of starter culture use is due to their capacity to induce the onset of fermentation. Probiotics seem to have positive effects on human health and they are mostly added in yogurts and supplementary food. Biopreservation helps in the extension of food shelf life while bacteriophages are capable of inactivating foodborne pathogens along with spoilage organisms (Verraes et al. 2013).

The problem of the transfer of antimicrobial resistance bacteria through food chain concerns both developed and developing world but the condition in the developing world is more serious because it affects mortality rates in comparison to the developed world where the losses are mostly financial due to the increased therapeutic costs (Founou et al. 2016; Padungtod et al. 2008). A global action plan was published in 2015 by the World Health Organization, Food and Agriculture Organization (FAO) of the United Nations, and World Organization for Animal Health (OIE). The main purpose of this plan was to increase knowledge and awareness of antibiotics use and developing antimicrobial resistance. It aims to the reduction of infectious diseases and the optimization of the rational use of antibiotics (Founou et al. 2016).

It is well known that the risk for transfer of antimicrobial resistance bacteria is extremely high with raw food consumption, while if heat treatments are applied the risk is reduced. Nevertheless, the probability of transfer of antimicrobial resistance bacteria seems to increase if minimum processes and preservation techniques are applied due to the existence of stressed bacteria (McMahon et al. 2007a, b). To ensure safe food production, good manufacturing, and hygienic practices should be used at all stages of the food production chain. Furthermore, heat treatments should be adjusted in temperature and duration which is recommended for different foods in order to be safe for consumption. At the same time, more research should be done on the subject of transmission of antimicrobial resistance bacteria through the food chain and new ways to cope with this problem must be found (Verraes et al. 2013). Until then, national systems should monitor antimicrobial usage in food animals, and guidelines should be developed and applied for veterinarians to reduce the improper use of antibiotics in livestock (WHO 2001b).

1.6.2 Antibiotic Stewardship

Antibiotics stewardship refers to a multidisciplinary program, which was developed to improve prescribing, to optimize clinical outcomes and at the same time decrease the adverse consequences of antimicrobial use. In 1997, the program of antibiotics stewardship was considered to be a key component for the prevention of the emergence of antimicrobial resistance in hospitals according to the guidelines of the joint committee of Society for Healthcare Epidemiology of America (SHEA) and Infectious disease Society of America (IDSA). Nowadays, due to the decrease in the discovery of new antibiotics along with the rapid development of antimicrobial resistance both in community settings and hospitals, the optimal use of the existing antibiotics is necessary to extend their effectiveness. This highlights the greater importance of antibiotics stewardship programs in the twenty-first century in comparison to the past. It should be mentioned that the antibiotics stewardship program is included in antimicrobial, infection prevention and diagnostic models (Hughes and Andersson 2015). The antibiotics stewardship program is based not only on American guidelines of SHEA and IDSA but also on German and Dutch guidelines for antibiotics stewardship programs. In 2016, the new guidelines for antibiotics stewardship program were published by SHEA and IDSA (Barlam et al. 2016; Dellit et al. 2007; Dik et al. 2016; Fishman 2006; Septimus 2018; Weber and Courvalin 2005).

The main purpose of antibiotics stewardship is to reassure the clinical success of the treatment with an antibiotic and to decrease the potential consequences as the development of antimicrobial resistance and collateral damage. The term collateral damage is used to describe the ecological adverse effects of antibiotic therapy, which include the selection of antimicrobial resistant bacteria and infections with multi drug resistant microorganisms.

For instance, the use of quinolones and cephalosporins is associated with collateral damage; therefore, they are not suitable for sustained use in hospitals. However, if the therapy, which causes collateral damage is discontinued or replaced, the antibiotic pressure against certain bacteria will be reduced which is called collateral benefit. The antibiotics stewardship programs involve a number of interventions and the use of evidence based treatment regimens, which aim to the optimal antimicrobial use and to the decrease of antimicrobial resistance development. In order to achieve these, specific indications and criteria for antibiotic use are needed before the start of the treatment. The implementation of antibiotics stewardship programs seems to contribute to the reduction of the mortality and recurrent infections rate, the length of hospital stay, the duration of the therapy, and superinfection with multi drug resistant bacteria.

An antimicrobial stewardship team that will be comprised of clinical microbiologists, infectious disease specialists, hospital pharmacists with the support of trained doctors and nurses in the hospital ward is needed. Although the financial cost of training is a barrier to the widespread implementation of antibiotics stewardship programs, it seems that there is a long term cost reduction. In cases where there is no possibility of rapid laboratory results that are needed to provide evidence for a bacterial infection, the choice of therapy is empiric and is based on the most likely diagnosis and the characteristics of the patient. The empiric therapy is also the choice in severely ill patients in whom it is proved that any delay in the start of the treatment results in poorer infection outcomes. When the laboratory results are available the initial empirical antibiotic regimen should be changed with a more appropriate one, based on the laboratory tests, culture results and the clinical status of the patient.

The optimization and personalization of the therapy are of vital importance. The appropriate antibiotic should be selected and it should be capable to act on the site of infection. The optimal dose, the route of administration and the duration of the treatment play also an important role in the therapy. Actually, the spectrum of the initial empiric therapy is usually broad so if the laboratory results indicate it, a change from a broad regimen to a narrower regimen is recommended. This will contribute to a decrease in the extended use of broad spectrum antibiotics. In cases, where the presence of an infection is not proved with a laboratory examination, the initial therapy should be discontinued. This method called de-escalation and its use seems to increase the likelihood of clinical success and considered to be another key strategy against antimicrobial resistance development.

Preauthorization is a method that also aims to the improvement of antibiotic use. According to this method, clinicians will need approval for the administration of certain antibiotics which also seems to lead in antimicrobial resistance reduction. The implementation of antibiotics stewardship programs should be combined with other methods that aim to the prevention of resistance development and should be integrated with other programs for pharmacy management, microbiology, diagnostics and laboratory quality control. Behavioral change strategies are also important especially those who target prescribers. Furthermore, the improvement of antibiotics stewardship programs in animals should not be neglected because human consumption of resistant bacteria which are found in animals leads to the development of infection (Allcock et al. 2017; Dik et al. 2016; Fishman 2006; Garau et al. 2014; Paskovaty et al. 2005; Paterson 2004; Septimus 2018).

1.6.3 Research and Development of New Antibacterial Drugs

It is widely known that the research and development of new antibiotics are urgently needed. Antimicrobial resistance appeared since the discovery of the first antibiotics. Although, during the last decades the rate of antimicrobial resistance increased rapidly and the main cause is considered to be the overuse along with the misuse of antibiotics. Indeed, the spread of resistance worldwide seems to be a threat to the well-being of many people. Unfortunately, the discovery of new drugs can not follow the rate of resistance development. During the period of time, drug development started to rely more on structural changes of antibiotics which already exist while there is a decline in the number of newly approved antibiotics in comparison with the past. There are many reasons which render difficult the success of the development of new antibiotics. Some of them concern the proper selection of the target which must fulfill some criteria. Especially, the target should be essential, and at the same time not susceptible to the rapid development of resistance. All these characteristics decrease the possibility of success and increase economic costs.

There is the conviction that the conventional pipelines for antibacterial drug discovery dried up. Therefore, new drug targets in conjunction with novel mechanisms of antibacterial drug action are needed to develop more timely modern classes of antibiotics which will be less susceptible to antimicrobial resistance development. Actually, the antibiotics that need to be developed should target the virulence potential of bacteria to induce few, if any antimicrobial resistance strains. To achieve these, new molecular tools and new molecular targets that have not been used before are needed. Some of the promising molecular tools are antisense oligonucleotides, nanoparticles (Shende et al. 2017), phage therapies, riboswitches, antimicrobial peptides, and other novel antibiotics (Allcock et al. 2017; Lewis 2013; Penchovsky and Stoilova 2013; Penchovsky and Traykovska 2015).

The antisense oligonucleotides offer many advantages for antibacterial drug development including fast, comprehensive, and accurate procedures of rational drug design. The antisense oligonucleotides are attached to a cell-penetrating peptide, such as pVEC, which delivers them into the bacterial cell (Penchovsky and Traykovska 2015). They are chemically modified to resist enzyme degradation. The chemical modifications of antisense oligonucleotides are classified into 3 different groups. The antisense oligonucleotides of the first group are recognized by the enzyme RNase, which cleaves targeted bacterial mRNA where the antisense oligonucleotide is hybridized to it (Fig. 1.2). In this way, we can inhibit the expression of any essential bacterial RNA and kill the bacteria.

As it is mentioned above, the use of antibiotics changes the microbiota which may have negative effects on human health. This is one of the main reasons why there is a great need in research and development of novel narrow spectrum antibiotics which will target only bacterial pathogens to decrease the effect that antibiotics exert to microbiota. A method, which can be implemented initially to prevent microbiota alterations, is the use of probiotics which most of the times are lactic acid bacteria and seem to produce various antibiotics that are capable of competing with

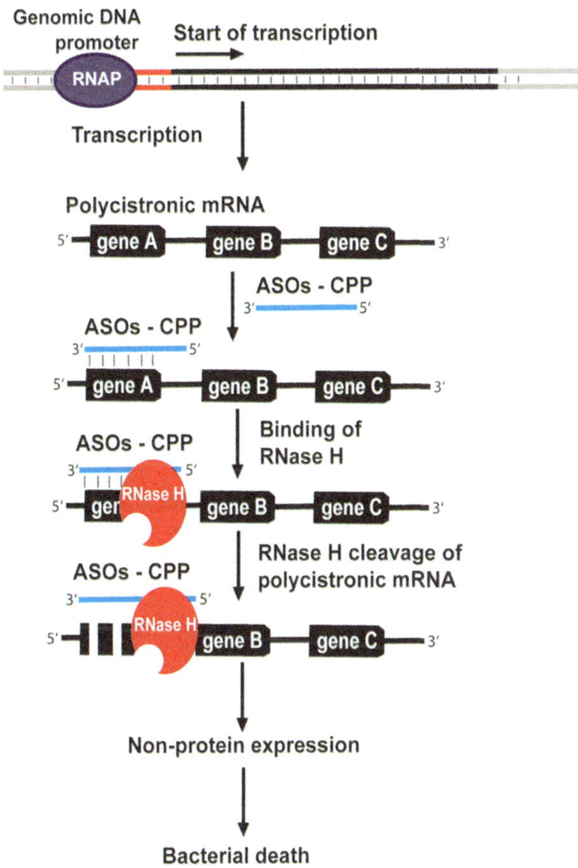

Fig. 1.2 Applying antisense oligonucleotides as novel antibiotics. The antisense oligonucleotides are attached to cell-penetrating peptides (CPPs) that deliver them into the bacterial cell

other gut microbes and at the same time they may inhibit the growth of some pathogenic bacteria. Based on a limited number of studies, fecal microbiota transplantation of fecal bacteria from a healthy individual seems to be effective in patients who suffered from *C. difficile* infections. Especially, in a study in which patients with recurrent *C. difficile* infections participated, fecal microbiota transplant was used successfully in an effort to treat the infections and considered to be more effective as a treatment in comparison with the use of vancomycin. However, the potential long term risks that fecal microbiota transplant may cause should not be neglected. It must also be mentioned that this method is not recommended for acutely ill patients (Cattoir and Felden 2019; Mantravadi et al. 2019; Penchovsky and Traykovska 2015; Raffatellu 2018; van Nood et al. 2013).

1.7 Conclusion

The reduction in antimicrobial resistance to an acceptable minimum is possible if measures described here are executed worldwide. From a practical point of view, it would be a great achievement if we manage to reverse the trend of ever increasing emergence of antimicrobial resistance. We cannot stop the development of antimicrobial resistance because it is an intrinsic part of nature. However, we can manage it much better if we use the antibiotics based on solid scientific guidelines as described. At the same time, we need to constantly develop new antibiotics against multi drug resistant bacterial strains.

Acknowledgments The research in the Robert Penchovsky laboratory is supported by a grant DN13/14/20.12.2017 awarded by the Bulgarian National Science Fund, and a grant 80-10-31/18.03.2020 awarded by the Science Fund of Sofia University.

References

Adams EJ, Garcia PJ, Garnett GP, Edmunds WJ, Holmes KK (2003) The cost-effectiveness of syndromic management in pharmacies in Lima, Peru. Sex Transm Dis 30(5):379–387

Aiello AE, Larson EL (2002) What is the evidence for a causal link between hygiene and infections? Lancet Infect Dis 2(2):103–110

Aiello AE, Larson E (2003) Antibacterial cleaning and hygiene products as an emerging risk factor for antibiotic resistance in the community. Lancet Infect Dis 3(8):501–506

Allcock S, Young EH, Holmes M, Gurdasani D, Dougan G, Sandhu MS et al (2017) Antimicrobial resistance in human populations: challenges and opportunities. Glob Health Epidemiol Genomics 2:e4. https://doi.org/10.1017/gheg.2017.4

Ande O, Oladepo O, Brieger WR (2004) Comparison of knowledge on diarrheal disease management between two types of community-based distributors in Oyo State, Nigeria. Health Educ Res 19(1):110–113. https://doi.org/10.1093/her/cyg004

Ball P, Baquero F, Cars O, File T, Garau J, Klugman K et al (2002) Antibiotic therapy of community respiratory tract infections: strategies for optimal outcomes and minimized resistance emergence. J Antimicrob Chemother 49(1):31–40. https://doi.org/10.1093/jac/49.1.31

Barker KF (1999) Antibiotic resistance: a current perspective. Br J Clin Pharmacol 48(2):109–124. https://doi.org/10.1046/j.1365-2125.1999.00997.x

Barlam TF, Cosgrove SE, Abbo LM, MacDougall C, Schuetz AN, Septimus EJ et al (2016) Implementing an antibiotic stewardship program: guidelines by the Infectious Diseases Society of America and the Society for Healthcare Epidemiology of America. Clin Infect Dis 62(10):e51–e77. https://doi.org/10.1093/cid/ciw118

Barocchi MA, Black S, Rappuoli R (2016) Multicriteria decision analysis and core values for enhancing vaccine-related decision-making. Sci Transl Med 8(345):345ps314. https://doi.org/10.1126/scitranslmed.aaf0756

Bassetti M, Poulakou G, Ruppe E, Bouza E, Van Hal SJ, Brink A (2017) Antimicrobial resistance in the next 30 years, humankind, bugs and drugs: a visionary approach. Intensive Care Med 43(10):1464–1475. https://doi.org/10.1007/s00134-017-4878-x

Bavestrello L, Cabello A, Casanova D (2002) Impact of regulatory measures in the trends of community consumption of antibiotics in Chile. Rev Med Chil 130(11):1265–1272

Bennadi D (2013) Self-medication: a current challenge. J Basic Clin Pharm 5(1):19–23. https://doi.org/10.4103/0976-0105.128253

Bennett KM, Scarborough JE, Sharpe M, Dodds-Ashley E, Kaye KS, Hayward TZ 3rd, Vaslef SN (2007) Implementation of antibiotic rotation protocol improves antibiotic susceptibility profile in a surgical intensive care unit. J Trauma 63(2):307–311. https://doi.org/10.1097/TA.0b013e318120595e

Bexell A, Lwando E, von Hofsten B, Tembo S, Eriksson B, Diwan VK (1996) Improving drug use through continuing education: a randomized controlled trial in Zambia. J Clin Epidemiol 49(3):355–357

Black S, Rappuoli R (2010) A crisis of public confidence in vaccines. Sci Transl Med 2(61):61mr61. https://doi.org/10.1126/scitranslmed.3001738

Black S, De Gregorio E, Rappuoli R (2015) Developing vaccines for an aging population. Sci Transl Med 7(281):281ps288. https://doi.org/10.1126/scitranslmed.aaa0722

Blair JM, Webber MA, Baylay AJ, Ogbolu DO, Piddock LJ (2015) Molecular mechanisms of antibiotic resistance. Nat Rev Microbiol 13(1):42–51. https://doi.org/10.1038/nrmicro3380

Bloom DE, Black S, Rappuoli R (2017) Emerging infectious diseases: a proactive approach. Proc Natl Acad Sci U S A 114(16):4055–4059. https://doi.org/10.1073/pnas.1701410114

Boyd N, Nailor MD (2011) Combination antibiotic therapy for empiric and definitive treatment of gram-negative infections: insights from the Society of Infectious Diseases Pharmacists. Pharmacotherapy 31(11):1073–1084. https://doi.org/10.1592/phco.31.11.1073

Brown EM, Nathwani D (2005) Antibiotic cycling or rotation: a systematic review of the evidence of efficacy. J Antimicrob Chemother 55(1):6–9. https://doi.org/10.1093/jac/dkh482

Carattoli A (2008) Animal reservoirs for extended spectrum beta-lactamase producers. Clin Microbiol Infect 14(Suppl 1):117–123. https://doi.org/10.1111/j.1469-0691.2007.01851.x

Cattoir V, Felden B (2019) Future antibacterial strategies: from basic concepts to clinical challenges. J Infect Dis 220:350–360. https://doi.org/10.1093/infdis/jiz134

Chuanchuen R, Beinlich K, Hoang TT, Becher A, Karkhoff-Schweizer RR, Schweizer HP (2001) Cross-resistance between triclosan and antibiotics in Pseudomonas aeruginosa is mediated by multidrug efflux pumps: exposure of a susceptible mutant strain to triclosan selects nfxB mutants overexpressing MexCD-OprJ. Antimicrob Agents Chemother 45(2):428–432. https://doi.org/10.1128/AAC.45.2.428-432.2001

Chuanchuen R, Narasaki CT, Schweizer HP (2002) The MexJK efflux pump of Pseudomonas aeruginosa requires OprM for antibiotic efflux but not for efflux of triclosan. J Bacteriol 184(18):5036–5044

Chuc NT, Larsson M, Do NT, Diwan VK, Tomson GB, Falkenberg T (2002) Improving private pharmacy practice: a multi-intervention experiment in Hanoi, Vietnam. J Clin Epidemiol 55(11):1148–1155

Cui J, Liu Y, Wang R, Tong W, Drlica K, Zhao X (2006) The mutant selection window in rabbits infected with Staphylococcus aureus. J Infect Dis 194(11):1601–1608. https://doi.org/10.1086/508752

de With K, Allerberger F, Amann S, Apfalter P, Brodt HR, Eckmanns T et al (2016) Strategies to enhance rational use of antibiotics in hospital: a guideline by the German Society for Infectious Diseases. Infection 44(3):395–439. https://doi.org/10.1007/s15010-016-0885-z

Dellit TH, Owens RC, McGowan JE Jr, Gerding DN, Weinstein RA, Burke JP et al (2007) Infectious Diseases Society of America and the Society for Healthcare Epidemiology of America guidelines for developing an institutional program to enhance antimicrobial stewardship. Clin Infect Dis 44(2):159–177. https://doi.org/10.1086/510393

Depoorter P, Persoons D, Uyttendaele M, Butaye P, De Zutter L, Dierick K et al (2012) Assessment of human exposure to 3rd generation cephalosporin resistant E. coli (CREC) through consumption of broiler meat in Belgium. Int J Food Microbiol 159(1):30–38. https://doi.org/10.1016/j.ijfoodmicro.2012.07.026

DeRyke CA, Lee SY, Kuti JL, Nicolau DP (2006) Optimising dosing strategies of antibacterials utilising pharmacodynamic principles: impact on the development of resistance. Drugs 66(1):1–14. https://doi.org/10.2165/00003495-200666010-00001

Dik JW, Poelman R, Friedrich AW, Panday PN, Lo-Ten-Foe JR, van Assen S et al (2016) An integrated stewardship model: antimicrobial, infection prevention and diagnostic (AID). Future Microbiol 11(1):93–102. https://doi.org/10.2217/fmb.15.99

Drlica K (2003) The mutant selection window and antimicrobial resistance. J Antimicrob Chemother 52(1):11–17. https://doi.org/10.1093/jac/dkg269

Enne VI, Livermore DM, Stephens P, Hall LM (2001) Persistence of sulphonamide resistance in Escherichia coli in the UK despite national prescribing restriction. Lancet 357(9265):1325–1328. https://doi.org/10.1016/S0140-6736(00)04519-0

Erbay A, Colpan A, Bodur H, Cevik MA, Samore MH, Ergonul O (2003) Evaluation of antibiotic use in a hospital with an antibiotic restriction policy. Int J Antimicrob Agents 21(4):308–312

Essack SY (2006) Strategies for prevention and containment of antibiotic resistance. S Afr Fam Pract 48(1):50

Fairchok MP, Ashton WS, Fischer GW (1996) Carriage of penicillin-resistant pneumococci in a military population in Washington, DC: risk factors and correlation with clinical isolates. Clin Infect Dis 22(6):966–972

Ferrer R, Martin-Loeches I, Phillips G, Osborn TM, Townsend S, Dellinger RP et al (2014) Empiric antibiotic treatment reduces mortality in severe sepsis and septic shock from the first hour: results from a guideline-based performance improvement program. Crit Care Med 42(8):1749–1755. https://doi.org/10.1097/CCM.0000000000000330

Fishman N (2006) Antimicrobial stewardship. Am J Med 119(6 Suppl 1):S53–S61; discussion S62–S70. https://doi.org/10.1016/j.amjmed.2006.04.003

Founou LL, Founou RC, Essack SY (2016) Antibiotic resistance in the food chain: a developing country-perspective. Front Microbiol 7:1881. https://doi.org/10.3389/fmicb.2016.01881

Fox W, Sutherland I, Daniels M (1954) A five-year assessment of patients in a controlled trial of streptomycin in pulmonary tuberculosis; report to the tuberculosis chemotherapy trials committee of the medical research council. Q J Med 23(91):347–366

Garau J, Nicolau DP, Wullt B, Bassetti M (2014) Antibiotic stewardship challenges in the management of community-acquired infections for prevention of escalating antibiotic resistance. J Glob Antimicrob Resist 2(4):245–253. https://doi.org/10.1016/j.jgar.2014.08.002

Geli P, Laxminarayan R, Dunne M, Smith DL (2012) "One-size-fits-all"? Optimizing treatment duration for bacterial infections. PLoS One 7(1):e29838. https://doi.org/10.1371/journal.pone.0029838

Griffiths AJF, Miller JH, Suzuki DT, Lewontin RC, Gelbart WM (2000) An introduction to genetic analysis, 7th edn. W. H. Freeman, New York

Guillemot D, Carbon C, Balkau B, Geslin P, Lecoeur H, Vauzelle-Kervroedan F et al (1998) Low dosage and long treatment duration of beta-lactam: risk factors for carriage of penicillin-resistant Streptococcus pneumoniae. JAMA 279(5):365–370

Gullberg E, Cao S, Berg OG, Ilback C, Sandegren L, Hughes D, Andersson DI (2011) Selection of resistant bacteria at very low antibiotic concentrations. PLoS Pathog 7(7):e1002158. https://doi.org/10.1371/journal.ppat.1002158

Gutierrez G, Guiscafre H, Bronfman M, Walsh J, Martinez H, Munoz O (1994) Changing physician prescribing patterns: evaluation of an educational strategy for acute diarrhea in Mexico City. Med Care 32(5):436–446

Harbarth S, Gundlapalli AV, Stockdale W, Samore MH (2003) Shortage of penicillin G: impact on antibiotic prescribing at a US tertiary care centre. Int J Antimicrob Agents 21(5):484–487

Hayes JD, Wolf CR (1990) Molecular mechanisms of drug resistance. Biochem J 272(2):281–295. https://doi.org/10.1042/bj2720281

Hermsen R, Deris JB, Hwa T (2012) On the rapidity of antibiotic resistance evolution facilitated by a concentration gradient. Proc Natl Acad Sci U S A 109(27):10775–10780. https://doi.org/10.1073/pnas.1117716109

Hudspeth MK, Smith TC, Barrozo CP, Hawksworth AW, Ryan MA, Gray GC, Streptococcus pneumoniae Surveillance G (2001) National Department of Defense Surveillance for Invasive Streptococcus pneumoniae: antibiotic resistance, serotype distribution, and arbitrarily

primed polymerase chain reaction analyses. J Infect Dis 184(5):591–596. https://doi.org/10.1086/322786
Hughes D, Andersson DI (2015) Evolutionary consequences of drug resistance: shared principles across diverse targets and organisms. Nat Rev Genet 16:459. https://doi.org/10.1038/nrg3922
Jampilek J (2018) Design and discovery of new antibacterial agents: advances, perspectives, challenges. Curr Med Chem 25(38):4972–5006. https://doi.org/10.2174/0929867324666170918122633
Jansen WT, van der Bruggen JT, Verhoef J, Fluit AC (2006) Bacterial resistance: a sensitive issue complexity of the challenge and containment strategy in Europe. Drug Resist Updat 9(3):123–133. https://doi.org/10.1016/j.drup.2006.06.002
Kagan LJ, Aiello AE, Larson E (2002) The role of the home environment in the transmission of infectious diseases. J Community Health 27(4):247–267
Kaku N, Yanagihara K, Morinaga Y, Yamada K, Harada Y, Migiyama Y et al (2014) Influence of antimicrobial regimen on decreased in-hospital mortality of patients with MRSA bacteremia. J Infect Chemother 20(6):350–355. https://doi.org/10.1016/j.jiac.2013.12.009
Kruse AB, Kristensen CS, Rosenbaum Nielsen L, Alban L (2019) A register-based study on associations between vaccination, antimicrobial use and productivity in conventional Danish finisher pig herds during 2011 to 2014. Prev Vet Med 164:33–40. https://doi.org/10.1016/j.prevetmed.2019.01.007
Kubin CJ (2002) Antimicrobial control programs. Semin Perinatol 26(5):379–386
Laing R, Hogerzeil H, Ross-Degnan D (2001) Ten recommendations to improve use of medicines in developing countries. Health Policy Plan 16(1):13–20. https://doi.org/10.1093/heapol/16.1.13
le Grand A, Hogerzeil HV, Haaijer-Ruskamp FM (1999) Intervention research in rational use of drugs: a review. Health Policy Plan 14(2):89–102. https://doi.org/10.1093/heapol/14.2.89
Levy SB (2000) Antibiotic and antiseptic resistance: impact on public health. Pediatr Infect Dis J 19(10 Suppl):S120–S122
Levy SB (2001) Antibacterial household products: cause for concern. Emerg Infect Dis 7(3 Suppl):512–515. https://doi.org/10.3201/eid0707.010705
Levy SB (2002) The 2000 Garrod lecture. Factors impacting on the problem of antibiotic resistance. J Antimicrob Chemother 49(1):25–30
Levy S (2014) Reduced antibiotic use in livestock: how Denmark tackled resistance. Environ Health Perspect 122(6):A160–A165. https://doi.org/10.1289/ehp.122-A160
Levy SB, Marshall B (2004) Antibacterial resistance worldwide: causes, challenges and responses. Nat Med 10(12 Suppl):S122–S129. https://doi.org/10.1038/nm1145
Lewis K (2013) Platforms for antibiotic discovery. Nat Rev Drug Discov 12(5):371–387. https://doi.org/10.1038/nrd3975
Lim VK, Cheong YM (1992) Bacteriology turnaround time in seven Malaysian general hospitals. Malays J Pathol 14(1):41–43
Mabadeje AF, Akintonwa AA, Ashorobi RB (1991) The value and effects of implementing an essential drugs list in the Lagos University Teaching Hospital. Clin Pharmacol Ther 50(2):121–124. https://doi.org/10.1038/clpt.1991.114
Mantravadi PK, Kalesh KA, Dobson RCJ, Hudson AO, Parthasarathy A (2019) The quest for novel antimicrobial compounds: emerging trends in research, development, and technologies. Antibiotics (Basel) 8(1). https://doi.org/10.3390/antibiotics8010008
Markou N, Markantonis SL, Dimitrakis E, Panidis D, Boutzouka E, Karatzas S et al (2008) Colistin serum concentrations after intravenous administration in critically ill patients with serious multidrug-resistant, gram-negative bacilli infections: a prospective, open-label, uncontrolled study. Clin Ther 30(1):143–151. https://doi.org/10.1016/j.clinthera.2008.01.015
Mayrhofer S, Paulsen P, Smulders FJ, Hilbert F (2006) Antimicrobial resistance in commensal Escherichia coli isolated from muscle foods as related to the veterinary use of antimicrobial agents in food-producing animals in Austria. Microb Drug Resist 12(4):278–283. https://doi.org/10.1089/mdr.2006.12.278

McEwen SA, Fedorka-Cray PJ (2002) Antimicrobial use and resistance in animals. Clin Infect Dis 34(Suppl 3):S93–S106. https://doi.org/10.1086/340246

McMahon MA, Blair IS, Moore JE, Mc Dowell DA (2007a) The rate of horizontal transmission of antibiotic resistance plasmids is increased in food preservation-stressed bacteria. J Appl Microbiol 103(5):1883–1888. https://doi.org/10.1111/j.1365-2672.2007.03412.x

McMahon MA, Xu J, Moore JE, Blair IS, McDowell DA (2007b) Environmental stress and antibiotic resistance in food-related pathogens. Appl Environ Microbiol 73(1):211–217. https://doi.org/10.1128/AEM.00578-06

McMurry LM, Oethinger M, Levy SB (1998) Overexpression of marA, soxS, or acrAB produces resistance to triclosan in laboratory and clinical strains of Escherichia coli. FEMS Microbiol Lett 166(2):305–309. https://doi.org/10.1111/j.1574-6968.1998.tb13905.x

Medeiros AA (1997) Evolution and dissemination of beta-lactamases accelerated by generations of beta-lactam antibiotics. Clin Infect Dis 24(Suppl 1):S19–S45

Mendelson M, Matsoso MP (2014) A global call for action to combat antimicrobial resistance: can we get it right this time? S Afr Med J 104(7):478–479. https://doi.org/10.7196/samj.8534

Mitchison DA (1954) Problems of drug resistance. Br Med Bull 10(2):115–124. https://doi.org/10.1093/oxfordjournals.bmb.a069388

Mitchison DA (1998) How drug resistance emerges as a result of poor compliance during short course chemotherapy for tuberculosis. Int J Tuberc Lung Dis 2(1):10–15

Munita JM, Arias CA (2016) Mechanisms of antibiotic resistance. Microbiol Spectr 4(2). https://doi.org/10.1128/microbiolspec.VMBF-0016-2015

Murphy GS Jr, Echeverria P, Jackson LR, Arness MK, LeBron C, Pitarangsi C (1996) Ciprofloxacin- and azithromycin-resistant Campylobacter causing traveler's diarrhea in U.S. troops deployed to Thailand in 1994. Clin Infect Dis 22(5):868–869

Mutanda LN, Omari AM, Wamola IA (1989) Adaptation of a method of measuring zone diameters of bacterial growth inhibition by antibiotics to suit developing countries. East Afr Med J 66(7):441–447

O'Brien TF, Stelling JM (1996) WHONET: removing obstacles to the full use of information about antimicrobial resistance. Diagn Microbiol Infect Dis 25(4):162–168

O'Neil J (2016) Tackling drug-resistant infections globally: final report amd recommendations. Retrieved from London, United Kingdom

Okeke IN, Lamikanra A (2003) Export of antimicrobial drugs by west African travelers. J Travel Med 10(2):133–135. https://doi.org/10.2310/7060.2003.31786

Okeke IN, Lamikanra A, Edelman R (1999) Socioeconomic and behavioral factors leading to acquired bacterial resistance to antibiotics in developing countries. Emerg Infect Dis 5(1):18–27. https://doi.org/10.3201/eid0501.990103

Okeke IN, Klugman KP, Bhutta ZA, Duse AG, Jenkins P, O'Brien TF et al (2005) Antimicrobial resistance in developing countries. Part II: strategies for containment. Lancet Infect Dis 5(9):568–580. https://doi.org/10.1016/S1473-3099(05)70217-6

Olofsson SK, Cars O (2007) Optimizing drug exposure to minimize selection of antibiotic resistance. Clin Infect Dis 45(Suppl 2):S129–S136. https://doi.org/10.1086/519256

Owens RC Jr, Shorr AF (2009) Rational dosing of antimicrobial agents: pharmacokinetic and pharmacodynamic strategies. Am J Health Syst Pharm 66(12 Suppl 4):S23–S30. https://doi.org/10.2146/090087d

Padungtod P, Kadohira M, Hill G (2008) Livestock production and foodborne diseases from food animals in Thailand. J Vet Med Sci 70(9):873–879

Pallin DJ, Ronan C, Montazeri K, Wai K, Gold A, Parmar S, Schuur JD (2014) Urinalysis in acute care of adults: pitfalls in testing and interpreting results. Open Forum Infect Dis 1(1):ofu019. https://doi.org/10.1093/ofid/ofu019

Parimi N, Pinto Pereira LM, Prabhakar P (2002) The general public's perceptions and use of antimicrobials in Trinidad and Tobago. Rev Panam Salud Publica 12(1):11–18

Paskovaty A, Pflomm JM, Myke N, Seo SK (2005) A multidisciplinary approach to antimicrobial stewardship: evolution into the 21st century. Int J Antimicrob Agents 25(1):1–10. https://doi.org/10.1016/j.ijantimicag.2004.09.001
Pastoret PP, Jones P (2004) Veterinary vaccines for animal and public health. Dev Biol (Basel) 119:15–29
Paterson DL (2004) "Collateral damage" from cephalosporin or quinolone antibiotic therapy. Clin Infect Dis 38(Suppl 4):S341–S345. https://doi.org/10.1086/382690
Pena C, Pujol M, Ricart A, Ardanuy C, Ayats J, Linares J et al (1997) Risk factors for faecal carriage of Klebsiella pneumoniae producing extended spectrum beta-lactamase (ESBL-KP) in the intensive care unit. J Hosp Infect 35(1):9–16
Penchovsky R, Stoilova CC (2013) Riboswitch-based antibacterial drug discovery using high-throughput screening methods. Expert Opin Drug Discovery 8(1):65–82. https://doi.org/10.1517/17460441.2013.740455
Penchovsky R, Traykovska M (2015) Designing drugs that overcome antibacterial resistance: where do we stand and what should we do? Expert Opin Drug Discovery 10(6):631–650. https://doi.org/10.1517/17460441.2015.1048219
Perencevich EN, Wong MT, Harris AD (2001) National and regional assessment of the antibacterial soap market: a step toward determining the impact of prevalent antibacterial soaps. Am J Infect Control 29(5):281–283
Perez A, Dennis RJ, Rodriguez B, Castro AY, Delgado V, Lozano JM, Castro MC (2003) An interrupted time series analysis of parenteral antibiotic use in Colombia. J Clin Epidemiol 56(10):1013–1020
Phillips-Howard PA, Wannemuehler KA, ter Kuile FO, Hawley WA, Kolczak MS, Odhacha A et al (2003) Diagnostic and prescribing practices in peripheral health facilities in rural western Kenya. Am J Trop Med Hyg 68(4 Suppl):44–49
Piddock LJ (2006) Clinically relevant chromosomally encoded multidrug resistance efflux pumps in bacteria. Clin Microbiol Rev 19(2):382–402. https://doi.org/10.1128/CMR.19.2.382-402.2006
Raffatellu M (2018) Learning from bacterial competition in the host to develop antimicrobials. Nat Med 24(8):1097–1103. https://doi.org/10.1038/s41591-018-0145-0
Rappuoli R, Del Giudice G, Nabel GJ, Osterhaus AD, Robinson R, Salisbury D et al (2009) Public health. Rethinking influenza. Science 326(5949):50. https://doi.org/10.1126/science.1179475
Rashid MU, Weintraub A, Nord CE (2012) Effect of new antimicrobial agents on the ecological balance of human microflora. Anaerobe 18(2):249–253. https://doi.org/10.1016/j.anaerobe.2011.11.005
Rhodes A, Evans LE, Alhazzani W, Levy MM, Antonelli M, Ferrer R et al (2017) Surviving sepsis campaign: international guidelines for management of sepsis and septic shock: 2016. Intensive Care Med 43(3):304–377. https://doi.org/10.1007/s00134-017-4683-6
Ross-Degnan D, Soumerai SB, Goel PK, Bates J, Makhulo J, Dondi N et al (1996) The impact of face-to-face educational outreach on diarrhoea treatment in pharmacies. Health Policy Plan 11(3):308–318
Rydberg J, Cederberg A (1986) Intrafamilial spreading of Escherichia coli resistant to trimethoprim. Scand J Infect Dis 18(5):457–460
Saez-Llorens X, Castrejon de Wong MM, Castano E, De Suman O, De Moros D, De Atencio I (2000) Impact of an antibiotic restriction policy on hospital expenditures and bacterial susceptibilities: a lesson from a pediatric institution in a developing country. Pediatr Infect Dis J 19(3):200–206
Santoso B, Suryawati S, Prawaitasari JE (1996) Small group intervention vs formal seminar for improving appropriate drug use. Soc Sci Med 42(8):1163–1168
Saul A, Rappuoli R (2009) The Novartis Vaccines Institute for Global Health: a new initiative for developing vaccines for neglected diseases in developing countries. J Infect Dev Ctries 2(2):154–155
Schuetz P, Albrich W, Mueller B (2011) Procalcitonin for diagnosis of infection and guide to antibiotic decisions: past, present and future. BMC Med 9:107. https://doi.org/10.1186/1741-7015-9-107

Selgelid MJ (2007) Ethics and drug resistance. Bioethics 21(4):218–229. https://doi.org/10.1111/j.1467-8519.2006.00542.x
Septimus EJ (2018) Antimicrobial resistance: an antimicrobial/diagnostic stewardship and infection prevention approach. Med Clin N Am 102(5):819–829. https://doi.org/10.1016/j.mcna.2018.04.005
Shapiro RL, Kumar L, Phillips-Howard P, Wells JG, Adcock P, Brooks J et al (2001) Antimicrobial-resistant bacterial diarrhea in rural western Kenya. J Infect Dis 183(11):1701–1704. https://doi.org/10.1086/320710
Shende S, Gade A, Rai M (2017) Large-scale synthesis and antibacterial activity of fungal-derived silver nanoparticles. Environ Chem Lett 15:7
Silbergeld EK, Graham J, Price LB (2008) Industrial food animal production, antimicrobial resistance, and human health. Annu Rev Public Health 29:151–169. https://doi.org/10.1146/annurev.publhealth.29.020907.090904
Singh M, Chaudhry MA, Yadava JN, Sanyal SC (1992) The spectrum of antibiotic resistance in human and veterinary isolates of Escherichia coli collected from 1984–86 in northern India. J Antimicrob Chemother 29(2):159–168
Soothill G, Hu Y, Coates A (2013) Can we prevent antimicrobial resistance by using antimicrobials better? Pathogens 2(2):422–435. https://doi.org/10.3390/pathogens2020422
Srinivasan V, Nam HM, Sawant AA, Headrick SI, Nguyen LT, Oliver SP (2008) Distribution of tetracycline and streptomycin resistance genes and class 1 integrons in Enterobacteriaceae isolated from dairy and nondairy farm soils. Microb Ecol 55(2):184–193. https://doi.org/10.1007/s00248-007-9266-6
Stine OC, Johnson JA, Keefer-Norris A, Perry KL, Tigno J, Qaiyumi S et al (2007) Widespread distribution of tetracycline resistance genes in a confined animal feeding facility. Int J Antimicrob Agents 29(3):348–352. https://doi.org/10.1016/j.ijantimicag.2006.11.015
Tagliabue A, Rappuoli R (2018) Changing priorities in vaccinology: antibiotic resistance moving to the top. Front Immunol 9:1068. https://doi.org/10.3389/fimmu.2018.01068
Tan L, Nielsen NH, Young DC, Trizna Z, Council on Scientific Affairs, American Medical Association (2002) Use of antimicrobial agents in consumer products. Arch Dermatol 138(8):1082–1086
Tenover FC (2006) Mechanisms of antimicrobial resistance in bacteria. Am J Med 119(6 Suppl 1):S3–S10; discussion S62–S70. https://doi.org/10.1016/j.amjmed.2006.03.011
Thampi N, Showler A, Burry L, Bai AD, Steinberg M, Ricciuto DR et al (2015) Multicenter study of health care cost of patients admitted to hospital with Staphylococcus aureus bacteremia: impact of length of stay and intensity of care. Am J Infect Control 43(7):739–744. https://doi.org/10.1016/j.ajic.2015.01.031
Traugott KA, Echevarria K, Maxwell P, Green K, Lewis JS 2nd. (2011) Monotherapy or combination therapy? The Pseudomonas aeruginosa conundrum. Pharmacotherapy 31(6):598–608. https://doi.org/10.1592/phco.31.6.598
Van Boeckel TP, Glennon EE, Chen D, Gilbert M, Robinson TP, Grenfell BT et al (2017) Reducing antimicrobial use in food animals. Science 357(6358):1350–1352. https://doi.org/10.1126/science.aao1495
van Nood E, Vrieze A, Nieuwdorp M, Fuentes S, Zoetendal EG, de Vos WM et al (2013) Duodenal infusion of donor feces for recurrent Clostridium difficile. N Engl J Med 368(5):407–415. https://doi.org/10.1056/NEJMoa1205037
Verraes C, Van Boxstael S, Van Meervenne E, Van Coillie E, Butaye P, Catry B et al (2013) Antimicrobial resistance in the food chain: a review. Int J Environ Res Public Health 10(7):2643–2669. https://doi.org/10.3390/ijerph10072643
Wayland C (2004) The failure of pharmaceuticals and the power of plants: medicinal discourse as a critique of modernity in the Amazon. Soc Sci Med 58(12):2409–2419. https://doi.org/10.1016/j.socscimed.2003.09.023
Weber JT, Courvalin P (2005) An emptying quiver: antimicrobial drugs and resistance. Emerg Infect Dis 11(6):791–793. https://doi.org/10.3201/eid1106.050471

Weinstein MP (2003) Blood culture contamination: persisting problems and partial progress. J Clin Microbiol 41(6):2275–2278

White DG, McDermott PF (2001) Biocides, drug resistance and microbial evolution. Curr Opin Microbiol 4(3):313–317

Whitehouse T (2014) National strategy for combating antibiotic resistant bacteria

WHO (2001a) Essential drugs monitor antimicrobila resistance: a global threat (editorial). World Health Organization

WHO (2001b) WHO global strategy for containment of antimicrobial resistance. World Health Organization - 2001, WHO/CDS/CSR/DRS/2001.2

WHO (2002) The selection and use of essential medicines. Report of the WHO expert commitee, Geneva

WHO (2015) WHO model list of essential medicines

Williams JD, Sefton AM (1999) The prevention of antibiotic resistance during treatment. Infection 27(Suppl 2):S29–S31

Woolhouse M, Waugh C, Perry MR, Nair H (2016) Global disease burden due to antibiotic resistance – state of the evidence. J Glob Health 6(1):010306. https://doi.org/10.7189/jogh.06.010306

World Health Organization, Food and Agriculture Organization of the United Nations and World Organisation for Animal Health (2018) Monitoring global progress on addressing antimicrobial resistance: analysis report of the second round of results of AMR country self-assessment survey 2018: World Health Organization

Wright GD (2011) Molecular mechanisms of antibiotic resistance. Chem Commun (Camb) 47(14):4055–4061. https://doi.org/10.1039/c0cc05111j

Zhao X, Drlica K (2001) Restricting the selection of antibiotic-resistant mutants: a general strategy derived from fluoroquinolone studies. Clin Infect Dis 33(Suppl 3):S147–S156. https://doi.org/10.1086/321841

Zhu YL, Hu LF, Mei Q, Cheng J, Liu YY, Ye Y, Li JB (2012) Testing the mutant selection window in rabbits infected with methicillin-resistant Staphylococcus aureus exposed to vancomycin. J Antimicrob Chemother 67(11):2700–2706. https://doi.org/10.1093/jac/dks280

Zirakzadeh A, Patel R (2005) Epidemiology and mechanisms of glycopeptide resistance in enterococci. Curr Opin Infect Dis 18(6):507–512

Chapter 2
Dietary Management by Probiotics, Prebiotics and Synbiotics for the Prevention of Antimicrobial Resistance

Fouad M. F. Elshaghabee and Namita Rokana

Abstract The increasing global threat of multi drug resistant pathogens is indicating that this is the time to put together our efforts to develop some approaches to turn down the spread of drug resistivity among the microbial world. The best way to reduce the evolution of antimicrobial resistance is to eliminate the heavy burden of antibiotics from our environment. The unfeasibility of elimination of antibiotics from our healthcare system directs us to develop some effective means to reduce their use at the least level. For this, we need to shift from completely antibiotic dependent therapeutic strategy to the multiple prophylactic and therapeutic approaches. Substantial efforts are being invested worldwide to find the sustainable line of defense against the rising pressure of antimicrobial resistance.

In this chapter we investigated the possible role of alternative multiple strategies using biologics such as probiotics, prebiotics, synbiotics and their metabolites in alleviation of the development of drug resistance. These environment and host friendly approaches could reduce the burden of infections by the means of direct or indirect mechanisms such as colonization interference, antimicrobial activity and stimulation of host defense system. Regardless of prompt research and substantial increase in clinical relevance, the approaches are still used as subsidiary or prophylactic strategy only. Advanced efforts are required to establish them as an absolute therapeutic alternative to reduce or replace the use of antibiotics.

Keywords Probiotics · Prebiotics · Synbiotics · Biologics · Antimicrobial resistance · Immunomodulation

---

F. M. F. Elshaghabee
Department of Dairy Science, Faculty of Agriculture, Cairo University, Giza, Egypt

N. Rokana (✉)
College of Dairy Science and Technology, Guru Angad Dev Veterinary and Animal Sciences University, Ludhiana, Punjab, India

H. Panwar et al. (eds.), *Sustainable Agriculture Reviews 49*, Sustainable Agriculture Reviews 49, https://doi.org/10.1007/978-3-030-58259-3_2

2.1 Introduction

Microbes play a vital role in the existence of human being. They shape our immune system from the very beginning of our life and mold our physiology and metabolism even before the birth (Swartwout and Luo 2018; Thompson 2019). The natural interdependence of humans and microbes also comprises the host pathogen interaction. In this context, microbes again save our life by providing a large range of antimicrobial substances (Mohanta et al. 2020). However, after few decades of the discovery of such antimicrobials, the development of antibiotic resistance has become a major challenge for the wellbeing of humankind. The inappropriate practice of over-prescription and taking incomplete course of antibiotic treatment have come out as the eventual development of antibiotic resistance against majority of novel antibiotics. Nowadays, multi drug resistance microbes have become a serious threat to the health and economy of global community (Nadimpalli et al. 2018; Tornimbene et al. 2018). Presence of multi drug resistant *Escherichia coli*, *Mycobacterium tuberculosis*, drug resistant *Streptococcus pneumoniae* and *Klebsiella pneumoniae*, methicillin resistant *Staphylococcus aureus*, multi drug and extensively drug resistant *Pseudomonas aeruginosa* and many others in our biosphere have augmented the struggle of health workers.

The quest of novel and sustainable strategies to combat multi drug resistance is constantly going on among world-wide researchers. In this way, multiple innovative approaches using different kind of biologics to target pathogens or host to treat infections are being explored. Biologics such as immunoglobulin, bioactive peptides, phage therapy, bacterial vaccines, probiotics and synbiotics have been proven to be an effective alternative for the prevention of several communicable or non-communicable diseases. These components attract the interest of researchers because of their sustainable capacity to fight directly (antimicrobial activity) or indirectly (immunomodulation of the host) against the development of antimicrobial resistance (Czaplewski et al. 2016). Apparently the alternative strategies seem less effective than antibiotics, but in long terms they may reduce the burden and selective pressure of antibiotics which ends up with the better health and less burden of antibiotics.

2.2 Dietary Management to Mitigate Antimicrobial Resistance

There is a continuous quest for "new" and unique antimicrobial strategies which could reduce the risk of antimicrobial resistance in natural way of living. In this regard the dietary management for prevention of common infections seems to be very promising approach. Consumers also demands for the natural food supplements which could provide additional health benefits and reduce the risk of infections in a synergistic way to reduce the need for antibiotics. Likewise, the antioxidant and antimicrobial activity of food from biological sources is being explored by some researchers. The functional foods having living or non-living biological elements could be instrumental for mitigation of antimicrobial resistance by means of direct inhibition of drug resistance pathogens or indirectly by reducing the risk of infections.

Supplement of probiotics with combination of some natural antimicrobials is being used to get more therapeutic benefits. A study by Ankolekar and coworkers (2011) explored the effect of cherry juice fermented with *Lactobacillus acidophilus* on inhibition of *Helicobacter pylori,* and proliferation of probiotic *Bifidobacterium longum.* Moreover, nowadays combination of probiotics with prebiotics is gaining more attraction because the presence of prebiotics stimulate and supplement the functionality of these beneficial microbes (Pandey et al. 2015; Markowiak and Śliżewska 2017). In this context, synbiotic based supplements could be explored as an effective strategy to reduce the burden of antibiotics among the population. In this chapter we will analyze the conjoining approaches of probiotics, prebiotics and synbiotics as a therapeutic substitution of antibiotics and as a preventive approach for the development of antimicrobial resistance.

2.3 How Probiotics Reduce the Risk of Antimicrobila Resistance

Probiotic microorganisms were defined as 'live microorganisms that, when administered in adequate amounts, confer a health benefit on the host' (Hill et al. 2014a). This definition evolved during the last decade. Probiotic microorganisms consists of a wide range of different genera mainly *Lactobacillus*, *Bifidobacterium*, *Pediococcus*, *Propionibacterium*, *Saccharomyces* and species of spore forming *Bacillus* (Ayeni et al. 2009; Czerucka et al. 2007; Hill et al. 2014b; Abdhul et al. 2015). Direct feed microbial strains with probiotics properties have been applied as feed or food supplement for both animals and humans as an alternative supplement to antibiotics, immune stimulator, growth promoters and enhancer of the host health (Tellez et al. 2015; Muñoz-Atienza et al. 2013; Retta 2016).

The two main criteria for probiotic microorganisms include (1) resistance to harsh condition during gastrointestinal tract transient (Schillinger et al. 2005; Kaushik et al. 2009) as well as manufacturing conditions (EL-Deib et al. 2012; El-Shafei et al. 2018) and (2) promotion of health benefits toward the host (de Waard et al. 2001; Amrouche et al. 2006; EL-Deib et al. 2012; Madhu et al. 2012; Sanchez et al. 2014). The health benefits of probiotics include conferring defense against infection, prevention of metabolic disorders, besides stabilizing or reconstituting the physiological balance between the intestinal microbiota and its host (Bhushan et al. 2019; Elshaghabee et al. 2019) (Fig. 2.1).

Besides their health benefits, probiotics have been found instrumental in reducing the risk of antimicrobial resistance in many ways (Table 2.1). The

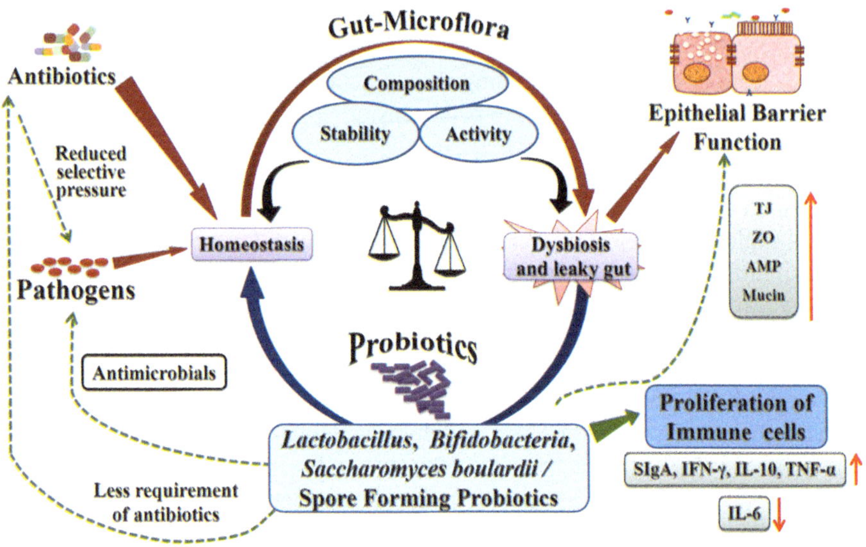

Fig. 2.1 Probiotic intervention against antimicrobial resistance. After colonization of probiotics into the intestine, they execute their beneficial effects using different pathways including immunomodulation, maintenance of epithelial barrier function, maintenance of intestinal microflora homeostasis and exclusion of pathogen. The beneficial activities of probiotics reduce the need and all over load of antibiotics in general population. Hence, reduced use of antibiotics pull down the selective pressure for the development of antimicrobial resistance among commensal microflora. Abbreviations: tight junction (TJ), zonula occludens (ZO), antimicrobial peptide (AMP), secretary immunoglobulin A (SIgA), interferon-γ (IFN- γ), interleukine-10 (IL-10), tumor necrosis fector-α (TNF-α), interleukine-6 (IL-6)

co-administration of probiotics with antibiotics can decline the development of drug resistance by diluting the selective pressure of antibiotic. The broad target range of antibiotics causes massive adverse effect on commensal microbial community of the host, sometime leading to secondary infections like diarrhea or yeast infection. Probiotics can also reduce the all over drug dependency by neutralizing many side effects caused by antibiotics such as distress, inflammation and electrolyte imbalance caused by gut microflora disturbance (Thiagarajah et al. 2015; Evans et al. 2016). There are different ways by which probiotics could cut down the use of antibiotics or combat the occurrence of antimicrobial resistance very efficiently. The mechanism of prevention of emergence of antimicrobial resistance using probiotic involves different direct and indirect interactions among host, probiotics and pathogens. Here we will go through the particulars of the beneficial actions of probiotics known to be useful against the battle with antimicrobial resistance.

Table 2.1 The antagonistic effect of probiotics against multi drug resistant (MDR) pathogens

MDR Pathogens	Probiotics	Type of study	Findings	Author(s)
S. aureus ATCC 25923, *E. coli* ATCC 25922	*L. acidophilus* ATCC3456, *L. casei* ATCC 39392, and *L. rhamnosus* ATCC 7469	*In vitro*	Cell free supernatant of *L. casei* was the most effective probiotic	Naderi et al. (2014)
Clinical isolates of *E. coli* and *K. pneumoniae*	Curd lactobacilli (*L. animalis, L. gasseri, L. acidophilus, L. rhamnosus*)	*In vitro*	Curd of lactobacilli alone or in combination with antibiotics had a therapeutic effects against infection	Halder and Mandal (2016)
Multi drug resistant isolates of *S. aureus* and *P. aeruginosa*	*L. paracasei*	*In vitro*	Combination of bacteriocins and Nano-silver particles could inhibit the multi drug resistant isolates	Gomaa (2018)
Thirty multi drug resistant isolates of *P. aeruginosa*	*L. reuteri* (DSM17938), *L. acidophilus* (DSM), *B. coagulans* (DSM1), *L. plantarum* 299v (DSM9843), and *B. bifidum* (DSM20456)	*In vitro*	Combination of probiotic strains with antibiotics could enhance the antagonistic effect	Moghadam et al. (2018)
Six multi drug resistant *E.coli* isolates	*L. acidophilus* EMCC 1324, *L. helveticus* EMCC 1654, *L. plantarum* EMCC 1027, *L. rhamnosus* EMCC 1105 *B. longum* EMCC 1547 *B. bifidum* EMCC 1334	*In vitro*	Cell free extract from skim milk by tested probiotics had strain specific antimicrobial activity against multi drug resistant *E. coli*	Abdelhamid et al. (2018)

(continued)

Table 2.1 (continued)

MDR Pathogens	Probiotics	Type of study	Findings	Author(s)
Multi drug resistant *S. typhimurium*	*L. acidophilus and S. cerevisiae*	*In vitro/In vivo*	Increased concentration of probiotic filtrate could increase the inhibition zone and oral administration of both probiotic isolates could decrease the counts of *S. typhimurium* in liver and spleen	Ibraheem et al. (2014)
Multi drug resistant isolates of *P. aeruginosa* and *E. coli*	LactoLevure® commercial probiotic product containing *L. plantarum, L. acidophilus, S. boulardii* and *B. lactis*	*In vivo*	Pretreatment of LactoLevure® could increase the survival rate, levels of cytokine e.g. TNF and IL-10 of mice under infection condition.	Machairas et al. (2015)
Multi drug resistant enteroaggregative *E. coli* and *E. coli* ATCC 25922	*L. plantarum* MTCC 1407 and *L. acidophilus* MTCC 10307	*In vivo*	Probiotic strains could be used as a therapeutic agent to curb multi drug resistant *E. coli.*	Kumar et al. (2016)
Multi drug resistant *E. coli*	*E. coli* Nissle 1913	Double blind, placebo-controlled trial	*E. coli* Nissle had not any inhibitory activity against MDR *E. coli*	Tannock et al. (2011)
K. pneumoniae	*L. casei* Shirota strain	Randomized, open-label controlled trial	Oral administration of probiotic *L. casei* Shirota strain could reduce the risk of Ventilator associated pneumonia (VAP) in patients	Rongrungruang et al. (2015)
K. pneumoniae	Lactocare capsules containing *Lactobacillus* species (*casei, acidophilus, rhamnosus, bulgaricus*), *Bifidobacterium* species (*breve, longum)*	Clinical	Adminstration of Lactocare could reduce the hospital stay of patients	Mahmoodpoor et al. (2019)

2.3.1 Establishment of Intestinal Homeostasis

Our intestine has been found to be structured in such a way that it is constantly in direct or indirect contact with both transient and resident microflora which is invariably exposed to a plethora of cytotoxins, antigens and pathogenic microbes to the epithelium. Humoral and immunological components of intestinal barrier function are continuously tailored to eliminate these factors from the lumen. Despite the backtracking efforts of barrier function elements, the dynamic homeostasis between intestinal barrier and enteric flora is often targeted by pathogens and several drugs (especially antibiotics and non-steroidal anti inflammatory drugs). The dysbiosis and inflammation in these conditions are consequences of the altered environment in the host physiological system which puts pressure on the gut microbial community to shift it towards an unfavourable composition for the enteric health (Fig. 2.1). This shift in microbiota leads to increased population of opportunistic pathogens and the ensuing loss of symbiotics or good bacteria from the gut.

The outcomes of a sizeable number of studies carried out on these lines have demonstrated the effect of probiotics on normalization of the composition of gut microbiota under several challenging condition. For example, Esaiassen and coworkers (2018) studied the effect of probiotics and antibiotic therapy on the developing gut microbiota and antibiotic resistome in extremely preterm infants in Norway. They found that supplement of probiotic (*Lactobacillus acidophilus* and *Bifidobacterium longum* subspecies *infantis;* Infloran®) could induce colonization, alleviate harmful effects of antibiotics and prevent the development of antibiotic resistome in infants. Similarly, Gao et al. (2019) observed that long term consumption of probiotics caused significant changes in the gut microbiota structure in elderly, including an increase in the composition of beneficial microorganisms. Authors stated that beneficial genus like *Blautia*, *Streptococcus*, *Enterococcus* and *Faecalibacterium* had higher abundance in the gut of probiotic group. In the same way, a number of studies (Doenyas 2018; Kong et al. 2019; Pérez-Burillo et al. 2019) have established the role of probiotics in maintenance of intestinal homeostasis. Hence, cumulatively probiotics support the growth and proliferation of other health promoting microorganisms. As a result, the population of opportunistic and potential pathogenic species remains under control and a healthy intestinal environment is maintained.

2.3.2 Modulation of Innate and Adaptive Immune System of Host

The complexity of relationship between intestinal microflora, immune system, inflammation and intestinal barrier is well recognized. The prophylactic and therapeutic effects of probiotics against dysbiosis and inflammation have also been established and proven clinically (Ducatelle et al. 2015). The therapeutic efficacy of probiotics has been found to be triggered by affecting gene expression of tight junction proteins, as well as increasing the secretion of mucus, modulating mucosal and systematic immunity, stimulating host antimicrobial peptides and IgA secretion and by improving the functionality of epithelial cells (Tsai et al. 2012; Nebot-Vivinus et al. 2014; Wang et al. 2014). The major advantage of probiotic interventions lies on their therapeutic action without provoking the host innate immunity that makes them more reliable among medical practitioners for the treatment of gut barrier related disorders. Hence, more in depth study to understand the mechanism involved in probiotic action in enhancing intestinal barrier are becoming the major focus of attention in the field of biotherapeutics as a safe and viable alternative to drugs.

Probiotic could enhance the immune response of host at different levels. Probiotics could regulate host innate immune response by activation of toll like receptors, dendritic cells, macrophages, and T and B lymphocytes (Vanderpool et al. 2008; Yan and Polk 2010). Long term effect of yoghurt consumption (200 g/day of yoghurt for 1 year) could decrease allergic symptoms and had little effect on levels of interferon gamma in young and senior adults (Van de Water et al. 1999). Kwon et al. (2010) demonstrated that a probiotic mixture consisting of *Lactobacillus acidophilus, Lactobacillus casei, Lactobacillus reuteri, Bifidobacterium bifidium*, and *Streptococcus thermophilus* stimulated regulatory dendritic cells and reduce the intestinal inflammation cascade. *Bifidobacterium breve* AH1205, *Bifidobacterium longum* and *Lactobacillus salivarius* AH102 were shown to reduce airway allergy (Lyons et al. 2010). *Lactobacillus acidophilus* Lafti L10 regulate genes involved in immune response including IL-23 signaling pathway (Van Baarlen et al. 2011). Microarray analysis of whole genome of *Lactobacillus acidophilus* NCFM resulted in regulation of different genes related to viral defense in murine bone-marrow derived dendritic cells including TLR-2, interferon-β, IL-12, and IL-10; however, these effects were not seen for *Bifidobacterium bifidum* Z9 and *Escherichia coli* Nissle 1917 (Weiss et al. 2010). Some active components of probiotic could regulate the immune system of the host. In this manner, *Lactobacillus rhamnosus* GG derived soluble protein p40 was noticed to reduce levels of tumor necrosis factor, IL-6, keratinocyte chemoattractant, and interferon-γ production indicating that p40 regulates innate immunity and Th1 immune response (Yan et al. 2011). Also, *Lactobacillus reuteri* RC-14 could produce cyclic dipeptides which could inhibit the staphylococcal accessory gene regulator (agr) quorum sensing system and decrease the expression of toxic shock syndrome toxin-1 in *Staphylococcus aureus* MN8 (Li et al. 2011).

Spore forming probiotic like *Bacillus coagulans* containing 1×10^9 CFU/g living bacteria could enhance the immune functions, spleen index and secretary immunoglobulin A (SIgA) of intestinal mucosa in Broilers (Xu et al. 2017). Also, inactivated *Bacillus coagulans* GBI-30 could enhance immune response by increasing levels of cytokines e.g. IL-1, tumor necrosis factor-α andinterferon-γ using *in vitro* model (Jensen et al. 2017). Different mechanisms by which spore forming probiotics (SFP) could enhance immune response of the host were reviewed by Elshaghabee et al. (2017). Non-commensal and non-pathogenic yeast *Saccharomyces boulardii* could inhibit the enterotoxigenic *Escherichia coli* (ETEC) induced expression of pro inflammatory cytokines and chemokines at both transcriptional and protein expression levels, including IL-6, IL-8 and IL-10 (Zanello et al. 2011). Figure 2.1 shows the immune modulation by different genera of probiotics.

Probiotics are weak inducers of pro inflammatory cytokines in comparison to pathogens because they could differentially stimulate the nuclear factor-kB (NF-kB) and the signal transducer and activator of transcription (STAT) (Sharma et al. 2010). It has been further noticed that probiotics can suppress the NF-kB pathway by blocking the degradation of inhibitor of NF-kB and prevent subsequent translocation of active NF-kB dimers to the nucleus (Bermudez-Brito et al. 2011). Probiotics also contribute towards reduction of inflammation by induction of T regulatory cells (T_{reg}) in the crypts that downregulate pro inflammatory signaling through production of interleukin-10 (IL-10) and transforming growth factor-β (Izcue et al. 2006; Jeon et al. 2012). A wide range of probiotics have been reported to inhibit T helper cell-1 (Th1) polarizing by activation of toll like receptor-2 (TLR2) mediated pathways (Evrard et al. 2011). The redirection of Th1/Th2 balance toward Th2 in inflamed gut encourage the expression of anti-inflammatory/regulatory cytokines like IL-10 and transforming growth factor-β associated with T_{reg} tolerance and IL-6, IL-12, interferon- γ and tumor necrosis factor-α suppression. Altogether, the inbuilt compositional properties of probiotics enable them to activate the immune cells towards adaptive or anti inflammatory mechanism. Even in the presence of pathogens, probiotics could modulate the infection derived inflammatory response to minimize damage to the host tissue.

2.3.3 Antimicrobial Activity Against Pathogens

Probiotic bacteria have antagonistic effect to control levels of pathogenic bacteria including opportunistic pathogen *Clostridium difficile* that is implicated in antibiotic associated diarrhea (Ouwehand et al. 2016). Also, probiotics could enhance the microbial balance in gut of the host and prevent gastrointestinal tract infections (such as stomach infections caused by *Helicobacter pylori*). This beneficial effect attributed to different probiotic strains could produce wide range of antimicrobial substances including bacteriocins, organic acids (mainly lactic and acetic acids) and hydrogen peroxide. Bacteriocins produced by different species of lactic acid bacteria were defined as small, heat stable, ribosomally synthesized bioactive peptide produced during growth of lactic acid bacteria (Gillor et al. 2008). Generally, most of bacteriocins except nisin and pediocin appear to be characterized as narrow spectrum of antimicrobial activity representing a major concern (Figueroa-González et al. 2011). Bacteriocins have been proven as the natural antimicrobial agents which are predominantly active against Gram positive pathogens and food spoilage bacteria, including *Listeria monocytogenes, Staphylococcus aureus, Bacillus cereus* and *Clostridium botulinum* (Chen and Hoover 2003).

Bacteriocins can be divided into two major classes according to their structure and mode of action; class I (lantibiotics) include nisin, which is active against Gram positive bacteria including food spoilage and pathogenic microbes. Nisin, which was mostly investigated, has a pentacyclic structure composed of 34 amino acids with one lanthionine residue. Another type of bacteriocins is class II peptides, which are heat stable and expressed from the bacterial cell without any post-translational modifications (Umu et al. 2016). Several types of bacteriocin were produced by lactic acid bacteria; nisin (*Lactococcus lactis*), reuterin (*Lactobacillus reuteri*), pediocin (*Pediococcus acidilactici*), acidophilin (*Lactobacillus acidophilus*), sacacin (*Lactobacillus sakei*), plantaricin (*Lactobacillus plantarum*), helveticin (*Lactobacillus helveticus*), curvacin (*Lactobacillus curvatus*), lactobin (*Lactobacillus amylovorus*). Bacteriocins based products could be used as an alternative therapy to classical antibiotics in order to reduce the risk of antimicrobial resistance; WipeOut® Dairy Wipes, and Mast Out® (Immucell Corporation) are already applied as an elective alternative for the treatment of mastitis (Pieterse et al. 2010). Recently, Sharma et al. (2018) reviewed several mechanisms by which probiotics and bacteriocins could decrease the antimicrobial resistance in dairy animals. These above mentioned examples shows that the production of growth inhibitory or bacteriostatic components (i.e. organic acids, H_2O_2) and bactericidal components (i.e. bacteriocins) are the key mechanisms of antimicrobial property of probiotics.

2.3.4 Interference with Colonization and Invasion of Pathogens

It is now well recognized that adhesion to the intestinal mucosa is a crucial step for transient colonization of microbes in the intestine (Carlson et al. 2009). In this context, one of the important prerequisites for probiotics to control the balance of the intestinal microbiota is to displace the pathogens from mucus layer and establish their own colonization to the mucosal surface. However, contrary to this, induction of alteration in mucus expression is an important strategy of the pathogens to induce infection in the target host tissue (Zarepour et al. 2013). Therefore, enhancement of the mucous layer is supposed to protect the host from attachment of hazardous molecules and pathogens to the epithelium. Thus, to facilitate the strengthening of mucosal layer, probiotics have evolved the ability to regulate mucin production by activating different signaling cascades and secretary elements (Caballero-Franco et al. 2007; Da Silva et al. 2014).

Intestinal epithelium has also been recognized as a delicate interphase between intestinal immune cells and their ligands. Any instability in this interphase is likely to expose a huge number of antigens to their reactive immune cells triggering acute pro inflammatory response at sub mucosal layer which eventually account for heavy structural and functional damage to the epithelial barrier. However, probiotics have the ability to restore the pathogens or allergen derived disturbances in intestinal permeability and immune homeostasis by evoking modulation of cytokine production either via immune activation or suppression. The initial stage of probiotic action includes reshaping the immune system to control the overgrowth of harmful microbes through stimulation of macrophages and natural killer cells and increasing IgA secretion by inducing secondary or adaptive immune system of the host (Sakai et al. 2014). In this context, probiotics and pathogens evoke opposite responses in the gut as they compete with each other for survival. Since the surface molecules of probiotic bacteria and pathogens are not easy to discriminate, when probiotics and pathogens both come in contact with intestinal epithelial cells, pathogenic microorganisms induce a strong host response because of presence of their additional virulent factors, while probiotics exhibit homeostatic control of the response and are able to competitively exclude enteropathogens (Lebeer et al. 2010; Rokana et al. 2016). Thus, we can say that probiotics could inhibit the colonization of pathogens into intestine by directly competing for space and nutrition or by indirectly stimulating the host mediated exclusion mechanisms.

2.3.5 Modulation of Intestinal Barrier Function

Probiotics have also been demonstrated to control or modulate the cytotoxic effect induced by the pathogens during infection by reinforcing the disrupted cellular permeability (Rokana et al. 2017). Quite a few previous studies have shown that pretreatment with probiotic bacteria could inhibit the decrease in resistance and alteration in tight junctions caused by stress, infection, or pro inflammatory cytokines (Karczewski et al. 2010; Wang et al. 2012). The outcome of few other reports (Mennigen et al. 2009; Anderson et al. 2010; Karczewski et al. 2010) have also shown that probiotics can subvert the deleterious effect of pathogens by stimulation of transcription and activation of myosin light chain kinase (MLCK), Rho GTPases signaling pathways besides regulating the arrangement of actomyosin ring, transmembrane tight junction proteins and finally reestablish the trans epithelial resistance of intestinal epithelium. The reversal of cytokine induced decrease in trans epithelial resistance and ion secretion is shown to be dependent on extracellular signal regulated kinase (ERK), p38, and phosphatidylinositol 3-kinase (PI3K) activation evoked by the probiotic bacteria (Resta-Lenert and Barrett 2006). Probiotics can also directly alter epithelial barrier function by influencing the structure of tight junctions also. These bacteria have been demonstrated to induce activation of occludin and zonula occludens (ZO-1) proteins, by increased levels of phosphorylated proteins without a significant change in the total levels. Increased permeability of the epithelial barrier can also be caused by apoptosis via activation of caspase-3. Probiotics can modulate the apoptosis cascade induced by harmful stimuli likely through inhibition of tumor necrosis factor-α production and secretion which is the main factor to induce the apoptosis in epithelial cells (Dalmasso et al. 2006).

Antimicrobial peptides, another important humoral element of epithelial barrier can also have a significant impact on host mucosal homeostasis. Several strains of probiotics have been reported to induce the secretion of antimicrobial agents for the management of dysbiosis. The antimicrobial potential of probiotics have been thoroughly investigated and have revealed that they are capable of inducing a diffused antimicrobial environment near epithelial cells by the mechanisms involving MAP kinases ERK ½ (microtubule associated protein kinase, extracellular signal regulated kinases), p38 and JNK (c-JUN N terminal kinase) signaling pathways which induce NF-kB and activator protein-1 transcription factors (Wehkamp et al. 2004; Froy 2005). Overall, probiotics strengthen the single layer of epithelial lining using variety of mechanisms. Broadly it includes reinforcement of structural components of cell-cell junction complex and stimulation of secretory antimicrobial components.

2.4 How Prebiotics and Synbiotics Reduce the Risk of Antimicrobial Resistance

Prebiotics are carbohydrate ingredients resistant to human gut digestive enzymes but get fermented by microflora of large intestine. Prebiotics are defined as "non digestible food ingredients that beneficially affect the host by selectively stimulating the growth and/or activity of one or a limited number of bacterial species already resident in the colon, and thus attempt to improve host health" (Gibson and Roberfroid 1995). The criteria for prebiotics are (1) resistance to gastric condition, (2) selective fermentation by beneficial microbes mainly probiotics, and (3) improve host health and well being (Roberfroid et al. 2010). Most of prebiotics (in other words, colonic foods) belong to dietary non-digestable polysaccharids such as galacto oligosaccharides, inulin, fructo oligosaccharides, raffinose, resistant starch, and resistant dextrins; non-starch polysaccharides (e.g., pectins, arabinogalactans, gum Arabic, gum guar and hemicellulose). Also, non-digestable oligosaccharides e.g. lactulose and sugar alcohol such as lactitol are considered as prebiotics (Yazawa et al. 1978; Gibson and Roberfroid 1999).

These substances induce selective stimulation of growth of specific groups of microflora which are devised with the capacity to metabolize them. Furthermore, consumption of prebiotics activates the metabolic pathways of health promoting bacteria and induces the production of beneficial metabolites thus ultimately improve the health of host (Holscher 2017). Hence, prebiotics could promote the health benefits of host by different mechanisms such as (1) modulation of gut microbiota and its metabolites (Viladomiu et al. 2013), (2) enhance the immune response (Nagura et al. 2002), (3) reduce the risk of hepatic encephalopathy (Dbouk and McGuire, 2006), (4) anti microbial activity and (Raafat et al. 2008) and anti obesity effect (Delzenne et al. 1993; Agheli et al. 1998; Daubioul et al. 2002; Sugatani et al. 2012). Prebiotics indirectly incite the protective mechanism against pathogenic infection by lowering the pH of intestinal milieu, improving the functionality of epithelial cells and by promoting the growth of competitive beneficial microbes in the intestine (Fig. 2.2). Moreover, prebiotics also have influence on nutrient

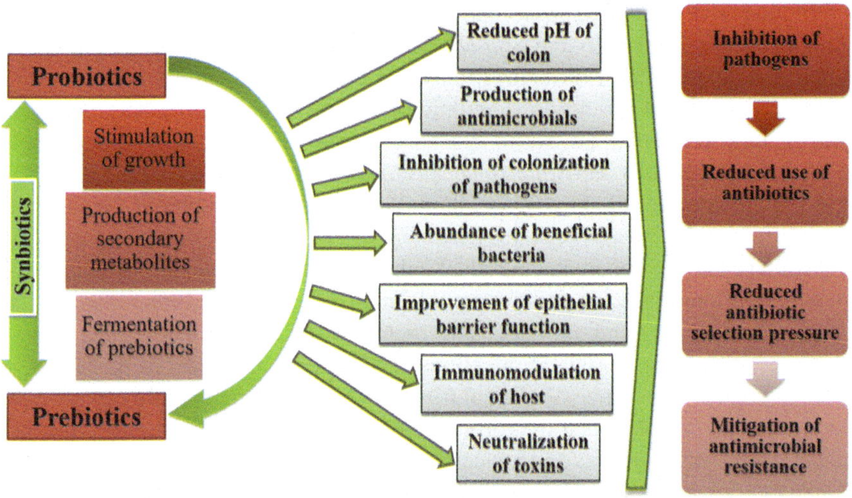

Fig. 2.2 Synbiotics and their mechanisms of action against antimicrobial resistant pathogens. Synbiotics collectively support intestinal homeostasis by stimulation of the growth of beneficial microflora. Production of metabolites such as short chain fatty acids also helps in modulation of immune system and neutralization of toxic components. Inhibition of pathogenesis in natural way results in reduced use of antibiotics and antibiotic generated selection pressure to cause antimicrobial resistance

absorption by intestinal epithelium and efficiency of host immune system (Scholz-Ahrens et al. 2007).

The concept of prebiotics also serves in combination of the activity of beneficial microbes in the intestine. Thereby, the combination of prebiotics and probiotics could aid sustainable improvement for the welfare of host. Gibson and Roberfroid introduced the term "synbiotics" for this concept and explained it as "mixtures of probiotics and prebiotics, growth promoter for probiotics, which beneficially affect the host by improving the survival and implantation of live microbial dietary supplements in the gastrointestinal tract."

2.5 Synbiotic Mechanism of Action

The gut environment has a range of nutrients which provide a favorable place for the colonization of different species of microorganisms. Presence of prebiotics gives an additional advantage to probiotics to compete out other organisms and pathogens in that space. The establishment and invasion of pathogens may also be hindered by lowering the pH of gut vicinity using fermentative metabolism of probiotics and synbiotics. This phenomenon has been evaluated by several researchers. For example, Kondepudi et al. (2012) examined antimicrobial activity of three strains of *Bifidobacterium* against *Clostridium difficile* in the presence of five different prebiotic non digestible oligosaccharides. Authors observed that in given conditions *Bifidobacterium breve* 46 and *Bifidobacterium lactis* 8:8 inhibited the growth and toxin production in four different strains of *Clostridium difficile*. In the same way, Koruri et al. (2016) reviewed the antimicrobial activity of *Pediococcus acidilactici* with natural prebiotics i.e. garlic and basil against *Escherichia coli*, *Salmonella*, *Enterococcus faecalis* and *Staphylococcus aureus*. The study showed that the presence of prebiotic resulted in enhanced inhibitory activity of probiotic strain against the pathogens.

Achievement of beneficial microbial balance in the intestine during and after illness is a difficult task. The restoration of imbalanced intestinal microbial community in both human and animals using prebiotics could be a better alternative to antibiotic treatment of several infections. The bifidogenic effect of prebiotics has been elucidated in a range of clinical trials and animal studies. In this context, prebiotic konjac glucomannan hydrolysate has reported to produce a favorable short chain fatty acid profile and selective stimulation of genus *Bifidobacterium*, *Lactobacillus-Enterococcus* group and Atopobium group in the batch culture inoculated with human faeces (Connolly et al. 2010). Correspondingly, a meta-analysis of controlled trials evaluating the effect of prebiotics on the composition of gut microbiota of healthy adults was done by So and coworkers (2018). This meta-analysis involved 64 studies and 2099 participants and revealed that the dietary fibers could increase the abundance of both *Bifidobacterium* spp. and *Lactobacillus* spp. and faecal short chain fatty acid concentration in healthy adults (So et al. 2018).

Some *in vivo* studies also shows the dynamic interactions between synbiotic and antibiotic interventions in reshaping the composition of intestinal microbiota. For instance, in a study conducted by Hammami et al. (2015), a synbiotic maple sap containing inulin and *Bifidobacterium lactis* Bb12 and *Lactobacillus rhamnosus* GG valio minimized the antibiotic induced breakdown of mice gut microbiota. Similarly, recently a more elaborated study of Jačan et al. (2019) exhibited that a synbiotic of nine probiotic strains and four types of prebiotics preserved the *Lactobacillales* and expanded the *Verrucomicrobiales* and *Bifidobacteriales* order in a mice model treated with antibiotic mix containing bacitracin, meropenem, neomycin, and vancomycin. In the same line, a positive effect of different concentrations of mannan oligosaccharides and fructo oligosaccharides was also observed on histo-morphometry and gut health status of broiler chickens (Biswas et al. 2018). Figure 2.2 shows the cumulative effect of synbiotics on the host including modulation of gut microbiota by inhibition of the growth of pathogens and improving the abundance of beneficial microbes.

Briefly, once prebiotic foods like inulin reached to colon, they fermented to different organic acids e.g. lactic, acetic acids and short chain fatty acids *i.e.* propionate and butyrate by beneficial microbes like *Bifidobacterium* spp. and resulted in increasing their abundance in gut. Lactate could be fermented to butyrate by lactate fermenting microbiota like *Anaerostipes caccae*/*Eubacterium hallii* (Belenguer et al. 2006). As stated previously, organic acids and short chain fatty acids work together in reducing the pH of colon resulting in reduced numbers of harmful and pathogenic microorganisms. These shifts in gut microbiota are useful for the public health including reducing the risk of antimicrobial resistance. A recent study by Perdijk et al. (2019) claims that in addition to differential promotion of the growth of *Bacteriodes* and *Bifidobacteria*, two human milk oligosaccharides namely sialyllactose and galactooligosaccharide can also induce the differentiation and repair of intestinal epithelial cells. Thereby, we can say that prebiotics could modulate the ecosystem of host intestine towards the population of beneficial microbes and helps in establishment of morphologically and physiologically healthy environment.

Prebiotics could also directly modulate the immune system of host by stimulating the expression of anti inflammatory cytokines (Shokryazdan et al. 2017). The modulation of host immune response is associated with modulation of gut microbiota through 1. Inhibition of pathogen colonization (Kogut 2013), and 2. Prebiotics act as non-pathogenic antigens where they can be recognized by different receptors of immune cells resulting in modulation of immune response (Teng and Kim 2018). Even prebiotics such as active hexose correlated compound is reported to attenuate the expression of different pro inflammatory cytokines including IL-1β, IL-1 receptor antagonist, tumor necrosis factor and monocyte chemoattractant protein-1 in colitis rat models (Daddaoua et al. 2007). Likewise, Bodera (2008) reviewed the influence of prebiotics on immune parameters in gut associated lymphoid tissue. In this review author deciphered that prebiotics could modulate various properties of the immune system of gut associated lymphoid tissue, secondary lymphoid tissues and peripheral circulation. Overall, prebiotics and synbiotics could indirectly reduce the resistivity to antibiotics by manipulating the gut health which will hinder the invasion of pathogen to intestinal epithelium; thus may lower the consumption of antibiotics and the positive selective pressure responsible for the development of antimicrobial resistance.

2.6 Antimicrobial Resistance in Probiotics: An Important Aspect to Be Considered

Antibiotic resistance of probiotic strains assures maintenance of healthy intestinal microbiota throughout antibiotic treatments of different microbial infections (Tuomola et al. 2001). Also, absence of "transferable" antibiotic resistance genes is a vital criterion for evaluation of safety of different probiotic strains (Franz et al. 2001; De Vuyst et al. 2003). The presence of highly antibiotic resistance strains among established probiotics raises the safety concern of the consumers. In this manner, a survey of susceptibility of 46 *Lactobacillus* strains to 44 antibiotics was assayed by Charteris et al. (1998). They found that all strains were resistant to a group of 14 antibiotics, which included inhibitors of cell wall synthesis (cefoxitin), protein synthesis (gentamycin), nucleic acid synthesis (nalidixic acid), and cytoplasmic membrane function (polymyxin B). Ispirli et al. (2017) also found that probiotic strains *Enterococcus durans* PY126 and *Enterococcus durans* PY146 possessed antibiotic resistance against number of common antibiotics including ampicillin, chloramphenicol, erythromycin, tetracycline hydrochloride, vancomycin, rifampicin, carbenicillin, amoxicillin and oxacillin. Thereby, it becomes essential to conduct an elaborated study on safety aspect of probiotic strains before establishing them for human consumption.

Currently, in market, many intrinsically vancomycin resistant strains of *Lactobacillus* have been safely used as probiotics without any indication of transferring this resistance to other species (Mattila-Sandholm et al. 1999). The natural resistance of probiotics to a wide range of clinically important antibiotics may enable the development of antibiotic/probiotic combination therapies for such conditions as diarrhea, female urogenital tract infection, and infective endocarditis (Charteris et al. 1998). But the potential and probable possibility of horizontal transfer of this trait should be evaluated carefully.

2.7 Conclusion

Probiotics and prebiotics or their combination positively improve the health of the host and contribute to control the invasion of pathogens. The mechanisms of prevention of infection involve interference with colonization and survival of pathogens, modulation of the composition of gut microflora, host immune system and epithelial barrier function. However the efficacy of these biologics as therapeutics largely depends on several factors such as the state of disease, mode of delivery and innate and physiological state of the host. Undoubtedly, probiotics and prebiotics extend a promising approach to lower the burden of antibiotics but further systemic studies to evaluate the direct interaction between multi drug resistant pathogens and probiotics/synbiotics are required to establish them as a reliable therapeutic alternative.

References

Abdelhamid AG, Esaam A, Hazaa MM (2018) Cell free preparations of probiotics exerted antibacterial and antibiofilm activities against multidrug resistant *E. coli*. Saudi Pharm J 26:603–607. https://doi.org/10.1016/j.jsps.2018.03.004

Abdhul K, Ganesh M, Shanmughapriya S, Vanithamani S, Kanagavel M, Anbarasu K et al (2015) Bacteriocinogenic potential of a probiotic strain *Bacillus coagulans* [BDU3] from Ngari. Int J Biol Macromol 79:800–806

Agheli N, Kabir M, Berni-Canani S, Petitjean E, Boussairi A, Luo J, Bornet F, Slama G, Rizkalla SW (1998) Plasma lipids and fatty acid synthase activity are regulated by short-chain fructo-oligosaccharides in sucrose-fed insulin-resistant rats. J Nutr 128(8):1283–1288. https://doi.org/10.1093/jn/128.8.1283

Amrouche T, Boutin Y, Priouit G, Fliss I (2006) Effects of bifidobacterial cytoplasm, cell wall and exopoly saccarides on mouse lymphocytes proliferation and cytokine production. Int Dairy J 16:70–80

Anderson RC, Cookson AL, McNabb WC, Park Z, McCann MJ, Kelly WJ, Roy NC (2010) *Lactobacillus plantarum* MB452 enhances the function of the intestinal barrier by increasing the expression levels of genes involved in tight junction formation. BMC Microbiol 10:316. https://doi.org/10.1186/1471-2180-10-316

Ankolekar C, Pinto M, Greene D, Shetty K (2011) Phenolic bioactive modulation by *Lactobacillus acidophilus* mediated fermentation of cherry extracts for anti-diabetic functionality, *Helicobacter pylori* inhibition and probiotic Bifidobacterium longum stimulation. Food Biotechnol 25(4):305–335. https://doi.org/10.1080/08905436.2011.617255

Ayeni FA, Adeniyi BA, Ogunbanwo ST, Tabasco R, Paarup T, Peláez C et al (2009) Inhibition of uropathogens by lactic acid bacteria isolated from dairy foods and cow's intestine in western Nigeria. Arch Microbiol 191(8):639–648. https://doi.org/10.1007/s00203-009-0492-9

Belenguer A, Duncan SH, Calder AG, Holtrop G, Louis P, Lobley GE, Flint HJ (2006) Two routes of metabolic cross-feeding between *Bifidobacterium adolescentis* and butyrate-producing anaerobes from the human gut. Appl Environ Microbiol 72:3593–3599. https://doi.org/10.1128/AEM.72.5.3593-3599.2006

Bermudez-Brito M, Plaza-Diaz J, Munoz-Quezada S, Gomez-Llorente C, Gil A (2011) Probiotic mechanisms of action. Ann Nutr Metab 61:160–174. https://doi.org/10.1159/000342079

Bhushan B, Singh BP, Saini K, Kumari M, Tomar SK, Mishra V (2019) Role of microbes, metabolites and effector compounds in host–microbiota interaction: a pharmacological outlook. Environ Chem Lett 1:1–20. https://doi.org/10.1007/s10311-019-00914-9

Biswas A, Messam R, Kumawat M, Namit M, Mandal AB, Mir NA (2018) Effects of prebiotics on intestinal histo-morphometry and gut microflora status of broiler chickens. Indian J Anim Res 8:1–5. https://doi.org/10.18805/ijar.B-3579

Bodera P (2008) Influence of prebiotics on the human immune system (GALT). Recent Patents Inflamm Allergy Drug Discov 2(2):149–153. https://doi.org/10.2174/187221308784543656

Caballero-Franco C, Keller K, De Simone C, Chadee K (2007) The VSL#3 probiotic formula induces mucin gene expression and secretion in colonic epithelial cells. Am J Physiol Gastrointest Liver Physiol 292:G315–G322. https://doi.org/10.1152/ajpgi.00265.2006

Carlson BA, Nightingale KK, Mason GL, Ruby JR, Choat WT, Loneragan GH, Smith GC, Sofos JN, Belk KE (2009) *Escherichia coli* O157: H7 strains that persist in feedlot cattle are genetically related and demonstrate an enhanced ability to adhere to intestinal epithelial cells. Appl Environ Microbiol 75:5927–5937. https://doi.org/10.1128/AEM.00972-09

Charteris W, Phillip MK, Morelli L, Collins JK (1998) Antibiotic susceptibility of potentially probiotic *Lactobacillus* species. J Food Prot 61:1636–1643. https://doi.org/10.4315/0362-028x-61.12.1636

Chen H, Hoover DG (2003) Bacteriocins and their food applications. Compr Rev Food Sci Food Saf 2(3):82–100. https://doi.org/10.1080/10408398.2015.1020918

Connolly ML, Lovegrove JA, Tuohy KM (2010) Konjac glucomannan hydrolysate beneficially modulates bacterial composition and activity within the faecal microbiota. J Funct Foods 2(3):219–224. https://doi.org/10.1016/j.jff.2010.05.001

Czaplewski L, Bax R, Clokie M, Dawson M, Fairhead H, Fischetti VA, Foster S, Gilmore BF, Hancock RE, Harper D, Henderson IR (2016) Alternatives to antibiotics—a pipeline portfolio review. Lancet Infect Dis 16(2):239–251. https://doi.org/10.1016/S1473-3099(15)00466-1

Czerucka D, Piche T, Rampal P (2007) Yeast as probiotics—*Saccharomyces boulardii*. Aliment Pharmacol Ther 26(6):767–778. https://doi.org/10.1111/j.1365-2036.2007.03442.x

Da Silva S, Robbe-Masselot C, Ait-Belgnaoui A, Mancuso A, Mercade-Loubière M, Salvador-Cartier C, Gillet M, Ferrier L, Loubière P, Dague E, Theodorou V, Mercier-Bonin M (2014) Stress disrupts intestinal mucus barrier in rats via mucin O-glycosylation shift: prevention by a probiotic treatment. Am J Physiol Gastrointest Liver Physiol 307:G420–G429. https://doi.org/10.1152/ajpgi.00290.2013

Daddaoua A, Martínez-Plata E, López-Posadas R, Vieites JM, González M, Requena P, Zarzuelo A, Suarez MD, de Medina FS, Martinez-Augustin O (2007) Active hexose correlated compound acts as a prebiotic and is anti-inflammatory in rats with hapten-induced colitis. J Nutr 137(5):1222–1228. https://doi.org/10.1093/jn/137.5.1222

Dalmasso G, Loubat A, Dahan S, Calle G, Rampal P, Czerucka D (2006) *Saccharomyces boulardii* prevents TNF-alpha-induced apoptosis in EHEC-infected T84 cells. Res Microbiol 157:456–465. https://doi.org/10.1016/j.resmic.2005.11.007

Daubioul C, Rousseau N, Demeure R, Gallez B, Taper H, Declerck B, Delzenne N (2002) Dietary fructans, but not cellulose, decrease triglyceride accumulation in the liver of obese Zucker fa/fa rats. J Nutr 132:967–973. https://doi.org/10.1093/jn/132.5.967

Dbouk N, McGuire BM (2006) Hepatic encephalopathy: a review of its pathophysiology and treatment. Curr Treat Opt Gastroenterol 9:464–474. https://doi.org/10.1007/s11938-006-0003-x

De Vuyst L, Foulquie-Moreno MR, Revets H (2003) Screening for enterocins and detection of hemolysin and vancomycin resistance in enterococci of different origins. Int J Food Microbiol 84:299–318. https://doi.org/10.1016/s0168-1605(02)00425-7

de Waard R, Garssen J, Snel J, Bokken GC, Sako T, Veld JH, Vos JG (2001) Enhanced antigen-specific delayed-type hypersensitivity and immunoglobulin G2b responses after oral administration of viable *Lactobacillus casei* YIT9029 in Wistar and Brown Norway rats. Clin Diagn Lab Immunol 8:762–767. https://doi.org/10.1128/CDLI.8.4.762-767.2001

Delzenne NM, Kok N, Fiordaliso MF, Deboyser DM, Goethals FM, Roberfroid MB (1993) Dietary fructooligosaccharides modify lipid metabolism in rats. Am J Clin Nutr 57:820S. https://doi.org/10.1093/ajcn/57.5.820S

Doenyas C (2018) Gut microbiota, inflammation, and probiotics on neural development in autism spectrum disorder. Neuroscience 374:271–286. https://doi.org/10.1016/j.neuroscience.2018.01.060

Ducatelle R, Eeckhaut V, Haesebrouck F, Van Immerseel F (2015) A review on prebiotics and probiotics for the control of dysbiosis: present status and future perspectives. Animal 9:43–48. https://doi.org/10.1017/S1751731114002584

EL-Deib SM, Abd Rabo FHR, Badran SM, Abd El-Fattah AM, Elshaghabee FMF (2012) The growth behavior and enhancement of probiotic viability in bio-yoghurt. Int Dairy J 22:44. https://doi.org/10.1016/j.idairyj.2011.08.003

El-Shafei K, Elshaghabee FMF, El-Sayed HS, Kassem JM (2018) Assessment the viability properties of *Lactobacillus casei* strain using Labneh as a carrier. Acta Sci Pol Technol Aliment 17(3):267–276. https://doi.org/10.17306/J.AFS.0583

Elshaghabee FMF, Rokana N, Gulhane R, Sharma C, Panwer H (2017) *Bacillus* as potential probiotics: status, concerns, and future perspectives. Front Microbiol 10:1490. https://doi.org/10.3389/fmicb.2017.01490

Elshaghabee FM, Rokana N, Panwar H, Heller KJ, Schrezenmeir J (2019) Probiotics for dietary management of non-alcoholic fatty liver disease. Environ Chem Lett 1:1–1. https://doi.org/10.1007/s10311-019-00896-8

Esaiassen E, Hjerde E, Cavanagh JP, Pedersen T, Andresen JH, Rettedal SI, Støen R, Nakstad B, Willassen NP, Klingenberg CA (2018) Effect of probiotic supplementation on the gut microbiota and antibiotic resistome development in preterm infants. Front Pediatr 6:347. https://doi.org/10.3389/fped.2018.00347

Evans M, Salewski RP, Christman MC, Girard SA, Tompkins TA (2016) Effectiveness of *Lactobacillus helveticus* and *Lactobacillus rhamnosus* for the management of antibiotic-associated diarrhoea in healthy adults: a randomised, double-blind, placebo-controlled trial. Br J Nutr 116(1):94–103. https://doi.org/10.1017/S0007114516001665

Evrard B, Coudeyras S, Dosgilbert A, Charbonnel N, Alamé J, Tridon A, Forestier C (2011) Dose-dependent immunomodulation of human dendritic cells by the probiotic *Lactobacillus rhamnosus* Lcr35. PLoS One 6(4):e18735. https://doi.org/10.1371/journal.pone.0018735

Figueroa-González I, Quijano G, Ramírez G, Cruz-Guerrero A (2011) Probiotics and prebiotics - perspectives and challenges. J Sci Food Agric 91(8):1341–1348. https://doi.org/10.1002/jsfa.4367

Franz CM, Muscholl-Silberhorn AB, Yousif NM, Vancanneyt M, Swings J, Holzapfel WH (2001) Incidence of virulence factors and antibiotic resistance among enterococci isolated from food. Appl Environ Microbiol 67:4385–4389. https://doi.org/10.1128/AEM.67.9.4385-4389.2001

Froy O (2005) Regulation of mammalian defense in expression by Toll-like receptor-dependent and independent signalling pathways. Cell Microbiol 7:1387–1397. https://doi.org/10.1111/j.1462-5822.2005.00590.x

Gao R, Zhang X, Huang L, Shen R, Qin H (2019) Gut microbiota alteration after long-term consumption of probiotics in the elderly. Probiotics Antimicrob Proteins 11:655–667. https://doi.org/10.1007/s12602-018-9403-1

Gibson GR, Roberfroid MB (1995) Dietary modulation of the human colonic microbiota: introducing the concept of prebiotics. J Nutr 125(6):1401–1412. https://doi.org/10.1093/jn/125.6.1401

Gibson GR, Roberfroid MB (1999) Prebiotics. In: Colonic microbiota, nutrition and health. Kluwer Academic, Dordrecht, pp 101–124. https://doi.org/10.1007/978-94-017-1079-4

Gillor O, Etion A, Riley MA (2008) The dual role of bacteriocins as anti- and probiotics. Appl Microbiol Biotechnol 81(4):591–606. https://doi.org/10.1007/s00253-008-1726-5

Gomaa EZ (2018) Synergistic antibacterial efficiency of bacteriocin and silver nanoparticles produced by probiotic *Lactobacillus paracasei* against multidrug resistant bacteria. Int J Pept Res Ther 2018:1–3. https://doi.org/10.1007/s10989-018-9759-9

Halder D, Mandal S (2016) Antibacterial potentiality of commercially available probiotic lactobacilli and curd lactobacilli strains, alone and in combination, against human pathogenic bacteria. Transl Biomed 7:2. https://doi.org/10.21767/2172-0479.100061

Hammami R, Ben Abdallah N, Barbeau J, Fliss I (2015) Symbiotic maple saps minimize disruption of the mice intestinal microbiota after oral antibiotic administration. Int J Food Sci Nutr 66(6):665–671. https://doi.org/10.3109/09637486.2015.1071340

Hill C, Guarner F, Reid G, Gibson GR, Merenstein DJ, Pot B et al (2014a) Expert consensus document: the International Scientific Association for Probiotics and Prebiotics consensus statement on the scope and appropriate use of the term probiotic. Nat Rev Gastroenterol Hepatol 11:506–514. https://doi.org/10.1038/nrgastro.2014.66

Hill C, Guarner F, Reid G, Gibson GR, Merenstein DJ, Pot B, Morelli L, Canani RB, Flint HJ, Salminen S, Calder PC (2014b) The International Scientific Association for Probiotics and Prebiotics consensus statement on the scope and appropriate use of the term probiotic. Nat Rev Gastroenterol Hepatol 11:506–514. https://doi.org/10.1038/nrgastro.2014.66

Holscher HD (2017) Dietary fiber and prebiotics and the gastrointestinal microbiota. Gut Microbes 8(2):172–184. https://doi.org/10.1080/19490976.2017.1290756

Ibraheem SK, Alshaibani AB, Ad'hiah AH (2014) Protective effect of *Lactobacillus acidophilus* and *Saccharomyces cerevisiae* against multi-drug resistant *Salmonella enterica* serovar typhimurium *in vitro* and *in vivo*. World J Pharm Res 3:193–203

Ispirli H, Demirbas F, Dertli E (2017) Characterization of functional properties of Enterococcus spp. Isolated from Turkish white cheese. LWT Food Sci Technol 75:358–368. https://doi.org/10.1016/j.lwt.2016.09.010

Izcue A, Coombes JL, Powrie F (2006) Regulatory T cells suppress systemic and mucosal immune activation to control intestinal inflammation. Immunol Rev 212:256–271. https://doi.org/10.1111/j.0105-2896.2006.00423.x

Jačan A, Kashofer K, Zenz G, Fröhlich EE, Reichmann F, Hassan AM, Holzer P (2019) Synergistic and antagonistic interactions between antibiotics and synbiotics in modifying the murine fecal microbiome. Eur J Nutr:1–14. https://doi.org/10.1007/s00394-019-02035-z

Jensen GS, Cash HA, Farmer S, Keller D (2017) Inactivated probiotic *Bacillus coagulans* GBI-30 induces complex immune activating, anti-inflammatory, and regenerative markers in vitro. J Inflamm Res 10:107. https://doi.org/10.2147/JIR.S141660

Jeon SG, Kayama H, Ueda Y, Takahashi T, Asahara T, Tsuji H, Tsuji NM, Kiyono H, Ma JS, Kusu T, Okumura R, Hara H, Yoshida H, Yamamoto M, Nomoto K, Takeda K (2012) Probiotic *Bifidobacterium breve* induces IL-10-producing Tr1 cells in the colon. PLoS Pathog 8:e1002714. https://doi.org/10.1371/journal.ppat.1002714

Karczewski J, Troost FJ, Konings I, Dekker J, Kleerebezem M, Brummer RJM, Wells JM (2010) Regulation of human epithelial tight junction proteins by *Lactobacillus plantarum in vivo* and protective effects on the epithelial barrier. Am J Physiol Gastrointest Liver Physiol 298:G851–G859. https://doi.org/10.1152/ajpgi.00327.2009

Kaushik JK, Kumar A, Duary RK, Mohanty AK, Grover S, Batish VK (2009) Functional and probiotic attributes of an indigenous isolate of *Lactobacillus plantarum*. PLoS One 4(12). https://doi.org/10.1371/journal.pone.0008099

Kogut MH (2013) The gut microbiota and host innate immunity: regulators of host metabolism and metabolic diseases in poultry? J Appl Poult Res 22:637–646. https://doi.org/10.3382/japr.2013-00741

Kondepudi KK, Ambalam P, Nilsson I, Wadstr T (2012) Prebiotic-non-digestible oligosaccharides preference of probiotic bifidobacteria and antimicrobial activity against *Clostridium difficile*. Anaerobe 18(5):489–497. https://doi.org/10.1016/j.anaerobe.2012.08.005

Kong C, Gao R, Yan X, Huang L, Qin H (2019) Probiotics improve gut microbiota dysbiosis in obese mice fed a high-fat or high-sucrose diet. Nutrition 60:175–184. https://doi.org/10.1016/j.nut.2018.10.002

Koruri SS, Chowdhury R, Bhattacharya P (2016) Potentiation of functional and antimicrobial activities through synergistic growth of probiotic *Pediococcus acidilactici* with natural prebiotics (garlic, basil). In: Microbes in the spotlight: recent progress in the understanding of beneficial and harmful microorganisms. BrownWlaker Press, Boca Raton, pp 219–224

Kumar M, Dhaka P, Vijay D, Vergis J, Mohan V, Kumar A, Kurkure NV, Barbuddhe SB, Malik SV, Rawool DB (2016) Antimicrobial effects of *Lactobacillus plantarum* and *Lactobacillus acidophilus* against multidrug-resistant enteroaggregative *Escherichia coli*. Int J Antimicrob Agents 48(3):265–270. https://doi.org/10.1016/j.ijantimicag.2016.05.014

Kwon HK, Lee CG, So JS et al (2010) Generation of regulatory dendritic cells and CD4+Foxp3+T cells by probiotics administration suppresses immune disorders. Proc Natl Acad Sci U S A 107:2159–2164. https://doi.org/10.1073/pnas.0904055107

Lebeer S, Vanderleyden J, De Keersmaecker SCJ (2010) Host interactions of probiotic bacterial surface molecules: comparison with commensals and pathogens. Nat Rev Microbiol 8:171–184. https://doi.org/10.1038/nrmicro2297

Li J, Wang W, Xu SX et al (2011) *Lactobacillus reuteri*-produced cyclic dipeptides quench agr-mediated expression of toxic shock syndrome toxin-1 in staphylococci. Proc Natl Acad Sci U S A 108:3360–3365. https://doi.org/10.1073/pnas.1017431108

Lyons A, O'Mahony D, O'Brien F et al (2010) Bacterial strain-specific induction of Foxp3+ T regulatory cells is protective in murine allergy models. Clin Exp Allergy 40:811–819. https://doi.org/10.1111/j.1365-2222.2009.03437.x

Machairas N, Pistiki A, Droggiti DI, Georgitsi M, Pelekanos N, Damoraki G, Kouraklis G, Giamarellos-Bourboulis EJ (2015) Pre-treatment with probiotics prolongs survival after experimental infection by multidrug-resistant *Pseudomonas aeruginosa* in rodents: an effect on sepsis-induced immunosuppression. Int J Antimicrob Agents 45(4):376–384. https://doi.org/10.1016/j.ijantimicag.2014.11.013

Madhu AN, Amrutha N, Prapulla SG (2012) Characterization and antioxidant property of probiotic and synbiotic yogurts. Probiotics Antimicrob Proteins 4:90–97. https://doi.org/10.1007/s12602-012-9099-6

Mahmoodpoor A, Hamishehkar H, Asghari R, Abri R, Shadvar K, Sanaie S (2019) Effect of a probiotic preparation on ventilator-associated pneumonia in critically ill patients admitted to the intensive care unit: a prospective double-blind randomized controlled trial. Nutr Clin Pract 34(1):156–162. https://doi.org/10.1002/ncp.10191

Markowiak P, Śliżewska K (2017) Effects of probiotics, prebiotics, and synbiotics on human health. Nutrients 9(9):1021. https://doi.org/10.3390/nu9091021

Mattila-Sandholm T, Matto J, Saarela M (1999) Lactic acid bacteria with health claims-ineractions and interference with gastrointestinal flora. Int Dairy J 9:25–35. https://doi.org/10.1016/S0958-6946(99)00041-2

Mennigen R, Nolte K, Rijcken E, Utech M, Loeffler B, Senninger N, Bruewer M (2009) Probiotic mixture VSL#3 protects the epithelial barrier by maintaining tight junction protein expression and preventing apoptosis in a murine model of colitis. Am J Physiol Gastrointest Liver Physiol 296:G1140–G1149. https://doi.org/10.1152/ajpgi.90534.2008

Moghadam SS, Khodaii Z, Zadeh SF, Ghooshchian M, Aghmiyuni ZF, Shabestari TM (2018) Synergistic or antagonistic effects of probiotics and antibiotics- alone or in combination- on antimicrobial-resistant *Pseudomonas aeruginosa* isolated from burn wounds. Arch Clin Infect Dis 13:e63121–e63125. https://doi.org/10.5812/archcid.63121

Mohanta D, Ghangal R, Solanki M, Patnaik S (2020) Delivery of microbial metabolites for human health care: a review. Environ Chem Lett 10:1–9. https://doi.org/10.1007/s10311-020-00967-1

Muñoz-Atienza E, Gómez-Sala B, Araújo C, Campanero C, Del Campo R, Hernández PE et al (2013) Antimicrobial activity, antibiotic susceptibility and virulence factors of lactic acid bacteria of aquatic origin intended for use as probiotics in aquaculture. BMC Microbiol 13(1):15. https://doi.org/10.1186/1471-2180-13-15

Naderi A, Kasra-Kermanshahi R, Gharavi S, Imani Fooladi AA, Abdollahpour Alitappeh M, Saffarian P (2014) Study of antagonistic effects of *Lactobacillus* strains as probiotics on multi drug resistant bacteria isolated from urinary tract infections. Iran J Basic Med Sci 17:201–208

Nadimpalli M, Delarocque-Astagneau E, Love DC, Price LB, Huynh BT, Collard JM, Lay KS, Borand L, Ndir A, Walsh TR, Guillemot D (2018) Combating global antibiotic resistance: emerging one health concerns in lower-and middle-income countries. Clin Infect Dis 66(6):963–969. https://doi.org/10.1093/cid/cix879

Nagura T, Hachimura S, Hashiguchi M, Ueda Y, Kanno T, Kikuchi H, Sayama K, Kaminogawa S (2002) Suppressive effect of dietary raffinose on T-helper 2 cell-mediated immunity. Br J Nutr 88:421–427. https://doi.org/10.1079/BJN2002666

Nebot-Vivinus M, Harkat C, Bzioueche H, Cartier C, Plichon-Dainese R, Moussa L, Eutamene H, Pishvaie D, Holowacz S, Seyrig C, Piche T, Theodorou V (2014) Multispecies probiotic protects gut barrier function in experimental models. World J Gastroenterol 20:6832–6843. https://doi.org/10.3748/wjg.v20.i22.6832

Ouwehand AC, Forssten S, Hibberd AA, Lyra A, Stahl B (2016) Probiotic approach to prevent antibiotic resistance. Ann Med 48(4):246–255. https://doi.org/10.3109/07853890.2016.1161232

Pandey KR, Naik SR, Vakil BV (2015) Probiotics, prebiotics and synbiotics-a review. J Food Sci Technol 52(12):7577–7587. https://doi.org/10.1007/s13197-015-1921-1

Perdijk O, van Baarlen P, Fernandez-Gutierrez MM, Van Den Brink E, Schuren FH, Brugman S, Savelkoul HF, Kleerebezem M, van Neerven RJ (2019) Sialyllactose and galactooligosaccharides promote epithelial barrier functioning and distinctly modulate microbiota composition and short chain fatty acid production *in vitro*. Front Immunol 10:94. https://doi.org/10.3389/fimmu.2019.00094

Pérez-Burillo S, Mehta T, Pastoriza S, Kramer DL, Paliy O, Rufián-Henares JÁ (2019) Potential probiotic salami with dietary fiber modulates antioxidant capacity, short chain fatty acid production and gut microbiota community structure. LWT 105:355–362. https://doi.org/10.1016/j.lwt.2019.02.006

Pieterse R, Todorov SD, Dicks LMT (2010) Mode of action and in vitro susceptibility of mastitis pathogens to macedocin ST91KM and preparation of a teat seal containing the bacteriocin. Braz J Microbiol 41:133–145. https://doi.org/10.1590/S1517-83822010000100020

Raafat D, von Bargen K, Haas A, Sahl HG (2008) Insights into the mode of action of chitosan as an antibacterial compound. Appl Environ Microbiol 74:3764–3773. https://doi.org/10.1128/AEM.00453-08

Resta-Lenert S, Barrett KE (2006) Probiotics and commensals reverse TNF-alpha and IFN-gamma-induced dysfunction in human intestinal epithelial cells. Gastroenterology 130:731–746. https://doi.org/10.1053/j.gastro.2005.12.015

Retta KS (2016) Role of probiotics in rumen fermentation and animal performance: a review. Int J Livest Prod 7(5):24–32. https://doi.org/10.5897/IJLP2016.0285

Roberfroid M, Gibson GR, Hoyles L, McCartney AL, Rastall R, Rowland I, Wolvers D, Watzl B, Szajewska H, Stahl B, Guarner F (2010) Prebiotic effects: metabolic and health benefits. Br J Nutr 104(S2):S1–S63. https://doi.org/10.1017/S0007114510003363

Rokana N, Singh R, Mallappa RH, Batish VK, Grover S (2016) Modulation of intestinal barrier function to ameliorate Salmonella infection in mice by oral administration of fermented milks produced with *Lactobacillus plantarum* MTCC 5690–a probiotic strain of Indian gut origin. J Med Microbiol 65(12):1482–1493. https://doi.org/10.1099/jmm.0.000366

Rokana N, Mallappa RH, Batish VK, Grover S (2017) Interaction between putative probiotic *Lactobacillus* strains of Indian gut origin and *Salmonella*: impact on intestinal barrier function. LWT Food Sci Technol 84:851–860. https://doi.org/10.1016/j.lwt.2016.08.021

Rongrungruang Y, Krajangwittaya D, Pholtawornkulchai K, Tiengrim S, Thamlikitkul V (2015) Randomized controlled study of probiotics containing *Lactobacillus casei* (shirota strain) for prevention of ventilator-associated pneumonia. J Med Assoc Thail 98(3):253–259

Sakai F, Hosoya T, Ono-Ohmachi A, Ukibe K, Ogawa A, Moriya T, Kadooka Y, Shiozaki T, Nakagawa H, Nakayama Y, Miyazaki T (2014) *Lactobacillus gasseri* SBT2055 induces TGF-β expression in dendritic cells and activates TLR2 signal to produce IgA in the small intestine. PLoS One 9:e105370. https://doi.org/10.1371/journal.pone.0105370

Sanchez M, Darimont C, Drapeau V, Emady-Azar S, Lepage M, Rezzonico E (2014) Effect of *Lactobacillus rhamnosus* CGMCC1.3724 supplementation on weight loss and maintenance in obese men and women. Br J Nutr 111:1507–1519. https://doi.org/10.1017/S0007114513003875

Schillinger U, Guigas C, Holzapfel WH (2005) *In vitro* adherence and other properties of lactobacilli used in probiotic yoghurt –like products. Int Dairy J 15:1289–1297. https://doi.org/10.1016/j.idairyj.2004.12.008

Scholz-Ahrens KE, Ade P, Marten B, Weber P, Timm W, Açil Y, Glüer CC, Schrezenmeir J (2007) Prebiotics, probiotics, and synbiotics affect mineral absorption, bone mineral content, and bone structure. J Nutr 137(3):838S–846S. https://doi.org/10.1093/jn/137.3.838S

Sharma R, Young C, Neu J (2010) Molecular modulation of intestinal epithelial barrier: contribution of microbiota. J Biomed Biotechnol 2010:305879. https://doi.org/10.1155/2010/305879

Sharma C, Rokana N, Chandra M, Singh BP, Gulhane RD, Gill JPS, Ray P, Puniya AK, Panwar H (2018) Antimicrobial resistance: its surveillance, impact, and alternative management strategies in dairy animals. Front Vet Sci 4:237. https://doi.org/10.3389/fvets.2017.00237

Shokryazdan P, Jahromi MF, Navidshad B, Liang JB (2017) Effects of prebiotics on immune system and cytokine expression. Med Microbiol Immunol 206(1):1–9. https://doi.org/10.1007/s00430-016-0481-y

So D, Whelan K, Rossi M, Morrison M, Holtmann G, Kelly JT, Shanahan ER, Staudacher HM, Campbell KL (2018) Dietary fiber intervention on gut microbiota composition in healthy adults: a systematic review and meta-analysis. Am J Clin Nutr 107(6):965–983. https://doi.org/10.1093/ajcn/nqy041

Sugatani J, Sadamitsu S, Wada T, Yamazaki Y, Ikari A, Miwa M (2012) Effects of dietary inulin, statin, and their co-treatment on hyperlipidemia, hepatic steatosis and changes in drug metabolizing enzymes in rats fed a high fat and high sucrose diet. Nutr Metab 9:23–41. https://doi.org/10.1186/1743-7075-9-23

Swartwout B, Luo XM (2018) Implications of probiotics on the maternal-neonatal interface: gut microbiome, immunomodulation, and autoimmunity. Front Immunol 9:2840. https://doi.org/10.3389/fimmu.2018.02840

Tannock GW, Tiong IS, Priest P, Munro K, Taylor C, Richardson A, Schultz M (2011) Testing probiotic strain *Escherichia coli* Nissle 1917 (Mutaflor) for its ability to reduce carriage of multidrug-resistant *E. coli* by elderly residents in long-term care facilities. J Med Microbiol 60:366–370. https://doi.org/10.1099/jmm.0.025874-0

Tellez G, Laukova A, Latorre JD, Hernandez-Velasco X, Hargis BM, Callaway T (2015) Food-producing animals and their health in relation to human health. Microb Ecol Health Dis 26:25876. https://doi.org/10.3402/mehd.v26.25876

Teng PY, Kim WK (2018) Roles of prebiotics in intestinal ecosystem of broilers. Front Vet Sci 5:245. https://doi.org/10.3389/fvets.2018.00245

Thiagarajah JR, Donowitz M, Verkman AS (2015) Secretory diarrhoea: mechanisms and emerging therapies. Nat Rev Gastroenterol Hepatol 12(8):446–457. https://doi.org/10.1038/nrgastro.2015.111

Thompson AL (2019) Early gut microbiome: a good start in nutrition and growth may have lifelong lasting consequences. In: How fermented foods feed a healthy gut microbiota. Springer, Cham, pp 239–258. https://doi.org/10.1007/978-3-030-28737-5_10

Tornimbene B, Eremin S, Escher M, Griskeviciene J, Manglani S, Pessoa-Silva CL (2018) WHO global antimicrobial resistance surveillance system early implementation 2016–17. Lancet Infect Dis 18(3):241–242. https://doi.org/10.1016/S1473-3099(18)30060-4

Tsai YT, Cheng PC, Pan TM (2012) The immunomodulatory effects of lactic acid bacteria for improving immune functions and benefits. Appl Microbiol Biotechnol 96:853–862. https://doi.org/10.1007/s00253-012-4407-3

Tuomola E, Crittenden R, Playne M, Isolauri E, Sakminen S (2001) Quality assurance criteria for probiotic bacteria. Am J Clin Nutr 73:393–398. https://doi.org/10.1093/ajcn/73.2.393s

Umu OC, Bauerl C, Oostindjer M, Pope PB, Hernández PE, Pérez-Martínez G et al (2016) The potential of class II bacteriocins to modify Gut microbiota to improve host health. PLoS One 11(10):e0164036. https://doi.org/10.1371/journal.pone.0164036

Van Baarlen P, Troost F, van der Meer C et al (2011) Human mucosal in vivo transcriptome responses to three Lactobacilli indicate how probiotics may modulate human cellular pathways. Proc Natl Acad Sci U S A 108(Suppl. 1):4562–4569. https://doi.org/10.1073/pnas.1000079107

Van de Water J, Ken CL, Gershwin ME (1999) The influence of chromic yogurt consumption on immunity. J Nutr 129:1492–1495. https://doi.org/10.1093/jn/129.7.1492S

Vanderpool C, Yan F, Polk DB (2008) Mechanisms of probiotic action: implications for therapeutic applications in inflammatory bowel diseases. Inflamm Bowel Dis 14:1585–1596. https://doi.org/10.1002/ibd.20525

Viladomiu M, Hontecillas R, Yuan L, Lu P, Bassaganya-Riera J (2013) Nutritional protective mechanisms against gut inflammation. J Nutr Biochem 24(6):929–939. https://doi.org/10.1016/j.jnutbio.2013.01.006

Wang Y, Liu Y, Sidhu A, Ma Z, McClain C, Feng W (2012) *Lactobacillus rhamnosus* GG culture supernatant ameliorates acute alcohol-induced intestinal permeability and liver injury. Am J Physiol Gastrointest Liver Physiol 303:G32–G41. https://doi.org/10.1152/ajpgi.00024.2012

Wang L, Cao H, Liu L, Wang B, Walker WA, Acra SA, Yan F (2014) Activation of epidermal growth factor receptor mediates mucin production stimulated by p40, a *Lactobacillus rhamnosus* GG derived protein. J Biol Chem 289:20234–20244. https://doi.org/10.1074/jbc.M114.553800

Wehkamp J, Harder J, Wehkamp K, Wehkamp-von Meissner B, Schlee M, Enders C, Sonnenborn U, Nuding S, Bengmark S, Fellermann K, Schröder JM, Stange EF (2004) NF-κB-and AP-1-mediated induction of human beta defensin-2 in intestinal epithelial cells by *Escherichia coli* Nissle 1917: a novel effect of a probiotic bacterium. Infect Immun 72:5750–5758. https://doi.org/10.1128/IAI.72.10.5750-5758.2004

Weiss G, Rasmussen S, Zeuthen LH, Zeuthen LH, Nielsen BN, Jarmer H, Jespersen L, Frøkiær H (2010) *Lactobacillus acidophilus* induces virus immune defence genes in murine dendritic cells by a Toll-like receptor-2-dependent mechanism. Immunology 131:268–281. https://doi.org/10.1111/j.1365-2567.2010.03301.x

Xu L, Fan Q, Zhuang Y, Wang Q, Gao Y, Wang C (2017) *Bacillus coagulans* enhance the immune function of the intestinal mucosa of yellow broilers. Rev Bras Ciência Avícola 19(1):115–122. https://doi.org/10.1590/1806-9061-2015-0180

Yan F, Polk DB (2010) Probiotics: progress toward novel therapies for intestinal diseases. Curr Opin Gastroenterol 26:95–101. https://doi.org/10.1097/MOG.0b013e328335239a

Yan F, Cao H, Cover TL, Washington MK, Shi Y, Liu L, Chaturvedi R, Peek RM, Wilson KT, Polk DB (2011) Colon-specific delivery of a probiotic-derived soluble protein ameliorates intestinal inflammation in mice through an EGFR-dependent mechanism. J Clin Invest 121:2242–2253. https://doi.org/10.1172/JCI44031

Yazawa K, Imai K, Tamura Z (1978) Oligosaccharides and polysaccharides specifically utilizableby bifidobacteria. Chem Pharm Bull 26:3306–3311. https://doi.org/10.1248/cpb.26.3306

Zanello G, Berri M, Dupont J, Sizaret PY, D'Inca R, Salmon H, Meurens F (2011) *Saccharomyces cerevisiae* modulates immune gene expressions and inhibits ETEC-mediated ERK1/2 and p38 signaling pathways in intestinal epithelial cells. PLoS One 6:e18573. https://doi.org/10.1371/journal.pone.0018573

Zarepour M, Bhullar K, Montero M, Ma C, Huang T, Velcich A, Xia L, Vallance BA (2013) The mucin Muc2 limits pathogen burdens and epithelial barrier dysfunction during *Salmonella enterica* serovar Typhimurium colitis. Infect Immun 81:3672–3683. https://doi.org/10.1128/IAI.00854-13

Chapter 3
Plant Natural Products for Mitigation of Antibiotic Resistance

Wen-Jie Ng, Chong-Seng Shit, Kah-Yaw Ee, and Tsun-Thai Chai

Abstract The emergence of antibiotic resistance and in particular multi drug resistance is of great threat to human health worldwide. Amid the ongoing efforts to search for novel antibacterial agents as alternatives to conventional antibiotics, researchers have intensively explored the potency of various antibacterial compounds derived from plant sources. In this chapter, we have summarised recent findings on five groups of plant natural products, namely flavonoids, phenolic acids, peptides, essential oils, and honey, as antibacterial agents. Research to date has demonstrated their effectiveness in combating various bacterial pathogens, including antibiotic resistant strains. These natural products exert their inhibitory effects through diverse mechanisms, for instance, perturbation of bacterial membrane integrity, inhibition of intracellular metabolism, in addition to interfering with quorum sensing and biofilm formation. Synergism between the aforementioned plant natural products and conventional antibiotics was established. Flavonoids and phenolic acids with superior inhibitory effects against human pathogenic bacteria, including relatively detailed understanding of their modes of action, have been documented.

Understanding of how endogenous plant peptides and protein hydrolysate-derived peptides of diverse structural complexities interact with the bacterial cell surface and exert their effects also continue to emerge. The potency of essential oils

W.-J. Ng
Department of Allied Health Sciences, Faculty of Science, Universiti Tunku Abdul Rahman, Jalan Universiti, Kampar, Malaysia

C.-S. Shit
Department of Biological Science, Faculty of Science, Universiti Tunku Abdul Rahman, Jalan Universiti, Kampar, Malaysia

K.-Y. Ee
Department of Agricultural and Food Science, Faculty of Science, Universiti Tunku Abdul Rahman, Jalan Universiti, Kampar, Malaysia

T.-T. Chai (✉)
Department of Chemical Science, Faculty of Science, Universiti Tunku Abdul Rahman, Jalan Universiti, Kampar, Malaysia
e-mail: chaitt@utar.edu.my

H. Panwar et al. (eds.), *Sustainable Agriculture Reviews 49*, Sustainable Agriculture Reviews 49, https://doi.org/10.1007/978-3-030-58259-3_3

as *in vivo* antibacterial agents was established in poultry and rat models. Notably, clinical studies have provided evidence that honey is an effective anti infective agent in the human body. Overall, the aforementioned plant natural products are not only potential alternatives to conventional antibiotics in the treatment of multi drug resistant bacterial infections, they are also promising candidates for future development of combination treatments with antibiotics.

Keywords Antibiotic resistance · Essential oil · Flavonoid · Honey · Peptide · Phenolic acid · Plant natural product

3.1 Introduction

The advent of antibiotics is widely regarded as a crucial medical breakthrough of the twentieth century. However, due to the emergence of bacteria that have developed or acquired resistance towards antibiotics, the application of antibiotics in modern medical practice may not be sustainable in future (Moore et al. 2017). In general, multi drug resistant bacteria, sometimes referred to as "superbugs", are resistant to three or more antibiotics (Styers et al. 2006), which makes standard treatments ineffective.

In 2017, the World Health Organization published a list of 12 families of antibiotic resistant "priority pathogens" that pose the greatest threat to human health (World Health Organization 2017). The World Health Organization list is divided into three categories according to the urgency of need for new antibiotics: critical, high and medium priority (Table 3.1). These bacteria are resistant to a large number of antibiotics, including carbapenems and third- generation cephalosporins, which are the best available antibiotics for targeting multi drug resistant bacteria.

The emergence of multi drug resistant bacteria increasingly limits the effectiveness of current antibiotics, leading to treatment failure. Owing to antibiotic resistance, more and more common diseases, including respiratory tract infections, sexually transmitted infections, and urinary tract infections have become untreatable. For instance, colistin is the last-resort treatment for life threatening infections caused by Enterobacteriaceae, which is resistant to carbapenems. Resistance to colistin has recently been detected in several countries, making infections caused by such bacteria untreatable. On the other hand, resistance of *Escherichia coli* to the fluoroquinolone antibiotics that are widely used for the treatment of urinary tract infections has been long established. There are countries in the world where fluoroquinolone treatment is now ineffective in more than half of the patients. Another example of antibiotic resistant bacteria is *Klebsiella pneumoniae*, a major cause of hospital acquired infections, such as pneumonia, bloodstream infections, and infections in new-borns and intensive care unit patients. Due to antibiotic resistance, carbapenem antibiotics, last-resort treatments, do not work in more than half of the people infected by *K. pneumoniae* (World Health Organization 2018).

Table 3.1 World Health Organization priority pathogens list for research and development of new antibiotics

Groups	Pathogens
Priority 1: Critical	1. *Acinetobacter baumannii*, carbapenem resistant
	2. *Pseudomonas aeruginosa*, carbapenem resistant
	3. Enterobacteriaceae, carbapenem resistant, extended spectrum β-lactamase producing
Priority 2: High	1. *Enterococcus faecium*, vancomycin resistant
	2. *Staphylococcus aureus*, methicillin resistant, vancomycin intermediate and resistant
	3. *Helicobacter pylori*, clarithromycin resistant
	4. *Campylobacter* spp., fluoroquinolone resistant
	5. *Salmonella*, fluoroquinolone resistant
	6. *Neisseria gonorrhoeae*, cephalosporin resistant, fluoroquinolone resistant
Priority 3: Medium	1. *Streptococcus pneumoniae*, penicillin non-susceptible
	2. *Haemophilus influenzae*, ampicillin resistant
	3. *Shigella* spp., fluoroquinolone resistant

According to the Centres for Disease Control and Prevention, each year in the United States of America, at least 2 million people get an antibiotic resistant infection, resulting in at least 23,000 deaths. The United Nations also reported that drug resistant diseases could cause 10 million deaths each year by 2050. Such public health threats will continue to worsen in the absence of effective strategies to treat multi drug resistant bacterial infection (Interagency Coordination Group on Antimicrobial Resistance 2019).

Living organisms produce primary and secondary metabolites. Primary metabolites are organic compounds that are essential for an organism to survive, whereas secondary metabolites are not directly involved in the growth, development and reproduction of the organism. Some secondary metabolites possess pharmacological and biological activities (Arshad and Batool 2017). Such natural products are important to the discovery and development of medicinal agents. Ever since the discovery of penicillin by Alexander Fleming, many more antibiotics were isolated from microorganisms. Afterwards, interest in antibiotics increased, leading to new waves of development of synthetic antibiotic. Mankind has relied more and more on synthetic and semi-synthetic antibiotics. Recently, the global issue of bacterial resistance to synthetic antibiotics has prompted researchers to consider the use of plant derived natural products which exert antibiotic actions (Abdallah 2011).

Plant products have been traditionally used as a therapeutic agents in folk medicine to treat various pathogenic diseases. Many scientists consider plant products to be important alternative sources of new and innovative antibacterial drugs against multi drug resistant bacteria. The potential of natural compounds derived from edible plant products, especially fruits, vegetables, herbs, spices and honey, for the prevention and even treatment of bacterial infections has now been extensively investigated. To date, more than 30,000 antimicrobial compounds have been identified from plants (Tajkarimi et al. 2010). Furthermore, plant natural products-antibiotic combinations are increasingly recognised as a promising strategy in tackling the issue of antibiotic resistance (Simões et al. 2009; Ayaz et al. 2019). In this chapter, we summarise recent findings on the potency of five groups of plant natural products, namely flavonoids, phenolic acids, peptides, essential oils, and honey, as antibacterial agents, especially for combating antibiotic resistant bacterial strains. Synergistic interactions between the aforementioned plant natural products and conventional antibiotics are highlighted. Emphasis is also given to their phytochemistry and modes of action underlying their antibacterial effects. Literature pertaining to antifungal plant natural products is not within the scope of this chapter. Concerning such discussion, we refer the reader to recent reviews by Daglia (2012); Lopes et al. (2017); Seleem et al. (2017); de Andrade Monteiro and dos Santos (2019). Figure 3.1 presents an overview of the mechanisms of action of five groups of plant natural products discussed in this chapter.

3.2 Flavonoids

Flavonoids are a class of natural secondary metabolites with the phenolic skeleton of C_6-C_3-C_6. According to their backbone structures, flavonoids can be categorised into major subclasses, which include aurones, flavones, isoflavones, neoflavones,

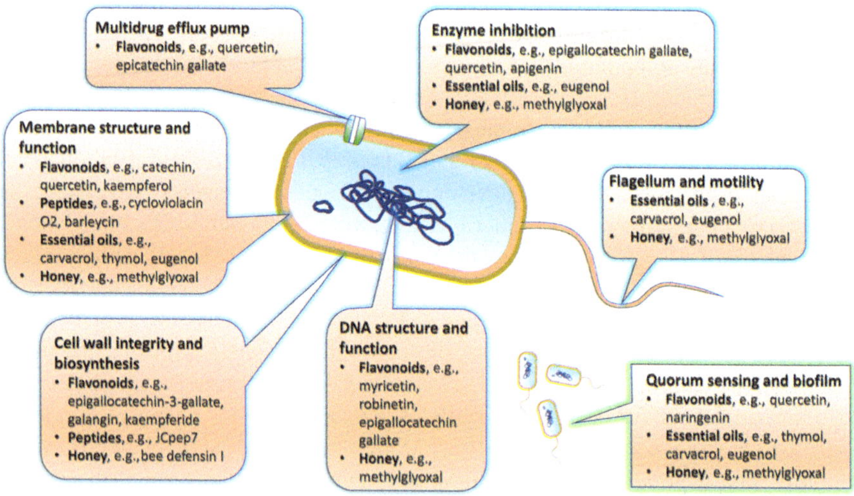

Fig. 3.1 An overview of the mechanisms of action of flavonoids, phenolic acids, peptides, essential oils, and honey. Such phytochemicals are able to target the metabolic functions and ultrastructural integrity of the bacterium cell. In addition, they could compromise cellular function, such as motility, and intercellular communication, which is key to biofilm formation. Some phytochemicals, e.g., quercetin and methylglyoxal, are capable of compromising multiple target sites

flavonols, flavans, flavanols (catechin), flavanones, flavanonols, chalcones, dihydrochalcones, anthocyanidins, proanthocyanidins, and leucoanthocyanidins (Cushnie and Lamb 2005; Rudrapal and Chetia 2017). Flavonoids are pharmacologically active compounds that exhibit various bioactivities, including antibacterial activity (Jaiswal and Kumar 2015). The therapeutic properties of flavonoids have also been shown in folk medicines. For example, the luteolin, quercetin-7-O-glucoside, kaempferol, kaempferol-7-O-glucoside, apigenin, and apigenin-7-O-glucoside isolated from a folk medicine *Tripleurospermum disciforme* exhibited antibacterial activities (Tofighi et al. 2015) (Fig. 3.2). In addition, the licoflavone C and derrone isolated from the *Retama raetam* flower were active against *P. aeruginosa* and *E. coli* (Edziri et al. 2012). A recent comprehensive review on the biosynthesis, structure-activity relationships, and medicinal potentials of plant chalcones demonstrates their diverse applications, which could inspire drug discovery in the future (Rammohan et al. 2020). Table 3.2 shows selected examples of plant flavonoids, their target bacterial species, and antibacterial activity.

Due to the increasing cases of infectious disease caused by antibiotic resistant bacteria and the need to search for novel bioactive compounds to target such bacteria, the antibacterial properties of plant flavonoids are attracting great attention in

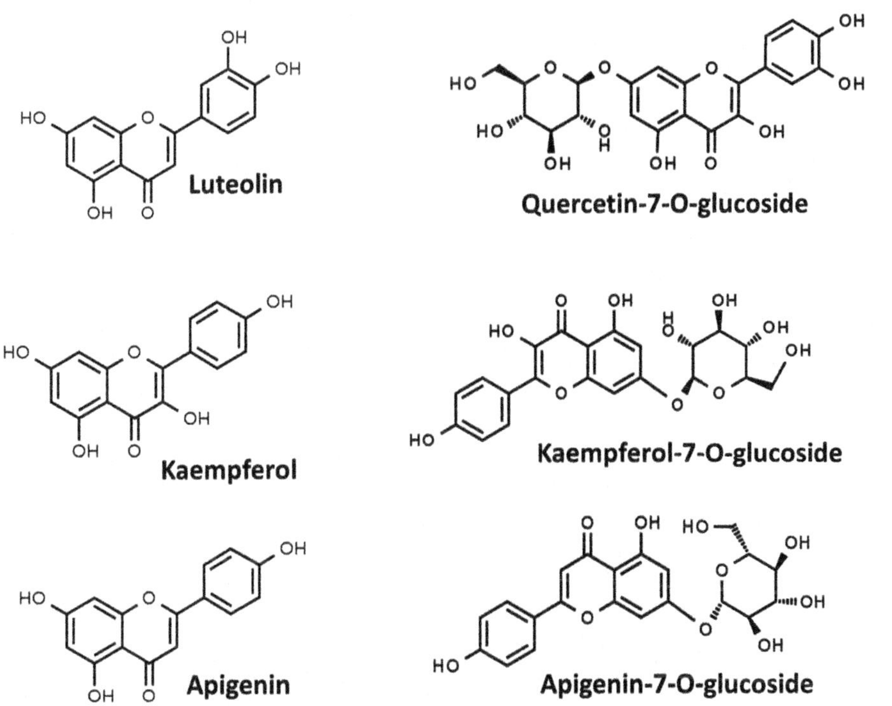

Fig. 3.2 Chemical structures of antibacterial flavonoids of medicinal plant *Tripleurospermum disciforme*. More details, including synonyms and chemical properties, of these flavonoids are available at ChemSpider (http://www.chemspider.com/)

Table 3.2 Examples of plant flavonoids and their antibacterial activities

Source	Flavonoids	Target species	Minimum inhibitory concentration	References
Alkanna orientalis	Sarothrin	*Mycobacterium smegmatis*	75–800 μg/mL	Bame et al. (2013)
		S. aureus		
Artocarpus anisophyllus	Artocarpin	*Bacillus cereus*	0.45 mg/mL	Jamil et al. (2014)
		E. coli		
		Pseudomonas putida		
Ficus sansibarica	Isovitexin	*S. aureus*	1.6–8 mg/mL	Awolola et al. (2014)
	Epicatechin			
	Trihydroxyflavanol			
Graptophyllum	Chrysoeriol xyloside	*Vibrio cholera*	0.25–2048 μg/mL	Tagousop et al. (2018)
Grandulosum	Luteolin apiofuranosyl xylopyranoside	*S. aureus*		
	Chrysoeriol apiofuranosyl xylopyranoside	*Candida albicans*		
	Chrysoeriol rhamnopyranosyl hydrogeno sulfate glucopyranoside	*Cryptococcus neoformans*		
	Isorhamnetin rhamnopyranosyl glucopyranoside			
Kalanchoe pinnata (lam.) Pers.	Quercetin	*E. coli*	50–100 μg/mL	Barboza et al. (2016)
Retama raetam flowers	Licoflavone C	*P. aeruginosa*	7.81–15.62 μg/mL	Edziri et al. (2012)
	Derrone	*E. coli*		
Terminalia arjuna bark	Free and bound	*Enterobector aerogens*	0.156–1.250 mg/mL	Jaiswal and Kumar (2015)
		B. subtilis		
		Routella planticola		
		Agrobacterium tumifacians		
		E. coli		
		P. aeruginosa		

(continued)

Table 3.2 (continued)

Source	Flavonoids	Target species	Minimum inhibitory concentration	References
Tripleurospermum disciforme	Luteolin	*S. aureus*	16–64 mg/mL	Tofighi et al. (2015)
	Quercetin-7-O-glucoside	*S. epidermidis*		
	Kaempferol			
	Kaempferol glucoside			
	Apigenin			
	Apigenin glucoside			
Black tea	Kaempferol	*Clostridium botulinum*	Not available	Sawamura et al. (2002)
	Kaempferitrin			
	Nicotiflorin			
	Quercetin glycoside			
Galangal	Galangin	*E. coli*	500–1000 μg/mL (synergistic with amoxicillin)	Eumkeb et al. (2012)
	Kaempferide			
	Kaempferol glucoside			
Grape seed extract	Catechin	*Streptococcus mutans*	5–15% (w/w)	El-Adawi (2012)
	Epicatechin			
Green tea	Catechin	*E. coli*	200 μM and above	Zhang and Rock (2004)
	Catechin gallate			
	Epicatechin			
	Epicatechin gallate			
	Epigallocatechin			
	Gallocatechin gallate			
	Epigallocatechin gallate			
Green tea	Epicatechin gallate	*E. coli*	100–500 mg/mL	Reygaert (2014)
	Epigallocatechin	*P. aeruginosa*		
	Epigallocatechin gallate	*S. aureus*		
		S. mutans		
		C. albicans		
Green tea	Epigallocatechin gallate	Enterohemorrhagic *E. coli*	0.05 mg/mL	Sugita-Konishi et al. (1999)
	Gallocatechin gallate			

research. The potential mechanisms of action of flavonoids against antibiotic resistant bacteria encompass (1) disruption of cytoplasmic membrane structure (Sanver et al. 2016; Tagousop et al. 2018); (2) inhibition of chemical modifying enzymes; (3) inhibition of nutrient and metabolite conveyance; (4) inhibition of nucleic acid synthesis (Wu et al. 2013); and (5) synergistic/potentiating effects (Górniak et al. 2019).

The effect of flavonoid-membrane interaction in the mitigation of antibiotic resistance has been documented, but the understanding on the complete mechanism remains controversial (Sanver et al. 2016). The presence of hydroxyl groups in flavonoids, especially in A ring at positions 5 and 7, B ring at 2 and 4, as well as C ring at position 3, has been suggested to increase the binding efficacy of flavonoids to negatively charged cell membranes, especially in Gram negative bacteria (Cushnie et al. 2008). The binding of some flavonoids, such as catechin, flavanone, and some flavonoid glycosides, to bacterial cell membrane was reported to damage membrane integrity and lead to leakage of intracellular substances in multi drug resistant *V. cholerae* (Tagousop et al. 2018) and methicillin resistant *S. aureus* (Cushnie et al. 2008; Reygaert 2014). In addition, green tea epigallocatechin gallate was reported as a potent inhibitor of both *trans*-2-enoyl-ACP and β-ketoacyl-ACP reductases in the bacterial type II fatty acid synthesis system. The inhibition of reductases interferes with acetate incorporation during the elongation cycle of fatty acid (Zhang and Rock 2004). Moreover, quercetin (a component of propolis), chrysin, and kaempferol were also reported to increase the permeability of the outer membrane of *B. subtilis*, *E. coli* and *Rhodobacter sphaeroides*, which further facilitates the absorption of flavonoids (Mirzoeva et al. 1997).

Flavonoids have also been reported to affect bacterial cell adhesion, quorum sensing and biofilm establishment, thus reducing the chance of mutation and inhibiting the establishment of antibiotic resistance (Borges et al. 2016; Babii et al. 2018). Many plant flavonoids, such as apigenin-6-C-glycoside, epicatechin (El-Adawi 2012; Nyila et al. 2012), 5,7,4′-trihydroxyflavanol (Awolola et al. 2014), quercetin, naringenin (Barboza et al. 2016) and synthetic tricyclic flavonoid (Babii et al. 2018) have been reported to be effective biofilm antagonists of *S. aureus*, *S. mutans*, *Listeria monocytogenes*, *K. pneumoniae*, and *E. coli*, although research on their mechanisms of action is rather limited (Borges et al. 2016; Babii et al. 2018). Flavonols, including galangin, kaempferol glucoside and kaempferide, have been reported to exert antibacterial activity against amoxicillin resistant *E. coli* and reverse its resistance by inhibiting ribosome and peptidoglycan synthesis (Eumkeb et al. 2012). In addition, direct and indirect interferences with the cell wall materials in methicillin resistant *S. aureus* by epigallocatechin-3-gallate were reported. Studies found that epigallocatechin-3-gallate interfered with the formation of glycocalyx, disrupted its interactions with the cell wall, and thus reducing the production of slime that accumulated to form biofilm. Epigallocatechin-3-gallate also bonded to peptidoglycan and induced the loss of the cell wall integrity (Zhao et al. 2001; Blanco et al. 2005).

Antibiotic resistant bacteria could employ chemical modification mechanism through certain aminoglycoside modifying enzymes, such as acetyltransferases, nucleotidytransferases, and phosphotransferaces, to degrade antibiotics (Ramirez and Tolmasky 2010). However, the literature on the inhibitory activity of flavonoids on these enzymes is currently limited. Quercetin and apigenin, for instance, were reported to inhibit the phosphotransferaces and related enzymes (Shakya et al. 2011).

Inhibition of nutrient and metabolite conveyance, through the formation of flavonoid-metal complexes, suppression of toxin production, and inhibition of efflux pumps, is one of the modes of antibacterial mechanisms. Flavonoid chelation of metal ions depends on the availability of metal ions, the binding sites of flavonoids, and the environmental pH (Kasprzak et al. 2015). Despite limited literature found on drug resistant bacteria species, bactericidal effects of flavone-metal complexes (Wang et al. 1992), quercetin-metal complexes (Bravo and Anacona 2001), and morin-metal complexes (Panhwar and Memon 2011) on other bacteria species have been reported. Studies suggested that the formation of these flavonoid-metal complexes halted the bioavailability of minerals which are required for the sustainability of bacterial metabolism. In the case of bacterial toxin production, similarly, many studies mainly focused on the inhibition of virulence factors, instead of the underlying mechanism. Typical examples are the inhibition effects of epigallocatechin-3-gallate and gallocatechin gallate on *E. coli* verotoxin (Sugita-Konishi et al. 1999), myricetin and quercetin on *Streptococcus agalactiae* hyaluronic acid lyase (Hertel et al. 2006), genistein on *S. aureus* exotoxin, kaempferol and quercetin glycoside on *C. botulinum* neurotoxin (Sawamura et al. 2002) and pinocembrin on *S. aureus* α-hemolysin (Soromou et al. 2013).

The ability of flavonoids to impair drug efflux system in bacterial cells has attracted significant attention in research. Effluence of antibiotics plays a key role in the ability of bacteria to resist antibiotic drugs. The down regulating and inhibitory effects of flavonoids on the efflux pumps of different bacteria have been reported. For examples, epicatechin gallate (minimum inhibitory concentration 64–512 μg/mL) and epigallocatechin gallate (minimum inhibitory concentration 32–64 μg/mL) possessed a fourfold higher inhibition activity than norfloxacin against norfloxacin resistant strain of *S. aureus*, which overexpressed the NorA multi drug efflux pump (Gibbons et al. 2004), sarothrin (minimum inhibitory concentration 75–800 μg/mL) inhibited the efflux pump NorA of drug resistant *S. aureus* (Bame et al. 2013), quercetin and epigallocatechin gallate inhibited the Mmr and EmrE efflux pumps of drug resistant *Mycobacterium tuberculosis*, *K. pneumoniae* and *E. coli* (Suriyanarayanan and Sarojini Santhosh 2015), and epigallocatechin gallate inhibited the CmeDEF efflux pumps of drug resistant *Campylobacter* spp. isolates (Kurinčič et al. 2012).

Topoisomerases are essential enzymes for DNA replication. Inhibition of these enzymes has been suggested as one of approaches to mitigate antibiotic resistance. The B ring of the flavonoids, including the 3-, 5-, 7-OH groups, plays a major role in bonding with the amino acid residues of topoisomerases, which explains the inhibitory action of flavonoids on DNA and RNA synthesis (Plaper et al. 2003; Wu et al. 2013). For examples, myricetin, robinetin and epigallocatechin gallate (components of *Elaeagnus glabra*) were reported to inhibit the synthesis of nucleic acids in bacteria (Cushnie and Lamb 2005). Besides, quercetin (a component of propolis), chrysin and kaempferol were reported to inhibit *E. coli* DNA gyrase B subunit (Wu et al. 2013). Baicalein, morin, epicatechin, silibinin, silymarin, quercetin and its derivatives inhibited the ATPase activity of gyrases and D-alanine-D-alanine ligase (Plaper et al. 2003; Wu et al. 2013) by blocking the ATP binding site (Wu et al. 2008), inhibiting ATP synthase, the rotation of the γ-subunit, and ATP hydrolysis (Chinnam et al. 2010). Furthermore, both helicases and dihydrofolate reductase are also common targets of antibacterial flavonoids. For examples, luteolin, morin and myricetin were revealed as the inhibitors of helicase RepA (Xu et al. 2001).

Epigallocatechin gallate was also shown to inhibit the activity of dihydrofolate reductase (Raju et al. 2015).

There have been many recent reports on synergistic and potentiating effects between flavonoids and conventional antibiotics (Górniak et al. 2019). These effects could be employed as mitigation tactics against antibiotic resistant bacteria. Synergistic effect is recognised when the fractional inhibitory concentration index is lower or equal to 0.5. When fractional inhibitory concentration index ranges from above 0.5 to 1.0, the effect is interpreted as potentiation (Górniak et al. 2019). To date, the five most vigorous flavonoid antibiotic synergistic combinations were demonstrated by Cushnie and Lamb (2011): (i) epicatechin gallate and oxacillin against methicillin resistant *S. aureus*; (ii) quercetin and β-lactam against penicillin resistant *S. aureus*; (iii) baicalein and β-lactam against methicillin-resistant *S. aureus*; (iv) myricetin and isoniazid against *Mycobacterium* spp.; (v) *Zanthoxylum piperitum* polymeric proanthocyanidin fraction (ZP-CT-A) and oxacillin against methicillin resistant *S. aureus*. Of all the flavonoid subclasses, the flavanol (catechin) subclass has been investigated most intensively. Potentiating effects were observed in different combinations of epicatechin, epigallocatechin gallates, and β-lactam antibiotics with regards to the inhibition of bacterial type II fatty acid synthesis and efflux activity in methicillin resistant *S. aureus* (Zhao et al. 2001). In addition, some other flavonoid subclasses also exhibit significant synergism with antibiotics. Examples include quercetin and its isomer morin in separate combination with either ciprofloxacin, tetracycline, or erythromycin against *S. aureus* strains (Abreu et al. 2015), and myricetin in different combinations with either cefoxitin, ampicillin/sulbactam, or amoxicillin/clavulanate against the pathogenic extended spectrum β-lactamase producing *K. pneumoniae* (Lin et al. 2005). Furthermore, synergism or potentiating effects were also reported for six types of isoflavonoids isolated from the root of *Erythrina* species in separate combinations with vancomycin against methicillin resistant *S. aureus* and vancomycin resistant enterococci (Sato et al. 2004). Fong et al. (2019) reported that oroxindin, rosmarinic acid and verbascoside acted as inhibitors of urease, shikimate kinase and aspartate-semialdehyde dehydrogenase, respectively, in the treatment of *H. pylori* infection. The study also revealed the potentiating effect of the combination of oroxindin and amoxicillin, with the fractional inhibitory concentration index value of 0.75 (Fong et al. 2019). Overall, further investigations on the detailed mechanisms underlying the aforementioned synergistic and potentiating effects, especially by using *in vivo* animal studies, for example suckling mice model and rabbit model of infection (Koley et al. 2019), are warranted.

3.3 Phenolic Acids

Phenolic acids occur in edible plant sources, which include various cereals and legumes, green and black teas, coffee, dark plum, and blueberry, as well as medicinal herbs (Wong et al. 2013; Miklasińska-Majdanik et al. 2018; Shahidi and Yeo 2018). Phenolic acids can be divided into two groups, (i) hydroxybenzoic acids, such as gallic, protocatechuic and *p*-hydroxybenzoic acids; (ii) hydroxycinnamic acids, such as caffeic, ferulic, chlorogenic and *p*-coumaric acids (Miklasińska-Majdanik et al. 2018; Shahidi and Yeo 2018). Figure 3.3 shows the structures of the aforementioned examples of phenolic acids.

The inhibitory effects of phenolic acids against multi drug resistant bacteria have been reported. Gallic acid and its derivatives exhibited antibacterial activity against multi drug resistant clinical isolate MDREC-KG4 of *E. coli*, with minimum inhibitory concentration ranging between 500 and 2000 μg/mL (Dwivedi et al. 2016). On the other hand, caffeic acid was inhibitory against methicillin resistant *S. aureus* reference and clinical strains, with minimum inhibitory concentration values ranging from 256 to 1024 μg/mL (Kępa et al. 2018). Greater lipophilicity and easier transport across the bacterial cell membrane may be accountable for the stronger antibacterial activity of caffeic acid relative to gallic, vanillic, and protocatechuic acids (Miklasińska-Majdanik et al. 2018).

Phenolic acids produced relatively high minimum inhibitory concentration values in comparison with conventional antibiotics. For example, the minimum inhibitory concentration values of caffeic, gallic and protocatechuic acids on strains of *A. baumannii*, a Gram negative pathogen known for multi drug resistance, ranged

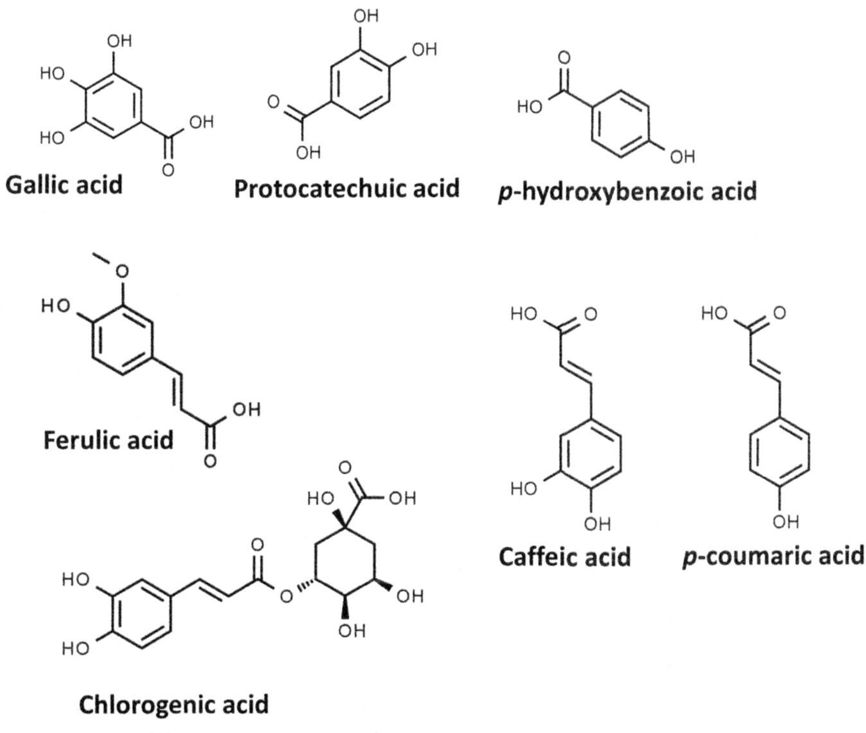

Fig. 3.3 Chemical structures of selected phenolic acids. More details, including synonyms and chemical properties, of these phenolic acids are available at ChemSpider (http://www.chemspider.com/)

between 32 and 256 μg/mL. By contrast, the minimum inhibitory concentration of antibiotic colistin on the same *A. baumannii* strains only ranged between 0.256 and 0.512 μg/mL (Ajiboye et al. 2018). Study on multi drug resistant clinical isolate of *E. coli* showed that gallic acid and its derivatives reduced the minimum inhibitory concentration of clinically used antibiotics (norfloxacin, ofloxacin, amikacin, tobramycin, ampicillin, cefoxitin, cefotaxime, tetracycline, and oxy-tetracycline) by two to eight folds when used in an antibiotic-phytochemical combination (Dwivedi et al. 2016). Thus, although not considered highly potent as antibacterial monotherapy, phenolic acids are promising candidates for combined therapy with antibiotics (Miklasińska-Majdanik et al. 2018). Recently, the synergy between caffeic acid and antibiotics (erythromycin, clindamycin, and cefoxitin) against methicillin resistant *S. aureus* reference and clinical strains has been demonstrated (Kępa et al. 2018).

The spread of *A. baumannii* is associated with nosocomial outbreaks, leading to high death rates. Development of resistance to colistin, a last-resort antibiotic against the pathogen, has been reported (Mohd. Rani et al. 2017; Almasaudi 2018). A recent study found that phenolic acids in combination with colistin may be an effective strategy in treating *A. baumannii* infections (Ajiboye et al. 2018). Caffeic, gallic, and protocatechuic acids were each able to enhance colistin mediated *A. baumannii* cell death. Acting in synergy, the phenolic acids and colistin exacerbated reactive oxygen species (ROS) mediated killing of the pathogen, as evidenced by elevated superoxide radical generation, as well as concomitant increase in NAD^+/NADH and ADP/ATP ratios, and decline in the level of reduced glutathione. The study suggested that the phenolic acids can potentiate the bactericidal action of colistin by compromising the pathogen's ability to detoxify H_2O_2. In addition, the phenolic acid colistin co-treatment can elevate superoxide radical production in the bacterial cells, likely a consequence of enhanced activities of the citric acid cycle and electron transport chains (Ajiboye et al. 2018).

3.4 Peptides

Antimicrobial peptides are small, compact peptides that exhibit microbicidal activity. They often comprise 15–100 amino acid residues and are normally cationic and cysteine rich. Antimicrobial peptides are key components of the innate immune system of plants. Thus they are ubiquitous in the plant kingdom and have been found in virtually every plant organ studied (Borges et al. 2015; Campos et al. 2018). Plant antimicrobial peptides may be broadly divided into three structural groups: cysteine-bond free, cysteine-rich, and cyclic families (Campos et al. 2018). Based on primary structure, molecular size, and cysteine content, plant antimicrobial peptides can be further classified into different families, which include glycine-rich proteins, cyclotides, defensins, knottin-like, hevein-like, lipid transfer proteins, snakins, myrosinase binding proteins, and short non-disulphide peptides (de Souza Cândido et al. 2014; Borges et al. 2015). Antibacterial activity of plant antimicrobial peptides against human pathogenic bacteria has been well documented. Table 3.3 shows some examples of plant antimicrobial peptides, their target bacterial species, and antibacterial activity.

Table 3.3 Examples of plant antimicrobial peptides

Source	Peptide	Size	Target species	Minimum inhibitory concentration	References
Guava (*Psidium guajava*)	Pg-AMP1	55 residues	*E. coli* *K. pneumoniae*	72, 32 μg/mL	Pelegrini et al. (2008)
Sweet violet (*Viola odorata*)	Cycloviolacin O2	30 residues	*E. coli* *P. aeruginosa* *S. aureus*	10–20 μM	Strömstedt et al. (2017)
Cowpea (*Vigna unguiculata*)	Cp-thionin II	47 residues	*S. aureus* *E. coli*	128, 64 μg/mL	Franco et al. (2006)
Green coconut (*Cocos nucifera*)	Cn-AMP1 Cn-AMP2 Cn-AMP3	8–11 residues	*E. coli* *B. subtilis* *P. aeruginosa* *S. aureus*	76–302 μg/mL	Mandal et al. (2009)
Jatropha curcas	JCpep7	7 residues	*Salmonella* Typhimurium *P. aeruginosa* *Shigella dysenteriae* *S. aureus* *B. subtilis* *S. pneumoniae*	24–64 μg/mL	Xiao et al. (2011)
Garden balsam (*Impatiens balsamina*)	Ib-AMP4	20 residues	Extended-spectrum β-lactamase-producing *E. coli* Methicillin-resistant *S. aureus*	4–16 μg/mL	Fan et al. (2013)
Wax gourd (*Benincasa hispida*)	Hispidalin	49 residues	*E. coli* *P. aeruginosa* *Salmonella enterica* *S. aureus*	80–120 μg/mL	Sharma et al. (2014)
Rapeseed (*Brassica napus*)	BnPRP1	35 residues	*E. coli* *Micrococcus luteus*	31.25, 62.5 μg/mL	Cao et al. (2015)
Alfalfa (*Medicago sativa*)	Met-Asp-Asn	3–8 residues	*B. subtilis*	2.45–5.27 mM	Kobbi et al. (2018)
	Gly-Asn-Ala-Pro-Gly-Ala-Val-Ala		*E. coli*	2.12–5.27 mM	
	Leu-Arg-Asp-Asp-Phe		*Listeria innocua*	2.00–3.12 mM	

(continued)

Table 3.3 (continued)

Source	Peptide	Size	Target species	Minimum inhibitory concentration	References
Highland barley (Tibetan barley)	Barleycin	9 residues	*B. subtilis*	4–16 μg/mL	Pei et al. (2018)
			S. aureus		
			L. innocua		
			E. coli		
			S. dysenteriae		

Note: Pg-AMP1, Cycloviolacin O2, Cp-thionin II, Cn-AMP1, Cn-AMP2, Cn-AMP3, JCpep7, Ib-AMP4, and BnPRP1 are names of antibacterial peptides designated by the respective authors

Pg-AMP1, isolated and identified from guava seeds, is an example of the glycine-rich proteins (Pelegrini et al. 2008). Such antimicrobial peptides are characterised by an abundance of glycine residues, up to about 70%, in the primary structure. They are also relatively hydrophobic owing to the occurrence of phenylalanine and tyrosinase residues (de Souza Cândido et al. 2014). Pg-AMP1 is the first glycine-rich protein which showed inhibition against Gram negative bacteria. The antimicrobial peptide inhibited the growth of *Klebsiella* sp. and *Proteus* sp., the principal human bacterial pathogens responsible for urinary and intestinal infections in immuno-suppressed patients. Pg-AMP1 is a monomer with a molecular mass of 6029.34 Da, but possibly requires homodimer formation for antibacterial activity (Pelegrini et al. 2008).

Cycloviolacin O2 is a cyclotide identified from the dried aerial plant materials of sweet violet (Strömstedt et al. 2017). Cyclotides are small, cyclic peptides comprising 28–37 amino acid residues. They are characterised by a cystine knot embedded in a macrocyclic backbone (de Souza Cândido et al. 2014; Strömstedt et al. 2017). Cycloviolacin O2 preferentially disrupts phosphatidylethanolamine-containing bacterial membranes, which may explain the potent antibacterial activity of Cycloviolacin O2 on Gram negative bacteria (Strömstedt et al. 2017).

Cp-thionin II is a 47-residue defensin identified from cowpea seeds. It has a molecular mass of 5.2 kDa, stabilised by four disulphide bonds. Cp-thionin II exhibited bactericidal activity against both Gram positive and Gram negative bacteria (Franco et al. 2006).

Cn-AMP1 (SVAGRAQGM, 858 Da), Cn-AMP2 (TESYFVFSVGM, 1249 Da), and Cn-AMP3 (YCSYTMEA, 950 Da) are three short non-disulphide peptides identified from green-coconut water (Mandal et al. 2009). Short non-disulphide peptides contain either no or very low cysteine content, unlike most plant antimicrobial peptides (de Souza Cândido et al. 2014). The three antimicrobial peptides showed bactericidal activities against *E. coli*, *B. subtilis*, *P. aeruginosa*, and *S. aureus*, with Cn-AMP1 being the most potent. Interestingly, Cn-AMP1 is cationic (net charge +1), whereas Cn-AMP2 and Cn-AMP3 are both anionic (net charge −1). Based on *ab-initio* molecular modelling, Cn-AMP1 has an alpha-helix structure. At the centre of the alpha-helix, an arginine residue occurs. The residue is believed to provide a positive charge, thus facilitating interaction with bacterial cell surface and contributing towards the antibacterial activity of Cn-AMP1 (Mandal et al. 2009).

JCpep7 (KVFLGLK) is another example of short non-disulphide antimicrobial peptides which exhibited antibacterial activity at low concentrations. JCpep7 is cationic, with total net charge of +2 and total hydrophobic ratio of 57%. It exhibited antibacterial activity against Gram negative and Gram positive bacteria. Analysis with fourier transform infrared spectroscopy and transmission electron microscopy techniques revealed that JCpep7 killed *S. aureus* mainly by breaking their cell walls and membranes, leading to cell lysis. After *S. aureus* was exposed to JCpep7 for 60 min, pores were found at the bacterial surface. Later, cell lysis was observed (Xiao et al. 2011).

Ib-AMP4 is a small cysteine-rich antimicrobial peptide identified from the seeds of *Impatiens balsamina.* IbAMP4 has been shown to be active against Gram positive and Gram negative bacteria at micromolar levels. Importantly, Ib-AMP4 efficiently targeted clinical multiresistant isolates, including methicillin resistant *S. aureus* and extended spectrum β-lactamase producing *E. coli*. Ib-AMP4 selectively targeted bacterial membranes and was inactive on sheep erythrocytes and A459 cancer cells. Such a lack of haemolysis and cytotoxicity is an advantage where clinical applications are concerned. It was proposed that Ib-AMP4 might be a potential candidate for clinical studies involving patients with septicaemia or for coating clinical devices. Furthermore, Ib-AMP4 may be combined with conventional antibiotics to treat antibiotic resistant pathogens (Fan et al. 2013).

Besides antimicrobial peptides that occur naturally or endogenously in plants, other antimicrobial peptides have also been discovered from the various plant protein hydrolysates (Xiao and Zhang 2012; Kobbi et al. 2018; Pei et al. 2018; Chai et al. 2019). These hydrolysate derived antimicrobial peptides, although not considered natural products in the strictest sense, are essentially fragments of natural plant proteins. Such peptides are short peptide sequences that are encrypted in the parent proteins and can be liberated through enzymatic hydrolysis. Antimicrobial peptides purified and identified from plant hydrolysates are often shorter than the naturally present plant antimicrobial peptides. For example, Met-Asp-Asn (378 Da), an antimicrobial peptide identified from the peptic hydrolysate of alfalfa ribulose-1,5-bisphosphate carboxylase/oxygenase, is only 3-residue long (Kobbi et al. 2018).

Barleycin (KIIIPPLFH, 1077.38 Da) is an antimicrobial peptide identified from the tryptic hydrolysate of highland barley proteins. Circular dichroism spectra indicated that barleycin had an alpha-helix conformation. The antimicrobial peptide is active against both Gram positive and Gram negative bacteria. It showed no cytotoxicity on human liver and renal cells. Furthermore, it was non-haemolytic against human red blood cells. The main mode of action of barleycin was proposed to be bacterial membrane permeabilisation, which may lead to the leakage of cytoplasmic contents and the death of sensitive bacteria (Pei et al. 2018).

JCpep8 (CAILTHKR) is an antimicrobial peptide identified from the protamex hydrolysate of *Jatropha curcas* meal protein isolate. JCpep8 was active against both

Gram negative and Gram positive bacteria, with minimum inhibitory concentration values of 29–68 μg/mL. Ultrastructural analysis of *S. aureus*, by transmission electron microscopy, indicated bacterial membrane disruption and cell lysis. JCpep8 has a total net charge of +3 and total hydrophobic ratio of 50%. Positive charge and hydrophobicity are believed to contribute to the binding of JCpep8 to the surface of bacterial membrane, which is important to its antibacterial effects (Xiao and Zhang 2012).

3.5 Essential Oils

"The essential oil is the product obtained from a vegetable raw material, either by steam distillation or by mechanical processes from the epicarp of Citrus, or dry distillation", according to a definition given by The French Agency for Normalisation: Agence Française de Normalisation (AFNOR) (Association francaise de normalisation 2000). These volatile oils are mainly colourless liquid with distinctive aroma. Plant essential oils may contain 20–60 lipophilic secondary plant metabolites at different concentrations. Two or three of the aforementioned components may be present at concentrations of up to 85%; these abundant components may be the main factors that exhibit antimicrobial activity (Bauer et al. 2001). Terpene derivatives and phenylpropenes are the main components in essential oils that exhibit antibacterial activity (Omonijo et al. 2018).

Terpenes are synthesised by the mevalonic acid pathway, requiring acetyl-CoA as the precursor (Chouhan et al. 2017); whereas phenylpropenes are produced via the shikimate pathway where phenylalanine is the precursor (Atkinson 2018). The main constituents in terpenes are monoterpenes ($C_{10}H_{16}$) and sesquiterpenes ($C_{15}H_{24}$). Thousands of monoterpenes and sesquiterpenes were discovered but only less than one hundred phenylpropenes were identified (Cooke et al. 1998; Lee et al. 2004; Omonijo et al. 2018).

Carvacrol is an example of monoterpenes that is present in most essential oils (Fig. 3.4). The essential oil of wild *Thymus* species contains 7–52% of carvacrol (Amiri 2012). The hydroxyl groups and the delocalised electrons present in carvacrol influence its antibacterial activity (Lambert et al. 2001; Ultee et al. 2002). For example, *p*-cymene, the precursor of carvacrol, had poorer antibacterial activity compared to carvacrol; *p*-cymene has a methyl ether instead of a hydroxyl group. The presence of hydroxyl group could greatly increase the hydrophobicity of monoterpenes, hence enhancing their antibacterial activity (Nazzaro et al. 2013). Carvacrol can target multiple cellular components in bacteria. In particular, it can bind to the surface of bacterial cell and accumulate in the phospholipid bilayer, causing cellular membrane expansion and membrane potential perturbation (Ultee et al. 2002). Following the accumulation of carvacrol, cell lysis may occur as the structural and functional properties of bacterial cellular membrane are compromised (Sikkema et al. 1995; Faleiro 2011; Yap et al. 2014).

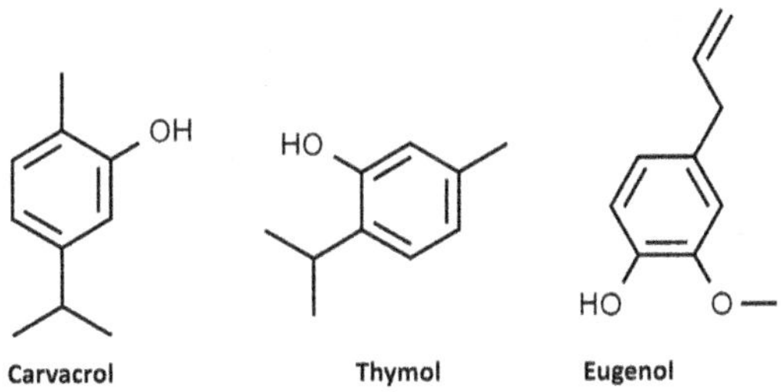

Fig. 3.4 Chemical structures of carvacrol, thymol and eugenol. More details, including synonyms and chemical properties, of these essential oil compounds are available at ChemSpider (http://www.chemspider.com/)

The sub-lethal effect of carvacrol may be attributed to errors during the folding of membrane proteins, resulting in the formation of defective proteins (Di Pasqua et al. 2010). *E. coli* cells upregulated the production of GroEL, a chaperone protein which assists in the proper folding of proteins, indicating that carvacrol compromised the process of membrane protein folding (Burt et al. 2007). Furthermore, the synthesis of flagellin, a microbial motility component, was inhibited by carvacrol, resulting in the production of bacterial cells without flagella (Gabel and Berg 2003).

Thymol is also a monoterpene that is present in most essential oils (Fig. 3.4). It is structurally similar to carvacrol; the difference between these two molecules is the position of their hydroxyl groups (Nazzaro et al. 2013). The essential oil of commercial *Thymus vulgaris* contains 20–60% of thymol (Satyal et al. 2016). Thymol diffuses into the bacterial cell membrane smoothly; due to its lipophilic property, thymol has great binding affinity to the components in bacterial cell membrane. Cell membrane dissociation happens as thymol partitions into the membrane lipids, destabilising the membrane structure (Sikkema et al. 1994; Nazzaro et al. 2013; Issa et al. 2019). On the other hand, cellular components present on bacterial cell membrane are also affected by thymol. For example, bacterial ATP synthesis is interfered as thymols bind to the ATP synthase (Denyer and Hugo 1991; Sikkema et al. 1995; Davidson 1997). Besides its effect on the bacterial membrane, thymol may also interrupt cellular metabolism, particularly by inhibiting mRNA transcription, thus leading to cell death (Benchaar et al. 2007; Lv et al. 2011; Bajpai et al. 2013; Nazzaro et al. 2013).

Generally, Gram positive bacteria are more sensitive to essential oils as their cell walls compose of peptidoglycan that allows rapid diffusion of hydrophobic essential oils into the bacterial cells. On the other hand, the outer membrane of Gram negative bacteria is rich in lipopolysaccharides, which reduces the diffusion of essential oils into the cells (Vaara 1992). Still, both thymol and carvacrol are able to overcome the Gram negative bacterial resistance by their lipopolysaccharides releasing properties. They cause damage to the outer bacterial membrane by releasing the lipopolysaccharides, thus sensitising the membrane (Omonijo et al. 2018). On the other hand, exposure to thymol and carvacrol altered the fatty acid composition of Gram negative bacterial cell membrane and outer membrane, which increased bacterial membrane fluidity (Di Pasqua et al. 2006; Di Pasqua et al. 2007; La Storia et al. 2011). Hence, a combination of thymol and carvacrol could be effective in combating multi drug resistant bacteria.

Essential oils rich in thymol and carvacrol, such as those extracted from the wild thyme, can also exert their antibacterial activity through the interruption of bacterial quorum sensing by inhibiting N-acyl homoserine lactones synthesis, and then interfering with biofilm production (MCetin et al. 2011; Magi et al. 2015; Joshi et al. 2016; Oh et al. 2017). A recent study revealed that quorum sensing activity of *Chromobacterium violaceum* was inhibited after exposure to thymol- and carvacrol-rich essential oils (Zhang et al. 2018). Both carvacrol and thymol, acting as quorum sensing inhibitors, interfered with intercellular communication among *C. violaceum* by inhibiting N-acyl homoserine lactones production and/or binding to the cognate receptor of N-acyl homoserine lactones (Myszka et al. 2016). The same essential oil also showed antibiofilm activity on a *Pseudomonas fluorescens* isolate (Zhang et al. 2018). Hence, to inhibit biofilm forming activity, the bacterial quorum sensing activity has to be interrupted.

The *in vivo* effectiveness of thymol- and carvacrol-rich essential oils was investigated, showing promising results. For example, mist generated from *Ocimum basilicum* essential oil cured 6–75% of pneumococci induced and 56–81% of *H. influenzae* induced acute otitis media in rats (Kristinsson et al. 2005). On the other hand, *Clostridium perfringens* induced intestinal lesions in broiler chickens were palliated by thymol- and carvacrol-rich supplements. The researchers postulated that the supplements interfered with the adhesion activity and/or toxin production of *C. perfringens*. Meanwhile, the total number of bacteria in the broiler chickens, especially the number of *E. coli*, decreased linearly after treatment with the supplements (Du et al. 2015).

Incorporation of essential oils into antibiotic treatments seems to be a promising strategy. At fairly low concentrations, 0.31 mM of thymol and 0.16 mM of carvacrol acted synergistically with penicillin to increase bacterial membrane permeability of *S. aureus*, which allowed the rapid penetration of penicillin into the bacterial cell (Lambert et al. 2001; Palaniappan and Holley 2010; Yap et al. 2013). On the other hand, a combination of thymol and carvacrol could act as extended spectrum β-lactamase-inhibitors in pathogens treated with fluoroquinolones (Si et al. 2008).

Eugenol is one of the well-studied phenylpropenes (Fig. 3.4). The antimicrobial activity of phenylpropenes is conferred by the free hydroxyl group and methyl group in their chemical structures (Jung and Fahey Jr 1983; Laekeman et al. 1990). The exceptionally great anti-cariogenic property of eugenol against the disease causing oral bacteria makes it a popular ingredient in oral care products (Zhang et al. 2009; Freires et al. 2015; Marchese et al. 2017). Meanwhile, eugenol is used as a dental filling component in dentistry (de Souza Costa et al. 2007). Surprisingly, eugenol exhibited greater antibacterial activity against Gram negative bacteria than against Gram positive bacteria (Hyldgaard et al. 2012). The growth of *H. pylori* was inhibited by eugenol even under low pH conditions (Ali et al. 2005). Eugenol disrupted the cellular membrane by altering the fatty acid profile of *Enterobacter aerogenes*, resulting in an increase of turgor pressure and thus collapsing the transport of ions and ATP. Eugenol also targeted bacterial enzymes, such as ATPase, histidine carboxylase, amylase and protease (Poolman et al. 1987; Thoroski et al. 1989; Trumpower and Gennis 1994; Wendakoon and Sakaguchi 1995). Like carvacrol, eugenol also exhibited anti-quorum sensing and anti biofilm properties. The levels of N-acyl homoserine lactones signalling molecules in *Pectobacterium* sp. decreased after the bacteria were treated with sub-lethal amount of eugenol (Joshi et al. 2016).

The addition of eugenol into poultry feed successfully reduced the number of *Salmonella* spp. by weakening the motility, adhesion, and colonisation of the bacteria in chicken oviduct epithelial cells (Upadhyaya et al. 2013). The genes responsible for the above mentioned activities were downregulated with the presence of eugenol (Kollanoor-Johny et al. 2012). In addition, the survival of *Salmonella enteritidis* in macrophages was reduced as eugenol interfered with the expression of its virulence genes (Upadhyaya et al. 2013).

3.6 Honey

Honey is produced by bees from plant nectars, plant secretions and excretions of plant-sucking insects. It is a mixture of natural macro- and micro-nutrients, consisting of a saturated solution of sugars and a wide range of minor phytochemical constituents (Alvarez-Suarez et al. 2010). It has been proposed that honey can serve as a vehicle for transferring phytomedicinal compounds. Due to the growing crisis of antibiotic resistance, there is a resurgence of interest in utilising honey to treat wound infections, especially those not responsive to conventional treatments. Several studies have confirmed the bactericidal effects of honey against several species of Gram positive and Gram negative bacteria, including antibiotic resistant strains. In a study conducted by Kwakman et al. (2011), all bacteria tested, including *B. subtilis*, methicillin resistant *S. aureus*, extended spectrum β-lactamase producing *E. coli*, ciprofloxacin resistant *P. aeruginosa*, and vancomycin resistant *E. faecium* were killed by 10–20% (v/v) honey.

Beside its effectiveness against the more vulnerable planktonic form of bacteria, honey also inhibit biofilm-embedded bacteria; the latter are 10–1000-fold more resistant to antibiotics than the free-floating planktonic bacteria (Ng et al. 2017; She et al. 2018). It has been reported that honey was able to repress curli genes (*csgBAC*), quorum sensing genes (AI-2 importer and indole biosynthesis), and virulence genes (*LEE* genes), thus reducing the biofilm colonisation and virulence of pathogenic *E. coli* O157:H7 (Lee et al. 2011). Honey can be used for prolonged infection treatments due to its low toxicity. Importantly, the risk of bacteria acquiring resistance to honey is low. A study showed reduced susceptibilities to Manuka honey in test bacteria, including two reference strains (*S. aureus* NCTC 10017 and *P. aeruginosa* ATCC 27853) and four clinical strains isolated from wounds (*E. coli*, methicillin resistant *S. aureus*, *P. aeruginosa* and *S. epidermidis*) during long term exposure. However, such changes were not permanent and honey resistant mutants were not detected (Cooper et al. 2010).

Besides hyperosmolality and acidity, the complex synergistic effect between hydrogen peroxide and phytochemicals, including phenolic compounds and methylglyoxal, also contributes to the overall antibacterial activity of honey. Table 3.4 summarises the antibacterial compounds present in honey and their mechanisms of action.

The hydrogen peroxide in honey is a by-product that arises during the conversion of glucose to gluconic acid by glucose oxidase. Brudzynski (2006) demonstrated that honey hydrogen peroxide exerted bacteriostatic and DNA degrading activities on *E. coli*. It was observed that in honey with high content of hydrogen peroxide, bacteria cannot respond normally to proliferative signals and their growth remains arrested. Pre-treatment of honey with catalase restored bacterial growth, thus suggesting that the endogenous hydrogen peroxide in honey was implicated in bacterial growth inhibition (Brudzynski 2006). The DNase-like activity was heat resistant but catalase sensitive, indicating that the hydrogen peroxide in honey participated in oxidative DNA damage. Although the hydrogen peroxide content in tested honey samples (0.248–2.68 mM) was over 900 fold lower than that in disinfectants (0.8–8 M) that kill bacteria on contact, the study concluded that honey hydrogen peroxide was involved in oxidative damage, causing bacterial growth inhibition and DNA degradation. Furthermore, these effects were clearly augmented by the action of other components in honey (Brudzynski et al. 2011).

The coupling chemistry between hydrogen peroxide and polyphenols in honey, rather than hydrogen peroxide alone, may exert oxidative effect causing bacterial growth arrest and DNA degradation (Brudzynski et al. 2012; Brudzynski and Lannigan 2012). Although polyphenols in honey are generally known to possess antioxidant activities, the same polyphenols could become powerful pro-oxidants when oxidised in the presence of oxygen. Oxidised polyphenols further generate hydrogen peroxide which, in the presence of transition metals such as Cu(II) or Fe(II), produces hydroxyl radicals through the Fenton reaction (Brudzynski and Lannigan 2012). Other than hydrogen peroxide, hydroxyl radicals are also powerful oxidants that can oxidise cellular biomolecules in a non-specific manner. A study has demonstrated for the first time that inhibitory effect of honey on methicillin resistant *S. aureus* and vancomycin resistant enterococci isolated from wounds was dose-dependently related to the generation of hydroxyl radicals from honey hydrogen peroxide (Brudzynski and Lannigan 2012). These observation indicates that honey induced oxidative stress in bacteria can be attributed to action of hydroxyl radicals, rather than from the action of molecular hydrogen peroxide per se. Thus, a functional link between the generation of hydroxyl radicals from honey hydrogen peroxide and bacterial growth inhibition has been established. In addition, the hydroxyl radical based mechanism of action of honey did not discriminate between antibiotic-sensitive and antibiotic-resistant bacteria (Brudzynski and Lannigan 2012).

Clumps of lysed *S. aureus* were observed under the electron microscope after they were treated with honey (Ng et al. 2017). The presence of phenolic acids in honey, including gallic, caffeic, ferulic, benzoic and cinnamic acids, was associated with the enhanced inhibitory activity against methicillin sensitive and resistant *S. aureus* (Aljadi and Yusoff 2003; Ng and Lim 2015). Among these phenolic acids,

Table 3.4 Antibacterial components in honey and their mechanisms of action

Component	Type of honey	Antibacterial action	References
Hydrogen peroxide	Most types	This compound is generated by glucose oxidase, an enzyme secreted by bee. Hydrogen peroxide is suggested to be a major antibacterial factor of many honeys. Despite occurring at low levels, hydrogen peroxide is capable of interacting with other antibacterial components of honey, producing radicals and causing bacterial DNA damage.	Brudzynski et al. (2011), Brudzynski and Lannigan (2012)
Phenolic compounds (Examples: gallic acid, caffeic acid, benzoic acid, ferulic acid, cinnamic acid, p-hydroxybenzoic acid, naringenin, pinocembrin and chrysin)	Most types	These compounds mainly originate from plant nectars. Other than antioxidant activities, some of them are potent against Gram positive and Gram negative bacteria, including antibiotic resistant strains.	Aljadi and Yusoff (2003), Estevinho et al. (2008)
Bee defensin I	Revamil honey	An antibacterial peptide secreted by bees into honey. This peptide is able to compromise bacterial membrane integrity by forming pores in the membranes, causing cell lysis. This peptide could prevent biofilm development either by (i) interfering with bacterial adhesion to a surface, (ii) inhibiting the growth of attached cells in the early biofilm stage, or (iii) altering polymeric substances production.	Klaudiny et al. (2005), Kwakman et al. (2010)
Jelleins	Buckwheat honey	This is an antibacterial peptide that was originally isolated from the royal jelly. It is a precursor of major royal jelly protein that is secreted by bees. This peptide plays a role in the destruction of the bacterial cell wall and the antibacterial effects of honey.	Brudzynski and Sjaarda (2015)
Leptosperin	Manuka honey	Formerly known as leptosin, this compound is a novel glycoside of methyl syringate. It is a naturally occurring chemical found only in the nectar of Manuka plants. Concentrations of leptosperin correlate positively with the antibacterial activity of Manuka honey. The antibacterial mechanism of action of leptosperin has not been elucidated.	Kato et al. (2014), Kato et al. (2012)

(continued)

Table 3.4 (continued)

Component	Type of honey	Antibacterial action	References
Methylglyoxal	Manuka honey	High level of methylglyoxal is found only in ripened Manuka honey. This compound is formed by non-enzymatic Maillard reactions. Methylglyoxal can disrupt the structure and function of bacterial DNA and proteins.	Adams et al. (2008), Adams et al. (2009), Weigel et al. (2004)

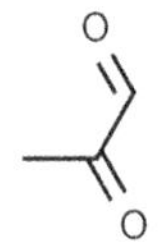

Fig. 3.5 Chemical structure of methylglyoxal. More details, including synonyms and chemical properties, are available at ChemSpider (http://www.chemspider.com/)

gallic and ferulic acids were believed to alter bacterial membrane properties irreversibly through hydrophobicity changes, decrease of negative surface charges, and pore formation, consequently causing leakage of essential intracellular constituents (Borges et al. 2013). According to Luís et al. (2014), the antibacterial mechanism of caffeic acid is associated with polyphenol membrane interaction. The study showed increased membrane permeability, depolarisation of cell membrane, and reduction of respiratory activity in *S. aureus* in the presence of caffeic acid. The authors suggested that caffeic acid may exert its effects by damaging cell membrane integrity and interfering with the aerobic metabolism of *S. aureus*. Furthermore, caffeic acid also shows relatively strong nucleophilic properties, thus it can donate an electron pair to electrophile functional groups of plasma membrane proteins and/or lipids, which may impair membrane function (Vaquero et al. 2007). Catechin, one of the flavonoids in honey, is known to damage bacterial membrane by penetrating directly into the lipid bilayer and perturb its barrier function. The flavonoid was able to damage the cytoplasmic membrane of *E. coli*. The bactericidal action of catechin is attributed to its ability to generate hydrogen peroxide, which damages the bacterial cell membrane (Arakawa et al. 2004).

Recent studies have focused on the antibacterial potential of methylglyoxal, a 1,2-dicarbonyl compound, in Manuka honey (*Leptospermum scoparium*) (Fig. 3.5). Methylglyoxal is believed to be the key factor for the non-peroxide mediated antibacterial activity of honey. The compound is present in Manuka honey in exceptionally high levels (38–725 mg/kg). It is formed from dihydroxyacetone, a nectar derived compound, via non-enzymatic Maillard reaction during the ripening of honey (Adams et al. 2008; Cokcetin et al. 2016). Methylglyoxal is a highly electrophilic molecule and can also bind to DNA and protein, thereby altering protein structure, function and synthesis. Booth et al. (2003) found that the adducts formed following cellular exposure to methylglyoxal reacted simultaneously with DNA guanine bases, subsequently activating the DNA repair systems. In addition, methylglyoxal reacts with the thiol groups of proteins, causing inhibition of enzyme activity (Booth et al. 2003). It has been proposed that methylglyoxal may disrupt the structural integrity and function of bacterial DNA and protein, such as the plasma membrane proteins, resulting in changes in permeability and cellular lysis. Methylglyoxal may also react with amino acids to produce free radicals. In a study conducted by Kang (2003), DNA strand was cleaved when plasmid DNA was incubated with methylglyoxal and lysine. Results of the study suggest that superoxide anion and hydrogen peroxide may be generated from a glycation reaction involving methylglyoxal and lysine. Furthermore, Cu(II) likely participates in a Fenton reaction with the reactive oxygen species to produce hydroxyl radicals, which in turn induces DNA cleavage.

Manuka honey can disrupt the regular cell division process of *S. aureus* (Jenkins et al. 2011). Cell division is complete when murein hydrolase degrades the cell wall between two daughter cells, allowing their separation (Priyadarshini et al. 2007). Manuka honey has been shown to inhibit the activity of murein hydrolase, causing a build-up of septated non-dividing cells (Jenkins et al. 2011). Another study has proposed an entirely different mechanism against *P. aeruginosa*. Reduced expression of outer membrane protein F (OprF), a key anchor protein of *P. aeruginosa*, has been observed after treatment with Manuka honey, along with membrane blebbing and cell lysis (Roberts et al. 2012). On the other hand, a study on the antibacterial action of Manuka honey on *E. coli* revealed up-regulation of stress response genes. In particular, the genes that encode products required for protein synthesis were down-regulated by at least two folds (Blair et al. 2009). Gene expression study also revealed that Manuka honey induced large-scale down-regulation of critical virulence genes (enterotoxins, fibronectin binding proteins, haemolysins, and lipases), with concomitant reductions in global regulators and quorum sensing genes, in *S. aureus* (Jenkins et al. 2013).

The methylglyoxal in Manuka honey compromised the morphology of bacteria by altering the structure of fimbriae and flagella, which are integral to bacterial adhesion, initiation of infection, and biofilm formation (Rabie et al. 2016). Exposure of *P. aeruginosa* to Manuka honey reduced both swarming and swimming motilities. This may be due to de-flagellation of the bacterial cell, which correlated with decreased expression of the major structural flagellin protein and concurrent suppression of flagellin associated genes (Roberts et al. 2014). Methylglyoxal also induced the loss of fimbriae and flagella in *B. subtilis* and *E. coli*; moreover, the bacteria were rounded and shrunken, with their membrane integrity lost (Rabie et al. 2016).

Hayashi et al. (2014) reported that the minimum inhibitory concentration values of methylglyoxal against both multi drug resistant strains and efflux deficient mutants of *P. aeruginosa*, *E. coli* and *S. enterica* were the same. This suggests that methylglyoxal is not recognised by the drug efflux systems in these antibiotic resistant bacteria (Hayashi et al. 2014). Chaki et al. (2010) demonstrated the ability of both methylglyoxal and honey added with methylglyoxal in inhibiting a wide range of Gram positive and Gram negative bacteria. Methylglyoxal exhibited antibacterial activity against antibiotic-sensitive and -resistant strains of *S. aureus*, *E. coli*,

Salmonella spp., *Shigella* spp., *K. pneumoniae* and *V. cholera* with minimum inhibitory concentration ranging from 0.5 to 2.0 mM. In addition, the antibacterial activity of methylglyoxal was increased by two to three folds when it was added with honey. This indicates potential synergistic antibacterial effect between methylglyoxal and other honey components (Chaki et al. 2010). Neutralisation reduced but did not diminish the antibacterial activity of methylglyoxal completely, which implies the presence of other antibacterial compounds in the Manuka honey (Chaki et al. 2010; Kwakman et al. 2011).

The diverse effects of Manuka honey in different bacteria species, including antibiotic resistant strains, highlight the potential for multiple modes of action and the presence of multiple antibacterial compounds in the honey. Overall, it is possible that the antibacterial activity of Manuka honey is attributable to synergism between methylglyoxal and other honey components, including hydrogen peroxide and phenolic compounds (Chaki et al. 2010).

Honey was shown to be an effective topical dressing for full-thickness burn wounds in animal models. Burn wound size was found to be markedly reduced and statistically smaller in the honey treated wounds than hydrofibre silver treated wounds. Moreover, honey treatment reduced bacterial growth in *P. aeruginosa* inoculated wounds in rats, with marked bacterial growth reduction on day 3, 12, 15, 18 and 21 of the experiment (Khoo et al. 2010). Another *in vivo* study also showed that topical application of honey on burn wounds contaminated with *P. aeruginosa* and *A. baumannii* gave the fastest healing rate than chitosan gel and hydrofibre silver treatments (Sukur et al. 2011). In a study conducted by Paramasivan et al. (2014), ovine frontal sinuses were irrigated with methylglyoxal augmented Manuka honey twice per day for 5 days. Both treatments of 0.9 mg/mL and 1.8 mg/mL of methylglyoxal reduced the biomass of *S. aureus* biofilm significantly. Besides, such treatments were found to be safe to mucosa with normal pseudostratified epithelium and cilia structure. Bacterial biofilms are involved in recalcitrance rhinosinusitis cases, thus methylglyoxal augmented Manuka honey was proposed to be a viable treatment option for chronic rhinosinusitis (Paramasivan et al. 2014).

The efficacy of honey in infection control and wound management was also proven in a clinical study which was conducted with 66 volunteers. The study revealed that honey was able to inhibit or reduce plaque formation in the mouth. Although 0.2% chlorhexidine (a disinfectant and antiseptic agent in mouthwash) was found to exhibit greater antiplaque efficacy (mean plaque score: 1.77 ± 0.86) than 1.8 mg/mL honey mouthwash (mean plaque score: 1.64 ± 0.90), the difference was not statistically significant. Besides, six tested oral bacteria (*Eubacterium nodatum*, *S. mutans*, *Campylobacter rectus*, *Streptococcus sanguinis*, *Aggregatibacter actinomycetemcomitans* and *Porphyromonas gingivalis*) were found to be inhibited by honey as well (Aparna et al. 2012).

On the other hand, in a surgical wound care clinical study, 20 patients with spinal cord injuries who had chronic pressure ulcers were treated with Manuka honey dressings. At the beginning of the honey treatment, various pathogenic bacteria were isolated from the pressure ulcers. These included Gram negative *K. pneumoniae*, *P. aeruginosa*, *E. coli*, *P. mirabilis*, *Providencia stuartii* and *Enterobacter cloacae*; Gram positive *S. epidermidis* and *S. aureus*; and methicillin resistant *S. aureus*. After a week of honey treatment, despite no antibiotic treatment, all wound swabs were void of bacterial growth. After 4 weeks of treatment, 90% of the patients showed complete wound healing. No negative effects, particularly no changes in blood sugar level, were observed in diabetic patients, even with large amounts of honey applied daily (Biglari et al. 2012). Hence, instead of viewing honey as an experimental treatment, clinicians should begin to consider honey as a safe and effective infection control.

3.7 Conclusion

There is a growing body of evidence that highlights the potency of plant natural products, particularly flavonoids, phenolic acids, peptides, essential oils and honey, as antibacterial agents. Research findings summarised in this chapter reveal that they exert their antibacterial activities through diverse modes of action, which encompass disruption of bacterial membrane integrity, interruption of intracellular metabolisms, and interference of quorum sensing and biofilm formation. Potency of some of these natural products in the elimination of pathogenic bacteria in animal models and in clinical studies was demonstrated. Notably, the inhibitory effects of the aforementioned natural products against multi drug resistant bacteria suggest that they are promising candidates for future development of therapeutics against antibiotic resistance. As substantiated by some encouraging findings discussed in this chapter, phytochemical-antibiotic combination treatment is a promising strategy to combat antibiotic resistance. Notwithstanding, issues such as bio-stability of the plant natural products, optimal phytochemical/antibiotic ratios, and potential side effects of phytochemical-antibiotic combination treatment warrant further research attention.

References

Abdallah E (2011) Plants: an alternative source for antimicrobials journal of applied pharmaceutical. Science 1:16–20

Abreu AC, Serra SC, Borges A, Saavedra MJ, Mcbain AJ, Salgado AJ, Simões M (2015) Combinatorial activity of flavonoids with antibiotics against drug-resistant *Staphylococcus aureus*. Microb Drug Resist 21:600–609. https://doi.org/10.1089/mdr.2014.0252

Adams CJ, Boult CH, Deadman BJ, Farr JM, Grainger MNC, Manley-Harris M, Snow MJ (2008) Isolation by HPLC and characterisation of the bioactive fraction of New Zealand manuka (*Leptospermum scoparium*) honey. Carbohydr Res 343:651–659. https://doi.org/10.1016/j.carres.2007.12.011

Adams CJ, Manley-Harris M, Molan PC (2009) The origin of methylglyoxal in New Zealand Manuka (*Leptospermum scoparium*) honey. Carbohydr Res 344:1050–1053. https://doi.org/10.1016/j.carres.2009.03.020

Ajiboye TO, Skiebe E, Wilharm G (2018) Phenolic acids potentiate colistin-mediated killing of *Acinetobacter baumannii* by inducing redox imbalance. Biomed Pharmacother 101:737–744. https://doi.org/10.1016/j.biopha.2018.02.051

Ali SM et al (2005) Antimicrobial activities of eugenol and cinnamaldehyde against the human gastric pathogen *Helicobacter pylori*. Ann Clin Microbiol Antimicrob 4:20

Aljadi AM, Yusoff KM (2003) Isolation and identification of phenolic acids in Malaysian honey with antibacterial properties. Turkish J Med Sci 33:229–236

Almasaudi SB (2018) *Acinetobacter* spp. as nosocomial pathogens: epidemiology and resistance features. Saudi J Biol Sci 25:586–596. https://doi.org/10.1016/j.sjbs.2016.02.009

Alvarez-Suarez JM, Tulipani S, Romandini S, Bertoli E, Battino M (2010) Contribution of honey in nutrition and human health: a review. Mediterr J Nutr Metab 3:15–23. https://doi.org/10.1007/s12349-009-0051-6

Amiri H (2012) Essential oils composition and antioxidant properties of three thymus species. Evid Based Complement Alternat Med 2012:728065–728065. https://doi.org/10.1155/2012/728065

Aparna S, Srirangarajan S, Malgi V, Setlur KP, Shashidhar R, Setty S, Thakur S (2012) A comparative evaluation of the antibacterial efficacy of honey in vitro and antiplaque efficacy in a 4-day plaque regrowth model in vivo: preliminary results. J Periodontol 83:1116–1121

Arakawa H, Maeda M, Okubo S, Shimamura T (2004) Role of hydrogen peroxide in bactericidal action of catechin. Biol Pharm Bull 27:277–281. https://doi.org/10.1248/bpb.27.277

Arshad MS, Batool SA (2017) Natural antimicrobials, their souces and food safety. In: Karunaratne DN, Pamunuwa G (eds) Food additives, IntechOpen, pp 87–102. https://doi.org/10.5772/intechopen.70197

Association francaise de normalisation (2000) Huiles essentielles, Tome 2, Monographies relatives aux huiles essentielles. AFNOR, Paris

Atkinson RG (2018) Phenylpropenes: occurrence, distribution, and biosynthesis in fruit. J Agric Food Chem 66:2259–2272. https://doi.org/10.1021/acs.jafc.6b04696

Awolola GV, Koorbanally NA, Chenia H, Shode FO, Baijnath H (2014) Antibacterial and anti-biofilm activity of flavonoids and triterpenes isolated from the extracts of *Ficus sansibarica* Warb. subsp. *sansibarica* (Moraceae) extracts. Afr J Tradit Comp Alter Med 11:124–131. https://doi.org/10.4314/ajtcam.v11i3.19

Ayaz M, Ullah F, Sadiq A, Ullah F, Ovais M, Ahmed J, Devkota HP (2019) Synergistic interactions of phytochemicals with antimicrobial agents: potential strategy to counteract drug resistance. Chem Biol Interact 308:294–303. https://doi.org/10.1016/j.cbi.2019.05.050

Babii C et al (2018) A novel synthetic flavonoid with potent antibacterial properties: *in vitro* activity and proposed mode of action. PLoS One 13:e0194898–e0194898. https://doi.org/10.1371/journal.pone.0194898

Bajpai VK, Sharma A, Baek K-H (2013) Antibacterial mode of action of *Cudrania tricuspidata* fruit essential oil, affecting membrane permeability and surface characteristics of food-borne pathogens. Food Control 32:582–590. https://doi.org/10.1016/j.foodcont.2013.01.032

Bame JR et al (2013) Sarothrin from *Alkanna orientalis* is an antimicrobial agent and efflux pump inhibitor. Planta Med 79:327–329. https://doi.org/10.1055/s-0032-1328259

Barboza TJS, Ferreira AF, Ignacio ACPR, Albarello N (2016) Cytotoxicity, antibacterial and anti-biofilm activities of aqueous extracts of leaves and flavonoids occurring in *Kalanchoe pinnata* (Lam.) Pers. J Med Plant Res 10:763–770

Bauer K, Garbe D, Surburg H (2001) Common fragrance and flavor materials: preparation, properties and uses. Wiley-VCH, Weinheim

Benchaar C, Chaves AV, Fraser GR, Beauchemin KA, McAllister TA (2007) Effects of essential oils and their components on *in vitro* rumen microbial fermentation. Can J Anim Sci 87:413–419. https://doi.org/10.4141/CJAS07012

Biglari B, Vd Linden P, Simon A, Aytac S, Gerner H, Moghaddam A (2012) Use of medihoney as a non-surgical therapy for chronic pressure ulcers in patients with spinal cord injury. Spinal Cord 50:165

Blair SE, Cokcetin NN, Harry EJ, Carter DA (2009) The unusual antibacterial activity of medical-grade Leptospermum honey: antibacterial spectrum, resistance and transcriptome analysis. Eur J Clin Microbiol Infect Dis 28:1199–1208. https://doi.org/10.1007/s10096-009-0763-z

Blanco AR, Sudano-Roccaro A, Spoto GC, Nostro A, Rusciano D (2005) Epigallocatechin gallate inhibits biofilm formation by ocular staphylococcal isolates. Antimicrob Agents Chemother 49:4339–4343. https://doi.org/10.1128/AAC.49.10.4339-4343.2005

Booth IR, Ferguson GP, Miller S, Li C, Gunasekera B, Kinghorn S (2003) Bacterial production of methylglyoxal: a survival strategy or death by misadventure? Biochem Soc Trans 31:1406–1408. https://doi.org/10.1042/bst0311406

Borges A, Ferreira C, Saavedra MJ, Simões M (2013) Antibacterial activity and mode of action of ferulic and gallic acids against pathogenic bacteria. Microb Drug Resist 19:256–265. https://doi.org/10.1089/mdr.2012.0244

Borges A, Saavedra MJ, Simoes M (2015) Insights on antimicrobial resistance, biofilms and the use of phytochemicals as new antimicrobial agents. Curr Med Chem 22:2590–2614. https://doi.org/10.2174/0929867322666150530210522

Borges A, Abreu AC, Dias C, Saavedra MJ, Borges F, Simões M (2016) New perspectives on the use of phytochemicals as an emergent strategy to control bacterial infections including biofilms. Molecules:21. https://doi.org/10.3390/molecules21070877

Bravo A, Anacona JR (2001) Metal complexes of the flavonoid quercetin: antibacterial properties. Transit Met Chem 26:20–23. https://doi.org/10.1023/A:1007128325639

Brudzynski K (2006) Effect of hydrogen peroxide on antibacterial activities of Canadian honeys. Can J Microbiol 52:1228–1237. https://doi.org/10.1139/w06-086

Brudzynski K, Lannigan R (2012) Mechanism of honey bacteriostatic action against MRSA and VRE involves hydroxyl radicals generated from honey's hydrogen peroxide. Front Microbiol 3:36–36. https://doi.org/10.3389/fmicb.2012.00036

Brudzynski K, Sjaarda C (2015) Honey glycoproteins containing antimicrobial peptides, Jelleins of the major Royal Jelly Protein 1, are responsible for the cell wall lytic and bactericidal activities of honey. PLoS One 10:e0120238. https://doi.org/10.1371/journal.pone.0120238

Brudzynski K, Abubaker K, St-Martin L, Castle A (2011) Re-examining the role of hydrogen peroxide in bacteriostatic and bactericidal activities of honey. Front Microbiol 2:213–213. https://doi.org/10.3389/fmicb.2011.00213

Brudzynski K, Abubaker K, Miotto D (2012) Unraveling a mechanism of honey antibacterial action: polyphenol/H_2O_2-induced oxidative effect on bacterial cell growth and on DNA degradation. Food Chem 133:329–336. https://doi.org/10.1016/j.foodchem.2012.01.035

Burt SA et al (2007) Carvacrol induces heat shock protein 60 and inhibits synthesis of flagellin in *Escherichia coli* O157:H7. Appl Environ Microbiol 73:4484–4490. https://doi.org/10.1128/AEM.00340-07

Campos ML, Lião LM, Alves ESF, Migliolo L, Dias SC, Franco OL (2018) A structural perspective of plant antimicrobial peptides. Biochem J 475:3359–3375. https://doi.org/10.1042/BCJ20180213

Cao H et al (2015) Identification of a novel proline-rich antimicrobial peptide from *Brassica napus*. PLoS One 10:e0137414. https://doi.org/10.1371/journal.pone.0137414

Chai T-T, Tan Y-N, Ee K-Y, Xiao J, Wong F-C (2019) Seeds, fermented foods, and agricultural by-products as sources of plant-derived antibacterial peptides. Crit Rev Food Sci Nutr 59:S162–S177. https://doi.org/10.1080/10408398.2018.1561418

Chaki S, Mukherjee S, Das S, Mookerjee M, Dastidar SG (2010) Evaluation of bactericidal action of methylglyoxal and its further potentiation in the presence of honey. Int J Biomed Pharm Sci 4:66–69

Chinnam N, Dadi PK, Sabri SA, Ahmad M, Kabir MA, Ahmad Z (2010) Dietary bioflavonoids inhibit *Escherichia coli* ATP synthase in a differential manner. Int J Biol Macromol 46:478–486. https://doi.org/10.1016/j.ijbiomac.2010.03.009

Chouhan S, Sharma K, Guleria S (2017) Antimicrobial activity of some essential oils-present status and future perspectives. Medicine 4:58. https://doi.org/10.3390/medicines4030058

Cokcetin NN, Pappalardo M, Campbell LT, Brooks P, Carter DA, Blair SE, Harry EJ (2016) The antibacterial activity of Australian Leptospermum honey correlates with methylglyoxal levels. PLoS One 11:e0167780–e0167780. https://doi.org/10.1371/journal.pone.0167780
Cooke CJ, Nanjee MN, Dewey P, Cooper JA, Miller GJ, Miller NE (1998) Plant monoterpenes do not raise plasma high-density-lipoprotein concentrations in humans. Am J Clin Nutr 68:1042–1045. https://doi.org/10.1093/ajcn/68.5.1042
Cooper RA, Jenkins L, Henriques AFM, Duggan RS, Burton NF (2010) Absence of bacterial resistance to medical-grade manuka honey. Eur J Clin Microbiol Infect Dis 29:1237–1241. https://doi.org/10.1007/s10096-010-0992-1
Cushnie TPT, Lamb AJ (2005) Antimicrobial activity of flavonoids. Int J Antimicrob Agents 26:343–356. https://doi.org/10.1016/j.ijantimicag.2005.09.002
Cushnie TPT, Lamb AJ (2011) Recent advances in understanding the antibacterial properties of flavonoids. Int J Antimicrob Agents 38:99–107. https://doi.org/10.1016/j.ijantimicag.2011.02.014
Cushnie TPT, Taylor PW, Nagaoka Y, Uesato S, Hara Y, Lamb AJ (2008) Investigation of the antibacterial activity of 3-O-octanoyl-(−)-epicatechin. J Appl Microbiol 105:1461–1469. https://doi.org/10.1111/j.1365-2672.2008.03881.x
Daglia M (2012) Polyphenols as antimicrobial agents. Curr Opin Biotechnol 23:174–181
Davidson PM (1997) Chemical preservatives and natural antimicrobial compounds. In: Doyle MP, Beuchat LR, Montville TJ (eds) Food microbiology: fundamentals and frontiers. ASM, Washington, DC, pp 520–556
de Andrade Monteiro C, dos Santos JRA (2019) Phytochemicals and their antifungal potential against pathogenic yeasts. In: Rao V, Mans DRA, Rao L (eds) Phytochemicals in human health. IntechOpen, pp 1–31
de Souza Costa CA, Teixeira HM, ABLD N, Hebling J (2007) Biocompatibility of resin-based dental materials applied as liners in deep cavities prepared in human teeth. J Biomed Mater Res Part B 81:175–184
de Souza Cândido E, Silva Cardoso MH, Sousa DA, Viana JC, de Oliveira-Júnior NG, Miranda V, Franco OL (2014) The use of versatile plant antimicrobial peptides in agribusiness and human health. Peptides 55:65–78. https://doi.org/10.1016/j.peptides.2014.02.003
Denyer SP, Hugo W (1991) Mechanisms of antibacterial action: a summary. In: Denyer SP, Hugo W (eds) Mechanisms of action of chemical biocides. Blackwell, Oxford, pp 331–334
Di Pasqua R, Hoskins N, Betts G, Mauriello G (2006) Changes in membrane fatty acids composition of microbial cells induced by addiction of thymol, carvacrol, limonene, cinnamaldehyde, and eugenol in the growing media. J Agric Food Chem 54:2745–2749. https://doi.org/10.1021/jf052722l
Di Pasqua R, Betts G, Hoskins N, Edwards M, Ercolini D, Mauriello G (2007) Membrane toxicity of antimicrobial compounds from essential oils. J Agric Food Chem 55:4863–4870. https://doi.org/10.1021/jf0636465
Di Pasqua R, Mamone G, Ferranti P, Ercolini D, Mauriello G (2010) Changes in the proteome of *Salmonella enterica* serovar Thompson as stress adaptation to sublethal concentrations of thymol. Proteomics 10:1040–1049. https://doi.org/10.1002/pmic.200900568
Du E, Gan L, Li Z, Wang W, Liu D, Guo Y (2015) In vitro antibacterial activity of thymol and carvacrol and their effects on broiler chickens challenged with *Clostridium perfringens*. J Anim Sci Biotechnol 6:58. https://doi.org/10.1186/s40104-015-0055-7
Dwivedi GR et al (2016) Gallic acid-based indanone derivative interacts synergistically with tetracycline by inhibiting efflux pump in multidrug resistant *E. coli*. Appl Microbiol Biotechnol 100:2311–2325. https://doi.org/10.1007/s00253-015-7152-6
Edziri H, Mastouri M, Mahjoub MA, Mighri Z, Mahjoub A, Verschaeve L (2012) Antibacterial, antifungal and cytotoxic activities of two flavonoids from *Retama raetam* flowers. Molecules 17:7284–7293. https://doi.org/10.3390/molecules17067284
El-Adawi H (2012) Inhibitory effect of grape seed extract (GSE) on cariogenic bacteria. J Med Plant Res 6:4883–4891

Estevinho L, Pereira AP, Moreira L, Dias LG, Pereira E (2008) Antioxidant and antimicrobial effects of phenolic compounds extracts of Northeast Portugal honey. Food Chem Toxicol 46:3774–3779. https://doi.org/10.1016/j.fct.2008.09.062

Eumkeb G, Siriwong S, Phitaktim S, Rojtinnakorn N, Sakdarat S (2012) Synergistic activity and mode of action of flavonoids isolated from smaller galangal and amoxicillin combinations against amoxicillin-resistant *Escherichia coli*. J Appl Microbiol 112:55–64. https://doi.org/10.1111/j.1365-2672.2011.05190.x

Falciro M (2011) The mode of antibacterial action of essential oils. In: Mendez-Vilas A (ed) Science against microbial pathogens: communicating current research and technological advances, vol 2. Formatex Research Center, Badajoz, pp 1143–1156

Fan X, Schäfer H, Reichling J, Wink M (2013) Bactericidal properties of the antimicrobial peptide Ib-AMP4 from *Impatiens balsamina* produced as a recombinant fusion-protein in *Escherichia coli*. Biotechnol J 8:1213–1220. https://doi.org/10.1002/biot.201300121

Fong P, Hao C-H, Io C-C, Sin P-I, Meng L-R (2019) *In silico* and *in vitro* anti-*Helicobacter pylori* effects of combinations of phytochemicals and antibiotics. Molecules 24:3608

Franco OL, Murad AM, Leite JR, Mendes PAM, Prates MV, Bloch C Jr (2006) Identification of a cowpea γ-thionin with bactericidal activity. FEBS J 273:3489–3497. https://doi.org/10.1111/j.1742-4658.2006.05349.x

Freires IA, Denny C, Benso B, De Alencar SM, Rosalen PL (2015) Antibacterial activity of essential oils and their isolated constituents against cariogenic bacteria: a systematic review. Molecules 20:7329–7358

Gabel CV, Berg HC (2003) The speed of the flagellar rotary motor of *Escherichia coli* varies linearly with protonmotive force. Proc Natl Acad Sci U S A 100:8748–8751. https://doi.org/10.1073/pnas.1533395100

Gibbons S, Moser E, Kaatz GW (2004) Catechin gallates inhibit multidrug resistance (MDR) in *Staphylococcus aureus*. Planta Med 70:1240–1242. https://doi.org/10.1055/s-2004-835860

Górniak I, Bartoszewski R, Króliczewski J (2019) Comprehensive review of antimicrobial activities of plant flavonoids. Phytochem Rev 18:241–272. https://doi.org/10.1007/s11101-018-9591-z

Hayashi K, Fukushima A, Hayashi-Nishino M, Nishino K (2014) Effect of methylglyoxal on multidrug-resistant *Pseudomonas aeruginosa*. Front Microbiol:5. https://doi.org/10.3389/fmicb.2014.00180

Hertel W, Peschel G, Ozegowski J-H, Müller P-J (2006) Inhibitory effects of triterpenes and flavonoids on the enzymatic activity of hyaluronic acid-splitting enzymes. Arch Pharm 339:313–318. https://doi.org/10.1002/ardp.200500216

Hyldgaard M, Mygind T, Meyer RL (2012) Essential oils in food preservation: mode of action, synergies, and interactions with food matrix components. Front Microbiol 3:12-12. https://doi.org/10.3389/fmicb.2012.00012

Interagency Coordination Group on Antimicrobial Resistance (2019) No time to wait: securing the future from drug-resistant infections. In: Report to the secretary-general of the United Nations. World Health Organization (WHO). https://www.who.int/antimicrobial-resistance/interagency-coordination-group/IACG_final_report_EN.pdf?ua=1

Issa D, Najjar A, Greige-Gerges H, Nehme H (2019) Screening of some essential oil constituents as potential inhibitors of the ATP synthase of *Escherichia coli*. J Food Sci 84:138–146. https://doi.org/10.1111/1750-3841.14421

Jaiswal P, Kumar P (2015) Antimicrobial screening of free and bound flavonoid from the bark of *Terminalia arjuna*. J Phytopharmacol 4:303–306

Jamil S, Lathiff SMA, Abdullah SA, Jemaon N, Sirat HM (2014) Antimicrobial flavonoids from *Artocarpus anisophyllus* Miq and *Artocarpus lowii*. King J Teknologi 71:95–99

Jenkins R, Burton N, Cooper R (2011) Manuka honey inhibits cell division in methicillin-resistant *Staphylococcus aureus*. J Antimicrob Chemother 66:2536–2542. https://doi.org/10.1093/jac/dkr340

Jenkins R, Burton N, Cooper R (2013) Proteomic and genomic analysis of methicillin-resistant *Staphylococcus aureus* (MRSA) exposed to manuka honey *in vitro* demonstrated down-regulation of virulence markers. J Antimicrob Chemother 69:603–615. https://doi.org/10.1093/jac/dkt430

Joshi JR, Khazanov N, Senderowitz H, Burdman S, Lipsky A, Yedidia I (2016) Plant phenolic volatiles inhibit quorum sensing in pectobacteria and reduce their virulence by potential binding to ExpI and ExpR proteins. Sci Rep 6:38126. https://doi.org/10.1038/srep38126

Jung HG, Fahey GC Jr (1983) Nutritional implications of phenolic monomers and lignin: a review. J Anim Sci 57:206–219. https://doi.org/10.2527/jas1983.571206x

Kang JH (2003) Oxidative damage of DNA induced by methylglyoxal *in vitro*. Toxicol Lett 145:181–187. https://doi.org/10.1016/S0378-4274(03)00305-9

Kasprzak MM, Erxleben A, Ochocki J (2015) Properties and applications of flavonoid metal complexes. RSC Adv 5:45853–45877. https://doi.org/10.1039/C5RA05069C

Kato Y, Umeda N, Maeda A, Matsumoto D, Kitamoto N, Kikuzaki H (2012) Identification of a novel glycoside, leptosin, as a chemical marker of Manuka honey. J Agric Food Chem 60:3418–3423. https://doi.org/10.1021/jf300068w

Kato Y, Fujinaka R, Ishisaka A, Nitta Y, Kitamoto N, Takimoto Y (2014) Plausible authentication of Manuka honey and related products by measuring leptosperin with methyl syringate. J Agric Food Chem 62:6400–6407. https://doi.org/10.1021/jf501475h

Kępa M, Miklasińska-Majdanik M, Wojtyczka RD, Idzik D, Korzeniowski K, Smoleń-Dzirba J, Wasik TJ (2018) Antimicrobial potential of caffeic acid against *Staphylococcus aureus* clinical strains. Biomed Res Int 2018. https://doi.org/10.1155/2018/7413504

Khoo Y-T, Halim AS, Singh K-KB, Mohamad N-A (2010) Wound contraction effects and antibacterial properties of Tualang honey on full-thickness burn wounds in rats in comparison to hydrofibre. BMC Complement Altern Med 10:48

Klaudiny J, Albert Š, Bachanová K, Kopernický J, Šimúth J (2005) Two structurally different defensin genes, one of them encoding a novel defensin isoform, are expressed in honeybee *Apis mellifera*. Insect Biochem Mol Biol 35:11–22. https://doi.org/10.1016/j.ibmb.2004.09.007

Kobbi S et al (2018) Synthesis and antibacterial activity of new peptides from Alfalfa RuBisCO protein hydrolysates and mode of action via a membrane damage mechanism against *Listeria innocua*. Microb Pathog 115:41–49. https://doi.org/10.1016/j.micpath.2017.12.009

Koley H, Howlader DR, Bhaumik U (2019) Chapter 21 – Assessment of antimicrobial activity of different phytochemicals against enteric diseases in different animal models. In: Ahmad Khan MS, Ahmad I, Chattopadhyay D (eds) New look to phytomedicine. Academic, pp 563–580. https://doi.org/10.1016/B978-0-12-814619-4.00022-7

Kollanoor-Johny A et al (2012) Reduction of *Salmonella enterica* serovar Enteritidis colonization in 20-day-old broiler chickens by the plant-derived compounds trans-cinnamaldehyde and eugenol. Appl Environ Microbiol 78:2981–2987

Kristinsson KG, Magnusdottir AB, Petersen H, Hermansson A (2005) Effective treatment of experimental acute otitis media by application of volatile fluids into the ear canal. J Infect Dis 191:1876–1880. https://doi.org/10.1086/430003

Kurinčič M, Klančnik A, Možina SS (2012) Effects of efflux pump inhibitors on erythromycin, ciprofloxacin, and tetracycline resistance in *Campylobacter* spp. isolates. Microb Drug Resist 18:492–501. https://doi.org/10.1089/mdr.2012.0017

Kwakman PHS, Velde AAT, Boer LD, Speijer D, Vandenbroucke-Grauls CMJE, Zaat SAJ (2010) How honey kills bacteria. FASEB J 24:2576–2582. https://doi.org/10.1096/fj.09-150789

Kwakman PHS, te Velde AA, de Boer L, Vandenbroucke-Grauls CMJE, Zaat SAJ (2011) Two major medicinal honeys have different mechanisms of bactericidal activity. PLoS One 6:e17709. https://doi.org/10.1371/journal.pone.0017709

La Storia A, Ercolini D, Marinello F, Di Pasqua R, Villani F, Mauriello G (2011) Atomic force microscopy analysis shows surface structure changes in carvacrol-treated bacterial cells. Res Microbiol 162:164–172. https://doi.org/10.1016/j.resmic.2010.11.006

Laekeman GM, van Hoof L, Haemers A, Berghe DAV, Herman AG, Vlietinck AJ (1990) Eugenol a valuable compound for *in vitro* experimental research and worthwhile for further *in vivo* investigation. Phytother Res 4:90–96. https://doi.org/10.1002/ptr.2650040304

Lambert RJW, Skandamis PN, Coote PJ, Nychas GJE (2001) A study of the minimum inhibitory concentration and mode of action of oregano essential oil, thymol and carvacrol. J Appl Microbiol 91:453–462. https://doi.org/10.1046/j.1365-2672.2001.01428.x
Lee KW, Everts H, Beynen AC (2004) Essential oils in broiler nutrition. Int J Poult Sci 3:738–752
Lee J-H, Park J-H, Kim J-A, Neupane GP, Cho MH, Lee C-S, Lee J (2011) Low concentrations of honey reduce biofilm formation, quorum sensing, and virulence in *Escherichia coli* O157:H7. Biofouling 27:1095–1104. https://doi.org/10.1080/08927014.2011.633704
Lin R-D, Chin Y-P, Lee M-H (2005) Antimicrobial activity of antibiotics in combination with natural flavonoids against clinical extended-spectrum β-lactamase (ESBL)-producing *Klebsiella pneumoniae*. Phytother Res 19:612–617. https://doi.org/10.1002/ptr.1695
Lopes G, Pinto E, Salgueiro L (2017) Natural products: an alternative to conventional therapy for dermatophytosis? Mycopathologia 182:143–167
Luís Â, Silva F, Sousa S, Duarte AP, Domingues F (2014) Antistaphylococcal and biofilm inhibitory activities of gallic, caffeic, and chlorogenic acids. Biofouling 30:69–79. https://doi.org/10.1080/08927014.2013.845878
Lv F, Liang H, Yuan Q, Li C (2011) *In vitro* antimicrobial effects and mechanism of action of selected plant essential oil combinations against four food related microorganisms. Food Res Int 44:3057–3064
Magi G, Marini E, Facinelli B (2015) Antimicrobial activity of essential oils and carvacrol, and synergy of carvacrol and erythromycin, against clinical, erythromycin-resistant group a streptococci. Front Microbiol 6:165–165. https://doi.org/10.3389/fmicb.2015.00165
Mandal SM, Dey S, Mandal M, Sarkar S, Maria-Neto S, Franco OL (2009) Identification and structural insights of three novel antimicrobial peptides isolated from green coconut water. Peptides 30:633–637. https://doi.org/10.1016/j.peptides.2008.12.001
Marchese A et al (2017) Antimicrobial activity of eugenol and essential oils containing eugenol: a mechanistic viewpoint. Crit Rev Microbiol 43:668–689
MCetin B, Cakmakci S, Cakmakci R (2011) The investigation of antimicrobial activity of thyme and oregano essential oils. Turk J Agric For 35:145–154
Miklasińska-Majdanik M, Kępa M, Wojtyczka RD, Idzik D, Wąsik TJ (2018) Phenolic compounds diminish antibiotic resistance of *Staphylococcus aureus* clinical strains. Int J Environ Res Public Health 15. https://doi.org/10.3390/ijerph15102321
Mirzoeva OK, Grishanin RN, Calder PC (1997) Antimicrobial action of propolis and some of its components: the effects on growth, membrane potential and motility of bacteria. Microbiol Res 152:239–246. https://doi.org/10.1016/S0944-5013(97)80034-1
Mohd. Rani FA, Rahman NI, Ismail S, Alattraqchi AG, Cleary DW, Clarke SC, Yeo CC (2017) *Acinetobacter* spp. infections in Malaysia: a review of antimicrobial resistance trends, mechanisms and epidemiology. Front Microbiol 8. https://doi.org/10.3389/fmicb.2017.02479
Moore BS, Carter GT, Brönstrup M (2017) Editorial: are natural products the solution to antimicrobial resistance? Nat Prod Rep 34:685–686. https://doi.org/10.1039/c7np90026k
Myszka K, Schmidt MT, Majcher M, Juzwa W, Olkowicz M, Czaczyk K (2016) Inhibition of quorum sensing-related biofilm of *Pseudomonas fluorescens* KM121 by *Thymus vulgare* essential oil and its major bioactive compounds. Int Biodeterior Biodegradation 114:252–259. https://doi.org/10.1016/j.ibiod.2016.07.006
Nazzaro F, Fratianni F, De Martino L, Coppola R, De Feo V (2013) Effect of essential oils on pathogenic bacteria. Pharmaceuticals (Basel) 6:1451–1474. https://doi.org/10.3390/ph6121451
Ng WJ, Lim MS (2015) Anti-staphylococcal activity of Melaleuca honey. Southeast Asian J Trop Med Public Health 46:472–479
Ng WJ, Chan YJ, Lau ZK, Lye PY, Ee KY (2017) Antioxidant properties and inhibitory effects of Trigona honey against *Staphylococcus aureus* planktonic and biofilm cultures. Int J GEOMATE 13:28–33. https://doi.org/10.21660/2017.37.2703
Nyila MA, Leonard CM, Hussein AA, Lall N (2012) Activity of South African medicinal plants against *Listeria monocytogenes* biofilms, and isolation of active compounds from *Acacia karroo*. S Afr J Bot 78:220–227. https://doi.org/10.1016/j.sajb.2011.09.001

Oh SY, Yun W, Lee JH, Lee CH, Kwak WK, Cho JH (2017) Effects of essential oil (blended and single essential oils) on anti-biofilm formation of *Salmonella* and *Escherichia coli*. J Anim Sci Technol 59:4. https://doi.org/10.1186/s40781-017-0127-7

Omonijo FA, Ni L, Gong J, Wang Q, Lahaye L, Yang C (2018) Essential oils as alternatives to antibiotics in swine production. Anim Nutr 4:126–136. https://doi.org/10.1016/j.aninu.2017.09.001

Palaniappan K, Holley RA (2010) Use of natural antimicrobials to increase antibiotic susceptibility of drug resistant bacteria. Int J Food Microbiol 140:164–168. https://doi.org/10.1016/j.ijfoodmicro.2010.04.001

Panhwar QK, Memon S (2011) Synthesis and evaluation of antioxidant and antibacterial properties of morin complexes. J Coord Chem 64:2117–2129. https://doi.org/10.1080/00958972.2011.590192

Paramasivan S, Drilling AJ, Jardeleza C, Jervis-Bardy J, Vreugde S, Wormald PJ (2014) Methylglyoxal-augmented manuka honey as a topical anti-*Staphylococcus aureus* biofilm agent: safety and efficacy in an *in vivo* model. In: International forum of allergy & rhinology, vol 3. Wiley Online Library, pp 187–195

Pei J et al (2018) Selectively screen the antibacterial peptide from the hydrolysates of highland barley. Eng Life Sci 18:48–54. https://doi.org/10.1002/elsc.201700118

Pelegrini PB et al (2008) Identification of a novel storage glycine-rich peptide from guava (*Psidium guajava*) seeds with activity against Gram-negative bacteria. Peptides 29:1271–1279. https://doi.org/10.1016/j.peptides.2008.03.013

Plaper A, Golob M, Hafner I, Oblak M, Šolmajer T, Jerala R (2003) Characterization of quercetin binding site on DNA gyrase. Biochem Biophys Res Commun 306:530–536. https://doi.org/10.1016/S0006-291X(03)01006-4

Poolman B, Driessen AJ, Konings WN (1987) Regulation of solute transport in streptococci by external and internal pH values. Microbiol Rev 51:498–508

Priyadarshini R, de Pedro MA, Young KD (2007) Role of peptidoglycan amidases in the development and morphology of the division septum in *Escherichia coli*. J Bacteriol 189:5334–5347. https://doi.org/10.1128/jb.00415-07

Rabie E, Serem JC, Oberholzer HM, Gaspar ARM, Bester MJ (2016) How methylglyoxal kills bacteria: An ultrastructural study. Ultrastruct Pathol 40:107–111. https://doi.org/10.3109/01913123.2016.1154914

Raju A, Degani MS, Khambete MP, Ray MK, Rajan MGR (2015) Antifolate activity of plant polyphenols against *Mycobacterium tuberculosis*. Phytother Res 29:1646–1651. https://doi.org/10.1002/ptr.5437

Ramirez MS, Tolmasky ME (2010) Aminoglycoside modifying enzymes. Drug Resist Updat 13:151–171. https://doi.org/10.1016/j.drup.2010.08.003

Rammohan A, Reddy JS, Sravya G, Rao CN, Zyryanov GV (2020) Chalcone synthesis, properties and medicinal applications: a review. Environ Chem Lett 18:433–458. https://doi.org/10.1007/s10311-019-00959-w

Reygaert WC (2014) The antimicrobial possibilities of green tea. Front Microbiol 5:434–434. https://doi.org/10.3389/fmicb.2014.00434

Roberts AEL, Maddocks SE, Cooper RA (2012) Manuka honey is bactericidal against *Pseudomonas aeruginosa* and results in differential expression of oprF and algD. Microbiology 158:3005–3013. https://doi.org/10.1099/mic.0.062794-0

Roberts AEL, Maddocks SE, Cooper RA (2014) Manuka honey reduces the motility of *Pseudomonas aeruginosa* by suppression of flagella-associated genes. J Antimicrob Chemother 70:716–725. https://doi.org/10.1093/jac/dku448

Rudrapal M, Chetia D (2017) Plant flavonoids as potential source of future antimalarial leads. Syst Rev Pharm 8:13–18

Sanver D, Murray BS, Sadeghpour A, Rappolt M, Nelson AL (2016) Experimental modeling of flavonoid–biomembrane interactions. Langmuir 32:13234–13243. https://doi.org/10.1021/acs.langmuir.6b02219

Sato M, Tanaka H, Oh-Uchi T, Fukai T, Etoh H, Yamaguchi R (2004) Antibacterial activity of phytochemicals isolated from *Erythrina zeyheri* against vancomycin-resistant enterococci and their combinations with vancomycin. Phytother Res 18:906–910. https://doi.org/10.1002/ptr.1556

Satyal P, Murray BL, McFeeters RL, Setzer WN (2016) Essential oil characterization of *Thymus vulgaris* from various geographical locations. Foods 5:70. https://doi.org/10.3390/foods5040070

Sawamura SI, Sakane I, Satoh E, Ishii T, Shimizu Y, Nishimura M, Umehara K (2002) Isolation and determination of an antidote for botulinum neurotoxin from black tea extract Folia. Pharmacologica Japonica 120:116P–118P

Seleem D, Pardi V, Murata RM (2017) Review of flavonoids: A diverse group of natural compounds with anti-*Candida albicans* activity *in vitro*. Arch Oral Biol 76:76–83

Shahidi F, Yeo J (2018) Bioactivities of phenolics by focusing on suppression of chronic diseases: a review. Int J Mol Sci 19. https://doi.org/10.3390/ijms19061573

Shakya T et al (2011) A small molecule discrimination map of the antibiotic resistance kinome. Chem Biol 18:1591–1601. https://doi.org/10.1016/j.chembiol.2011.10.018

Sharma S, Verma HN, Sharma NK (2014) Cationic bioactive peptide from the seeds of *Benincasa hispida*. Int J Pept 2014:156060–156060. https://doi.org/10.1155/2014/156060

She P, Wang Y, Luo Z, Chen L, Tan R, Wang Y, Wu Y (2018) Meloxicam inhibits biofilm formation and enhances antimicrobial agents efficacy by *Pseudomonas aeruginosa*. MicrobiologyOpen 7:e00545. https://doi.org/10.1002/mbo3.545

Si H, Hu J, Liu Z, Zeng Z-I (2008) Antibacterial effect of oregano essential oil alone and in combination with antibiotics against extended-spectrum β-lactamase-producing *Escherichia coli*. FEMS Immunol Med Microbiol 53:190–194. https://doi.org/10.1111/j.1574-695X.2008.00414.x

Sikkema J, de Bont JA, Poolman B (1994) Interactions of cyclic hydrocarbons with biological membranes. J Biol Chem 269:8022–8028

Sikkema J, de Bont JA, Poolman B (1995) Mechanisms of membrane toxicity of hydrocarbons. Microbiol Rev 59:201–222

Simões M, Bennett RN, Rosa EAS (2009) Understanding antimicrobial activities of phytochemicals against multidrug resistant bacteria and biofilms. Nat Prod Rep 26:746–757. https://doi.org/10.1039/B821648G

Soromou LW et al (2013) Subinhibitory concentrations of pinocembrin exert anti-*Staphylococcus aureus* activity by reducing α-toxin expression. J Appl Microbiol 115:41–49. https://doi.org/10.1111/jam.12221

Strömstedt AA, Park S, Burman R, Göransson U (2017) Bactericidal activity of cyclotides where phosphatidylethanolamine-lipid selectivity determines antimicrobial spectra. Biochim Biophys Acta Biomembr 1859:1986–2000. https://doi.org/10.1016/j.bbamem.2017.06.018

Styers D, Sheehan DJ, Hogan P, Sahm DF (2006) Laboratory-based surveillance of current antimicrobial resistance patterns and trends among *Staphylococcus aureus*: 2005 status in the United States. Ann Clin Microbiol Antimicrob 5:2-2. https://doi.org/10.1186/1476-0711-5-2

Sugita-Konishi Y, Hara-Kudo Y, Amano F, Okubo T, Aoi N, Iwaki M, Kumagai S (1999) Epigallocatechin gallate and gallocatechin gallate in green tea catechins inhibit extracellular release of Vero toxin from enterohemorrhagic *Escherichia coli* O157:H7. Biochim Biophys Acta Gen Subj 1472:42–50. https://doi.org/10.1016/S0304-4165(99)00102-6

Sukur SM, Halim AS, Singh KKB (2011) Evaluations of bacterial contaminated full thickness burn wound healing in Sprague Dawley rats Treated with Tualang honey. Indian J Plastic Surg 44:112

Suriyanarayanan B, Sarojini Santhosh R (2015) Docking analysis insights quercetin can be a non-antibiotic adjuvant by inhibiting Mmr drug efflux pump in *Mycobacterium* sp. and its homologue EmrE in *Escherichia coli*. J Biomol Struct Dyn 33:1819–1834. https://doi.org/10.1080/07391102.2014.974211

Tagousop CN, Tamokou J-D-D, Ekom SE, Ngnokam D, Voutquenne-Nazabadioko L (2018) Antimicrobial activities of flavonoid glycosides from *Graptophyllum grandulosum* and their mechanism of antibacterial action. BMC Complement Altern Med 18:252–252. https://doi.org/10.1186/s12906-018-2321-7

Tajkarimi MM, Ibrahim SA, Cliver DO (2010) Antimicrobial herb and spice compounds in food. Food Control 21:1199–1218. https://doi.org/10.1016/j.foodcont.2010.02.003

Thoroski J, Blank G, Biliaderis C (1989) Eugenol induced inhibition of extracellular enzyme production by *Bacillus subtilis*. J Food Prot 52:399–403. https://doi.org/10.4315/0362-028x-52.6.399

Tofighi Z, Molazem M, Doostdar B, Taban P, Shahverdi AR, Samadi N, Yassa N (2015) Antimicrobial activities of three medicinal plants and investigation of flavonoids of *Tripleurospermum disciforme*. Iran J Pharm Res 14:225–231

Trumpower BL, Gennis RB (1994) Energy transduction by cytochrome complexes in mitochondrial and bacterial respiration: The enzymology of coupling electron transfer reactions to transmembrane proton translocation. Annu Rev Biochem 63:675–716. https://doi.org/10.1146/annurev.bi.63.070194.003331

Ultee A, Bennik MHJ, Moezelaar R (2002) The phenolic hydroxyl group of carvacrol is essential for action against the food-borne pathogen *Bacillus cereus*. Appl Environ Microbiol 68:1561–1568. https://doi.org/10.1128/aem.68.4.1561-1568.2002

Upadhyaya I, Upadhyay A, Kollanoor-Johny A, Darre M, Venkitanarayanan K (2013) Effect of plant derived antimicrobials on *Salmonella* enteritidis adhesion to and invasion of primary chicken oviduct epithelial cells *in vitro* and virulence gene expression. Int J Mol Sci 14:10608–10625

Vaara M (1992) Agents that increase the permeability of the outer membrane. Microbiol Rev 56:395–411

Vaquero MJR, Alberto MR, de Nadra MCM (2007) Antibacterial effect of phenolic compounds from different wines. Food Control 18:93–101. https://doi.org/10.1016/j.foodcont.2005.08.010

Wang S-X, Zhang F-J, Li Y-L, Feng Q-P (1992) Synthesis, characterization, and antibacterial activity of transition metal complexes with 5-hydroxy-7,4′-dimethoxyflavone. J Inorg Biochem 46:251–257. https://doi.org/10.1016/0162-0134(92)80035-T

Weigel KU, Opitz T, Henle T (2004) Studies on the occurrence and formation of 1,2-dicarbonyls in honey. Eur Food Res Technol 218:147–151. https://doi.org/10.1007/s00217-003-0814-0

Wendakoon CN, Sakaguchi M (1995) Inhibition of amino acid decarboxylase activity of *Enterobacter aerogenes* by active components in spices. J Food Prot 58:280–283. https://doi.org/10.4315/0362-028x-58.3.280

Wong F-C, Yong A-L, Ong H-C, Chai T-T (2013) Evaluation of the antibacterial activities of selected medicinal plants and determination of their phenolic constituents. Sci Asia 39:591–595

World Health Organization (2017) WHO publishes list of bacteria for which new antibiotics are urgently needed. https://www.who.int/en/news-room/detail/27-02-2017-who-publishes-list-of-bacteria-for-which-new-antibiotics-are-urgently-needed. Accessed 13 June 2019

World Health Organization (2018) Antimicrobial resistance. https://www.who.int/news-room/fact-sheets/detail/antimicrobial-resistance

Wu D, Kong Y, Han C, Chen J, Hu L, Jiang H, Shen X (2008) D-Alanine:D-alanine ligase as a new target for the flavonoids quercetin and apigenin. Int J Antimicrob Agents 32:421–426. https://doi.org/10.1016/j.ijantimicag.2008.06.010

Wu T, Zang X, He M, Pan S, Xu X (2013) Structure–activity relationship of flavonoids on their anti-*Escherichia coli* activity and inhibition of DNA gyrase. J Agric Food Chem 61:8185–8190. https://doi.org/10.1021/jf402222v

Xiao J, Zhang H (2012) An *Escherichia coli* cell membrane chromatography-offline LC-TOF-MS method for screening and identifying antimicrobial peptides from *Jatropha curcas* meal protein isolate hydrolysates. J Biomol Screen 17:752–760. https://doi.org/10.1177/1087057112442744

Xiao J, Zhang H, Niu L, Wang X (2011) Efficient screening of a novel antimicrobial peptide from jatropha curcas by cell membrane affinity chromatography. J Agric Food Chem 59:1145–1151. https://doi.org/10.1021/jf103876b

Xu H et al (2001) Flavones inhibit the hexameric replicative helicase RepA. Nucleic Acids Res 29:5058–5066. https://doi.org/10.1093/nar/29.24.5058

Yap PSX, Lim SHE, Hu CP, Yiap BC (2013) Combination of essential oils and antibiotics reduce antibiotic resistance in plasmid-conferred multidrug resistant bacteria. Phytomedicine 20:710–713. https://doi.org/10.1016/j.phymed.2013.02.013

Yap PSX, Yiap BC, Ping HC, Lim SHE (2014) Essential oils, a new horizon in combating bacterial antibiotic resistance. Open Microbiol J 8:6–14. https://doi.org/10.2174/1874285801408010006

Zhang Y-M, Rock CO (2004) Evaluation of epigallocatechin gallate and related plant polyphenols as inhibitors of the FabG and FabI reductases of bacterial type II fatty-acid synthase. J Biol Chem 279:30994–31001. https://doi.org/10.1074/jbc.M403697200

Zhang H, Chen X, He J (2009) Pharmacological action of clove oil and its application in oral care products. Oral Care Ind 19:23–24

Zhang Y, Kong J, Xie Y, Guo Y, Cheng Y, Qian H, Yao W (2018) Essential oil components inhibit biofilm formation in *Erwinia carotovora* and *Pseudomonas fluorescens* via anti-quorum sensing activity. LWT Food Sci Technol:133–139

Zhao WH, Hu ZQ, Okubo S, Hara Y, Shimamura T (2001) Mechanism of synergy between epigallocatechin gallate and beta-lactams against methicillin-resistant *Staphylococcus aureus*. Antimicrob Agents Chemother 45:1737–1742. https://doi.org/10.1128/AAC.45.6.1737-1742.2001

Chapter 4
Essential Oils as Potential Antimicrobial Agents

Disha Varijakzhan, Shun-Kai Yang, Chou Min Chong, Riaz Akseer, Maryam Sultan Alhosani, Warren Thomas, Kok Song Lai, and Swee Hua Erin Lim

Abstract Antimicrobial resistance has been reported since the discovery of antibiotics; the microorganisms which have been exposed to antibiotics are continuously and rapidly evolving to overcome the effect of antimicrobial agents. This has made antimicrobial resistance a major public health issue. In order to overcome antimicrobial resistance, various alternatives are being explored; this includes the utilization of plant essential oils, which are mixtures of secondary metabolites produced by plants that have antimicrobial activity. Essential oils have proven to be effective against various pathogens such as, *Klebsiella pneumoniae*, *Campylobacter jejuni*, *Staphylococcus aureus* and others.

This chapter aims to briefly discuss resistance mechanisms employed by microorganisms and alternative methods used to overcome antimicrobial resistance. Then, the chemistry of essential oils and the effects these essential oils have on the

---

D. Varijakzhan
Aquatic Animal Health and Therapeutics Laboratory, Institute of Bioscience, Universiti Putra Malaysia, Serdang, Selangor, Malaysia

Perdana University – Royal College of Surgeons in Ireland, Serdang, Selangor, Malaysia

S.-K. Yang · R. Akseer · M. S. Alhosani · K. S. Lai
Division of Health Sciences, Abu Dhabi Women's College, Higher Colleges of Technology, Abu Dhabi, United Arab Emirates

C. M. Chong
Aquatic Animal Health and Therapeutics Laboratory, Institute of Bioscience, Universiti Putra Malaysia, Serdang, Selangor, Malaysia

W. Thomas
Perdana University – Royal College of Surgeons in Ireland, Serdang, Selangor, Malaysia

S. H. E. Lim (✉)
Perdana University – Royal College of Surgeons in Ireland, Serdang, Selangor, Malaysia

Division of Health Sciences, Abu Dhabi Women's College, Higher Colleges of Technology, Abu Dhabi, United Arab Emirates
e-mail: erinlimsh@gmail.com

H. Panwar et al. (eds.), *Sustainable Agriculture Reviews 49*, Sustainable Agriculture Reviews 49, https://doi.org/10.1007/978-3-030-58259-3_4

genomes and proteomes of the treated microorganisms has also been reviewed. These essential oils should be further explored in the future to examine their toxicity and side effects through *in vitro* and clinical studies.

Keywords Antimicrobial resistance · Antimicrobial activity · Combination therapy · Drug resistant pathogens · Essential oil · Extraction methods · Gene regulation · Plant metabolites · Proteomic analysis · Terpenes

4.1 Introduction

Antimicrobial resistance occurs when microorganisms such as bacteria, fungi, viru ses and parasites evolve so that the antimicrobials (antibiotics, antifungals, antivirals, antimalarials and anthelmintics) which were used to control the infections have become ineffective (World Health Organization 2017). The idea of the modern "antibiotic era" began with the principle of a "magic bullet" defined by Paul Ehrlich whereby the antibiotic selectively targets only disease causing microbes, but not the host (Aminov 2010). The first antibiotic, penicillin, was discovered by Alexander Fleming in 1928 (Aminov 2010; Ventola 2015). During the period between 1950s and 1970s, various novel antibiotics were discovered; these new treatments resulted in a decrease in the mortality and morbidity rates of the most serious infectious diseases. However, the discoveries of new classes of antibiotics have significantly declined since then (Fig. 4.1). Currently, modifications of the existing classes of antibiotics are the main approach used to combat antimicrobial resistance.

Since the introduction of antibiotics, microorganisms have continued to evolve to resist these agents, leading to the development of antimicrobial resistant strains that pose a significant risk to human health. The Centers for Disease Control and Prevention reported that in the European Union, antibiotic resistance caused 25,000 deaths annually; whereas in the United States, there were approximately 23,000 deaths annually due to infection by resistant bacterial strains (Centers for Disease Control and Prevention 2017). The massive expansion of bacterial genomic sequencing in recent years has led to the identification of 20,000 potential resistance genes, grouped into a lesser number of functional resistance determinants in diverse pathogenic species (Davies and Davies 2010; Aslam et al. 2018).

All antibiotics identified since the initial discovery of penicillin can be classified into one of 20 different classes. Table 4.1 describes several of these classes of antibiotics which are commonly used and their mode of action against bacterial cells.

The global rise in the number of antimicrobial resistance cases is alarming, and priority has been given to identifying new antimicrobial alternatives such as natural products for clinical application in infection control (Yap et al. 2014). Plant extracts used medicinally contain various constituents, and this diverse assembly of secondary metabolites can be tested for antimicrobial activity and also for synergistic

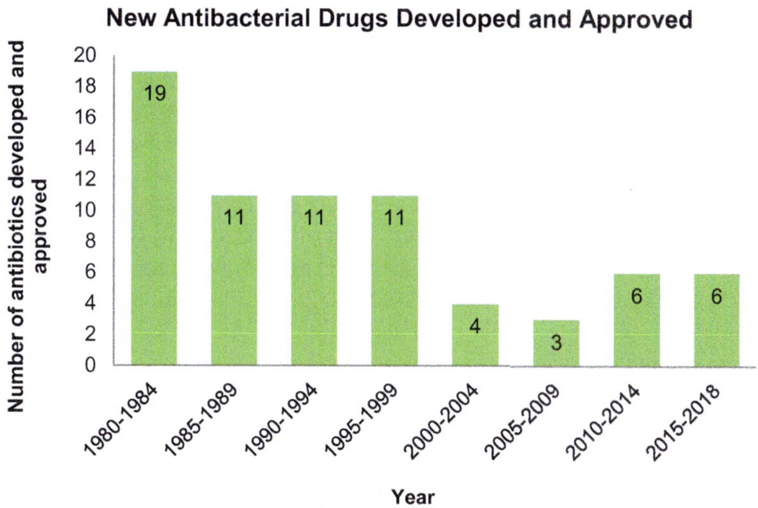

Fig. 4.1 The number of antibiotics discovered and approved showing a decrease over time. The number in the bar chart represents the number of antibiotics discovered over the years (Centers for Disease Control and Prevention 2013; Ventola 2015; Andrei et al. 2018)

Table 4.1 Groups of antibiotics commonly used and their mode of action against bacteria

Antibiotic Class	Example(s)	Target	Reference
β-lactam	Penicillin, Cephalosporin, Carbapenems and Monobactams	Biosynthesis of peptidoglycan	Etebu and Arikekpar (2016), Yap et al. (2017)
Aminoglycoside	Gentamicin, Streptomycin	Translation	Davies and Davies (2010), Yap et al. (2017)
Glycopeptide	Vancomycin	Biosynthesis of peptidoglycan	Davies and Davies (2010), Yap et al. (2017)
Macrolide	Erythromycin, Azithromycin	Translation	Leclercq (2002), Davies and Davies (2010), Etebu and Arikekpar (2016)
Lincosamide	Clindamycin	Translation	Leclercq (2002), Davies and Davies (2010), Etebu and Arikekpar (2016)
Quinolone	Ciprofloxacin	Deoxyribonucleic acid (DNA) replication	Davies and Davies (2010), Etebu and Arikekpar (2016)
Rifamycin	Rifampin	Transcription	Wehrli and Staehelin (1971), Davies and Davies (2010)
Cationic peptides	Colistin	Cell membrane	Davies and Davies (2010)

effects when combined with antibiotics. Essential oils are aromatic, oily liquids synthesized by different parts of plants and have been widely used in different fields such as the perfumery industry, cosmetics, aroma therapy and pharmaceutical development. The use of essential oils has been recorded in traditional medicines such as Ayurveda, traditional Iranian medicine and traditional Korean medicine for centuries (Sharifi-Rad et al. 2017; Varijakzhan et al. 2020). Essential oils consist of complex mixtures of hydrocarbons and oxygenated hydrocarbons; these are produced and secreted by specialized secretory plant tissues called glandular trichomes. The essential oils diffuse onto the surface of the plant organs such as the flowers and leaves (Semeniuc et al. 2017; Sharifi-Rad et al. 2017). Essential oils have the ability to inhibit the growth of microbes in plants by acting as an antibacterial, antiviral and also as antifungal agents in the control of phytopathogens (Fürstenberg-Hägg et al. 2013; Moo et al. 2020).

The objective of this chapter is to describe the chemistry of essential oils and the effect of the essential oils on the genomes and proteomes of the targeted pathogens.

4.2 Overview of Antimicrobial Resistance

Over time, bacteria have evolved to resist the activity of antibiotics, and the decline in efficacy has resulted in increased mortality and morbidity rates in hospital and community settings. In this subsection, we are going to discuss briefly the mechanisms developed by bacteria to tolerate and counter the growth inhibitory effects of antibiotics and the more effective strategies that have been developed to overcome antibacterial resistance in clinical practice.

4.2.1 Mechanisms of Antimicrobial Resistance

In general, microorganisms develop resistance towards antimicrobials when they are exposed to the same antimicrobials continuously at low, sub-inhibitory concentrations. Microorganisms are evolving to counter an environmental challenge in the manner of any other evolutionary driver for survival. Antimicrobial resistance can be developed naturally in the environment due to the intense competition between various microorganisms in mixed ecosystems. Most of the antimicrobial compounds used clinically are molecules produced naturally by microorganisms that live in these complex ecosystems. Therefore, natural environments such as the soil act as a potential reservoir of resistance genes in the armory of competing microorganisms (Stokes and Gillings 2011; Perry and Wright 2013; Chamosa et al. 2017). The resistance mechanisms that are used by bacteria to counter antibiotic activity can be categorized as intrinsic, acquired or adaptive (Hollenbeck and Rice 2012; Munita and Arias 2016; Pang et al. 2019). These will be discussed in the following sections.

4.2.2 *Intrinsic Resistance*

Gram positive and Gram negative bacteria are able to exhibit intrinsic resistance towards antibiotics. Intrinsic resistance is archaically integrated within the genome of a bacterial species or may be due to a critical structural feature of bacterial cells; either condition is not dependent on antibiotic selective pressure or horizontal gene transfer (Hollenbeck and Rice 2012; Kostyanev and Can 2017). Resistance towards β-lactams, fluoroquinolones and aminoglycosides for example, may be due to the intrinsic resistance found in the bacteria. *Pseudomonas aeruginosa* (Gram negative) and Enterococci (Gram positive) to name few, possess high levels of intrinsic resistance towards most classes of antibiotics. The principal mechanisms involved are reduction in outer membrane permeability, expression of efflux pump system and the production of enzymes that inactivate the antibiotic molecules (Fig. 4.2) (Breidenstein et al. 2011; Paraje 2011; Hollenbeck and Rice 2012; Pang et al. 2019). An example of intrinsic resistance based on structural feature is the inability of penicillin to kill *Mycoplasma*, a bacterium that lacks cell wall around the membrane.

4.2.2.1 Restriction of Outer Membrane Permeability and the Efflux System

The vast majority of antibiotics used clinically are able to pass through the cell membrane to reach their respective targets within bacterial cells (Mingeot-Leclercq et al. 1999; Lambert 2002). Aminoglycosides and polymyxins enter the bacterial cells by interacting with lipopolysaccharide on the outer membrane of Gram

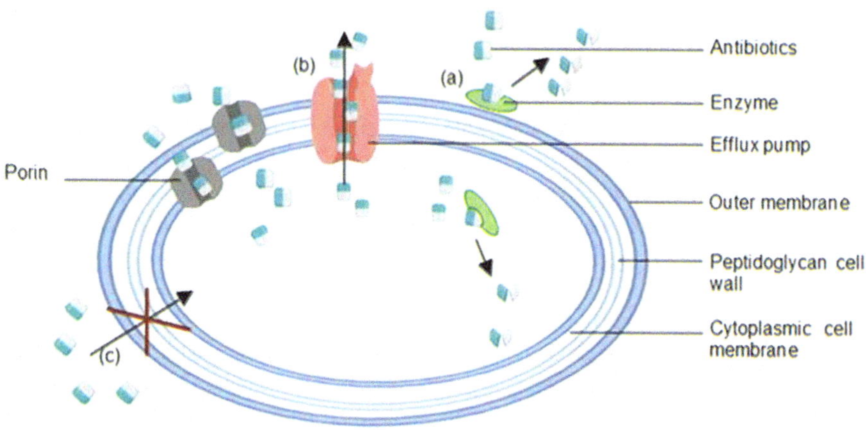

Fig. 4.2 intrinsic antibiotic resistance mechanisms in bacteria. (**a**) Enzymes such as β-lactamase break down antibiotics (penicillin) and inactivate the antibiotic. (**b**) Antibiotics that enter the bacteria cells through porins are pumped out of the cells through the efflux pump. (**c**) Antibiotics are not able to enter the cell due to lower outer membrane permeability of the membrane. (Figure adapted from Moo et al. 2019)

negative bacteria (Pang et al. 2019). The lipopolysaccharide structure is made up of Lipid A; central core oligosaccharide region and outermost O-antigen (Nishino et al. 2006). Calcium and magnesium cations act as a bridge between nearby lipopolysaccharide molecules to stabilize the monolayer (Hancock and Chapple 1999; Velkov et al. 2010; Yu et al. 2014). Polymyxin B antibiotic displaces the divalent cations (calcium and magnesium cations) thus weakening the packing of the adjacent lipid A molecules of the lipopolysaccharide; hence, inducing the expansion of the outer membrane (Yu et al. 2014). Due to the instability of the outer membrane, polymyxin B will cross the outer membrane, leading to the destruction of the integrity of the phospholipid bilayer of the inner membrane, so causing death of the bacterial cells. Bacterial cells achieve resistance to polymyxin B through lipid A modification by reducing the net negative charge of the outer membrane, and the dependence on cationic interaction for stability (Kato et al. 2012; Yu et al. 2014). This is achieved by shielding the phosphate group on Lipid A by positively charged groups such as phosphoethanolamine.

The function of bacterial efflux pumps is to expel toxic compounds out of the cells, which can be enhanced by the over-expression of the efflux pumps (Yang et al. 2018a, b). The efflux pumps can be classified into five families: resistance-nodulation-division family, major facilitator superfamily, Adenosine triphosphate (ATP) binding cassette superfamily, small multi drug resistance family and the multi drug and toxic compound extrusion family (Sun et al. 2014; Chakraborty 2017). In *P. aeruginosa*, the efflux pumps belong to the resistance-nodulation-division family and have an important role in antimicrobial resistance (Pang et al. 2019). Over-expression of more than one efflux pump in bacteria can result in the development of multi drug resistant bacterial strains such as multi drug resistant *P. aeruginosa* (Yang et al. 2018a, b; Pang et al. 2019).

4.2.2.2 Antibiotic Inactivating Enzymes

Antibiotic inactivating enzymes are able to inactivate antibiotics through the cleavage of hydrolysable chemical bonds such as amide and ester bonds. Enzymes such as β-lactamases, aminoglycoside modifying enzymes and enzyme superoxide dismutase are a few examples of enzymes that inactivate antibiotics (Hollenbeck and Rice 2012; Álvarez-Cisneros and Ponce-Alquicira 2018). β-lactamases can be grouped into classes A, B, C and D whereby enzymes from classes A, C and D hydrolyze β-lactams through an active serine site, while the class B enzymes are metalloenzymes that require zinc ions for activity (Bush and Jacoby 2010). Gram negative bacteria have the *ampC* gene (Class C β-lactamase) which encodes a hydrolytic β-lactamase that confers resistance to all penicillins and cephalosporins (Munita and Arias 2016).

4.2.3 *Acquired Resistance*

Bacteria are able to gain resistance through mutational changes or by acquisition of resistance genes, the latter occur *via* horizontal gene transfer between strains or species. Acquired resistance will only initially be found in a particular bacterial subpopulation (Hollenbeck and Rice 2012; Munita and Arias 2016; Álvarez-Cisneros and Ponce-Alquicira 2018). However, this resistant population may subsequently become predominant in a particular case or disease outbreak.

4.2.3.1 Horizontal Gene Transfer

Horizontal gene transfer in bacteria is the ability to acquire new genes through the uptake of broad host range plasmids or through the integration of transposons or integrons (Breidenstein et al. 2011). Horizontal gene transfers can be classified as: transformation (naked deoxyribonucleic acid (DNA) incorporation); transduction (phage mediated); or conjugation (bacterial "sex"). Resistance among pathogenic bacteria can be achieved through conjugation, which is a very efficient method to transfer genes and involves direct cell-to-cell contact between bacteria (Munita and Arias 2016). β-lactamases such as imipenemases, Verona integron-encoded metallo-β-lactamase, Sao Paulo metallo-β-lactamase, Germany imipenemase, New Delhi metallo-β-lactamase and Florence imipenenmase belong to class B β-lactamase enzymes which are metalloenzymes that require zinc ions for the hydrolysis of β-lactams (Bush and Jacoby 2010). They are carried by genetic elements such as integrons and plasmids and these genes have been identified in *P. aeruginosa* demonstrating the incredibly broad range of antimicrobial resistance mechanisms that are found in this organism (Khajuria et al. 2013; Hong et al. 2015; Pang et al. 2019).

4.2.3.2 Resistance by Gene Mutation

For this type of resistance, a group of bacterial cells from a susceptible population may undergo mutation in specific genes that will suppress the activity of antibiotic compound applied at sub-lethal concentrations. The resistant bacterial population will dominate as the antibiotic will suppress the growth or eliminate the susceptible bacterial cells. One example of an antimicrobial resistance mechanism affected by the mutation of genes would be a modification of the antibiotic that reduces its affinity for its target or decreases the rate of antibiotic uptake (Munita and Arias 2016). The modification of an antibiotic affecting its activity can also be achieved through the addition of a chemical moiety to the antibiotic which will inactivate it. This activity can be conferred by enzymes synthesized by the bacteria and is commonly found in both Gram positive and Gram negative species. Biochemical modifications that are catalyzed by these modifying enzymes include acetylation, adenylation and phosphorylation (Munita and Arias 2016). Aminoglycoside modifying enzymes modify the aminoglycoside molecule by changing the hydroxyl or amino groups present in the molecule. Aminoglycoside modifying enzymes can be classified into three groups: aminoglycoside phosphotransferase, aminoglycoside acetyltransferase and aminoglycoside nucleotidyl transferase (Ramirez and Tolmasky 2010; Munita and Arias 2016). Antibiotics are prevented from accumulating in the cytoplasm by energy-dependent efflux systems, while entry may be affected by the physical properties of trans-membrane pores. For example, clinical isolates of *Klebsiella pneumoniae* showed a shift in a porin expression from OmpK35 to OmpK36, where the latter possesses a smaller channel pore size that prevents antibiotic entry (Doménech-Sánchez et al. 2003; Hasdemir et al. 2004; Munita and Arias 2016).

4.2.4 Adaptive Resistance

Adaptive resistance can be defined as a reduction in antibiotic killing in an originally susceptible bacteria population after exposure to the antibiotic. The adaptive resistance increases the resistance of bacterial cells through changes in the expression of proteins or by alteration in genes as a response towards an environmental stimulus. In the absence of the stimulus, the mechanism is reversible (Pang et al. 2019). The ability to form biofilms is an example of adaptive resistance. Approximately 65% of infections are associated with biofilm formation (Paraje 2011). A biofilm is an organized community of bacteria whereby they collaborate amongst themselves, attaching to a surface through a polymeric matrix which is primarily made up of exopolysaccharide (Donlan 2002). Bacteria that are able to form biofilms are highly resistant towards antibiotics due to the structure of the biofilm and also the presence of sessile cells which act as a sink for antibiotic sequestration, thus leading to a protected environment (Costerton et al. 2003; Vuong et al. 2004; Patel 2005). The biofilm matrix acts as a diffusion barrier and in a biofilm, the degradation of antibiotics may be achieved in discrete parts of the biofilm, resulting in the formation of persister cells (Patel 2005; Paraje 2011). Some antibiotics may enter the biofilm without achieving the effective concentration required to suppress bacterial growth. Bacteria that occupy the peripheral layers of the biofilm can be killed by the antibiotics but the innermost population of bacterial cells will be exposed to a lower antibiotic concentration and will adapt to the evolutionary pressure and acquire antibiotic resistance (Patel 2005; Paraje 2011).

4.3 Strategies to Counteract Antimicrobial Resistance

To tackle the issue of increased antimicrobial resistance, alternative strategies have been evaluated. In this section, we will briefly discuss strategies that are used to overcome antimicrobial resistance.

4.3.1 Combination Drug Therapy

Combination drug therapy is the use of two or more agents to treat the same condition, in this context, bacterial infection. There are two factors that need to be taken into consideration when using a combination of drugs: (1) the mechanisms of action of the drugs should not be overlapping, and (2) the drugs should not have antagonistic interaction (Fischbach 2011). The treatment of *Mycobacterium tuberculosis* is an example of established combination therapy. The treatment relies upon a combination of four drugs: isoniazid which inhibits the enoylreductase subunit of fatty acid synthase; ethambutol which inhibits the arabinosyl transferases involved in cell wall biosynthesis; rifampicin and pyrazinamide which are ribonucleic acid (RNA) polymerase inhibitors (Fischbach 2011; Moo et al. 2019). A combination of these drugs is much more effective in preventing the development of resistance in *M. tuberculosis* as compared to monotherapy.

4.3.2 Bacteriophage Therapy

Bacteriophages are bacteria infecting viruses that kill bacteria by causing cell lysis (Clokie et al. 2011). Every bacteriophage, due to its highly specific surface molecules, can only bind to a narrow range of bacteria, possibly even a single subgroup within a species. Multiple bacteriophages may target one bacterium and the affinity of binding for each phage may vary. For example, there are approximately 137 different bacteriophages characterized as targeting the *Pseudomonas* genus (Pang et al. 2019). Importantly, bacteriophage therapy has been recorded to have potent activity against *Pseudomonas* or *Burkholderia* biofilms (Hughes and Webber 2017; Pang et al. 2019). The bacteriophages will invade the biofilm and move through the bacterial population within the biofilm resulting in a reduction in the number of viable cells within the biofilm (Hughes and Webber 2017). A study was conducted on a mouse model of chronic lung infection with *P. aeruginosa*. *P. aeruginosa* strain LESB65 was isolated from cystic fibrosis patients in an artificial sputum medium biofilm and was effectively killed by bacteriophage PELP20 indicated by enhanced clearance of the bacterial cells in the mouse model (Waters et al. 2017).

One advantage of using bacteriophage therapy includes the high specificity towards the target bacteria, so not affecting the commensal flora found in the human host. Bacteriophages are able to replicate at the site of infection, and have minimal systemic side effects compared with other treatments such as antibiotic therapy. Bacteriophages are able to exhibit bactericidal effects against antibiotic resistant bacteria and are easily administered to patients (Ly-Chatain 2014). To avoid the development of resistance towards bacteriophages, a cocktail of bacteriophages is used for the treatment of bacterial infections where possible (Ly-Chatain 2014; Moo et al. 2019).

4.3.3 Use of Nanoparticles

Nanoparticles are tiny materials which are less than 100 nm in size and have a large surface area to mass ratio (Pang et al. 2019). Antibiotics can be loaded into the nanoparticles by physical encapsulation, adsorption or chemical conjugation (Karaman et al. 2017). Nanoparticles are able to increase the efficacy of established antibiotics; this enables reduction in the dose administered. This limits the toxicity associated with the antibiotics used, such as aminoglycoside associated nephrotoxicity (Karaman et al. 2017; Kumar et al. 2018). When nanoparticles such as silver are used together with antibiotics, a synergistic interaction has been observed. For example, when tetracycline was attached to the surface of silver nanoparticles this resulted in an increase in anti-bacterial activity against *Salmonella* Typhimurium (Deng et al. 2016). Tetracycline-silver nanoparticle complexes accumulated around the bacterial cells and enhanced contact of the antibiotic with the cell wall, thus increasing the inhibition of bacterial growth.

4.4 Chemistry of Essential Oils

Essential oils are complex mixtures of hydrocarbons and oxygenated hydrocarbons; they are made up of over 300 different compounds whereby each organic volatile compound has a molecular weight of less than 300 Daltons (Da) (Dhifi et al. 2016; Swamy et al. 2016; Morsy 2017; Sharifi-Rad et al. 2017). The aroma and bioactive properties of essential oils, such as antimicrobial activity and anti-cancer, are dependent upon the chemical compounds found in the particular essential oils and whether they are present in their oxygenated or active form (Swamy et al. 2016). In general, an essential oil will have about 20–100 different bioactive compounds whereby only two or three of these compounds will be found as major fractions ranging from 20 to 70% of the total volume (Swamy et al. 2016; Moghaddam and Mehdizadeh 2017). Another important property of essential oil is its hydrophobicity and high solubility in alcohol, ether and fixed oils, but insolubility in water (Dhifi et al. 2016).

Different species of plants produce essential oils with different chemical constituents where in the chemical composition of the essential oils of a single plant are influenced by geographical location of cultivation, the immediate environment surrounding the plants, the harvesting conditions such as the season and climate, stage of maturity of the plant and the extraction methods used to prepare the essential oils (Lahlou 2004; Swamy et al. 2016; Morsy 2017). In a single species study conducted by Zheljazkov et al. (2008), significant variation was found in the essential oil chemical composition of 38 sub-types of sweet basil (*Ocimum basilicum* L). They categorized the sweet basil varieties into seven groups based on the oil composition: high–linalool chemotype; linalool-eugenol chemotype; methyl chavicol chemotype; methyl chavicol-linalool chemotype; methyl eugenol- linalool chemotype; methyl cinnamate-linalool chemotype and bergamotene chemotype (Zheljazkov et al. 2008).

Essential oils are primarily made up of terpenes and also other chemical classes such as alcohols, ethers or oxides, aldehydes, ketones, esters, amines, amides, phenols and heterocycles (Dhifi et al. 2016; Moghaddam and Mehdizadeh 2017; Morsy 2017; Mahizan et al. 2019). Terpenes can be further categorized as monoterpenes, sesquiterpenes, diterpenes and triterpenes where monoterpenes are the major component (~90% by volume) contributing to the bioactivity in an essential oil (Bakkali et al. 2008; Mahizan et al. 2019). Terpenes are synthesized through the mevalonic acid pathway and they are essentially polymers of isoprene joined in a repetitive head-to-tail manner (Bakkali et al. 2008) (chemical formula of C_5H_8) as shown in Fig. 4.3.

Monoterpenes are the product of the combination between two isoprene units and they can be easily oxidized on exposure to air and or heat sources. Monocyclic monoterpenes are found abundantly in essential oils, however, linear and bicyclic monoterpenes can also be found. Sesquiterpenes are terpenoid molecules made up of three isoprene units and when a functional group is added to a monoterpene or sesquiterpenes, it is known as a terpenoid (Zuzarte and Salgueiro 2015). Limonene is an example of a monoterpene which is a compound found in citrus fruits while zingiberene is an example of sesquiterpene compound which is commonly found in the essential oil of ginger (Table 4.2).

Many studies have reported that essential oils have antimicrobial activity where the evaluation of antimicrobial activities of the essential oils in a biological system is complicated by the fact that a mixture of compounds is being analyzed and that a number of the constituents in the mixture may have different biological activities (Yanishlieva et al. 2006; Souza et al. 2007). Any specific biological activity such as antimicrobial activity is usually conferred by only one or two main compounds found in the essential oil (Bakkali et al. 2008). However, at times, overall activity of the essential oil cannot be credited to one specific compound, instead a diverse combination of molecules may be needed to exert a significant antimicrobial activity (Isman et al. 2008). Therefore, the antimicrobial activity of an essential oil may be the consequence of synergistic effects between several chemical compounds. The activity of an essential oil is due to the presence of active constituents such as monoterpenes, sesquiterpenes, alcohols and phenols. However, the rate of diffusion of an essential oil into the bacterial cell varies not only due to the differences in the composition of essential oil but also due to the difference in the structure of cell walls of Gram positive and Gram negative bacteria (Nazzaro et al. 2013).

Gram positive bacteria consist of a thick peptidoglycan layer and molecules such as teichoic acid and proteins are attached to it. This allows hydrophobic molecules to penetrate the cells easily and to act on both the cell wall and cytoplasmic targets

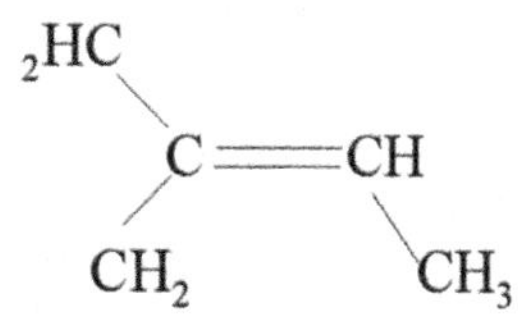

Fig. 4.3 Isoprene unit of terpene. (Figure adapted from Moghaddam and Mehdizadeh 2017)

Table 4.2 Chemical structures of compounds found in essential oils and their categorization

Plant	Chemical structure	Name of the compound	Reference
Citrus fruit such as lemon	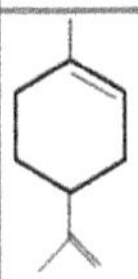	Limonene (Monoterpene)	Zuzarte and Salgueiro (2015)
Ginger	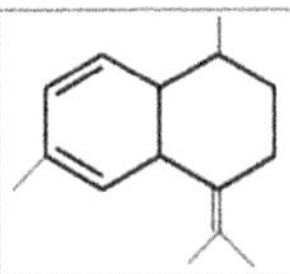	Zingiberene (Sesquiterpene)	Zuzarte and Salgueiro (2015)
Cinnamon	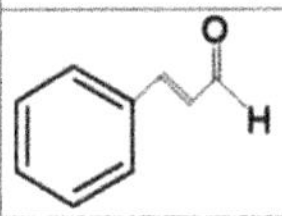	Cinnamaldehyde (Aldehyde)	Ashakirin et al. (2017)
Peppermint	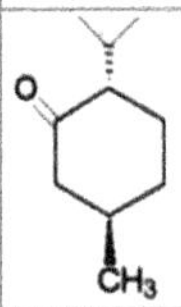	Menthone (Monoterpene)	Loolaie et al. (2017)
	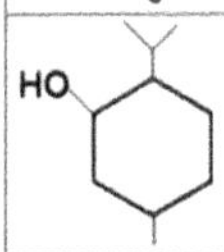	Menthol (Monoterpene alcohol)	Loolaie et al. (2017)
	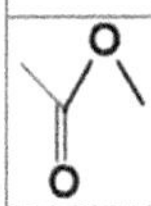	Methyl acetate (Monoterpene)	Loolaie et al. (2017)
	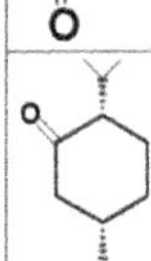	Iso-menthone (Monoterpene)	Loolaie et al. (2017)

(continued)

Table 4.2 (continued)

Plant	Chemical structure	Name of the compound	Reference
Oregano	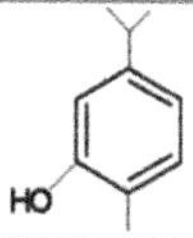	Carvacrol (Monoterpene)	Bokov et al. (2015)
	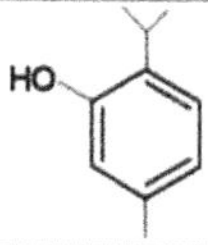	Thymol (Monoterpenoid phenol)	Bokov et al. (2015)
	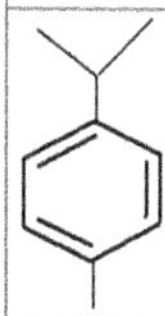	γ-terpinene (Monoterpene)	Bokov et al. (2015)
	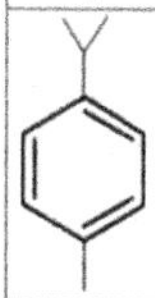	p-cymene (Monoterpene alkylbenzene)	Bokov et al. (2015)

(Nazzaro et al. 2013). Essential oils contains phenolic compounds which have antimicrobial activity against Gram positive bacteria that depends on the concentration of the phenolic compound within the essential oil (Tiwari et al. 2009). Phenolic compounds at low concentrations interfere with enzymes involved in the production of energy (adenosine triphosphate synthesis) whereas at a higher concentration, these compounds can cause protein denaturation. Gram negative bacteria have a thinner peptidoglycan layer compared to the Gram positive bacteria and also have an outer membrane layer surrounding the peptidoglycan layer. The outer membrane of Gram negative bacteria cells contains lipopolysaccharide (Nazzaro et al. 2013; Aljaafari et al. 2019). The structure of the Gram negative cell wall is one of the reasons for Gram negative bacteria to be more resistant to some essential oils. Only small hydrophilic molecules are able to pass through the outer membrane layer through porin proteins which are hydrophilic trans-membrane channels. This is also another reason why Gram negative bacteria are relatively resistant to hydrophobic compounds (Aljaafari et al. 2019). However, the outer membrane of Gram negative bacteria is partially permeable to the hydrophobic molecules because some small molecules are able to slowly transverse through the porins (Vaara and Nurminen 1999).

4.5 Essential Oils as Combination Therapy

Essential oils have been described as improving the effectiveness of various antibiotics to which various pathogens have become resistant. In this section, we will discuss a few of the essential oils that are commonly used and demonstrate the ability to improve the efficacy of the antibiotics. The interaction between the essential oil and the antibiotics can be categorized into three types: (1) synergistic; (2) antagonistic and (3) additive. The interaction can be identified by conducting checkerboard assays and from the values obtained through the addition of fractional inhibitory concentrations of each of the drugs. This is known as the fractional inhibitory concentration index (FICI). The interaction is categorized as synergistic if the FICI is less than or equal to 0.5; additive if the FICI greater than 0.5 but less than or equal to 1.0; and antagonistic if the FICI is greater than 2.0 (Moon et al. 2011; Yang et al. 2017).

Cinnamon bark essential oil enhances the effectiveness of the antibiotic meropenem through an additive interaction in combinatory therapy (Yang et al. 2017). Cinnamon bark essential oil and meropenem in combination were tested against *K. pneumoniae* BAA-1705 and was found to have an additive interaction. The minimum inhibitory concentration of the cinnamon bark essential oil was 0.16%, whereas the minimum inhibitory concentration of meropenem was 32 µg/mL. Cinnamon bark essential oil and meropenem used in combination resulted in a fractional inhibitory concentration index of 1.00 indicating an additive interaction. Time-kill analysis was performed on *K. pneumoniae* to determine the complete killing analysis. The combination of meropenem and cinnamon bark essential oil, both at sub-inhibitory concentrations of 16 µg/mL and 0.08% respectively, were able to kill the bacterial cells completely within 1.5 hours. The meropenem-cinnamon bark essential oil combination also increased the zeta potential value, indicating an increase in the charge of the membrane of the bacterial cells. This was also indicated when the cells treated with this combination of compounds displayed extensive corrugation and distortion to the bacterial cell envelope. Thus, it can be concluded that meropenem-cinnamon bark essential oil combination is more effective in killing the *K. pneumoniae* than individual compounds and this may have implications for clinical application.

Rosemary essential oil has been tested for its synergistic effects with antibiotics against eight clinical isolates of *E. coli* from urine (Abdulhasan 2017). Among these eight strains, six strains of the *E. coli* were moderate biofilm formers whereas the other two strains were strong biofilm formers. These strains were tested for sensitivity to gentamicin, trimethoprim/sulfamethoxazole, ciprofloxacin and the rosemary essential oil. The minimum inhibitory concentration of gentamicin, trimethoprim/sulfamethoxazole, ciprofloxacin and the rosemary essential oil for strong biofilm producing *E. coli* were 256 µg/mL, 2000 µg/mL, 500 µg/mL and 10^4µg/mL respectively whereas for the moderate biofilm producing *E. coli* were 512 µg/mL, 2000 µg/mL, 1000 µg/mL and 10^4µg/mL respectively. The combination of the antibiotic gentamicin with the rosemary essential oil indicated a synergistic effect when used against both types of the strains. The fractional inhibitory concentration for the gentamicin and the essential oil combination was 0.257 for strong biofilm producers whereas 0.263 for moderate biofilm producing strains. The synergistic effect was determined when the fractional inhibitory concentration is less than 0.5. The ciprofloxacin and rosemary essential oil combination also exhibited a synergistic interaction where the strong biofilm producing strains exhibited a value of 0.065 whereas the moderate biofilm producing strains exhibited 0.034.

Clove essential oil is another example of essential oil that has antibacterial activity and has been as an antiseptic of oral infection (Nuñez and D'Aquino 2012). Clove essential oil has a high concentration of eugenol which is responsible for the antimicrobial activity. Both the essential oil and eugenol are able to inhibit the growth of both Gram positive and Gram negative bacteria (Nuñez and D'Aquino 2012). Apart from the antibacterial activity, clove essential oil and the compound eugenol are also able to exhibit synergistic effects with antibiotics such as ampicillin and gentamicin to suppress the growth of oral pathogens (Moon et al. 2011). Clove essential oil and ampicillin combination treatment resulted in a synergistic effect when tested against the oral pathogens *Streptococcus mutans*, *Streptococcus sobrinus* and *Streptococcus gordonii* where the cell counts were reduced by more than four-fold when ampicillin and clove essential oil were used in combination. The combination of clove essential oil with gentamicin also achieved a synergistic action and was more effective against the pathogens *S. mutans*, *Streptococcus sanguinis*, *S. sobrinus*, *Streptococcus criceti*, *Streptococcus anginosus*, *S. gordonii*, *Actinobacillus actinomycetemcomitans*, *Fusobacterium nucleatum*, *Prevotella intermedia*, and *Porphylomonas gingivalis* but not for *Streptococcus ratti* which showed an additive effect. Similarly, eugenol in combination with gentamicin exhibited a synergistic effect against all the bacteria tested except for *S. mutans* and *S. ratti* which showed an additive effect. The combination of clove oil or eugenol with the antibiotics demonstrated a higher rate of killing in the bacterial cells within 1 h of exposure.

Lemon grass is a plant widely found in regions with a warm tropical climate and exhibits antibacterial activity (Langeveld et al. 2014). The essential oil is also able to improve the efficacy of antibiotics such as streptomycin and kanamycin against *Salmonella* Typhimurium KCMM 11862 (Shin 2005). A checkerboard assay testing lemon grass essential oil and its major compound citral showed a significant synergism with streptomycin and kanamycin, displaying fractional inhibitory concentration indices in range of 0.28–0.67. The essential oil individually had an average minimum inhibitory concentration of 1 μg/mL; the citral average minimum inhibitory concentration was 0.5 μg/mL; whereas the average minimum inhibitory concentration of streptomycin and kanamycin were 64 μg/mL and 8 μg/mL respectively.

4.6 Studies of Genomic and Proteomic of Microorganisms Treated with Essential Oils

There are various studies that have been conducted providing evidence of essential oils' antimicrobial activity. Figure 4.4 illustrates the mode of action of essential oil against bacteria cells. However, fewer studies have been done to explain the changes that microorganisms' cells undergo when they are exposed to the essential oil. In this section, we will be discussing the changes experienced by these cells in terms of genomic and protein expression when the cells are exposed to the essential oil. We will be focusing on a few essential oils which are being widely studied and have demonstrated efficacy in antimicrobial activity against pathogenic microorganisms. They are: (1) cinnamon essential oil, (2) peppermint essential oil, (3) oregano essential oil, (4) rosemary essential oil, (5) thyme essential oil, and (6) *Eucalyptus* essential oil.

4.6.1 Effects of Essential Oils on Genome Expression

Cinnamon is commonly used in food preservation and for flavoring purposes. The major component of the essential oil is cinnamaldehyde which is an aldehyde compound (Raeisi et al. 2015). A study was conducted to determine the effect of

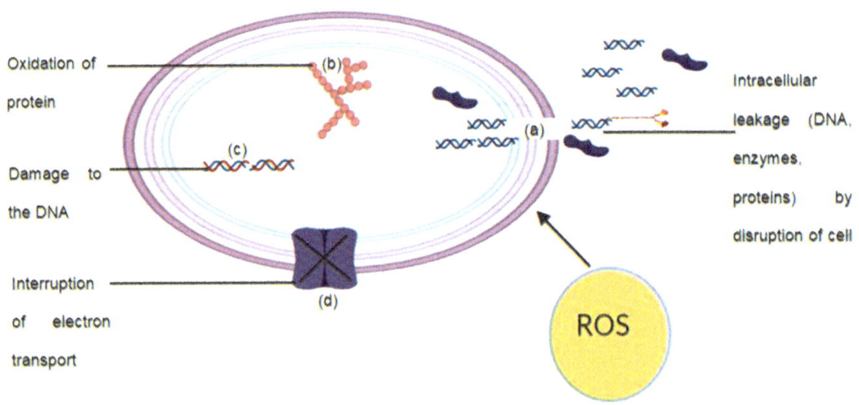

ROS: Reactive oxygen species

Fig. 4.4 Proposed antimicrobial mechanism of essential oils in bacteria. The diagram above illustrates several modes of action exhibited by essential oils against bacterial cells. Reactive oxygen species are generated by antioxidants found in an essential oil. The mechanism involves (**a**) disruption of the cell membrane of the bacteria resulting in the leakage of the cell's content; (**b**) oxidation of the proteins by modifying the covalent bonds involved in maintaining the structure of the proteins; (**c**) damage to the deoxyribonucleic acid (DNA) and (**d**) interruption of the electron transport chain. The mechanisms represented are adapted from Benzaid et al. 2019; Yang et al. 2019, 2020

cinnamon essential oil on *icaA* gene expression by *Staphylococcus epidermidis* (Nuryastuti et al. 2009). *S. epidermidis* is a Gram positive bacterium which is an important nosocomial infectious agent. The gene *icaA* is responsible for the production of polysaccharide intercellular adhesion protein which is required for the formation of a biofilm (Namvar et al. 2013) and it belongs to *ica* operon. Sixteen clinical isolates of *S. epidermidis* were tested for the effect of cinnamon essential oil. The *icaA* gene was overexpressed when *S. epidermidis* was exposed to a 0.01% concentration of the essential oil. However, when *S. epidermidis* was exposed to the cinnamon essential oil at 2%, expression of gene *icaA* was inhibited which is responsible for the synthesis of polysaccharide intercellular adhesion protein, thus preventing the formation of a biofilm. However, low level exposure to the cinnamon essential oil promoted *icaA* expression and enhanced biofilm formation.

Peppermint (*Mentha piperita*) is another essential oil that has been recorded to have antimicrobial activity. There are four main constituents that have been identified from peppermint essential oil: menthone, menthol, iso-menthone and methyl acetate (Mahboubi and Kazempour 2014; Yang et al. 2018a, b; Kovács et al. 2019). There was a study conducted to investigate the effect of peppermint essential oil on bacterial motility of *Campylobacter jejuni* as a reflection of its antibacterial effects (Kovács et al. 2019). *C. jejuni* are highly motile bacteria; the bacterial cells were tested for the effect of peppermint essential oil on their motility. After 24-hour treatment with peppermint essential oil at a concentration 150 μg/mL, there was no swarming activity. In this study, 44 genes were analyzed to examine the impact of peppermint essential oil on the *C. jejuni*. Most of the changes were observed in general stress genes, such as *dnaK, groEL* and *groES* which are responsible for the synthesis of chaperones that are responsible for the folding of other proteins in the cell (Lund 2001; Stintzi 2003). Gene *fliA* was up-regulated when treated with peppermint essential oil, whereas genes *rpoN* and *rpoD* were down-regulated which functions as RNA polymerase sigma factor.

Peppermint essential oil was tested against *Candida* sp., an opportunistic fungal pathogen in human in relative to an antifungal agent, Amphotericin B (Benzaid et al. 2019). The study was conducted to investigate the effect of the essential oil in regulating expression of *SAP* and *HWP1* genes. The peppermint essential oil was able to down-regulate significantly the genes *SAP1, SAP2, SAP3, SAP9, SAP10* and *HWP-1* which are responsible for the virulence of the *C. albicans* cells. The essential oil was also able to distort the shape of the cells which was due to the loss of cytosolic volume. The effect of the essential oil on the surface was similar to that seen in *C. albicans* cells treated with Amphotericin B. Other than affecting the gene regulation, the essential oil was also able to cause cytolysis or disruption of the cell membrane which led to the death of the cells.

Besides, a study was conducted on enterohaemorrhagic *E. coli* serotype O157:H7 to determine the effect of oregano essential oil and its main constituent compound carvacrol on the expression of genes involved in enterohaemorrhagic *E. coli* O157:H7 virulence (Mith et al. 2015). The virulence genes which were monitored in this study were genes *ler, stx2B, fliC* and *luxS*. The gene *ler* is located in the *LEE1* operon which encodes a type III secretion system important for injecting effector proteins into epithelial cells, causing secretory diarrhea (Berdichevsky et al. 2005; Mellies et al. 2011). The *ler* gene acts as an anti-silencer of multiple LEE operons genes. Gene *stx2B* produces Shiga toxin (Wang et al. 2002) and gene *fliC* is responsible for the synthesis of flagellin, a subunit protein which will polymerize to form the filament of bacterial flagella (Wang et al. 2000). Gene *luxS* is involved in the biosynthesis of auto-inducer AI-2 which is involved in regulating quorum sensing (Mith et al. 2015). This study found that exposure of enterohaemorrhagic *E. coli* O157:H7 to oregano essential oil and carvacrol at a sub-growth inhibitory concentration (0.005% and 0.008% respectively) caused the down-regulation of *luxS* gene followed by the genes *ler, stx2B* and *fliC* without affecting bacterial growth. This could indicate that the virulence of enterohaemorrhagic *E. coli* O157:H7 can be controlled with oregano essential oil or carvacrol treatment.

Rosemary (*Rosemarinus officinalis L.*) essential oil consists of cineole as the major constituent, followed by camphor and α-pinene (Elyemni et al. 2019). Other compounds which were found in the essential oil at significant abundance were linalool, borneol, α-terpinene and β-caryophyllene. Rosemary essential oil was tested against clinically isolated extended spectrum β-lactamase positive *E. coli*; whereby standard strain *E. coli* ATCC 2 combination therapy 922 was used as control (Sienkiewicz et al. 2013). The essential oil was tested against *E. coli* F'lac K12 LE140 to investigate its effect on plasmid transfer (Schelz et al. 2006; Yu et al. 2019). From this study, it was found that the essential oil was able to inhibit the replication of the F'lac metabolic plasmid by 3.1% at a 1.09 mg/mL concentration, thus preventing the vertical transfer of the antibiotic resistance gene carried by the plasmid during bacterial growth. The ability of the essential oil to inhibit the transfer of resistance gene ensures the *Enterobacteriaceae* pathogens will not emerge to be multi drug resistance pathogens. The probable mechanism which prevents the transfer and replication of the resistance genes through plasmid would be the complex formation with the guanine-cytosine rich regions in the plasmid, which is required for the replication of the plasmid (Schelz et al. 2006).

Thyme (*Thymus vulgaris*) essential oil is known to be effective against both Gram positive and Gram negative bacteria and multi drug resistant strains, such as *E. coli, S. aureus, E. faecalis* and *E. faecium* (Sienkiewicz et al. 2012). The essential oil and its major components, both thymol and carvacrol have been reported to have the ability to inhibit the quorum sensing involved in the formation of biofilms by down-regulating the gene expression involved in the synthesis of flagellar proteins, which suppresses the motility of the bacterium and reduce viability.

A study was conducted by Myzka et al. (2016) on *Pseudomonas fluorescens* KM121, a biofilm producing organism to determine the effect of thyme essential oil and its major compounds thymol and carvacrol on the inhibition of quorum sensing, thus preventing the formation of a biofilm (Myszka et al. 2016). Thyme essential oil and its major compounds were able to suppress flagellum related movement in *P. fluorescens* KM121. The essential oil itself was more potent than the two individual compounds in the inhibition of bacterial cell motility. The motility assay was validated by performing quantitative real time polymerase chain reactions (qRT-PCR). Quantitative real time polymerase chain reaction analysis showed that thyme essential oil exhibited the greatest reduction in the abundance of messenger ribonucleic acid (mRNA) for the gene *flgA*. The alteration in transcription of gene flgA was mainly caused by carvacrol. The down-regulation in *flgA* gene synthesis resulted to the inhibition of the swarming by bacterial cells, thus resulting to the loss of motility resulting to the inhibition of the biofilm formation by *P. fluorescens*.

Eucalyptus essential oil obtained from *Eucalyptus globulus* Labill was tested against three *Aspergillus* sp., namely *Aspergillus parasiticus* (KMi-220-LR), *Aspergillus parasiticus* (KMi-227-LR) and *Aspergillus flavus* (KMi-202-LR), which are capable of producing mycotoxins (Císarová et al. 2016). From the study, it was found that the essential oil resulted in the significant growth antagonism of the mycelium of the fungi. The fungal strains were treated with *Eucalyptus* essential oil at a concentration of 500 μL/mL and resulted to the inhibition in the synthesis of fungal toxic aflatoxin B_1 which is carcinogenic and one of the four major aflatoxins synthesized by *Aspergillus* sp. (Yu et al. 2004). The proposed mechanism which inhibits the synthesis of aflatoxin B_1 would be by down-regulation of genes *nor-1, ver-1, omtA, aflR* and *pksA* (Jahanshiri et al. 2015). Gene *aflR* is a positive regulatory gene which involves in the biosynthesis of the aflatoxin, therefore, the low expression of this gene resulted to the down-regulation of other genes which are involved in the biosynthesis of aflatoxin (Jahanshiri et al. 2015). The essential oil was able to inhibit the growth of the *Aspergillus* sp. and also capable of inhibiting the synthesis of aflatoxin B_1.

4.6.2 Effects of Essential Oils on Proteomic Expression

A study conducted by Yang et al. (2019) on carbapenemase producing *K. pneumoniae* (Gram negative bacteria) and cinnamon bark (*Cinnamomum verum* J. Presl) essential oil, found that the oil exhibited antimicrobial activity against *K. pneumoniae*. The bacterial cells, untreated and treated with cinnamon bark essential oil were subjected to proteomic analysis. From the study, it was found out that *K. pneumoniae* treated with cinnamon bark essential oil expressed 242 detectable proteins, where 10 proteins out of the 242 proteins were uniquely expressed by the cinnamon bark essential oil treated bacterial cells. Non-treated *K. pneumoniae* expressed 384 detectable proteins, where 152 proteins were uniquely expressed by the non-treated bacterial cells. In the essential oil treated cells, proteins involved in biological processes, cellular components and molecular functions were down-regulated. Cinnamon bark essential oil acted on *K. pneumoniae* by disrupting the membrane of the bacterial cells resulting in the loss of the plasma membrane protein complexes involved in energy generation that are embedded in the plasma membrane such as the adenosine triphosphate (ATP) synthase, the electron transport complex and the nicotinamide adenine dinucleotide hydrogen (NADH)-quinone oxidoreductases which were lost completely (Yang et al. 2019). In addition, the bacterial cells also underwent oxidative stress when treated with the cinnamon bark essential oil. This was identified by the presence of proteins such as autonomous glycyl radical cofactor and catalase peroxidase. The glycyl radical cofactor affects pyruvate formate lyase which is involved in glucose metabolism (Yang et al. 2019). The presence of reactive oxygen species at a high concentration will lead to oxidative damage to the nucleic acids in the bacterial cells.

Other than affecting genome expression, peppermint essential oil is also able to affect the expression of proteins in *C. jejuni*. There were decrease in the expression of proteins involved in the synthesis of virulence associated factors such as PEB4 (a temperature dependent colonization factor) and HtrA (a serine protease which is involved in adherence and invasion). However there were very few proteins with an elevated expression, but these included adhesion factors (PEB1 and PEB3), the stress response protein (DnaK), the elongation factor (Tu) and oxidoreductase, adenylate kinase, enzymes involved in energy metabolism, succinyl CoA and thiol peroxidase that indicates the bacterial cells are undergoing stress when exposed to the peppermint essential oil (Kovács et al. 2019).

Peppermint essential oil has also been reported to have antifungal property and is able to affect the expression of protein. The essential oil was tested against *Candida* sp., an opportunistic fungal pathogen in human in relative to an antifungal agent, Amphotericin B (Benzaid et al. 2019). Benzaid and colleague also tested the effect of the peppermint essential oil on the secreted aspartyl proteinases enzymes. The enzymes secreted aspartyl proteinases includes 10 types of enzymes which are involved in the degradation of the proteins of the host and also to invade tissues and organs of the human host. *C. albicans* treated with peppermint essential oil resulted to the decrease in the synthesis of secreted aspartyl proteinase enzymes. Apart from that, the effectiveness of the essential oil to inhibit the formation of biofilm also was tested. From the study, it was found that the peppermint essential oil was able to inhibit the formation of biofilm of *C. albicans* by producing low density biofilm similar to the Amphotericin B treated biofilms compared to the non-treated biofilms. The decrease in the biofilm formation is due to the down-regulation of hyphal cell wall protein which is responsible for the formation of biofilm and also pathogenesis (Benzaid et al. 2019).

Other than affecting genomic expression, oregano essential oil and its main compound carvacrol, are capable of affecting the proteomic expression. Carvacrol was tested for antibacterial activity against *E. coli* K12, where the minimum inhibitory concentration obtained was 256 mg/L (Božik et al. 2018). The mode of action of carvacrol was through disruption of the plasma membrane of the bacterial cells, thus increasing membrane permeability resulting in the leakage of protons and potassium, leading to the loss of membrane potential (Xu et al. 2008). In the study conducted by Božik et al. (2018), matrix-assisted laser desorption/ionization-time of flight- mass spectrometry (MALDI-TOF-MS) was used in the proteomic analysis of the stress response induced by exposure of *E. coli* K12 cells for 0, 90 and 120 min. After treatment with carvacrol, protein YthA, a stress response protein was expressed at greater abundance compared to non-treated samples and the histone-like DNA-binding protein HU-alpha was also highly induced by carvacrol. The function of this protein is to stabilize the DNA by wrapping around it to prevent denaturation. The 30S ribosomal proteins S15 and S19 were moderately expressed in the treated sample. Both these proteins enable RNA binding and are part of the small ribosomal subunit in the cytosol. The 50S ribosomal protein L30 was also induced by carvacrol. The function of this protein is to aggregate, arrange and promote the binding of RNAs and proteins to form the large ribosomal subunit (Božik et al. 2018).

Rosemary essential oil has been shown to have antiviral property. β-caryophyllene, a compound found in the rosemary essential oil can be used as an anti-viral for the treatment of herpes simplex virus type 1. This virus has been reported to have become resistant to some of the anti-herpes virus drugs (Astani et al. 2011). The compound acts by directly inactivating and interfering with the virion envelope structure or by masking the viral structure required for adsorption or entry into the host cells. This is achieved by inhibiting the glycosylation of viral proteins. The virion envelope structure is made up of proteins which enable the virus itself to bind to the host cells. However, the mechanism that interferes with the protein structure of the virion envelope is still not defined.

Apart from its antibacterial activity, thyme essential oil have also been shown to exhibit antiviral properties on acyclovir-resistant herpes simplex virus-type 1 and on acyclovir-sensitive herpes simplex virus-type 1 (Schnitzler et al. 2007). Acyclovir-sensitive and resistant herpes simplex virus pre-treated before infection with thyme essential oil showed a significant reduction in infectivity. This indicates that the thyme essential oil affected the virus before adsorption; however the essential oil is less effective if the virus is replicating within the cells and also when the virus is spreading from cell-to-cell. The thyme essential oil acts on the virion envelope structure that contains proteins responsible for the virus to enter into the host cells for multiplication. Preliminary electron microscope studies have also shown that there was disruption of the viral envelope of the herpes simplex virus after treatment with thyme essential oil, therefore resulting in its inability to infect the host cells. However, more studies are required to understand the mechanism that results to the down-regulation of the proteins on the viral envelope of the virus by thyme essential oil.

Other than exhibiting anti-fungal properties, *Eucalyptus* essential oil, is also able to inhibit the growth of bacteria. A study was conducted to test antibacterial activity on Gram positive bacteria, Gram negative bacteria and on multi drug resistant *E. faecalis* and antibiofilm activity of the essential oil on multi drug resistant *E. faecalis* (Correa et al. 2019). From the study, it was found that the essential oil exhibited *in vitro* activity against Gram positive bacteria (*S. aureus* ATCC 4163, *S. epidermidis* ATCC 35984, *E. faecalis* ATCC 29212, *S. gallolyticus* ATCC 9809, *S. agalactiae* ATCC 13813, *Listeria monocytogenes* ATCC 7644, *Bacillus pumilus* IA/ICBS and *Bacillus cereus* ATCC 14579). The *Eucalyptus* essential oil was able to inhibit the biofilm formation by multi drug resistant *E. faecalis* strains (Correa et al. 2019). Treatment of the bacterial cells before formation of the biofilm enables the essential oil to interact with the surface proteins Esp, which are found on the bacterial surface, thus affecting the initial phase in biofilm formation which involves the adhesion of bacterial cells to the surface and also interferes with the quorum sensing systems. The biofilm formation by *E. faecalis* clinical strains showed a decrease when the cells were pre-treated with the essential oil prior to the formation of the biofilm. Table 4.3 summarizes the effects of various essential oils on the expressions of both genome and proteome of various pathogens.

Table 4.3 Summary of effects of various essential oils on the genome and proteome expressions of target pathogens

Essential oil	Genome expression	Proteome expression
Cinnamon	*Staphylococcus epidermidis* when treated with cinnamon essential oil at 2% prevented the formation of biofilm by inhibiting the expression of gene *icaA* (Nuryastuti et al. 2009).	Carbapenemase producing *K. pneumoniae* expressed 10 unique proteins such as autonomous glycyl radical cofactor, catalase peroxidase, bifunctional protein GlmU, carbon storage regulator homolog, cobalamin biosynthesis protein CobD, DNA ligase, ferrochelatase, hydroxyacylglutathione hydrolase, integration host factor subunit beta, probable malate: quinone oxidoreductase and tRNA-2thiocytidine biosynthesis protein TtcA when treated with cinnamon bark essential oil compared to the non-treated *K. pneumoniae* cells (Yang et al. 2019).
Peppermint	*Campylobacter jejuni* treated with peppermint essential oil resulted to the expression of general stress genes such as *dnaK*, *groEL* and *groES* which are responsible for the synthesis of chaperones (Kovács et al. 2019).	*C. jejuni* treated with peppermint essential oil also showed a decrease in the expression of proteins involved in the synthesis of virulence associated factors. However, few proteins showed an increase in expression, which are adhesion factors, the stress response protein, the elongation factor and oxidoreductase, adenylate kinase, enzymes involved in energy metabolism Kovács et al. 2019).
	Peppermint essential oil also was able to decrease the expression of genes *SAP1*, *SAP2*, *SAP3*, *SAP9*, *SAP10* and *HWP-1* which are responsible for the virulence of *Candida albicans* (Benzaid et al. 2019).	
Oregano	Oregano essential oil and its main compound carvacrol were tested against enterohaemorrhagic *E. coli* O157:H7 virulence and resulted to the down-regulation of *luxS* gene followed by the genes *ler*, *stx2B* and *fliC* without affecting bacterial growth (Mith et al. 2015).	Carvacrol, a major compound found in oregano, when treated against *E. coli* K12, resulted to over expression of protein YthA, a stress response protein and the histone-like RNA-DNA-binding protein HU-alpha (Božik et al. 2018).
Rosemary	Rosemary essential oil was able to inhibit replication of the F'lac metabolic plasmid of multi drug resistant strain *E. coli* by preventing the vertical transfer of the antibiotic resistance gene carried by the plasmid (Sienkiewicz et al. 2013).	β-caryophyllene, a compound found in rosemary essential oil inactivates and interferes with the virion envelope structure of herpes simplex virus 1 or masks the viral structure required for adsorption or entry into the host cells (Astani et al. 2011).

(continued)

Table 4.3 (continued)

Essential oil	Genome expression	Proteome expression
Thyme	The quantitative real time polymerase chain reaction analysis showed that thyme essential oil exhibited decrease in the messenger ribonucleic acid (mRNA) for the gene *flgA* of *Pseudomonas fluorescens* KM121 resulting to the loss of motility (Myszka et al. 2016) .	Thyme essential oil and the major compounds thymol and carvacrol were tested against *Pseudomonas fluorescens* KM121. The essential oil and compounds resulted to reduction in N-acyl-homoserine lactone which is a signaling molecule in the quorum sensing (Myszka et al. 2016).
Eucalyptus	The *Eucalyptus* essential oil inhibited the synthesis of fungal toxic aflatoxin B_1 in *Aspergillus* sp. (Císarová et al. 2016).	*Eucalyptus* essential oil when treated with multi drug resistant *E. faecalis* strains enables the essential oil to interact with the proteins which are found on the bacterial surface, thus affecting the initial phase in biofilm formation (Correa et al. 2019).

4.7 Conclusion and Future Prospects

There is an evident and worrying increase in antimicrobial resistance cases worldwide resulting in the search for alternative approaches for the treatment of infection. Essential oils, a mixture of secondary metabolites that are produced by plants as a defense mechanism against pathogens, have been used as a treatment for infection in traditional medicines even before the discovery of antibiotics. Hence, essential oil is being explored as a potential alternative intervention. At present, different types of essential oils are being tested for antimicrobial activity from a variety of plants species. The compounds responsible for antimicrobial activities are being identified and tested against various pathogens individually and also tested for their combinatory effect with antimicrobials which might result in reversion back to their original sensitivity level. Unfortunately, there have been limited studies done to understand the precise mechanisms by which essential oils act as antimicrobial agents thus far. It is hoped that proteomic and genomic analyses will be able to provide the missing links in mechanistic determination, thus, providing a fuller picture of the pathways involved.

Essential oils are currently being widely used not only in aromatherapy, but also in hospital environments to manage stress and to reduce patients' anxiety (Allard and Katseres 2018). The use of essential oil in aromatherapy has been approved by the Food and Drug Administration (Nuñez and D'Aquino 2012). However, the antimicrobial activity of essential oil has not been subject to extensive animal testing and human clinical trials. Currently, there are no essential oils that have been tested for their antimicrobial activity in human subjects or in animal models and so studies on their efficacy against pathogenic microorganisms has all been done *in vitro* (Koley et al. 2019). Based on data from the website clinicaltrials.gov, essential oils are widely undergoing clinical trials for the efficacy of aromatherapy in overcoming sleep disorders, in addition to incorporation within perineal towels for women (an anti-bacterial feminine hygiene wipe) as well as, the effects on the cardiovascular system of using *Eucalyptus* essential oil. However, studies relating to oral health such as treatment of gingivitis and dental plaque are also being studied (Quintas et al. 2015).

As various essential oils are identified to have antimicrobial activity, they will proceed to future testing in appropriate animal models for toxicity and side effects following consumption. Essential oils and compounds that have been identified as non-toxic and safe may ultimately proceed to the human trials to test for efficacy and safety towards humans subject to proper regulation. It is likely to be some time before essential oils finds their way into normal clinical practice as a treatment for infection.

Essential oils have been found to be able to interact synergistically or additively with the currently used antibiotics where the development of resistance by pathogens has been reported. By furthering studies in interactions between essential oils and antibiotics, currently redundant antibiotics can be revived for clinical use. Furthermore, the knowledge acquired about the mechanisms of essential oils' action on microorganisms through proteomic and genomic analyses and the effect of the essential oils and the compounds on the humans through clinical trials can be utilized to design and develop new antimicrobial agents. Through these methods, it is hoped that we will be better equipped to tackle antimicrobial resistance.

Acknowledgement We would like to acknowledge Higher College of Technologies (HCT) Interdisciplinary Grant 1319 for supporting this work.

References

Abdulhasan GA (2017) Synergism effect of rosemary essential oil and some antibiotic against *Escherichia coli* isolated from clinical samples. IOSR J Pharm Biol Sci 12(02):39–42. https://doi.org/10.9790/3008-1202033942

Aljaafari M, Alhosani M, Abushelaibi A, Lai KS, Lim SHE (2019) Essential oils: partnering with antibiotics. In: El-Shemy H (ed) Essential oils-oils of nature. InTechOpen, p 13. https://doi.org/10.5772/57353

Allard ME, Katseres J (2018) Using essential oils to enhance nursing practice and for self-care. Nurse Pract 43(5):39–46. https://doi.org/10.1097/01.NPR.0000531915.69268.8f

Álvarez-Cisneros YM, Ponce-Alquicira E (2018) Antibiotic resistance in lactic acid bacteria. In: Kumar Y (ed) Antimicrobial resistance-a global threat. InTechOpen. https://doi.org/10.5772/intechopen.80624

Aminov RI (2010) A brief history of the antibiotic era: lessons learned and challenges for the future. Front Microbiol 1(DEC):1–7. https://doi.org/10.3389/fmicb.2010.00134

Andrei S, Valeanu L, Chirvasuta R, Stefan MG (2018) New FDA approved antibacterial drugs: 2015-2017. Discoveries 6(1):1–10. https://doi.org/10.15190/d.2018.1

Ashakirin SN, Tripathy M, Patil UK, Majed ABA (2017) Chemistry and bioactivity of cinnamaldehyde: a natural molecule of medicinal importance. Int J Pharm Sci Res 8(6):2333–2340. https://doi.org/10.13040/IJPSR.0975-8232.8(6).2333-40

Aslam B, Wang W, Arshad MI, Khurshid M, Muzammil S, Rasool MH, Nisar MA, Alvi RF, Aslam MA, Qamar MU, Salamat MKQ, Baloch Z (2018) Antibiotic resistance: a rundown of a global crisis. Infect Drug Resist 11:1645–1658. https://doi.org/10.2147/IDR.S173867

Astani A, Reichling J, Schnitzler P (2011) Screening for antiviral activities of isolated compounds from essential oils. Evid Based Complement Alter Med. https://doi.org/10.1093/ecam/nep187

Bakkali F, Averbeck S, Averbeck D, Idaomar M (2008) Biological effects of essential oils – a review. Food Chem Toxicol 46(2):446–475. https://doi.org/10.1016/j.fct.2007.09.106

Benzaid C, Belmadani A, Djeribi R, Rouabhia M (2019) The effects of *mentha* × *piperita* essential oil on *C. albicans* growth, transition, biofilm formation, and the expression of secreted aspartyl proteinases genes. Antibiotics 8(10):1–15. https://doi.org/10.3390/antibiotics8010010

Berdichevsky, T., Friedberg, D., Nadler, C., Rokney A., Oppenheim, A. and Rosenshine, I. (2005) '*Ler* is a negative autoregulator of the LEE1 operon in enteropathogenic *Escherichia coli.*', J Bacteriol Am Soc Microbiol, 187(1), pp. 349–357. doi: https://doi.org/10.1128/JB.187.1.349-357.2005

Bokov DO, Morokhina SL, Popov DM (2015) Phytochemical study of essential oil from Turkish oregano (*Origanum Onites L.*) by gas chromatography/mass spectrometry. Pharm Chem J 49(4):259–267. https://doi.org/10.1007/s11094-015-1267-z

Božik M, Cejnar P, Šašková M, Nový P, Maršík P, Klouček P (2018) Stress response of *Escherichia coli* to essential oil components-insights on low-molecular-weight proteins from MALDI-TOF. Nature 8(13042). https://doi.org/10.1038/s41598-018-31255-2

Breidenstein EBM, de la Fuente-Núñez C, Hancock REW (2011) *Pseudomonas aeruginosa*: all roads lead to resistance. Trends Microbiol 19(8):419–426. https://doi.org/10.1016/j.tim.2011.04.005

Bush K, Jacoby GA (2010) Updated functional classification of-lactamases. Antimicrob Agents Chemother 54(3):969–976. https://doi.org/10.1128/AAC.01009-09

Centers for Disease Control and Prevention (2013) Antibiotic/Antimicrobial Resistance | CDC. Available at https://www.cdc.gov/drugresistance/. Accessed 7 Apr 2019

Centers for Disease Control and Prevention (2017) CDC Global Health – infographics – antibiotic resistance. The Global Threat. Available at https://www.cdc.gov/globalhealth/infographics/antibiotic-resistance/antibiotic_resistance_global_threat.htm. Accessed: 29 Mar 2019

Chakraborty AK (2017) Mechanisms of AMR: Bacteria won the battle against antibiotics. Insights Biomed 2(4):18. https://doi.org/10.21767/2572-5610.100034

Chamosa LS, Álvarez VE, Nardelli M, Quiroga MP, Cassini MH, Centrón D (2017) Lateral antimicrobial resistance genetic transfer is active in the open environment. Nature Sci Rep 7(513). https://doi.org/10.1038/s41598-017-00600-2

Císarová M, Tančinová D, Medo J, Kačániová M (2016) The in vitro effect of selected essential oils on the growth and mycotoxin production of *Aspergillus* species. J Environ Sci Health Part B Pest Food Contaminants Agric Wastes 51(10):668–674. https://doi.org/10.1080/03601234.2016.1191887

Clokie MR, Millard AD, Letarov AV, Heaphy S (2011) Phages in nature. Bacteriophage. Taylor & Francis 1(1):31–45. https://doi.org/10.4161/bact.1.1.14942

Correa MS, Schwambach J, Mann MB, Frazzon J, Frazzon APG (2019) Antimicrobial and antibiofilm activity of the essential oil from dried leaves of *Eucalyptus staigeriana*. Pharmacology 86:1–7. https://doi.org/10.1590/1808-1657000202018

Costerton W, Veeh R, Shirtliff M, Pasmore M, Post C, Ehrlich G (2003) The application of biofilm science to the study and control of chronic bacterial infections. J Clin Investig 112(10):1466–1477. https://doi.org/10.1172/JCI20365

Davies J, Davies D (2010) Origins and evolution of antibiotic resistance. Microbiol Mol Biol Rev 74(3):417–433. https://doi.org/10.1128/MMBR.00016-10

Deng H, McShan D, Zhang Y, Sinha SS, Arslan Z, Ray PC, Yu H (2016) Mechanistic study of the synergistic antibacterial activity of combined silver nanoparticles and common antibiotics graphical abstract HHS Public Access Author manuscript. Environ Sci Technol 50(16):8840–8848. https://doi.org/10.1021/acs.est.6b00998

Dhifi W, Bellili S, Jazi S, Bahloul N, Mnif W (2016) Essential oils' chemical characterization and investigation of some biological activities: a critical review. Medicines 3(25):1–16. https://doi.org/10.3390/medicines3040025
Doménech-Sánchez A, Martínez-Martínez L, Hernández-Allés S, Conejo MDC, Pascual Á, Tomás JM, Albertí S, Benedí VJ (2003) Role of *Klebsiella pneumoniae* OmpK35 porin in antimicrobial resistance. Antimicrob Agents Chemother 47(10):3332–3335. https://doi.org/10.1128/AAC.47.10.3332-3335.2003
Donlan RM (2002) Biofilms: microbial life on surfaces. Emerg Infect Dis. Available at http://www.microbelibrary.org/. Accessed 24 Apr 2019
Elyemni M, Louaste B, Nechad I, Elkamli T, Bouia A, Taleb M, Chaouch M, Eloutassi N (2019) Extraction of essential oils of *Rosmarinus officinalis L.* by two different methods: hydrodistillation and microwave assisted hydrodistillation. Sci World J 2019:1–6. https://doi.org/10.1155/2019/3659432
Etebu E, Arikekpar I (2016) Antibiotics: classification and mechanisms of action with emphasis on molecular perspectives. Int J Appl Microbiol Biotechnol Res 4:90–101
Fischbach MA (2011) Combination therapies for combating antimicrobial resistance. Curr Opin Microbiol 14(5):519–523. https://doi.org/10.1016/j.mib.2011.08.003
Fürstenberg-Hägg J, Zagrobelny M, Bak S (2013) Plant defense against insect herbivores. Int J Mol Sci 14(5):10242–10297. https://doi.org/10.3390/ijms140510242
Hancock RE, Chapple DS (1999) 'Peptide antibiotics.', Antimicrobial agents and chemotherapy. Am Soc Microbiol J 43(6):1317–1323. https://doi.org/10.1128/AAC.43.6.1317
Hasdemir UO, Chevalier J, Nordmann P, Pagès JM (2004) Detection and prevalence of active drug efflux mechanism in various multidrug-resistant *Klebsiella pneumoniae* strains from Turkey. J Clin Microbiol 42(6):2701–2706. https://doi.org/10.1128/JCM.42.6.2701-2706.2004
Hollenbeck BL, Rice LB (2012) Intrinsic and acquired resistance mechanisms in enterococcus. Virulence 3(5):421–569. https://doi.org/10.4161/viru.21282
Hong DJ, Bae IK, Jang IH, Jeong SH, Kang HK, Lee K (2015) Epidemiology and characteristics of metallo-β-lactamase-producing *Pseudomonas aeruginosa*. Infect Chemother. Korean Soc Infect Dis 47(2):81–97. https://doi.org/10.3947/ic.2015.47.2.81
Hughes G, Webber MA (2017) Novel approaches to the treatment of bacterial biofilm infections. Br J Pharmacol 174(14):2237–2246. https://doi.org/10.1111/bph.13706
Isman MB, Wilson JA, Bradbury R (2008) Insecticidal activities of commercial rosemary oils (Rosmarinus officinalis.) against larvae of *Pseudaletia unipuncta*. and Trichoplusia ni. in relation to their chemical compositions. Pharm Biol 46(1–2):82–87. https://doi.org/10.1080/13880200701734661
Jahanshiri Z, Shams-Ghahfarokhi M, Allameh A, Razzaghi-Abyanneh M (2015) Inhibitory effect of eugenol on aflatoxin B1 production in *Aspergillus parasiticus* by downregulating the expression of major genes in the toxin biosynthetic pathway. World J Microbiol Biotechnol. Springer Netherlands 31(7):1071–1078. https://doi.org/10.1007/s11274-015-1857-7
Karaman, D. Ş., Manner, S., Fallarero, A. and Rosenholm, J.M.(2017) 'Current approaches for exploration of nanoparticles as antibacterial agents', in Kumavath, RN. (ed.) Antibacterial agents. InTechOpen, pp. 61–86. doi: https://doi.org/10.5772/68138
Kato A, Chen HD, Latifi T, Groisman EA (2012) Reciprocal control between a bacterium's regulatory system and the modification status of its lipopolysaccharide. Mol Cell 47(6):897–908. https://doi.org/10.1016/j.molcel.2012.07.017
Khajuria A, Praharaj AK, Kumar M, Grover N (2013) Emergence of NDM – 1 in the clinical isolates of *Pseudomonas aeruginosa* in India. J Clin Diagnostic Res: JCDR. JCDR Research & Publications Private Limited 7(7):1328–1331. https://doi.org/10.7860/JCDR/2013/5509.3137
Koley H, Howlader DR, Bhaumik U (2019) Assessment of antimicrobial activity of different phytochemicals against enteric diseases in different animal models. New Look Phytomed Elsevier Inc. https://doi.org/10.1016/b978-0-12-814619-4.00022-7
Kostyanev T, Can F (2017) The global crisis of antimicrobial resistance. Antimicrobial Stewardship. Academic Press 1:3–12. https://doi.org/10.1016/B978-0-12-810477-4.00001-5

Kovács JK, Felső P, Horváth G, Schmidt J, Dorn Á, Ábráham H, Cox A, Márk L, Emődy L, Kovács T, Schneider G (2019) Stress response and virulence potential modulating effect of peppermint essential oil in *Campylobacter jejuni*. BioMed Res Int. Hindawi 2019:1–11. https://doi.org/10.1155/2019/2971741

Kumar M, Curtis A, Hoskins C (2018) Application of nanoparticle technologies in the combat against anti-microbial resistance. Pharmaceutics 10(1):1–17. https://doi.org/10.3390/pharmaceutics10010011

Lahlou M (2004) Methods to study the phytochemistry and bioactivity of essential oils. Phytother Res 18(6):435–448. https://doi.org/10.1002/ptr.1465

Lambert PA (2002) Mechanisms of antibiotic resistance in *Pseudomonas aeruginosa*. J R Soc Med. Royal Society of Medicine Press 95(41):22–26. Available at http://www.ncbi.nlm.nih.gov/pubmed/12216271. Accessed: 23 Apr 2019

Langeveld WT, Veldhuizen EJA, Burt SA (2014) Synergy between essential oil components and antibiotics: a review. Crit Rev Microbiol 40(1):76–94. https://doi.org/10.3109/1040841X.2013.763219

Leclercq R (2002) Mechanisms of resistance to macrolides and lincosamides: nature of the resistance elements and their clinical implications. Clin Infect Dis 34(4):482–492. https://doi.org/10.1086/324626

Loolaie M, Moasefi N, Rasouli H, Adibi H (2017) Peppermint and its functionality: a review. Arch Clin Microbiol 08(04):1–16. https://doi.org/10.4172/1989-8436.100053

Lund PA (2001) Microbial molecular chaperones. Adv Microbial Physiol 44:93–140. Available at http://www.ncbi.nlm.nih.gov/pubmed/11407116. Accessed: 30 Apr 2019

Ly-Chatain MH (2014) The factors affecting effectiveness of treatment in phages therapy. Front Microbiol 5(51). https://doi.org/10.3389/fmicb.2014.00051

Mahboubi M, Kazempour N (2014) Chemical composition and antimicrobial activity of peppermint (*Mentha piperita L.*) essential oil. Songklanakarin J Sci Technol 36(1):83–87

Mahizan NA, Yang SK, Moo CL, Song AAL, Chong CM, Chong CW, Abushelaibi A, Lim SHE, Lai KS (2019) Terpene derivatives as a potential agent against antimicrobial resistance (AMR) pathogens. Molecules 24(14):1–21. https://doi.org/10.3390/molecules24142631

Mellies JL, Benison G, McNitt W, Mavor D, Boniface C, Larabee FJ (2011) *Ler* of pathogenic *Escherichia coli* forms toroidal protein-DNA complexes. Microbiology. Microbiology Society 157(4):1123–1133. https://doi.org/10.1099/mic.0.046094-0

Mingeot-Leclercq MP, Glupczynski Y, Tulkens PM (1999) Aminoglycosides: activity and resistance. Antimicrob Agents Chemother 43(4):727–737. https://doi.org/10.1128/AAC.43.4.727

Mith H, Clinquart A, Zhiri A, Daube G, Delcenserie V (2015) The impact of oregano (*Origanum heracleoticum*) essential oil and carvacrol on virulence gene transcription by *Escherichia coli* O157:H7. FEMS Microbiol Lett. Narnia 362(1):1–7. https://doi.org/10.1093/femsle/fnu021

Moghaddam M, Mehdizadeh L (2017) Chemistry of essential oils and factors influencing their constituents. Soft Chem Food Ferment. Elsevier Inc:379–419. https://doi.org/10.1016/B978-0-12-811412-4/00013-8

Moo CL, Yang SK, Yusoff K, Ajat M, Thomas W, Abushelaibi A, Lim SHE, Lai KS (2019) Mechanisms of antimicrobial resistance (AMR) and alternative approaches to overcome AMR. Curr Drug Discov Technol 16. https://doi.org/10.2174/1570163816666190304122219

Moo CL, Yang SK, Osman MA, Yuswan MH, Loh JY, Lim WM, Lim SHE, Lai KS (2020) Antibacterial activity and mode of action of β-caryophyllene on *Bacillus cereus*. Polish J Microbiol 69(1):49–54. https://doi.org/10.33073/pjm-2020-007

Moon SE, Kim HY, Cha JD (2011) Synergistic effect between clove oil and its major compounds and antibiotics against oral bacteria. Arch Oral Biol. Elsevier Ltd 56(9):907–916. https://doi.org/10.1016/j.archoralbio.2011.02.005

Morsy, N. F. S. (2017) 'Chemical structure, quality indicces and bioactivity of essential oil constituents', El-Shemy, H. (ed.) Active ingredients from aromatic and medicinal plants. InTechOpen, pp. 175–206. doi: https://doi.org/10.5772/67161

Munita JM, Arias CA (2016) Mechanisms of antibiotic resistance. Microbiol Spectr 4(2). https://doi.org/10.1128/microbiolspec.VMBF-0016-2015

Myszka K, Schmidt MT, Majcher M, Juzwa W, Olkowicz M, Czaczyk K (2016) Inhibition of quorum sensing-related biofilm of *Pseudomonas fluorescens* KM121 by *Thymus vulgare* essential oil and its major bioactive compounds. Int Biodeterior Biodegrad 114:252–259. https://doi.org/10.1016/j.ibiod.2016.07.006

Namvar AE, Asghari B, Ezzatifar F, Azizi G, Lari AR (2013) Detection of the intercellular adhesion gene cluster (*ica*) in clinical *Staphylococcus aureus* isolates. GMS Hygiene Infect Control. German Medical Science 8(1). https://doi.org/10.3205/dgkh000203

Nazzaro F, Fratianni F, Martino LD, Coppola R, De Feo V (2013) Effect of essential oils on pathogenic bacteria. Pharmaceuticals (Basel, Switzerland). Multidisciplinary Digital Publishing Institute (MDPI) 6(12):1451–1474. https://doi.org/10.3390/ph6121451

Nishino K, Hsu FF, Turk J, Cromie MJ, Wösten MMSM, Groisman EA (2006) Identification of the lipopolysaccharide modifications controlled by the *Salmonella* PmrA/PmrB system mediating resistance to Fe(III) and Al(III). Mol Microbiol 61(3):645–654. https://doi.org/10.1111/j.1365-2958.2006.05273.x

Nuñez L, D'Aquino M (2012) Microbicide activity of clove essential oil (*Eugenia caryophyllata*). Braz J Microbiol 43(4):1255–1260. https://doi.org/10.1590/S1517-83822012000400003

Nuryastuti T, Van der Mei HC, Busscher HJ, Iravati S, Aman AT, Krom BP (2009) Effect of cinnamon oil on *icaA* expression and biofilm formation by *Staphylococcus epidermidis*. Appl Environ Microbiol 75(21):6850–6855. https://doi.org/10.1128/AEM.00875-09

Pang Z, Raudonis R, Glick BR, Lin TJ, Cheng Z (2019) Antibiotic resistance in *Pseudomonas aeruginosa*: mechanisms and alternative therapeutic strategies. Biotechnol Adv 37(1):177–192. https://doi.org/10.1016/j.biotechadv.2018.11.013

Paraje MG (2011) Antimicrobial resistance in biofilms. Available at: http://www.formatex.info/microbiology3/book/736-744.pdf. Accessed: 21 Apr 2019

Patel R (2005) Biofilms and antimicrobial resistance. Clin Orthop Relat Res 437:41–47. https://doi.org/10.1097/01.blo.0000175714.68624.74

Perry JA, Wright GD (2013) The antibiotic resistance "mobilome": searching for the link between environment and clinic. Front Microbiol. Frontiers 4(138). https://doi.org/10.3389/fmicb.2013.00138

Quintas V, Prada-López I, Donos N, Suárez-Quintanilla D, Tomás I (2015) Antiplaque effect of essential oils and 0.2% chlorhexidine on an in situ model of oral biofilm growth: a randomised clinical trial. PLoS One 10(2):1–18. https://doi.org/10.1371/journal.pone.0117177

Raeisi M, Tajik H, Yarahmadi A, Sanginabadi S (2015) Antimicrobial effect of cinnamon essential oil against *Escherichia coli* and *Staphylococcus aureus*. Health Scope 4(4). https://doi.org/10.17795/jhealthscope-21808

Ramirez MS, Tolmasky ME (2010) Aminoglycoside modifying enzymes. Drug resistance updates : reviews and commentaries in antimicrobial and anticancer chemotherapy. NIH Public Access 13(6):151–171. https://doi.org/10.1016/j.drup.2010.08.003

Schelz Z, Molnar J, Hohmann J (2006) Antimicrobial and antiplasmid activities of essential oils. Fitoterapia 77(4):279–285. https://doi.org/10.1016/j.fitote.2006.03.013

Schnitzler P, Koch C, Reichling J (2007) Susceptibility of drug-resistant clinical herpes simplex virus type 1 strains to essential oils of ginger, thyme, hyssop, and sandalwood. Antimicrob Agents Chemother 51(5):1859–1862. https://doi.org/10.1128/AAC.00426-06

Semeniuc CA, Pop CR, Rotar AM (2017) Antibacterial activity and interactions of plant essential oil combinations against Gram-positive and Gram-negative bacteria. J Food Drug Anal 25(2):403–408. https://doi.org/10.1016/j.jfda.2016.06.002

Sharifi-Rad J, Sureda A, Tenore GC, Daglia M, Sharifi-Rad M, Valussi M, Tundis R, Sharifi-Rad M, Loizzo MR, Ademiluyi AO, Sharifi-Rad R, Ayatollahi SA, Iriti M (2017) Biological activities of essential oils: from plant chemoecology to traditional healing systems. Molecules 22(70):1–55. https://doi.org/10.3390/molecules22010070

Shin S (2005) Anti-Salmonella activity of lemongrass oil alone and in combination with antibiotics. *Natural Product Sciences*, pp:160–164

Sienkiewicz M, Łysakowska M, Denys P, Kowalczyk E (2012) The antimicrobial activity of thyme essential oil against multidrug resistant clinical bacterial strains. Microb Drug Resist 18(2):137–148. https://doi.org/10.1089/mdr.2011.0080

Sienkiewicz M, Łysakowska M, Pastuszka M, Bienias W, Kowalczyk E (2013) The potential of use basil and rosemary essential oils as effective antibacterial agents. Molecules 18:9334–9351. https://doi.org/10.3390/molecules18089334

Souza EL, Stamford TLM, Lima EO, Trajano VN (2007) Effectiveness of *Origanum vulgare L.* essential oil to inhibit the growth of food spoiling yeasts. Food Control 18:409–413. https://doi.org/10.1016/j.foodcont.2005.11.008

Stintzi A (2003) Gene expression profile of *Campylobacter jejuni* in response to growth temperature variation. J Bacteriol. Am Soc Microbiol (ASM) 185(6):2009–2016. https://doi.org/10.1128/JB.185.6.2009-2016.2003

Stokes HW, Gillings MR (2011) Gene flow, mobile genetic elements and the recruitment of antibiotic resistance genes into Gram-negative pathogens. FEMS Microbiol Rev 35(5):790–819. https://doi.org/10.1111/j.1574-6976.2011.00273.x

Sun J, Deng Z, Yan A (2014) Bacterial multidrug efflux pumps: mechanisms, physiology and pharmacological exploitations. Biochem Biophys Res Commun 453(2):254–267. https://doi.org/10.1016/j.bbrc.2014.05.090

Swamy MK, Akhtar MS, Sinniah UR (2016) Antimicrobial properties of plant essential oils against human pathogens and their mode of action : an updated review. Evid Based Complement Alter Med. Hindawi Publishing Corporation. https://doi.org/10.1155/2016/3012462

Tiwari B, Valdramidis VP, Donnell CPO, Muthukumarappan K, Bourke P, Cullen PJ (2009) Application of natural antimicrobials for food preservation. J Agric Food Chem 57(14):5987–6000. https://doi.org/10.1021/jf900668n

Vaara M, Nurminen M (1999) Outer membrane permeability barrier in *Escherichia coli* mutants that are defective in the late acyltransferases of Lipid A biosynthesis. Antimicrob Agents Chemother. Available at: https://www.ncbi.nlm.nih.gov/pmc/articles/PMC89296/pdf/ac001459.pdf. Accessed: 29 Apr 2019

Varijakzhan D, Chong CM, Abushelaibi A, Lai KS, Lim SHE (2020) Middle eastern plant extracts: an alternative to modern medicine problems. Molecules 25:1–19. https://doi.org/10.3390/molecules25051126

Velkov T, Thompson PE, Nation RL, Li J (2010) Structure-activity relationships of polymyxin antibiotics. J Med Chem 53(5):1898–1916. https://doi.org/10.1021/jm900999h

Ventola CL (2015) The antibiotic resistance crisis Part 1: causes and threats. 40(4):277–283. Available at https://www.ncbi.nlm.nih.gov/pmc/articles/PMC4378521/

Vuong C, Kocianova S, Voyich JM, Yao Y, Fischer ER, Deleo FR, Otto M (2004) A crucial role for exopolysaccharide modification in bacterial biofilm formation, immune evasion, and virulence. Biol Chem. JBC Papers in Press 279(52):54881–54886. https://doi.org/10.1074/jbc.M411374200

Wang L, Rothemund D, Curd H, Reeves PR (2000) Sequence diversity of the *Escherichia coli* H7 *fliC* genes: implication for a DNA-based typing scheme for *E. coli* O157:H7. J Clin Microbiol 38(5):1786–1790. Available at https://www.ncbi.nlm.nih.gov/pmc/articles/PMC86588/pdf/jm001786.pdf. Accessed 1 May 2019

Wang G, Clark CG, Rodgers FG (2002) Detection in *Escherichia coli* of the genes encoding the major virulence factors, the genes defining the O157:H7 serotype, and components of the type 2 Shiga toxin family by multiplex PCR. J Clin Microbiol. Am Soc Microbiol (ASM) 40(10):3613–3619. https://doi.org/10.1128/JCM.40.10.3613-3619.2002

Waters EM, Neill DR, Kaman B, Sahota JS, Clokie MRJ, Winstanley C, Kadioglu A (2017) Phage therapy is highly effective against chronic lung infections with *Pseudomonas aeruginosa*. Thorax 72:666–667. https://doi.org/10.1136/thoraxjnl-2016-209265

Wehrli W, Staehelin M (1971) Actions of the rifamycins. Bacteriol Rev 35(3):290–309. Available at http://www.ncbi.nlm.nih.gov/pubmed/5001420%0A, http://www.pubmedcentral.nih.gov/articlerender.fcgi?artid=PMC378391

World Health Organization (2017) What is antimicrobial resistance? WHO. World Health Organization. Available at https://www.who.int/features/qa/75/en/. Accessed: 30 Apr 2019

Xu J, Zhou F, Ji BP, Pei RS, Xu N (2008) The antibacterial mechanism of carvacrol and thymol against *Escherichia coli*. Lett Appl Microbiol. John Wiley & Sons, Ltd 47(10.1111):174–179. https://doi.org/10.1111/j.1472-765X.2008.02407.x

Yang SK, Yusoff K, Mai CW, Lim WM, Yap WS, Lim SHE, Lai KS (2017) Additivity vs. synergism: investigation of the additive interaction of cinnamon bark oil and meropenem in combinatory therapy. Molecules 22(11):1–14. https://doi.org/10.3390/molecules22111733

Yang SK, Low LY, Yap PSX, Yusoff K, Mai CW, Lai KS, Lim SHE (2018a) Plant-derived antimicrobials: insights into mitigation of antimicrobial resistance. Rec Nat Prod 12(4):295–316. https://doi.org/10.25135/rnp.41.17.09.058

Yang SK, Polly SXY, Krishnan T, Yusoff K, Chan KG, Yap WS, Lai KS, Lim SHE (2018b) Mode of action: synergistic interaction of peppermint (*Mentha x piperita L. Carl*) essential oil and meropenem against plasmid-mediated resistant *E. coli*. Rec Nat Prod 12(6):582–594. https://doi.org/10.25135/rnp.59.17.12.078

Yang SK, Yusoff K, Ajat M, Thomas W, Abushelaibi A, Akseer R, Lim SHE, Lai KS (2019) Disruption of KPC-producing *Klebsiella pneumoniae* membrane via induction of oxidative stress by cinnamon bark (*Cinnamomum verum* J. Presl) essential oil. PLoS One 14(4):1–20. https://doi.org/10.1371/journal.pone.0214326

Yang SK, Yusoff K, Thomas W, Akseer R, Alhosani MS, Abushelaibi A, Lim SHE, Lai KS (2020) Lavender essential oil induces oxidative stress which modifies the bacterial membrane permeability of carbapenemase producing *Klebsiella pneumoniae*. Sci Rep 10(1):1–14. https://doi.org/10.1038/s41598-019-55601-0

Yanishlieva NV, Marinova E, Pokorný J (2006) Natural antioxidants from herbs and spices. Eur J Lipid Sci Technol. https://doi.org/10.1002/ejlt.200600127

Yap PSX, Yiap BC, Ping HC, Lim SHE (2014) Essential oils, a new horizon in combating bacterial antibiotic resistance. Open Microbiol J 8(1):6–14. https://doi.org/10.2174/1874285801408010006

Yap, P. S. X., Yang, S.K., Lai, K.S. and Lim, S.H.E. (2017) Essential oils: the ultimate solution to antimicrobial resistance in *Escherichia coli*?', In Samie, A. (ed.) *Escherichia coli* – recent advances on physiology, pathogenesis and biotechnological applications. InTechOpen, pp. 299–313. Doi: https://doi.org/10.5772/57353

Yu J, Chang PK, Ehrlich KC, Cary JW, Bhatnagar D, Cleveland TE, Payne GA, Linz JE, Woloshuk CP, Bennett JW (2004) Clustered pathway genes in aflatoxin biosynthesis. Appl Environ Microbiol 70(3):1253–1262. https://doi.org/10.1128/AEM.70.3.1253-1262.2004

Yu Z, Qin W, Lin J, Fang S, Qiu J (2014) Antibacterial mechanisms of polymyxin and bacterial resistance. BioMed Res Int. Hindawi 2015:1–11. https://doi.org/10.1155/2015/679109

Yu Z, Tang J, Khare T, Kumar V (2019) The alarming antimicrobial resistance in ESKAPEE pathogens: Can essential oils come to the rescue? Fitoterapia. Elsevier 140(October 2019):104433. https://doi.org/10.1016/j.scitotenv.2019.133588

Zheljazkov VD, Cantrell CL, Evans WB, Ebelhar MW, Coker C (2008) Yield and composition of *Ocimum basilicum L.* and *Ocimum sanctum L.* grown at four locations. HortScience 43(3):737–741. https://doi.org/10.21273/HORTSCI.43.3.737

Zuzarte M, Salgueiro L (2015) Essential oils chemistry. In: de Sousa DP (ed) Bioactive essential oils and cancer. Springer, pp 19–28. https://doi.org/10.1007/978-3-319-19144-7

Chapter 5
Polymeric Antimicrobials with Quaternary Ammonium Moieties

Anca Giorgiana Grigoras

Abstract Pathogenic microorganisms develop over time a resistance especially to the antimicrobial substances used abusively. Medical education and preventive medicine practiced by doctors is complemented by the research activity of chemists, pharmacists and physicists regarding the discovery of new antimicrobial substances. In order to minimize environmental toxicity and short duration of action characteristic of antimicrobial agents with low molecular weights, specialists focused over last few years on conceiving and studying of polymeric materials with antimicrobial properties.

This updated review refers to certain quaternary ammonium compounds synthesized based on natural or synthetic polymers, especially to those biocompatible. Polymers like cellulose, chitosan, dextran, pullulan, starch, cashew gum, poly(lactide), poly(amidoamine), poly(urethane), poly(siloxane), poly(methacrylate) or poly(ethylene) were modified with cationic quaternary ammonium moieties by different methods. Due to physicochemical properties of polymers or microenvironment factors, these quaternary ammonium containing polymers specifically interfere with the metabolism of a wide range of bacteria and fungi. Often, in order to increase the efficiency of these antimicrobial polymeric materials, the synergistic action of the quaternary ammonium groups with other groups or chemical compounds is considered.

Keywords Antimicrobials · Polymers · Quaternary ammonium · Bacteria · Fungi

---

A. G. Grigoras (✉)
"Petru Poni" Institute of Macromolecular Chemistry, Iasi, Romania
e-mail: angrig@icmpp.ro

H. Panwar et al. (eds.), *Sustainable Agriculture Reviews 49*, Sustainable Agriculture Reviews 49, https://doi.org/10.1007/978-3-030-58259-3_5

5.1 Introduction

Control and prevention of microbial contamination represent major challenges for researchers, doctors, and population. Over time, pathogenic microorganisms have developed some features that have helped them to survive even to the most aggressive antimicrobials of time. Usually, after a long period of efficient usage of new antimicrobials, resistance to those substances develops. Antimicrobial agents with low molecular weight generally have a series of disadvantages like environmental toxicity and short term antimicrobial capacity (Kenawy et al. 2007). In order to minimize these problems, specialists have focused in last years on design and study of polymeric materials with enhanced antimicrobial efficacy, reduced toxicity toward organisms or environment, and prolonged action time, compared with their small molecular weight counterparts (Jain et al. 2014). In this respect, various methods of introducing atoms or functional groups on polymer chain in order to obtain materials able to destroy structural integrity of the bacteria, fungi or algae have been tested. Antimicrobial macromolecular substances have been classified as: quaternary ammonium polymers, guanidine polymers, polymers designed to mimic natural peptides, halogenated macromolecules, polymers containing phosphonic or sulfonic derivatives and silver ion bearing polymers (Munoz-Bonilla and Fernandes-Garcia 2012; Siedenbiedel and Tiller 2012).

Attachment of substances with potential antimicrobial activity to the surface of microorganisms is possible due to the specific interactions between extracellular polymeric components like exopolysaccharides, proteins, lipids or humic substances, and reactive functional groups of antimicrobials. After cell surface adhesion, antimicrobial agents can act by various mechanisms: breakdown of cell membrane structure, inhibition of protein synthesis or metabolic pathways, interference with synthesis of nucleic acids, etc. Due to the surface negative charge of microbial entities, the most probable and efficient interactions will be with cationic contact surfaces. This category also includes quaternary ammonium compounds. Cationic quaternary ammonium antimicrobial agents are part of some formulations used as disinfectants, which act through electrostatic attraction, infiltration and diffusion (Rajkowska et al. 2016).

Importance of this type of materials is evidenced by a large number of reviews that generally discussed various aspects of mechanism of action and medical applications of antimicrobial polymers, as well as of quaternary ammonium based materials (Kenawy et al. 2007; Timofeeva and Kleshcheva 2011; Kenawy et al. 2014; Xue et al. 2015; Santos et al. 2016; Francolini et al. 2017; Jiao et al. 2017).

Present chapter covers most recent studies, predominantly over past 5 years, focused on natural or synthetic quaternary ammonium polymeric compounds and factors that influence their antimicrobial activity. It is generally assumed that molecular weight variation of polymers, hydrophilic-hydrophobic balance, conformation of polymer chain in solution, strength and type of intramolecular and intermolecular interactions will influence antimicrobial efficacy of polymers containing quaternary ammonium moieties. Also, this chapter highlighted the diversity of polymers, especially those biocompatible that can be modified with quaternary ammonium groups to create new antimicrobial materials.

5.2 Polymeric Antimicrobials with Quaternary Ammonium Moieties

Specialized literature reports that various modifications of polymers in solution or in bulk, enhance their antimicrobial activity. From this point of view, antimicrobial applications of polymers with quaternary ammonium moieties are represented by coatings, modified surfaces and solutions. If, in some cases, coating implies application of electrospinning, dip-coating and polyelectrolyte complex formation onto polymeric support; in other ones, modified surfaces resulted from covalent linkage of quaternary ammonium salts directly onto polymeric support. Polymers with quaternary ammonium moieties and potential antimicrobial properties were synthesized from solution, purified by dialysis, concentrated and precipitated in non-solvent, filtered, dried for solvent removal, stored and then dispersed or dissolved in suitable solvent for antimicrobial tests.

In order to prevent biofouling phenomenon, researchers use different strategies to improve antibacterial properties of surfaces *via* creation of superhydrophobic surfaces; incorporation and controlled diffusion over time of biocide compounds from surfaces; and conjugation of antibiotic functional groups on surfaces. By such modifications, bacterial adhesion is suppressed, biocide leaching is initiated, and contact killing is activated (Lichter et al. 2009). Cationic quaternary ammonium groups could be immobilized or anchored onto polymeric chains *via* different approaches: chemical coupling reactions, surface initiated polymerization of monomers bearing antibacterial moieties and post-polymerization modifications to synthesize surface-tethered antimicrobial polymer brush (Gettings and White 1987; Lee et al. 2004; Lenoir et al. 2006; Wiarachai et al. 2012; Yao et al. 2010). In next sections, polymeric antimicrobials with quaternary ammonium moieties are classified and analyzed according to the nature of polymer matrix: natural or synthetic.

5.3 Antimicrobials Based on Natural Polymers

Natural polymers like cellulose, chitosan, dextran, starch, pullulan, gum, poly(lactic acid) are suitable for chemical modifications with quaternary ammonium moieties. The new polymers are characterized by improved biological, chemical and physical properties compared with their precursors *viz* better water solubility, moisture absorption, flocculation, nontoxicity, biocompatibility and antimicrobial activity.

5.3.1 Cellulose Type Antimicrobials

Cellulose is a polysaccharide with linear chain structure consisting of $\beta(1\rightarrow4)$ linked D-glucose units, and is a suitable macromolecule for chemical changes for applications in pharmaceutical industry in form of membrane, fibers or hydrogels. Meng et al. (2015) described a one-step modification method for direct covalent linking of quaternary ammonium salts onto membrane surface of regenerated cellulose, based on alkoxy silane polycondensation reaction and silane coupling agents like trimethoxysilylpropyl trimethyl ammonium chloride and trimethoxysilylpropyl octadecyldimethyl ammonium chloride. Reaction mechanism ensured chemical coupling of cationic antibacterial alkyl groups responsible for enhanced hydrophobicity of regenerated cellulose membrane and infiltration of ammonium groups through hydrophobic membranes of tested microorganisms. In same culture conditions, it was reported that *Staphylococcus aureus* ATCC 6538 more easily formed colonies on modified cellulose membrane compared with *Escherichia coli* DH5α. In addition, length of hydrophobic alkyl chains from regenerated cellulose membranes modified with trimethoxysilylpropyl trimethyl ammonium chloride or trimethoxysilylpropyl octadecyldimethyl ammonium chloride induced different behavior against the viability of bacteria. Thus, viability of *S. aureus* or *E. coli* was about 99% in presence of membrane modified with trimethoxysilylpropyl trimethyl ammonium chloride, while membrane modified with trimethoxysilylpropyl octadecyldimethyl ammonium chloride reduced the cell viabilities up to about 0.5%.

In order to avoid growth of pathogenic microorganisms on skin, researchers designed a hydrogel as a component of diapers, based on blending of native cellulose solution with quaternized cellulose solution (Peng et al. 2016). In this way, novel hydrogel formed by chemical cross-linking in aqueous solution of NaOH-urea mixture and in presence of epichlorohydrin, represented a potential antimicrobial material with improved mechanical properties, too. Varying molecular weight and substitution degree of quaternized cellulose (M_w = 94000 g/mol or 256000 g/mol; DS = 0.23–0.69), different hydrogels encoded as Gel9–2, Gel9–4, Gel9–6, Gel25–2, Gel25–4, and Gel25–6 were prepared and microbiologically tested. Quaternary ammonium groups introduced in hydrogel network by quaternization reaction of cellulose with 3-chloro-2-hydroxypropyl-trimethylammoniumchloride were responsible for inhibition of *Saccharomyces cerevisiae* cultures. The best antibacterial activity of Gel25–6 sample compared with other hydrogel samples suggested that a higher substitution degree of quaternized cellulose has intensified electrostatic type interactions between polycationic quaternary ammonium groups of cellulosic hydrogel and anionic components of microbial membranes leading to disruption and death of cells.

5.3.2 Chitosan Type Antimicrobials

As a natural material derived from chitin, chitosan is a non-toxic, biodegradable and linear macromolecule with cationic behaviour and comprises of β-(1 $\rightarrow$ 4) linked copolymer of 2-acetamido-2-deoxy-D-glucopyranose units and 2-amino-2-deoxy-D-glucopyranose, often used to design biocompatible materials. Even if it has antimicrobial properties, opportunity to enhance them was exploited by insertion of quaternary ammonium groups. Usually, chitosan is functionalized by quaternization, carboxymethylation, acylation or sulfhydrylation of amino groups in C_2 position of glucopyranose unit. Chitosan based materials with quaternary ammonium moieties are diverse in shape, state or functionality: hydrogels (Mohamed et al. 2015; Fan et al. 2015), fibers based on polyelectrolyte complexes (Ignatova et al. 2016), chitosan ammonium salts (Tang et al. 2015; Li et al. 2015; Tan et al. 2016; Li et al. 2016; Wang et al. 2016; Tang et al. 2016; Chen et al. 2016; Oyervides-Munoz et al. 2017) or copolymers (Song et al. 2016).

Hydrogels represent 3-D networks able to retain large amounts of biological fluids or water, being used in different fields such as biomedical devices, food packing or water purification. Also, quaternized chitosan based hydrogels serve as antimicrobial or wound healing materials. When Mohamed et al. (2015) designed hydrogels based on *N*-trimethyl ammmonium chitosan chloride and poly(vinyl alcohol) in weight ratios of 1:3, 1:1 and 3:1, they used glutaraldehyde in weight ratio of 1–5% as chemical cross-linking agent to ensure formation of chemical bonds between glutaraldehyde and hydroxyl groups of poly(vinyl alcohol) or residual amino groups from *N*-trimethyl ammmonium chitosan chloride. Beside different physico-mechanical properties, resulted materials exhibited specific antibacterial or antifungal activities. Thus, antimicrobial activity of *N*-trimethyl ammmonium chitosan chloride/poly(vinyl alcohol) hydrogels was higher than *N*-trimethyl ammmonium chitosan chloride itself, while antimicrobial effect increased with glutaraldehyde concentration.

Fan et al. (2015) performed gamma radiation-crosslinking to prepare hydrogels based on solution of hyaluronic acid and quaternary ammonium chitosan, poly(ethylene oxide) and poly(vinyl alcohol). Preliminary, quaternary ammonium chitosan was synthesized from chitosan and *N*-(3-chloro-2-hydroxypropyl)trimethyl ammonium chloride in NaOH solution. Then, solution of quaternary ammonium chitosan mixed with poly(vinyl alcohol)/poly(ethylene oxide) solution was subjected to irradiation with a ^{60}Co source. The sample irradiated with a dose of 40 kilograys was tested against *E. coli* RCMB 000107 and *S. aureus* RCMB 000106. In both cases, polymeric hydrogels containing quaternary amino $N^{+}(CH_3)_3$ groups showed a clear inhibition zone compared with poly(vinyl alcohol)/poly(ethylene oxide) hydrogel. Due to excellent moisture properties, these hydrogels were proposed as valuable materials for wound dressing applications.

By applying electrospinning, dip-coating and polyelectrolyte complex formation, Ignatova et al. (2016) designed various fibrous materials with antimicrobial and antioxidant properties, based on quaternized chitosan derivative named

N-trimethyl ammonium chitosan iodide, poly(3-hydroxybutyrate), caffeic acid and *k*-carrageenan. Thus, system represented by caffeic acid /poly(3-hydroxybutyrate) fibers was coated with *N*-trimethyl ammonium chitosan iodide/*k*-carrageenan polyelectrolyte complex, while system based on poly(3-hydroxybutyrate) fibers was coated with *N*-trimethyl ammonium chitosan iodide/*k*-carrageenan complex containing caffeic acid. Ability of fibrous materials containing *N*-trimethyl ammonium chitosan iodide and/or caffeic acid to inhibit the growth of *E. coli* and *S. aureus* was due to the fact that caffeic acid and *N*-trimethyl ammonium chitosan iodide exercised synergic antibacterial activity (bacteriostatic or bactericidal). Both materials containing caffeic acid and quaternized chitosan suppressed bacteria growth after 3–4 h of exposure. In addition, by studying *S. aureus* cells adhesion to the surface of fibrous materials, it was observed from scanning electron microscopy images that a large number of viable *S. aureus* cells with unaltered morphology adhered on surface of hydrophobic neat poly(3-hydroxybutyrate) fibers. In return, on contact with surface of treated poly(3-hydroxybutyrate) fibers, adhesion of pathogenic *S. aureus* bacteria was suppressed such that no bacteria or only a limited number of adhered bacteria were observed.

When antimicrobial properties of molecular iodine were combined with those of *N*-(2-hydroxy) propyl-3-trimethylammonium chitosan chloride, a new material with stronger antimicrobial activity was obtained (Tang et al. 2015). Thus, a stable charge transfer complex of *N*-(2-hydroxy) propyl-3-trimethylammonium chitosan chloride with iodine resulted by combination of those two components in a molar ratio of 1:1.33, due to the attraction between large electron cloud density of iodine and positive charge of quaternary ammonium salt. By testing antibacterial efficacies of samples against *S. aureus* and *E. coli*, it was observed that the antibacterial inhibitory effect increased in order: chitosan > *N*-(2-hydroxy) propyl-3-trimethylammonium chitosan chloride > *N*-(2-hydroxy) propyl-3-trimethylammonium chitosan chloride-iodide. Other approach to improve antimicrobial activity of chitosan consisted of synthesis of chitosan quaternary ammonium salts with halogens: chitosan halo-acetates and chitosan halo-1,2,3-triazoles (Tan et al. 2016; Li et al. 2016). In this way, electronegativity of halogenic substituent groups in chitosan ammonium salts enriched positive charge density of cationic amino groups, and antimicrobial activity of chitosan derivatives, consequently.

Antifungal activity of a series of water soluble chitosan ammonium salts with halogens namely, chitosan-bromoacetate, chitosan-chloroacetate, chitosan-dichloroacetate, chitosan-trichloroacetate and chitosan-trifluoroacetate was evaluated *in vitro* by hypha measurement of three phytopathogens *viz. Fusarium oxysporum*, *Phomopsis asparagi* and *Colletotrichum lagenarium*. For example, in case of 1.0 mg/mL of potential antimicrobial agent, and in presence of *F. oxysporum*, inhibitory index values of 55.8%, 69.6%, 71.0%, 73.9% and 78.5% were reported for chitosan-bromoacetate, chitosan-chloroacetate, chitosan-dichloroacetate, chitosan-trichloroacetate and chitosan-trifluoroacetate, respectively. These increased values compared with respect to chitosan (11.8%) were in relation with substitution degree of polysaccharide and protonation degree of amino groups. As electronegativity of halogenic substituent groups in chitosan ammonium salts decreased in order trifluoromethyl > trichloromethyl > dichloromethyl > chloromethyl > – bromomethyl, the antifungal activity followed same tendency: chitosan-trifluoroacetate > chitosan-trichloroacetate > chitosan-dichloroacetate > chitosan-chloroacetate > chitosan-bromoacetate > chitosan); such that a stronger adherence of antimicrobials to outer membranes of fungi produced more damage to fungal integrity and transport of nutrients was affected (Tan et al. 2016).

Starting from 6-bromo-6-deoxy-*N*-phthaloyl-chitosan, Li et al. (2016) synthesized triazole chitosan quaternary ammonium iodide, chloro-1,2,3-triazole chitosan quaternary ammonium iodide and bromo-1,2,3-triazole chitosan quaternary ammonium iodide. In case of chloro-1,2,3-triazole chitosan quaternary ammonium iodide and bromo-1,2,3-triazole chitosan quaternary ammonium iodide, the growth inhibition of phytopathogens like *F. oxysporum f. sp. niveum* ATCC36116, *F. oxysporum. f. sp. cucumebrium* Owen ATCC42357 and *C. lagenarium* (Pass) Ell.et halst ATCC30016 was due to an interactive effect of halogen and triazole moieties. Chitosan quaternization by chemical grafting reactions with different low molecular weight quaternary ammonium salts represents a usual practice to obtain chitosan derivatives. In this way, limited antibacterial and antifungal activities of chitosan which are related to its cationic character below pH 6.5, were improved. In addition, even solubility of new chitosan derivatives was better compared with pure chitosan.

Later, Overvidez-Munoz et al. (2017) functionalized amine groups of chitosan with different quaternary ammonium salts such as 4-bromobutyl-benzalkonium bromide, 4-bromobutyl-triethylammonium bromide or 4-bromobutyl-pyridinium bromide, resulting in following derivatives of chitosan: 4-bromobutyl-benzalkonium bromide chitosan, 4-bromobutyl-triethylammonium bromide chitosan and 4-bromobutyl-pyridinium bromide chitosan. Amongst these modified chitosan samples, 4-bromobutyl-pyridinium bromide chitosan showed highest antibacterial activity, while 4-bromobutyl-triethylammonium bromide chitosan was the least active. Chitosan bearing benzalkonium, triethylammonium and pyridinium moieties, resulting from mixing of 4-bromobutyl-benzalkonium bromide, 4-bromobutyl-triethylammonium bromide and 4-bromobutyl-pyridinium bromide in a weight ratio of 1:1:1, was less soluble, and displayed a reduced antimicrobial activity due to an improper contact of insoluble material with bacterial cells.

Wang et al. (2016) intended to modify the hydroxyl group of chitosan from C_2 position, and prepared five water-soluble *O*-quaternary ammonium salt-chitosans bearing *N*-methyl-*N*-R-*N*, *N*-bis(2-hydroxyethyl) ammonium bromides where radical R represented benzyl, dodecyl, tetradecyl, hexadecyl or octadecyl. Because the new amphiphilic chitosan derivatives presented lipotropic character due to long carbon chains, and hydrophilic character due to quaternary ammonium salt moiety within *O*-quaternary ammonium salt-chitosan backbone, its antibacterial abilities and cytotoxicity were consistently improved compared to their low molecular weight quaternary ammonium salt homologues. In other works, a chitosan quaternary ammonium salt, named *N*-(2-hydroxyl)propyl-3-trimethyl ammonium chitosan chloride, obtained by grafting glycidyl trimethylammonium chloride on chitosan, was the subject of subsequent transformations: combination with commercial-grad Reactive Red x-3b (Tang et al. 2016) or phthalic anhydride (Chen et al. 2016). Using Reactive Red x-3b, a color reactive bearing sulfonic groups, suitable for textile and wood, a biopolymer dye with improved water solubility and antibacterial properties compared with pure low molecular weight dye was achieved. It was observed that in presence of new biopolymer dye, number of bacterial colony was reduced from 79% to 99% in case of *E. Coli*, and from 73% to 99% in case of *S. aureus* due to a synergic effect of quaternary ammonium and sulfonic groups from structure of biopolymer dye (Tang et al. 2016).

Following esterification reaction of *N*-(2-hydroxyl)propyl-3-trimethyl ammonium chitosan chloride with phthalic anhydride, subsequent introduction of NCO-sulfobetaine onto OH position of *N*-phathaloyl quaternized chitosan derivative were confirmed. Amine groups of resulting *N*-phathaloyl quaternized betainized chitosan were recovered using an aqueous solution of hydrazine monohydrate (Chen et al. 2016). The final zwitterionic product (*O*-sulfobetaine-*N*-(2-hydroxyl)propyl-3-trimethyl ammonium chitosan chloride) fulfilled role of materials with enhanced antibacterial activity and biocompatibility based on synergic action of sulfobetaine and quaternary ammonium groups. Improved water solubility, low cytotoxicity and hemolytic activity of zwitterionic chitosan derivatives are among the necessary parameters for their application under *in vitro* and *in vivo* condition. Beside sulfonic and sulfobetaine groups, thiourea may synergistically act, potentiating the antimicrobial properties of the compound carrying quaternary ammonium groups. Usually, benzoyl thiourea and acyl thiourea derivatives of chitosan display antifungal activity (Eweis et al. 2006; Mohamed and El-Ghany 2012). Earlier, Li et al. (2015) introduced double antibacterial groups, namely *O*-quaternary ammonium and *N*-acyl thiourea, onto OH and NH_2 positions of macromolecular chains of chitosan following few steps: synthesis of *N*-benzylidene-chitosan; quaternization of *N*-benzylidene-chitosan with glycidyl trimethylammonium chloride resulting in *O*-quaternary ammonium *N*-benzylidenechitosan; synthesis of *O*-quaternary ammonium chitosan; reaction of acyl thiocyanate with *O*-quaternary ammonium chitosan resulting in *O*-quaternary ammonium-*N*-acyl thiourea chitosan. In case of *S. aureus*, *Bacillus subtilis, E. coli*, *Pseudomonas aeruginosa* and *Aspergillus niger*, antibacterial activity increased in order: *O*-quaternary ammonium-*N*-acyl thiourea chitosan > *O*-quaternary ammonium chitosan > chitosan. Zeta potential measurements and transmission electron microscopy images confirmed hypothesis related to electrostatic interactions between cationic amino groups and negative charged cell membranes. Thus, higher values of zeta potential in case of quaternized chitosans compared with pure chitosan indicated an increase in positive charge of chitosan derivatives and an increased number of electrostatic interactions. Also, changes in bacterial morphology after treatment with *O*-quaternary ammonium-*N*-acyl thiourea chitosan were due to the rupture of cell membranes and modification of cell metabolism as a result of quaternized chitosan infiltration.

Knowing that chitosan quaternary ammonium salt has antimicrobial and good antioxidant properties, Song et al. (2016) attempted to integrate it in a traditional dental material in order to form a resin base which could improve the overall oral health. They used *N*-trimethyl ammmonium chitosan chloride, denture water (containing methyl methacrylate monomer, cross-linking agent, inhibitor and an UV absorber) and denture powder (containing poly(methyl methacrylate)), and prepared two types of formulations in accordance with order of material mixing. Material 1 was prepared physically by adding varying amount of chitosan quaternary ammonium salt directly to denture powder, and then denture water. Material 2 was prepared chemically by adding variable amount of *N*-trimethyl ammmonium chitosan chloride to denture water, which determined the graft copolymerization of methyl methacrylate monomer with the chitosan quaternary ammonium salt. Both formulations presented low cytotoxicity and insignificantly modified tensile strength. In contrast, these materials recorded different antimicrobial properties and degrees of corrosion resistance. Antimicrobial tests were carried out with microorganisms specific to oral cavity: *Streptococcus mutans* and *Candida albicans*. In case of both materials, antibacterial rate increased with concentration of chitosan quaternary ammonium salt. As material 1 may have higher specific surface area over chemically produced material 2; it recorded a better performance in both antibacterial and antifungal tests as compared to material 2. In addition, material 2 did not recorded any antifungal property.

5.3.3 Dextran Type Antimicrobials

Naturally synthesized by *Leuconostoc mesenteroides* and *S. mutans* bacteria, dextrans are complex glucans composed of glucose molecules linked by α-1,6 glycosidic linkages in main chain or by α-1,3 glycosidic linkages in branching points. These polysaccharides with various molecular weights due to branched glucose chains of variable lengths are intensively used in medicine and laboratory as anticoagulants, size-exclusion chromatography matrices, cell osmotic pressure or blood sugar level regulators, and components of biosensors or bioreactors. To diversify its degree of application, dextran could be chemically modified such that to obtain cationic amphiphilic dextran derivatives with potential application as broad spectrum external biocides.

Quaternary ammonium groups were attached to dextran main chain bearing alkyl or dialkyl end groups by reaction of modified polysaccharide with an equimolar mixture of a tertiary amine (*N,N*-dimethyl-*N*-benzylamine, *N,N*-dimethyl-*N*-octylamine or 1-methylimidazol) and epichlorohydrin. Obtained cationic amphiphilic dextran derivatives were tested from microbiological point of view (Tuchilus et al. 2017). It was observed that all samples were ineffective against *P. aeruginosa* ATCC 27853, but displayed antimicrobial activity against *E. coli* ATCC 25922, *S. aureus* ATCC 25923, *Sarcina lutea* ATCC 9341, *Candida glabrata* ATCC MYA2950, *C. albicans* ATCC 90028 and *C. parapsilosis* ATCC 22019. Besides type of microbes, antimicrobial activity of samples was correlated with polymer chemical composition. Thus, self-assembling properties, and consequently interactions with microbial cellular components, were tuned by dextran with relative molar mass of 6000 or 10,000, chemical structure of ammonium groups e.g. R_3 = benzyl, octyl; R_2 = dimetyl-R_3-quaternary ammonium, imidazol; R_1 = dodecyl, octadecyl, and length of end alkyl group, meaning by hydrophilic/hydrophobic balance. Even that length of alkyl or dialkyl chains like C_{12}, C_{18} or $(C_{12})_2$ did not significantly influenced antimicrobial activity of samples originating from dextran with the same molecular mass, modified polymers based on dextran 10,000 recorded lower activity compared with those coming from dextran 6000. In addition, polymers with *N,N*-dimetyl-*N*-benzyl-quaternary ammonium groups showed the best results in case of all tested microorganisms, while samples with *N,N*-dimetyl-*N*-octyl-quaternary ammonium groups have a preference for *E. coli*, and imidazolium based polymers induced only a weak antifungal activity.

5.3.4 Pullulan Type Antimicrobials

Pullulan is a neutral homopolysaccharide with linear chain consisting of almost regularly repeating α-(1 $\rightarrow$ 4)–maltotriosyl units (3-D-glucopyranosyl) joined through α-(1 $\rightarrow$ 6) linkages. It looks like an amorphous slime formed by aerobic fermentation of *Aureobasidium pullulans* polymorphic fungus (Singh et al. 2008; Cheng et al. 2011). Molecular weight of this exopolysaccharide is from 4.5×10^4 to 6×10^5 Da and varies with yeast cultivation parameters. Hydroxyl functional groups as a part of flexible polysaccharide chain are the subject for chemical modifications and can result into a series of derivatives: pullulan succinylate, pullulan acetate, pullulan amine, carboxymethyl pullulan, cholesterol bearing pullulan (Singh et al. 2015). In this way, chemical and physical properties of pullulan such as hygroscopicity, biodegradability, viscosity, non-reducing agent, water solubility, formation of oxygen impermeable films are improved due to solubility in organic solvents or enrichment with new reactive functional groups.

Since its introduction as food additive by the Japanese, pullulan and its derivatives recorded numerous applications in foods, pharmaceutical and medical industries. Exploiting antimicrobial potential of quaternary ammonium groups, Grigoras et al. (2013) designed three pullulan derivatives. Length and frequency of grafts influenced all solutions properties, and consequently antimicrobial activity. Diameter of inhibition zones, recorded in presence of *S. aureus* ATCC 25923 strains and salted aqueous polymer solutions, varied from 7 mm to 10 mm in accordance with solution concentration and poly(3-acrylamidopropyl) trimethylammonium chloride content in grafted polymer. Antibacterial activity of grafted pullulans was due to electrostatic interactions between quaternary ammonium cation of poly(3-acrylamidopropyl)trimethylammonium chloride and phosphatidylethanolamine, a negatively charged component from bacterial cell wall.

5.3.5 Starch Type Antimicrobials

Starch (amylum) is a polysaccharide synthesized by plants and structurally formed from amylase and amylopectin molecules in variable proportions. Because of their widespread availability, biodegradability and environmental friendliness, this macromolecule and its derivatives frequently are used as flocculants and disinfectants in water treatment industry. Cationic starch based flocculants possessing quaternary ammonium functional groups on backbone have been developed by grafting reaction or esterification, a more convenient, cost saving, and reliable reaction. Huang et al. (2017) synthesized four different starch-graft-poly(2-methacryloyloxyethyl) trimethyl ammonium chlorides with various grafting ratios, while Liu et al. (2017) reported synthesis of four starch-3-chloro-2-hydroxypropyl triethylammonium chlorides having various quaternary ammonium salt groups on starch backbone. Tests on synthetic turbid and microbiological contaminated waters revealed that starch based derivatives have dual functionality: flocculation effect and antimicrobial performance. Three dimensional excitation emission matrix fluorescence *spectra* of supernatants of bacterial cultures and scanning electron microscopy images of *E. coli* CMCC 44102 and *S. aureus* CMCC 26003 before and after flocculation using cationic starch based flocculants are used to represent antibacterial properties of these starch derivatives. Fluorescence signals from wavelength intervals of 200–240 nm and 280–380 nm, attributed to protein like extracellular organic matters, were more intense for *E. coli* than for *S. aureus* suggesting the higher breakdown of *E. coli* cells. Also, after flocculation, treatment with cationic starch based derivatives, changed shape of bacteria from uniform elliptical to anamorphic one in case of *E. coli*, while most of *S. aureus* cells preserved their spherical shape or appeared “pinched”. The study suggested that due to synergistic effect from inorganic particles of kaolin and cationic starch based flocculants, bacterial cell walls were effectively destroyed through strong electrostatic interactions.

5.3.6 Cashew Gum Type Antimicrobials

Cashew gum is a chemical constituent of *Anacardium occidentale* L. tree stem, extracted in order to prepare viscous and emulsifying suspensions for food and pharmaceutical industries. This anionic heteropolysaccharide is composed of β-D-galactose, α-D-glucose, arabinose, rhamnose and glucuronic acid in proportion of 72%, 14%, 4.6%, 3.2% and 4.6%, respectively. Galactose units are joined by β $(1 \rightarrow 3)$ links in main chain of macromolecule or by β $(1 \rightarrow 6)$ links in side chain (de Paula et al. 1998). To improve its weak antimicrobial activity (Campos et al. 2012), Quelemes et al. (2017) chemically modified cashew gum by quaternization reaction. Firstly, cashew gum alkoxide was reacted with epoxide- or

N-(3-chloro-2-hydrohypropyl) trimethylammonium chloride. In this way, alkoxide groups of cashew gum were nucleophilic substituted by cationic quaternary ammonium moieties. All three resulted quaternized cashew gum derivatives with degree of substitution of 42%, 68% and 73% were tested against eleven strains of *Staphylococcus* genus. Generally, it was observed that minimum inhibitory concentration and minimum bactericidal concentration values decreased with the increase in degree of substitution; anti-staphylococcal activity was enhanced due to more incorporated positive charges in quaternized cashew gum. Influence of the most promising derivative on bacterial morphology was evaluated using atomic force microscopy. After a 24 h exposure of methicilin sensitive *S. aureus* ATCC 29213 culture to solution of quaternized cashew gum having 73% degree of substitution, mean height of cells changed from 0.9 μm (in case of untreated cultures) to 1.4 μm or 1.3 μm at minimum inhibitory concentration or minimum bactericidal concentration. In addition, integrity of cell wall was gradually affected due to partial damage of bacterial cell. Also, all quaternized cashew gum derivatives showed good biocompatibility on erythrocytes, fibroblasts and keratinocytes which recommended them as promising agents against skin pathogens.

5.3.7 Poly(lactide) Type Antimicrobials

Being a non-toxic, biodegradable and bioactive bioplastic intensively used globally, poly(lactic acid) or poly(lactide) represents a thermoplastic aliphatic polyesther extracted from natural sources like sugarcane, corn starch or cassava roots, and used as fibers or films. Thus, poly(lactide) fibers could be more sustainable compared with other polyesther fibers derived from petroleum.

Usually, finishing of poly(lactide) fibers is carried out by their treatment with an antimicrobial film of silver or zinc oxide nanoparticles, essential oils, antibiotics or chitosan. Some of these antimicrobial coatings operate by mechanism of controlled release or by formation of a biological barrier. To increase the effectiveness of antimicrobial protection in case of poly(lactide) fibers, Logar et al. (2016) tailored antimicrobial coatings with dual and synergistic activities using silver and quaternary ammonium functional groups. They developed a three-stage finishing procedure which involved creation of a silica matrix (I), in situ synthesis of AgCl from silver nitrate and sodium chloride (II) and in third stage, application of silver chloride and 3-(trimethoxysilyl)-propyldimethyltetradecyl ammonium chloride. Even though application of this coating generated some esthetic disadvantages for poly(lactide) fibers such as reduced lightness and increased yellowing; from microbiological point of view it displayed excellent bactericidal activity with a 99.99% reduction in *S. aureus* and *E. coli* colonies.

A water soluble cationic benzanthrone derivative namely 1-[(7-oxo-7H-benzo[de]anthracen-3-ylcarbamoyl)-methyl]-triethylammonium chloride was synthesized and incorporated into a poly(lactide) thin film in order to test its antimicrobial activity (Staneva et al. 2015). The compound was observed to be very photostable and exhibited a prolonged release of benzanthrone derivative into aqueous solution. The system composed of poly(lactide) matrix and benzanthrone derivative was tested against a wide spectra of microorganisms (*Bacillus cereus*, *B. subtilis*, *S. lutea*, *Micrococcus luteus*, *E. coli*, *Pseudomonas aeruginosa*, *Acinetobacter johnsonii*, *S. cerevisiae*, *Xanthomonas oryzae*, *Candida lipolytica*), and minimum inhibitory concentration was in range of 48–125 μg/mL and zones of inhibition were in range of 12–24 mm. Also, optical densities of growth media for *E. coli* and *P. aeruginosa* strains decreased in the presence of composite material compared with untreated poly(lactide) matrix. Authors attributed the antimicrobial activity of new system to action of cationic quaternary ammonium groups onto plasma membrane of yeasts and cytoplasmic (inner) membrane of bacteria.

5.4 Antimicrobials Based on Synthetic Polymers

Because natural sources are limited, sometimes researchers attempt to design synthetic polymers with antimicrobial activities. Biocompatible synthetic polymers like poly(amidoamine), poly(urethane)s, poly(siloxane)s, poly(methacrylate)s and poly(ethylene) have found applications in various medical subdomains. In addition, these have efficient antimicrobial properties and are non-toxic for rest of cells, too.

5.4.1 Poly(amidoamine) Type Antimicrobials

A new trend to enhance the contact surface between pathogenic cells and antimicrobial substances involves the use of tree like branched polymers, with a sphere like shape, named dendrimers. Modulating synthesis conditions of these molecules, the number of branches could exponentially increase with each new generation of branches. Poly(amidoamine) is a representative of dendrimer class, composed of repetitively branched subunits of amide and amine functionality. Because it is biocompatible, easy to synthesize and has similar properties with globular proteins, some researchers had functionalized this macromolecule in order to fabricate novel antibacterial agent for water treatment. Thus, Maleki et al. (2017) modified poly(amidoamine) dendrimers (generations G2 and G4) into quaternary ammonium salts using Cl, Br, I halogens groups. Then, antimicrobial activity was determined against *E. coli*, *Klebsiella oxytoca*, *B. subtilis*, and *S. aureus* isolated from contaminated water samples. Compared with unmodified polymers, quaternary ammonium salts exhibited an enhanced antimicrobial efficacy against bacteria, the most effective being G4 generation of poly(amidoamine) modified with iodine.

5.4.2 Poly(urethane) Type Antimicrobials

Versatile materials like poly(urethane)s, intensively applied in medical and automotive fields as biomaterials or coatings, are synthesized in forms of foams, starting from di- or triisocyanates and polyols. To avoid potential leaching of physically bonded biocides from polyurethane matrix, some authors chosed chemically bonded cationic groups like imidazolium, pyrrolidonium or ammonium to design antimicrobials with prolonged usage. Thus, Udabe et al. (2017) prepared porous materials with antibacterial properties using glycerol propoxilate, tri- or tetra-hydroxyl functionalized quaternary ammonium compounds, and poly(hexamethylene diisocyanate) or toluene diisocyanate in different compositions. They observed that poly(urethane) ability to grow was enhanced in accordance with amount of quaternary ammonium compound in foam formulation. Also, 20% of quaternary ammonium component in poly(urethane) foams ensured a high antimicrobial activity. Chemically incorporated ammonium groups into poly(urethane) backbone were responsible for killing of *S. aureus* ATCC 29737 and *E. coli* ATCC 25922. In case of *E. coli*, an efficiency of 89% was observed for poly(urethane) formulation with 16% quaternary ammonium content. However, in case of *S. aureus*, maximum killing efficiency was observed with 7% of quaternary ammonium content. Besides, different chemical composition of microorganism structure and different content of reactive antimicrobial groups, type of isocyanate was another influencing factor for antibacterial behavior. In comparison with poly(hexamethylene diisocyanate), the more hydrophobic molecule toluene diisocyanate ensured a higher antimicrobial rate.

In another study, dressings based on poly(urethane) foams containing poly(diallyl-dimethylammonium chloride), known as polyquaternium-6, were applied on wounds infected with different microorganisms: *S. aureus* AH133; *P. aeruginosa* strain PAO1 Lux; a clinical isolate of *Acinetobacter baumannii*; *S. aureus* Lux; MRSA strains of *S. aureus* (Tran et al. 2017). Wound dressing material was placed on back of laboratory animals and bacterial biofilm formation in tissue under bandage was evaluated. It was observed that poly(diallyl-dimethylammonium chloride) containing poly(urethane) dressings totally inhibited biofilm formation, for all test organisms, reducing wound overinfection.

To endow them with antimicrobial properties, the biodegradable and biocompatible poly(urethane) coatings were successfully prepared by Liu et al. (2015) starting from a mixture of terpene-based polyol, various quaternary ammonium salts and hydrophilically modified hexamethylene diisocyanate tripolymer. In this case, quaternary ammonium salts were synthesized by quaternization reaction of terpene-based carbamate with alkyl bromides. Beside excellent mechanical properties and water resistance, resulted products recorded considerable antimicrobial activities against both *E. coli* and *S. aureus* even at reduced concentrations (5 wt%). As expected, antimicrobial activity of poly(urethane) coatings was improved by introduction of quaternary ammonium groups.

In order to prevent damage of medical devices covered by antimicrobials, but subsequently overpopulated with dead microorganisms, a research team designed a complex reverse surface structure, composed of an contact-active antibacterial upper-layer and a long-lasting antifouling sub-layer (He et al. 2016). Thus, gemini quaternary ammonium salt waterborne poly(urethane) films casted from solutions have been prepared using: isophorone diisocyanate, poly(tetramethylene glycol), poly(ethylene glycol), *N,N,N′,N′*-tetramethyl-*N,N′*-bisdodecyl-2,6-bis(ammonium bromide)–*L*–lysine-(1′,3′-propylene diamide)-*L*-lysine, and *L*-lysine. Poly(tetramethylene glycol) soft segment of modified poly(urethane) films and isophorone diisocyanate were hydrophobic, while soft segment poly(ethylene glycol) and *L*-lysine formed anti-fouling sub-layer, and *N,N,N′,N′*-tetramethyl-*N,N′*-bisdodecyl-2,6-bis(ammonium bromide)–*L*–lysine-(1′,3′-propylene diamide)-*L*-lysine antibacterial brushes formed upper layer. By varying molar fraction of components, different gemini quaternary ammonium salt waterborne poly(urethane) samples were obtained. Killing efficiency of this novel surface structure was tested against both types of Gram bacteria. It was observed that after a critical concentration of *N,N,N′,N′*-tetramethyl-*N,N′*-bisdodecyl-2,6-bis(ammonium bromide)–*L*–lysine-(1′,3′-propylene diamide)-*L*-lysine (4.96 wt%), all gemini quaternary ammonium salt waterborne poly(urethane) samples displayed strong antibacterial activity. Simultaneously, antifouling properties were related with surface hydrophilicity determined by contact angle measurements. Decreasing of time related water contact angle and enhancing of hydrophilicity at the same time with increase in *N,N,N′,N′*-tetramethyl-*N,N′*-bisdodecyl-2,6-bis(ammonium bromide)–*L*–lysine-(1′,3′-propylene diamide)-*L*-lysine, were attributed to the cationic nature of gemini quaternary ammonium fragments from modified poly(urethane)s.

5.4.3 Poly(siloxane) Type Antimicrobials

Poly(siloxane)s, generically called silicones, are biocompatible and biodurable materials widely applied in healthcare industry. State of aggregation of final products could be tuned by varying –Si–O– chain length, side organic groups attached to silicon atoms and crosslinking degree. Thus, silicones with properties characteristic to liquids or hard plastics such as thermal and chemical stability, hydrophobicity or low surface tension, represented matrix for various medical equipment and instruments. When the latter are to be used for therapeutic purposes, conditions of sterility and asepsis should also be considered. In this regard, antimicrobial materials based on silicones and quaternary ammonium moieties were designed.

Starting from poly(siloxane)s containing tertiary amino group and epichlorohydrin, Cui et al. (2015) obtained poly(siloxane) quaternary ammonium salts containing epoxy group with different molecular weights (M_w = 3150–13,000 g/mol) by a quaternization reaction in ethanol. It was observed that the new products spontaneously formed micelles in aqueous solutions and exhibited surfactant properties, as well as thermal and chemical stabilies. From microbiological point of view, poly(siloxane) quaternary ammonium salts containing epoxy group were active against *S. aureus*, *B. subtilis*, and *E. coli* such that increased molecular weight of polymers led to a high antibacterial activity. In addition, sensitivity of microorganisms in relation to poly(siloxane) quaternary ammonium salts containing epoxy group decreased in order: *B. subtilis* (most sensitive) > *S. aureus* (less sensitive) > *E. coli* (most insensitive).

Beside better wetting, emulsifying and solubilization properties, and lower critical micelle concentration, compared with conventional surfactants, gemini surfactants (molecules composed of two hydrophilic headgroups and two hydrophobic tails connected through a spacer unit) could have antimicrobial properties, especially when they have cationic or zwitterionic character. Taking into account all these advantages, Bao et al. (2017) synthesized some cationic gemini surfactants with poly(ether siloxane) linked group (C_m-PSi-C_m, m = 8, 10, 12, 14, 16, 18). Qualitative and quantitative antimicrobial tests revealed that C_{10}-PSi-C_{10} polymeric surfactants have strongest antimicrobial ability against *E. coli* and *S. aureus*, while C_{14}-PSi-C_{14} possessed the strongest antimicrobial activity against *A. flavus*. As expected, antimicrobial activities of C_8-PSi-C_8 and C_{18}-PSi-C_{18} compounds were insignificant, because the inadequate length of hydrophobic chain (too long or too short) from structure of polymeric gemini surfactants was unfavorable to interactions with tested pathogenic microorganisms.

Another approach to improve antimicrobial properties of biocompatible synthetic polymers involves synthesis of copolymers, especially block copolymers. Because pure poly(dimethylsiloxane) has tendency to form a brittle silica like layer, it was chosen as candidate for blending with antimicrobial agents and subsequently chemical surface modifications. Thus, Qin et al. (2015) designed an antibacterial coating from block copolymers of poly(dimethylsiloxane) with quaternized poly(*N,N*-dimethylaminoethyl methacrylate). In this study, hydrophilic poly(*N,N*-dimethylaminoethyl methacrylate) was converted into cationic form by quaternization of tertiary amino groups with n-octyliodide. Spin coated copolymer films were obtained from acetonitrile solution of block copolymers mixed with hexamethylene diisocyanate. A different chemical composition of quaternized block copolymers was related with variable Si/N ratio: 1.5/1, 0.6/1, 0.7/1 and 1.1/1. In case of some films, mobility of poly(dimethylsiloxane) chains and intermolecular ionic interactions between alkyl side chains and positively charged groups in quaternary ammonium salts have favored appearance of microphase separations. So, surface roughness determined interaction with bacteria such that heterogeneous surfaces ensured an increased contact area with microorganisms and improved antimicrobial activity. From entire series of quaternized block copolymers, the exponent with the higher content of N^+ showed antimicrobial activity towards both *B. subtilis* and *E. coli*. In contrast, the other three were insensitive towards Gram negative bacteria.

Self-assembling capacity of block copolymers was exploited by Zhou et al. (2015) in order to design new fluorosilicone copolymers containing bloks of dithiocarbonate terminated poly(dimethylsiloxane), poly(2-(dimethylamino)ethyl methacrylate) quaternized with n-octyliodide, poly(hexafluorobutyl methacrylate) and hydroxyethyl methacrylate, respectively. The new quaternized multi block copolymers contained different mass percentages of poly(2-(dimethylamino)ethyl methacrylate) and poly(hexafluorobutyl methacrylate). Visualization of inhibition zones around multi block copolymer films, in presence of representative Gram positive bacteria (*B. subtilis* ATCC 63501) and Gram negative bacteria (*E. coli* ATCC 44752), helped to correlate antimicrobial activities of these quaternized multi block copolymers with the stronger tendency of poly(dimethylsiloxane) and quaternary ammonium salts related blocks to migrate to surface of films, compared with poly(hexafluorobutyl methacrylate) blocks. Thus, fluorosilicone multi block copolymer containing appropiate amount of poly(hexafluorobutyl methacrylate), usually lower than 26.1 wt%, recorded antibacterial activity due to a higher C-N$^+$ content and ability to form films with relatively smooth morphology.

5.4.4 Poly(methacrylate) Type Antimicrobials

Monomethacrylates and di-methacrylates are monomers intesivelly used in polymerization reactions resulting in thermoplastic materials with excellent weatherability, good mechanical properties and chemical resistance. Makvandi et al. (2018) reviewed antibacterial properties of dental composite materials composed of a quaternary ammonium modified methacrylate resin matrix, beside inorganic microfillers or nanofillers, coupling agents, and an initiator–accelerator system. Even that dental restoration materials incorporated with quaternary ammonium compounds exert a long time antibacterial effect compared with other antimicrobials, e.g. silver or zinc oxide nanoparticles, a balance between antimicrobial properties and mammalian cell cytotoxicity must always be considered.

Lv and team (2018) designed an electrochemical biosensor for immobilization of redox protein, which possesed antimicrobial properties, too. They used positively charged polymeric quaternary ammonium salts of dimethylaminoethyl methacrylate and negatively charged hemoglobin for constructing a film onto a glassy carbon electrode. Catalytic activity of immobilized hemoglobin was evaluated toward peroxide of hydrogen, and antimicrobial properties were tested against *E. coli* (ATCC 25922), *S. aureus* (ATCC 6538), *Candida albicans* (ATCC 14053) and *Aspergillus fumigatus* (Af 293). Both properties were influenced by the length of alkyl chain or type of methacrylate molecule (macromolecule or monomer).

5.4.5 Poly(ethylene) Type Antimicrobials

Beside well-known plastics like poly(urethane), poly(styrene), poly(propylene) or poly(vinyl chloride), being intensively used in daily life, poly(ethylene) is another thermoplastic semicrystalline polymer usually applied in packaging industry or medical instruments and devices. Because most of poly(ethylene) type materials come into contact with living beings, it is necessary to ensure their sterility. Thus, Rossetti et al. (2017) mixed poly(ethylene) from melt with mono- and bicationic quaternary ammonium salts. They used nine different salts: benzyldimethylstearylammonium chloride; trimethylstearylammonium chloride; dimethyldistearylammonium chloride; methyltristearylammonium bromide; tetrastearylammonium bromide; 1,12-bis(dimethyloctylammonium)dodecane dibromide; 1,20-bis(dimethyloctylammonium)eicosane dibromide; 1,30-bis(dimethyloctylammonium) triacontane dibromide; bis(dimethyloctylammonium)PEG(400) ditosylate. Resulted antimicrobial poly(ethylene)s were self-organized in such a way that quaternary ammonium salts bounded by Vander-Waals forces were displayed to the surface of polymer, forming nonleaching, permanent biocidal surfaces.

5.5 Target Microorganisms Affected by Polymeric Antimicrobials Containing Quaternary Ammonium Moieties

Eradication of various pathogens such as viruses, bacteria, fungi, algae from surrounding world, or of opportunistic germs from living organisms, involves the use of more or less aggressive physical or chemical methods. Each method is chosen according to the main structural features of target microorganism. In this regard, it takes in consideration hydrophilic character of Gram positive bacteria or hydrophobic character of Gram negative bacteria. This difference is due to synergic action of main components of cells. Thus, murein layer in Gram positive bacteria cell wall is thick, cross-linked and reinforced with teichoic and lipoteichoic acids, and displayed to external part of cell wall. In return, in case of Gram negative bacteria, thin layer of murein is located in periplasmic space between outer and inner membranes. If membrane of Gram positive bacteria is composed of cardiolipin, predominant phospholipids in inner membrane of Gram-negative bacteria are phospahtidylethanolamine and phosphatidylglycerol. In addition, outer membrane of Gram negative bacteria is covered with a lypopolysaccharides layer, while in case of Gram positive bacteria, outer membrane is missing. Even chemical structure of fungi is variable. For example, mycelium hyphae consisting of branched filament tubes are surrounded by a rigid cell wall with variable chemical composition, most of fungi containing chitin and glucan. Some fungus like organisms have a cell wall made up of considerable amounts of cellulose, while cell surface of *Candida albicans* is negatively charged due to terminal sialic acid, which is found on the surface of the membrane. There is a wide spectrum of pathogens studied by researchers, but representative microorganisms tested in the presence of polymers containing quaternary ammonium moieties are limited and grouped in Table 5.1 or schematically represented in Fig. 5.1 and Table 5.2, respectively.

A possible lower antimicrobial activity of quaternary ammonium polymers compared with standard antibiotics is balanced by their broader activity. Bacteriostatic/fungistatic and bactericidal/fungicidal effects of quaternary ammonium polymers are related to passive or active mechanism of action of substances in the presence of microorganisms. If a passive action of antimicrobials is supposed to repel pathogenic entity due to hydrophilic/hydrophobic/electrostatic repulsion or low surface energy, an active action involves microorganism killing by electrostatic or biocidal interaction (Huang et al. 2016). In depth, molecular mechanism of antimicrobial action is carried out along several stages: adsorption of antimicrobial agent onto cell surface/to outer membrane; formation of interface complexes between

Table 5.1 Representative microorganisms tested in presence of polymers with quaternary ammonium moieties

Microorganisms	*Species*	References
Gram positive bacteria	*Staphylococcus aureus, S. epidermidis*	Meng et al. (2015), Mohamed et al. (2015), Fan et al. (2015), Ignatova et al. (2016), Tang et al. (2015), Oyervides-Munoz et al. (2017), Wang et al. (2016), Tang et al. (2016), Chen et al. (2016), Li et al. (2015), Tuchilus et al. (2017), Grigoras et al. (2013), Quelemes et al. (2017), Logar et al. (2016), Maleki et al. (2017), Udabe et al. (2017), Liu et al. (2015), He et al. (2016), Cui et al. (2015), Bao et al. (2017), Lv et al. (2018), Rossetti et al. (2017)
	Streptococcus mutans	Song et al. (2016)
	α-Hemolytic Streptococcus	Wang et al. (2016)
	β-Hemolytic Streptococcus	Wang et al. (2016)
	Bacillus subtilis	Li et al. (2015), Maleki et al. (2017), Cui et al. (2015), Qin et al. (2015), Zhou et al. (2015)
	Enterococcus faecalis	Mohamed et al. (2015)
	Sarcina lutea	Tuchilus et al. (2017)
Gram negative bacteria	*Escherichia coli*	Meng et al. (2015), Mohamed et al. (2015), Fan et al. (2015), Ignatova et al. (2016), Tang et al. (2015), Oyervides-Munoz et al. (2017), Wang et al. (2016), Tang et al. (2016), Chen et al. (2016), Li et al. (2015), Tuchilus et al. (2017), Logar et al. (2016), Staneva et al. (2015), Maleki et al. (2017), Udabe et al. (2017), Liu et al. (2015), He et al. (2016), Cui et al. (2015), Bao et al. (2017), Qin et al. (2015), Zhou et al. (2015), Lv et al. (2018), Rossetti et al. (2017)
	Pseudomonas aeruginosa	Wang et al. (2016), Li et al. (2015), Tuchilus et al. (2017), Staneva et al. (2015), Rossetti et al. (2017)
	Proteus vulgaris	Wang et al. (2016)
	Klebsiella pneumoniae, K. oxytoca	Mohamed et al. (2015), Maleki et al. (2017)
Fungi	*Saccharomyces cerevisiae*	Peng et al. (2016)
	Aspergillus niger, A. fumigatus, A. flavus	Mohamed et al. (2015), Wang et al. (2016), Li et al. (2015), Bao et al. (2017), Lv et al. (2018)
	Candida albicans, C. glabrata, C. parapsilosis	Wang et al. (2016), Song et al. (2016), Tuchilus et al. (2017), Lv et al. (2018)
	Colletotrichum lagenarium (Pass) Ell. et halst	Tan et al. (2016), Li et al. (2016)
	Fusarium oxysporum f.sp.niveum	Tan et al. (2016), Li et al. (2016)
	Fusarium oxysporum.f.sp. cucumebrium Owen	Tan et al. (2016), Li et al. (2016)
	Phomopsis asparagi	Tan et al. (2016)
	Geotricum candidum	Mohamed et al. (2015)

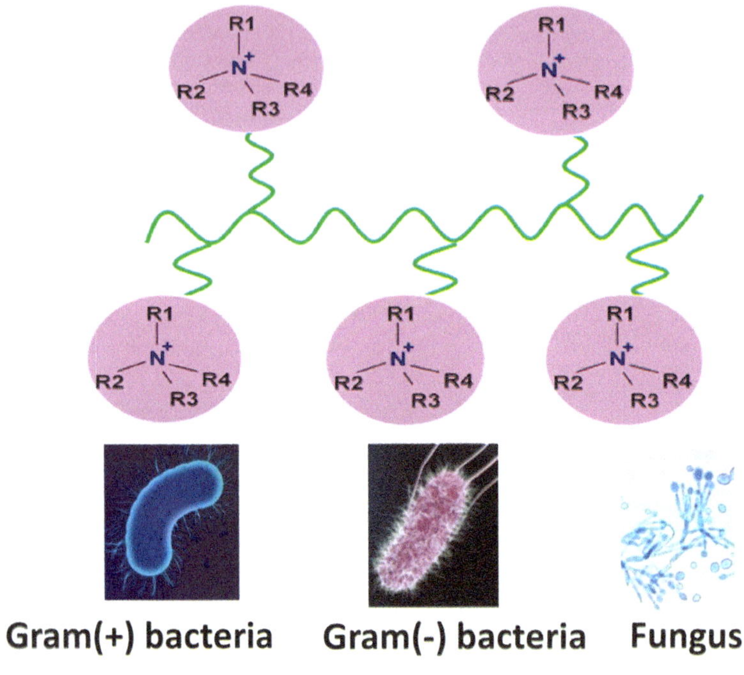

Fig. 5.1 Schematic representation of microorganisms and polymer chain bearing quaternary ammonium moieties. Under favorable conditions, macromolecular chains bearing positive charged groups of quaternary ammonium can interact with components of microbial entities

microorganism membrane and antimicrobial substance by diffusion through cell wall and binding of substances to cytoplasmic membrane; cytoplasmic membrane disruption; translocation of negatively charged lipids of membrane from inside part to outside part of membrane and lateral segregation of membrane lipids; destabilization of outer membrane by releasing cytoplasmic constituents like potassium ions, DNA and RNA; interaction of genetic material with biocidal agent; cell death (Munoz-Bonilla and Fernandes-Garcia 2012; Timofeeva and Kleshcheva 2011).

Preliminary qualitative microbiological tests and extensive quantitative microbiological methods are used in order to evaluate antimicrobial activity of substances. Some of parameters directly refer to microorganism number affected by potential antimicrobials; others are indirectly related with the effect of antimicrobials. Usually, colony forming units are counted, while cell viability, inhibitory index, bacterial reduction, and antimicrobial efficiency are assessed in percentage. Other parameters are also estimated from microbiological tests: bactericidal activity in time (h), bacteriostatic efficiency (log reduction), minimum inhibitory concentration, minimum bactericidal concentration and minimum fungicidal concentration. There are different approaches to evaluate inhibition zone; some authors include in diameter of zone of inhibition, even the size of cylinder or disk containing or immersed with antimicrobial solution; while others calculate zone of inhibition (in mm) by separating support "imprinted" with antimicrobial solution from diameter of transparent zone. Table 5.3 presents the antimicrobial activity of polymers

Table 5.2 Chemical formulas of polymers with quaternary ammonium moieties and antimicrobial activity (selected from literature)

Quaternary ammonium polymers	Chemical formulas	References
Regenerated cellulose (RC) membrane surface croslinked with trimethoxysilylpropyl trimethyl ammonium chloride ($QASC_0$) or trimethoxysilylpropyl octadecyldimethyl ammonium chloride ($QASC_{18}$)	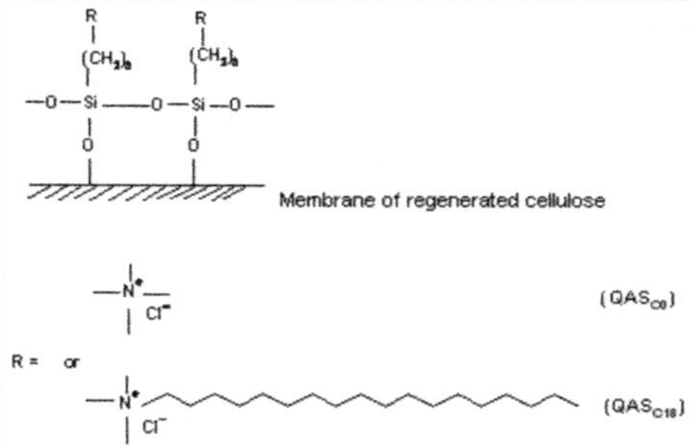	Meng et al. (2015)
Chitosan reacted with with glycidyl trimethylammonium chloride and dye	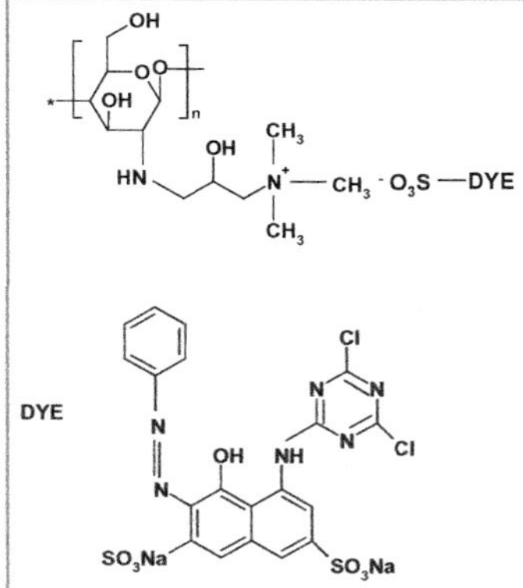	Tang et al. (2015)

(continued)

Table 5.2 (continued)

Quaternary ammonium polymers	Chemical formulas	References
N-(2-hydroxyl)propyl-3-trimethyl ammonium chitosan *N*-QxCS (x = 1–3) as of N-quaternary chitosan derivatives	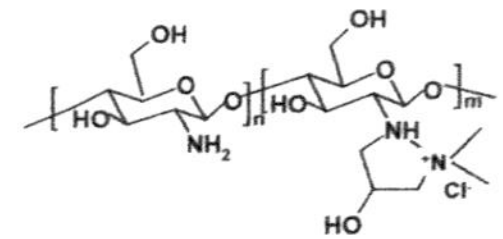 N-Q_xCS (x=1-3)	Chen et al. (2016)
O-sulfobetaine-*N*-(2-hydroxyl)propyl-3-trimethyl ammonium chitosan chloride Q3ByCS (y = 1–3) as zwitterionic chitosan derivatives	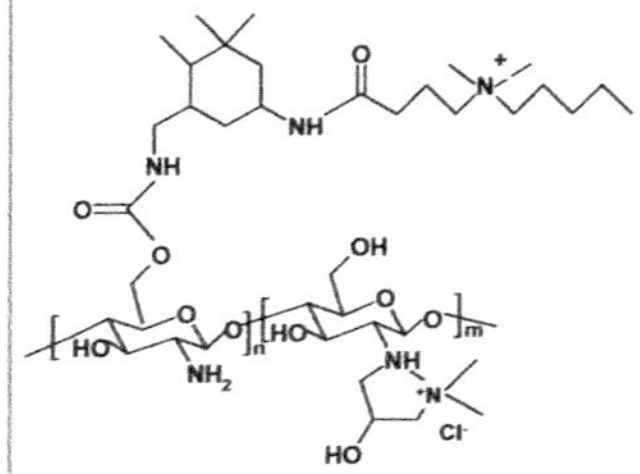 Q_3B_yCS (y=1-3)	
Cationic amphiphilic dextran derivatives	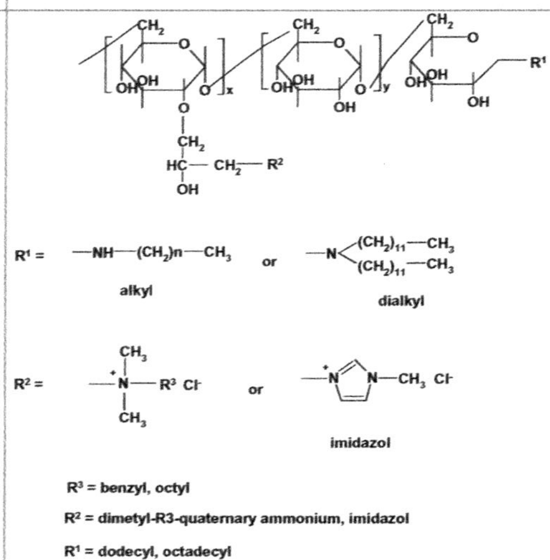	Tuchilus et al. (2017)

Cashew gum quaternized with (3-chloro-2-hydroxypropyl) trimethylammonium chloride	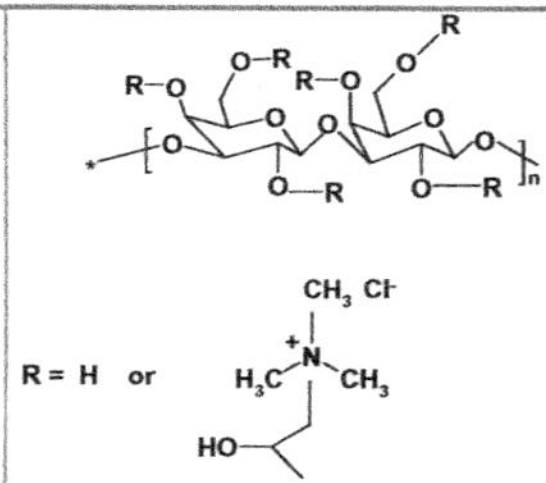	Quelemes et al. (2017)
Polyurethane bearing *N*-tetraethanolammonium bromide	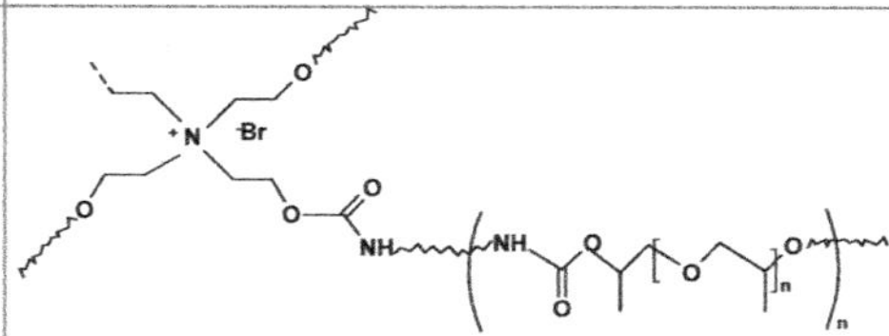	Udabe et al. (2017)
Poly(siloxane) quaternary ammonium salts containing epoxy group	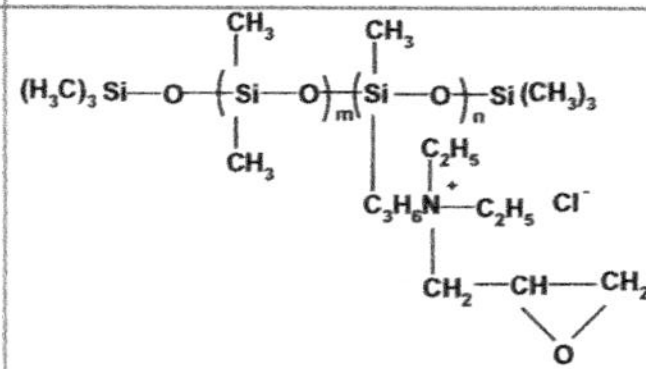	Cui et al. (2015)
Quaternized multi block copolymers composed of dithiocarbonate-terminated poly(dimethylsiloxane) PDMS, poly(2-(dimethylamino)ethyl methacrylate) quaternized with n-octyliodide, poly(hexafluorobutyl methacrylate) and hydroxyethyl methacrylate	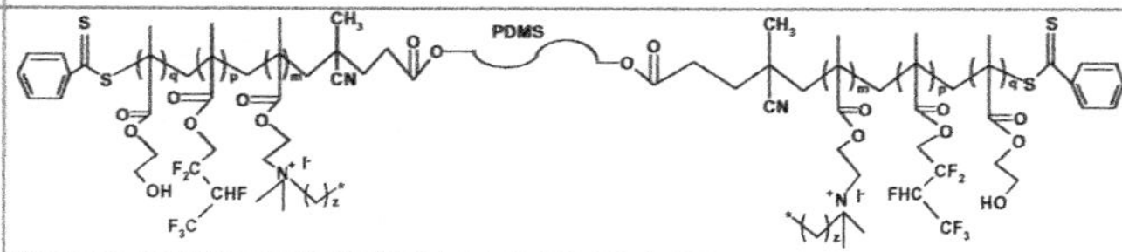	Zhou et al. (2015)

Table 5.3 Antimicrobial activity of polymers with quaternary ammonium moieties

Polymeric antimicrobials	Tested microorganisms	Microbiological parameters/tests			References
Natural polymers					
$RC\text{-}QAS_{(C0)}$ membrane	*E. coli* (DH5α)				Meng et al. (2015)
	S. aureus (ATCC 6538)	Cell viability (%)			
			$RC\text{-}QAS_{(C0)}$	$RC\text{-}QAS_{(C18)}$	
$RC\text{-}QAS_{(C18)}$ membrane	Original inoculum:				
	1× 10^6 CFU/mL	*E. coli*	~99.9	0.4	
		S. aureus	~99.9	0.5	
Hydrogels containing quaternized cellulose (QC) and native cellulose:	*Saccharomyces cerevisiae* N85	Cell viability (%)			Peng et al. (2016)
	Original inoculum:	Gel9-2	88		
	10^6–10^7CFU/mL	Gel9-4	33.3		
		Gel9-6	33.6		
Gel9-2 (D.S. 0.23)		Gel25-2	87.1		
Gel9-4 (D.S. 0.42)		Gel25-4	66.9		
Gel9-6 (D.S. 0.61)		Gel25-6	19.9		
Gel25-2 (D.S. 0.28)					
Gel25-4 (D.S. 0.44)					
Gel25-6 (D.S. 0.69)					
NQC	S1: *B. subtilis* RCMB 010067	Diameter of inhibition zone (mm)			Mohamed et al. (2015)
Q1P3	S2: *S. aureus* RCMB 010028				

Q1P1	S3: *Klebsiella pneumoniae* RCMB 0010093		NQC	Q1P3	Q1P1	Q3P1	Genta micin	Ampi cilin	Amphotericin B
Q3P1	S4: *E. coli* RCMB 010052	S1	8	13–17	15–19	12–16	26	–	
	S5: *Aspergillus fumigatus* RCMB 02568	S2	11	15–19	16–20	14–17	22	–	
	S6: *Geotricum candidum* RCMB 05097	S3	11	16–20	17–20	15–18	–	28	
		S4	13	17–22	17–25	16–20	–	32	
		S5	11	13–20	15–20	13–18			24
		S6	10	13–21	13–23	13–19			29
HACC/PVA/PEO hydrogel	*S. aureus* RCMB 000106	Diameter of inhibition zone (qualitative test)							Fan et al. (2015)
	E. coli RCMB 000107	*S. aureus*				*E. coli*			
		++				++			
QCh	*S. aureus* 749	Bactericidal activity in time (h)							Ignatova et al. (2016)
Car	*E. coli* 3588 (National Bank for Industrial Microorganisms and Cell Cultures, Sofia, Bulgaria)					*S. aureus*		*E. coli*	
CA/PHB		CA (1800 mg/mL)				24		–	
QCh/Car-coated PHB		CA/PHB				24		24	
QCh/Car-(CA/PHB)		QCh (3000 mg/mL)				1		2	
CA/QCh/Car-PHB		QCh/Car-coated PHB				4		6	
		QCh/ Car-(CA/PHB)				3		4	
		CA/QCh/Car-PHB				3		4	

(continued)

Table 5.3 (continued)

Polymeric antimicrobials	Tested microorganisms	Microbiological parameters/tests					References
CTS	*E. coli*	Diameter of inhibition zone (mm)					Tang et al. (2015)
CTS–CTA	*S. aureus*						
(CTS–CTA)–I_2					*E. coli*	*S. aureus*	
		CTS			0	0	
		CTS–CTA			11	14	
		(CTS–CTA)–I_2			23	23	
CS		Inhibitory index (%) at 1.0 mg/mL polymer					Tan et al. (2016)
CSB	S1: *Fusarium oxysporum*						
CSC			S1	S2	S3		
CSDC	S2: *Colletotrichum lagenarium*						
CSTC		CS	11.8	25	–		
CSTF		CSB	55.8	69.1	–		
	S3: *Phomopsis asparagi*	CSC	69.6	73.5	–		
		CSDC	71	76.5	~ 80		
		CSTC	73.9	77.9	~ 80		
		CSTF	78.5	82.4	~ 80		

CS		Inhibitory index (%) at 1.0 mg/mL polymer				Li et al. (2016)
TCTS	S1:*Colletotrichum lagenarium*					
CTCTS	(Pass) Ell.et halst ATCC30016		S1	S2	S3	
BTCTS						
	S2:*Fusarium oxysporum f.sp. niveum* ATCC 36116	CS	30	24.2	14.7	
		TCTS	85.1	58.5	86.1	
		CTCTS	93.2	84	91.7	
	S3:*Fusarium oxysporum.f.sp. cucumebrium* Owen ATCC 42357	BTCTS	88.1	81.8	91.7	
Cs	*E. coli* 25922	Diameter of inhibition zone (mm)			Minimum inhibitory concentration (μg/mL)	Oyervides-Munoz et al. (2017)
BZK-Cs	*S. aureus* 25923					
TEA-Cs			*E. coli*	*S. aureus*	*E. coli* / *S. aureus*	
PYA-Cs	Original inoculum:					
BTP-Cs	10^8 CFU/mL	Cs	21	21	256 / 256	
		BZK-Cs	25	24	128 / 128	
		TEA-Cs	23	22	128 / 128	
		PYA-Cs	27	26	128 / 64	
		BTP-Cs	27	24	128 / 512	

(continued)

Table 5.3 (continued)

Polymeric antimicrobials	Tested microorganisms	Microbiological parameters/tests							References
CS		Diameter of inhibition zone (mm)							Wang et al. (2016)
BNQAS-CS			CS	BNQAS-CS	C12QAS-CS	C14QAS-CS	C16QAS-CS	C18QAS-CS	
C12QAS-CS									
C14QAS-CS	S1: *S. aureus* ATCC 6538	S1	6.5–11	8–14	8–17	8–15	8–14	7–12	
C16QAS-CS	S2: α-*Hemolytic Streptococcus* (α-H-tococcus, CMCC(B) 31005)	S2	8–12	7–11	9–10	8–12	8–15	7–13	
C18QAS-CS	S3: *β-Hemolytic Streptococcus* (β-H-tococcus, ATCC 21059)	S3	–	7–11	10–16	9–14	9–14	9–14	
	S4: *E.coli* ATCC 25922	S4	7–12	7–12	6–11	7–11	7–11	7–11	
	S5: *P. aeruginosa* ATCC 9027	S5	–	–	8–10	7–11	6–10	–	
	S6: *Proteus vulgaris* CMCC(B) 49027	S6	–	–	7–10	8–12	7–9	–	
	S7: *Aspergillus* CMCC(F) 98003	S7	7	8–16	8–16	7–13	8–16	7–13	
	S8: *C. albicans* ATCC 10231	S8	7–9.5	8–12	8–12	10–14	11–15	8–13	
Chitosan biopolymer dye	*E. coli*	Cell viability (%)							Tang et al. (2016)
	S. aureus	*E. coli*		*S. aureus*					
	Original inoculum:	< 0.1 (after 24 h)		< 0.1 (after 24 h)					
	2.3x 10^8 CFU/mL								

CS	*S. aureus* (ATCC 6538)	Diameter of inhibition zone (mm)			Chen et al. (2016)
N-QCS	*E. coli* (ATCC 25922)				
N-Q2CS			*S. aureus*	*E. coli*	
N-Q3CS	Original inoculum:				
Q3BCS	10^8 CFU/mL	CS	6	6	
Q3B2CS		N-QCS	6	6	
Q3B3CS		N-Q2CS	9	10	
		N-Q3CS	15	15	
		Q3BCS	15	16	
		Q3B2CS	17	17	
		Q3B3CS	18	18	
CS	*S. aureus* ATCC 6538	MIC (w/v %) for tested microorganisms			Li et al. (2015)
OQCS	*E. coli* ATCC 8739				
OQCATUCS-1	*A. niger* ATCC 16404	OQCS		0.025–0.06	
OQCATUCS-3	*P. aeruginosa* ATCC 9027				
OQCATUCS-5	*B. subtilis* ATCC 6633	OQCATUCS		0.0125–0.025	
	Original inoculum:				
	10^8 CFU/mL				

(continued)

Table 5.3 (continued)

Polymeric antimicrobials	Tested microorganisms	Microbiological parameters/tests												References
QCS-*co*-MMA copolymers:	*Streptococcus mutans* ATCC 25175	Inhibition rate (%)												Song et al (2016)
Material 1 (physically prepared)	*C. albicans* ATCC 90028		*S.mutans*							*C.albicans*				
	Original inoculum:													
	5–10 × 10^5 CFU / mL	Material 1	70–85							20–65				
Material 2 (chemically prepared)		Material 2	25–70							0				
A1-A8	S1: *S. aureus* ATCC 25923		DIZ (mm)							MIC and MBC/MFC (mg/mL)				Tuchilus et al. (2017)
	S2: *Sarcina lutea* ATCC 9341		S1	S2	S3	S4	S5	S6	S7	S1		S5		
										MIC	MBC	MIC	MFC	
	S3: *E. coli* ATCC 25922	A1	14	14	0	0	11	13	13	1.25	2.5	2.5	5	
	S4: *P. aeruginosa* ATCC 27853	A2	14	15	11	0	12	13	20	1.25	2.5	2.5	5	
	S5: *C. albicans* ATCC 90028	A3	13	14	11	0	12	12	20	1.25	2.5	2.5	5	
	S6: *C. glabrata* ATCC MYA2950	A4	13	13	0	0	12	12	20	1.25	2.5	2.5	5	
	S7: *C. parapsilosis* ATCC 22019	A5	10	14	0	0	13	12	20	1.25	2.5	2.5	5	
		A6	15	14	0	0	15	13	22	0.6	1.25	1.25	2.5	
		A7	15	18	11	0	14	15	23	0.6	1.25	1.25	2.5	
		A8	0	0	0	0	10	11	15	–	–	–	–	

P-*g*-pAPTAC1	*S. aureus* ATCC 25923		Diameter of inhibition zone (mm)							Grigoras et al. (2013)
P-*g*-pAPTAC2		P-*g*-pAPTAC1	8.5 -10							
P-*g*-pAPTAC3		P-*g*-pAPTAC2	7 – 9							
		P-*g*-pAPTAC3	9 – 10							
QCG-1	S1: *S. aureus* ATCC 29213 (MSSA)	MIC (μg/mL) and MBC (μg/mL) of QCG derivatives against *Staphylococcus sp.*								Quelemes et al. (2017)
			QCG-1		QCG-2		QCG-3		Control	
QCG-2	S2: *S. aureus* ATCC 25923 (MSSA)		MIC	MBC	MIC	MBC	MIC	MBC	MIC	
QCG-3	S3: *S. aureus* MS52 (MSSA) (skin burn)	S1	1000	1000	250	250	125	125	< 0.25	
	S4: *S. aureus* ATCC 43300 (MRSA)	S2	1000	1000	125	125	125	125	< 0.25	
	S5: *S. aureus*-Col (MRSA)	S3	1000	1000	250	500	125	250	0.25	
	S6: *S. aureus* MR17 (MRSA) (surgical wound)	S4	500	1000	62.5	62.5	62.5	62.5	0.5	

(continued)

Table 5.3 (continued)

Polymeric antimicrobials	Tested microorganisms	Microbiological parameters/tests								References
	S7: *S. aureus* MR359 (MRSA) (surgical wound)	S5	1000	1000	125	125	62.5	125	0.5	
	S8: *S. aureus* MR0405 (MRSA) (nasal secretion)	S6	500	1000	62.5	125	31.25	62.5	0.5	
	S9: *S. epidermidis* ATCC 12228 (MSSE)	S7	1000	1000	125	250	125	125	0.5	
	S10: *S. epidermidis* MR 111 (MRSE) (blood culture)	S8	1000	>1000	125	250	62.5	125	0.5	
	S11: *S. epidermidis* 70D (MRSE) (blood culture)	S9	62.5	1000	31.25	250	31.25	250	0.5	
	Original inoculum:	S10	1000	1000	125	500	125	250	1.0	
	5×10^5 CFU/mL	S11	1000	1000	125	250	125	125	1.0	

PLA-N	*E. coli* ATCC 25922	Bacterial reduction R (%) in the presence of PLA derivatives				Logar et al. (2016)
PLA-Ag	*S. aureus* ATCC 6538					
PLA-SiQAC			c_{Ag} (mg/kg)	R (%)		
PLA-RV-Ag				*E.coli*	*S.aureus*	
PLA-RV-Ag-SiQAC	Original inoculum:	PLA-N	0	–	–	
		PLA-Ag	9	50	59	
	1–2 × 10^5 CFU / mL	PLA-SiQAC	0	68	78	
		PLA-RV-Ag	140	100	100	
		PLA-RV-Ag-SiQAC	53	100	100	
PLA film	*P. aeruginosa*	Bacterial reduction R (%) in the presence of PLA derivatives				Staneva et al. (2015)
B-PLA film	*E. coli*		R (%)			
			P. aeruginosa	*E. coli*		
		PLA film	7	19		
		B-PLA film	31	25		
Synthetic polymers						
Modified PAMAM dendrimers	*S. aureus*		MIC (μg/mL)	MBC (μg/mL)	DIZ (mm)	Maleki et al. (2017)
	B. subtilis					
(G4I)	*Klebsiella oxytoca*	*S. aureus*	52	64	31	
	E. coli	*B. subtilis*	50	67	28	
		Klebsiella oxytoca	55	71	26	
		E. coli	57	75	25	

(continued)

Table 5.3 (continued)

Polymeric antimicrobials	Tested microorganisms	Microbiological parameters/tests			References
PU foams	*E. coli* ATCC 25922	Antimicrobial efficiency (%) of PU foams toward bacteria strain			Udabe et al. (2017)
	S. aureus ATCC 29737		*E. coli*	*S.aureus*	
		PU foam 1	36	61	
		PU foam 2	38	1	
		PU foam 3	11	90	
		PU foam 4	2	4	
		PU foam 6	66	0	
QASs: 3a, 3b, 3c, 3d	*S. aureus*	MIC (μg/mL) for QASs			Liu et al. (2015)
PU=PU coating without QAS	*E. coli*		*S. aureus*	*E.coli*	
QAS-containing PU coatings:		3a	62.5	500	
PU(1)=compound 3b, 5 wt%		3b	31.25	250	
PU(2)= compound 3b, 9 wt%		3c	31.25	62.5	
PU(3)= compound 3b, 13 wt%		3d	15.63	62.5	
PU(4)= compound 3b, 16 wt%		Bacterial reduction R (%) in the presence of QAS-containing PU coatings			
PU(5)= compound 3a, 5 wt%			*S.aureus*	*E.coli*	
PU(6)= compound 3c, 5 wt%		PU	0	0	

PU(7)= compound 3d, 5 wt%		PU(1)		29.4			25.3		
		PU(2)		30.4			28.5		
		PU(3)		36.3			35.0		
		PU(4)		55			45.2		
		PU(5)		27.5			23.6		
		PU(6)		36.7			29.7		
		PU(7)		37.8			32.2		
P(SiO) m(SiOQAEp): P1 (M_w = 3150 g/mol)	*E. coli*	MBC (× 10^{-5} mol/L)							Cui et al. (2015)
P2 (M_w = 4670 g/mol)	*S. aureus*		P1	P2		P3	P4		
P3 (M_w = 7520 g/mol)	*Bacillus subtilis*	*E. coli*	1.4	0.5		0.65	0.1		
P4 (M_w = 13000 g/mol)		*S. aureus*	1.75	0.7		0.45	0.2		
		B. subtilis	2.7	1.5		0.25	0.3		
C_m-PSi-C_m (m= 8, 10, 12, 14, 16, 18)	*E. coli*	Zones of inhibition R (in mm) of 1.0 wt% C_m-PSi-C_m against microorganisms							Bao et al. (2017)
	S. aureus *Aspergillus flavus*		m= 8	m= 10	m= 12	m= 14	m= 16	m= 18	
		E. coli	-	3.5	3	2	1.5	1.5	
		S. aureus	2	4	3.5	3	2.5	2.5	
		A. flavus	–	2	2.5	3	2.5	–	

(continued)

Table 5.3 (continued)

Polymeric antimicrobials	Tested microorganisms	Microbiological parameters/tests					References
PDMS-*b*-QPDMAEMA40	*B. subtilis*	Antimicrobial activity of block copolymer films					Qin et al. (2015)
PDMS-*b*-QPDMAEMA60	*E. coli*		P-*b*-Q40	P-*b*-Q60	P-*b*-Q80	P-*b*-Q100	
PDMS-*b*-QPDMAEMA80		*B. subtilis*	+	+	+	+	
PDMS-*b*-QPDMAEMA100		*E. coli*	–	–	–	+	
Quaternized CBABC copolymers	*B. subtilis* ATCC 63501	Antimicrobial activity of the multi-block copolymer films					Zhou et al. (2015)
	E. coli ATCC 44752						
	Original inoculum:		*B. subtilis*		*E. coli*		
	10^5–10^6 CFU/mL	PDMS-QPM_{80}	+		+		
		PDMS-QPM_{80}-PF_{30}	+		+		
		PDMS-QPM_{80}-PF_{52}	+		+		
		PDMS-QPM_{80}-PF_{70}	–		–		

Quat-modified PE 1-9	*S. aureus*	Antibacterial activity of modified PE samples containing 5 wt-% quat (after leaching)				Rossetti et al. (2017)
		Quat-PE	*S. aureus*	*E. coli*	*P. aeruginosa*	
	E. coli	1	++	++	n.a.	
	P. aeruginosa	2	–	n.a.	n.a.	
		3	–	n.a.	n.a.	
		4	++	+/–	++	
		5	–	n.a.	–	
		6	++	++	++	
		7	+	+	++	
		9	+	–	++	
		Notes: The amount of quat 8 available was not sufficient for a thorough investigation; however, in preliminary experiments it was found to have good antibacterial activity against *S. aureus*; ++: most bacteria are dead; +: proportion of dead bacteria clearly increased compared to PE reference; +/–: different results with different samples; –: proportion of dead bacteria not increased compared to PE reference.				

Legend: CFU = colony forming units; CV = cell viability (%); DIZ = diameter of inhibition zone (mm); MIC = minimum inhibitory concentration; MBC = minimum bactericidal concentration; MFC = minimum fungicidal concentration;

Inhibitory index (%) = $(1 - D_a/D_b) \times 100$ (1)

where D_a is the diameter of the growth zone in the test plates and D_b is the diameter of the growth zone in the control plate

Zones of inhibition R (mm) = $(D_1 - D_2)/2$ (2)

where D_1 is diameter of transparent zone in mm, D_2 is diameter of 20 mm filter paper

$RC\text{-}QAS_{(C0)}$ = regenerated cellulose (RC) membrane including trimethoxysilylpropyl trimethyl ammonium chloride

$RC\text{-}QAS_{(C18)}$ = regenerated cellulose (RC) membrane including trimethoxysilylpropyl octadecyldimethyl ammonium chloride

CS; Cs; CTS; Ch = chitosan

NQC = N-trimethyl ammmonium chitosan chloride

Q1P3, Q1P1 and Q3P1 = hydrogels composed of N-quaternized chitosan (NQC) and poly(vinyl alcohol) (PVA) in different weight ratios (1:3), (1:1) and (3:1) chemically crosslinked by glutaraldehyde (GA) in different weight ratios (1.0 and 5.0%)

HACC/PVA/PEO hydrogel = hybrid hydrogel based on quaternary ammonium chitosan (HACC) combined with poly(vinylalcohol) (PVA) and poly(ethylene oxide) (PEO) obtained by γ-irradiated crosslilnking

QCh = *N,N,N*-trimethylchitosan iodide (quaternized chitosan)

Car = *k*-carrageenan

(continued)

Table 5.3 (continued)

CA/PHB = poly(3-hydroxybutyrate) PHB fibers containing caffeic acid CA
QCh/Car-coated PHB = PHB fibers coated with QCh/Car complex
QCh/Car-(CA/PHB) = CA/PHB fibers coated with QCh/Car polyelectrolyte complex
CA/QCh/Car-PHB = PHB fibers coated with QCh/Car complex containing CA
CTS–CTA = N-(2-hydroxy) propyl-3-trimethylammonium chitosan chloride
(CTS–CTA)–I_2 = complex of CTS–CTA with iodine (1: 1.33 molar ratio)
CSB = chitosan-bromoacetate
CSC = chitosan-chloroacetate
CSDC = chitosan-dichloroacetate
CSTC = chitosan-trichloroacetate
CSTF = chitosan-trifluoroacetate
TCTS = chitosan derivative containing 1,2,3- triazole without halogen
CTCTS, BTCTS = chitosan derivatives containing 1,2,3- triazole with halogen (Cl or Br)
BZK-Cs = chitosan grafted with 4-bromobutyl-benzalkonium bromide (BZK-Br)
TEA-Cs = chitosan grafted with 4-bromobutyl-triethylammonium bromide (TEA-Br)
PYA-Cs = chitosan grafted with 4-bromobutyl-pyridinium bromide (PYA-Br)
BTP-Cs = chitosan grafted with a mixture of 1.5 mmol each of BZK-Br, TEA-Br and PYA-Br (1:1:1 M_w ratio)
QAS-CS = *O*-quaternary ammonium salt-chitosans bearing *N*-methyl-N-R-N, N-bis(2-hydroxyethyl) ammonium bromides (R = –benzyl (chloride, BNQAS-CS), –dodecyl (C12QAS-CS), –tetradecyl (C14QAS-CS), –hexadecyl (C16QAS-CS), –octadecyl (C18QAS-CS))
Chitosan biopolymer dye = obtained by insertion of Reactive red x-3b (dye containing sulfonate groups) in chitosan quaternary ammonium salt (*N*-(2-hydroxyl)propyl-3-trimethyl ammonium chitosan chloride)
N-Q_xCS (x = 1–3) = *N*-quaternary ammonium chitosan derivatives from quaternization of CS with glycidyl trimethylammonium chloride GTMAC
Q_3B_yCS (y = 1–3) = *O*-sulfobetaine-N-Q_3CS = *N*-quaternary ammonium-*O*-sulfobetaine-chitosan (zwitterionic compounds)
OQCS = *O*-quaternary ammonium chitosan
OQCATUCS-1, OQCATUCS-3, OQCATUCS-5 = *O*-quaternary ammonium *N*-acyl thiourea chitosan derivatives with 77% degree of quaternization substitution DSQ and different degree of acyl thiourea DSAT substitution of chitosan (81%, 87% and 93%, respectively)
QCS-*co*-MMA copolymers = copolymers of chitosan quaternary ammonium salt (QCS) and methyl methacrylate (MMA)
Material 1 = composite prepared by directly adding of QCS to Denture Powder (containing polyMMA) followed by adding of then the Denture Water (containing MMA monomer and trace amount of the cross-linking agent, inhibitor and UV absorber)
Material 2 = composite prepared by adding varying amount of QCS to the Denture Water, allowing QCS and MMA monomer to engraft
A1-A8 = cationic amphiphilic dextran derivatives with a long alkyl group (dodecylamine, octadecylamine or di-*N*-dodecylamine type) attached to the reductive end of the polysaccharide chain and quaternary ammonium groups (*N,N*-dimethyl-*N*-octylamine, *N,N*-dimethyl-*N*-benzylamine or 1-methylimidazol type) attached as pendent groups in the presence of epichlorohydrin ECH to the main dextran backbone (with variable molecular mass: M_n (GPC) = 8000 or 4500 g/mol)
P-*g*-pAPTAC1–3 = grafted pullulans (P) with 22.53, 29.05, and 34.51 (wt.%) content of poly(3-acrylamidopropyl) trimethylammonium chloride pAPTAC

QCG1–3 = quaternized cashew gum with different substitution degree (0.42, 0.68 and 0.73) of 3-chloro-2-hydroxypropyl) trimethylammonium chloride CHPTAC

PLA-N = non-treated poly(lactic acid) fabrics

PLA-Ag = poly(lactic acid) fabrics physically bonded with Ag

PLA-SiQAC = poly(lactic acid) fabrics chemically bonded with 3-(trimethoxysilyl)-propyldimethyltetradecyl ammonium chloride

PLA-RV-Ag = poly(lactic acid) fabrics coated with crosslinked Si-matrix and Ag

PLA-RV-Ag-SiQAC = poly(lactic acid) fabrics coated with crosslinked Si-matrix, Ag and 3-(trimethoxysilyl)-propyldimethyltetradecyl ammonium chloride

PLA film = polylactic acid film

B-PLA film = cationic water soluble fluorescent B possessing amino groups (1-[(7-oxo-7H-benzo[de]anthracen-3-ylcarbamoyl)-methyl]-triethylammonium chloride) incorporated into thin polylactic acid film

Modified PAMAM dendrimers = modified poly(amidoamine) PAMAM dendrimers (generations G2 and G4) into quaternary ammonium salts using Cl, Br, I halogens groups (G2Cl, G2Br, G2I, G4Cl, G4Br, and G4I)

PU foams = poly(urethane) PU foams 1–9 with different quatermary ammonium content: PU foam 1 (5.4% quaternary ammonium content); PU foam 2 (7.2% quaternary ammonium content); PU foam 3 (containing poly(hexamethylene diisocyanate) pHDI and 16% quaternary ammonium content); PU foam 4 (containing toluene diisocyanate TDI); PU foam 6 (0% quaternary ammonium content)

3a-d = terpene-based carbamate group-containing QASs synthesized through the quaternization of terpene-based carbamate with alkyl bromides

QAS-containing PU coatings = polyurethane coatings containing quaternary ammonium salts; QASs incorporated into PU through crosslinking with terpene-based polyol and polyisocyanate (hydrophilically modified hexamethylene diisocyanate (HDI) tripolymer)

$P(SiO)_m(SiOQAEp)$ = P1-P4 polysiloxane quaternary ammonium salt containing epoxy group obtained from polysiloxane containing tertiary amino group $P(SiO)_m(SiOTA)n$ and epichlorohydrin by quaternization (where m is the length of hydrophobic (organosilicon group) chains, and n is the length of hydrophilic (quaternary ammonium group) chains) with $n = 7.86–20.14$, and $m/n = 1.67–2.67$

C_m-PSi-C_m = cationic gemini surfactants with polyether siloxane linked group and quaternary ammonium hydrophilic head group (C_m-PSi-C_m, m = 8, 10, 12, 14, 16, 18)

PDMS-b-QPDMAEMA = block copolymers based on poly(dimethylsiloxane) PDMS macro-chain transfer agent and poly(N,N-dimethylaminoethyl methacrylate (DMAEMA) quaternized with n-octyliodide

Quaternized CBABC copolymers = CBABC-type fluorosilicone multi-block copolymers (containing dithiocarbonate-terminated PDMS, PDMAEMA and PHFBMA) quaternized with n-octyliodide

PDMS-PM_{80} = BAB-type triblock copolymer PDMS-*b*-[PDMAEMA-*b*-P(DMAEMA-*co*-HEMA)]$_2$ containing poly(dimethylsiloxane) PDMS, poly(2-(dimethylamino)ethyl methacrylate) PDMAEMA and hydroxyethyl methacrylate HEMA

PDMS-QPM = quaternized copolymer PDMS-*b*-[PDMAEMA-*b*-P(DMAEMA-*co*-HEMA)]$_2$

PDMS-PM_{80}-PF_{30}, PDMS-PM_{80}-PF_{52} and PDMS-PM_{80}-PF_{70} = CBABC-type multi-block copolymers PDMS-*b*-[PDMAEMA-*b*-PHFBMA-*b*-P(HFBMA-*co*-HEMA)]$_2$ with three different contents of the poly(hexafluorobutyl methacrylate) PHFBMA blocks

PDMS-QPM-PF = quaternized multi-block copolymer PDMS-*b*-[PDMAEMA-*b*-PHFBMA-*b*-P(HFBMA-*co*-HEMA)]$_2$

Quat-modified PE 1–9 = composites of poly(ethylene) PE with mono- or bifunctional quaternary ammonium salts (benzyldimethylstearylammonium chloride (1); trimethylstearylammonium chloride (2); dimethyldistearylammonium chloride (3); methyltristearylammonium bromide (4); tetrastearylammonium bromide (5); 1,12-bis(dimethyloctylammonium)dodecane dibromide (6); 1,20-bis(dimethyloctylammonium)eicosane dibromide (7); 1,30-bis(dimethyloctylammonium)triacontane dibromide (8); bis(dimethyloctylammonium)PEG(400) ditosylate (9)) containing quaternary ammonium moieties. It could be observed that diameter of inhibition had values of 6–25 mm for quaternized compounds compared with their precursors characterized by lower or nonexistent antimicrobial activity. Also, for a constant concentration of potential biocidal polymer, diameter of inhibition zone increased in accordance with quaternization degree of polymers. In some cases, values of diameter of inhibition zone were lower than those recorded in presence of standard antibiotics (22–32 nm).

After a variable time of microorganisms incubation in presence of polymeric antimicrobials containing quaternary ammonium moieties, e.g. 4 h for hydrogels containing quaternized cellulose and native cellulose (Peng et al. 2016); 12 h for regenerated cellulose membranes including trimethoxysilylpropyl trimethyl ammonium chloride or trimethoxysilylpropyl octadecyldimethyl ammonium chloride (Meng et al. 2015) or 24 h for chitosan biopolymer dye (Tang et al. 2016), cell viability (%) was considerably reduced. This decrease in cell viability was inversely proportional to the alkyl chain dimension, substitution degree of ionizable groups in polymer chain and incubation time period. A similar behavior was observed in case of bacterial reduction. For example, for poly(urethane) coatings containing quaternary ammonium salts, this parameter had the highest value in case of compound with the longest hydrophobic alkyl chains of the whole series (Liu et al. 2015). In other case, if poly(lactic acid) fabrics coated with crosslinked Si-matrix contained 3-(trimethoxysilyl)-propyldimethyltetradecyl ammonium chloride and silver nanoparticles, the bacterial reduction represented a synergistic effect of quaternary ammonium groups and silver (Logar et al. 2016).

Because the quality and antiseptic properties of a substance are not assured only by a bacteriostatic effect, usually bactericidal activity is also examined (https://emerypharma.com/biology/minimum-inhibitory-concentration/). Literature reports that bacteriostatic activity is associated with a ratio of minimum bactericidal concentration to minimum inhibitory concentration greater than 4, although determination of this ratio is affected by numerous factors and technical problems. Regarding *in vitro* microbiological activity, it has been found that, at high concentrations, some antibacterial agents considered bacteriostatic are often bactericidal towards some susceptible organisms, while at low concentrations, other bactericidal drugs simply exhibit bacteriostatic effect. *In vitro* bacteriostatic or bactericidal data provide information about potential action of antimicrobial agents because only clinical results are relevant in treatment of bacterial infections. Thus, presumption that bactericidal agents are superior compared with bacteriostatic agents was invalidated by clinical results: meningitis, usually treated with bactericidal drugs, was effectively cured with bacteriostatic agents (Pankey and Sabath 2004).

In case of cationic amphiphilic dextran derivatives with a long alkyl group and quaternary ammonium moieties, minimum bactericidal concentration was two times lower than minimum inhibitory concentration; same results was recorded between minimum fungicidal concentration and minimum inhibitory concentration (Tuchilus et al. 2017). In the same time, values of minimum inhibitory concentration were insignificantly different from minimum bactericidal concentration values for the most quaternized cashew gums with different substitution degree of

(3-chloro-2-hydroxypropyl) trimethylammonium chloride (Quelemes et al. 2017), while for poly(amidoamine) dendrimers modified with halogenated quaternary ammonium salts, values of minimum bactericidal concentration were slightly higher than minimum inhibitory concentration values (Maleki et al. 2017). Study about antimicrobial activity of poly(siloxane) quaternary ammonium salts containing epoxy group revealed that microbiological parameters indirectly have been influenced by concentration of quaternary ammonium groups such that minimum bactericidal concentration values generally decreased with increase of molecular weight of polymers (Cui et al. 2015).

5.6 Factors That Influence Antimicrobial Activity

Beside already presented heterogeneous chemical composition of microorganisms responsible for hydrophilic, hydrophobic, lipophilic or amphiphilic character of microbial entities, there are other factors that influence antimicrobial activity of substances (Table 5.4). Higher is the *degree of substitution* of ionizable groups, more potent is the antimicrobial activity. Because of a large number of incorporated positive charges in modified polymers, *charge density* increases with increase in zeta potential values for macromolecules in solution. *Molecular weight of polymer* is another characteristic that could indirectly influence charge density. By increasing degree of substitution, molecular weight of polymer increase and more electrostatic interactions are established between biomembranes and antimicrobial substances (Wang et al. 2016; Quelemes et al. 2017). A higher antimicrobial activity was recorded with an increase in molecular weight, in case of poly(siloxane) quaternary ammonium salts containing epoxy group compared with their precursor (Cui et al. 2015).

Depending on *position of the biological active quaternary ammonium groups* in polymer structure (usually pendant, and rarely in side chain) and their *steric hindrance*, the *flexibility* and *conformation* of macromolecular chains may vary, influencing thus probability of interactions between cationic quaternary ammonium groups and anionic components of microorganisms (Bao et al. 2017). Flexible chains bearing quaternary ammonium groups have a facile access to components of microorganisms, while an extended conformation enhances antimicrobial effect (Grigoras et al. 2013). Also, *probability of electrostatic interactions* depends on *density/concentration of quaternary ammonium bearing grafts* on polymer backbone which is indirectly related to degree of substitution of ionizable groups (Grigoras et al. 2013). For example, in case of wastewater treatment industry, the number of grafts on polymeric backbone is important. Thus, flocculation properties of some quaternary ammonium type materials were enhanced with increase of grafting ratio, because cell wall of pathological *E. coli* was destroyed by electrostatic interactions established between modified starches and biomembranes (Huang et al. 2017).

Table 5.4 Physical, chemical and physicochemical factors that influence antimicrobial activity of compounds bearing quaternary ammonium moieties

Factors	References
Degree of substitution of macromolecules	Peng et al. (2016), Li et al. (2015)
Molecular weight of polymers	Wang et al. (2016), Quelemes et al. (2017), Cui et al. (2015)
Charge density of macromolecular chain	Chen et al. (2016), Tuchilus et al. (2017)
Zeta potential of antimicrobials	Chen et al. (2016), Tuchilus et al. (2017)
Position of biological active quaternary ammonium groups in polymer structure: pendant or lateral	Tuchilus et al. (2017)
Steric hindrance of quaternary ammonium groups	Bao et al. (2017)
Flexibility of macromolecular chains	Grigoras et al. (2013), Lv et al. (2018)
Conformation of polymer chains	Grigoras et al. (2013)
Pendant chain dimensions or length of alkyl chains between quaternary ammonium groups and polymer backbone	Tuchilus et al. (2017)
Hydrophilic–hydrophobic balance	Tuchilus et al. (2017)
Critical micelle concentration	Tuchilus et al. (2017)
Density of the grafts on polymer backbone	Grigoras et al. (2013)
Chemical structure of polymer; polyampholyte or polyzwitterionic character of antimicrobials	Chen et al. (2016), Tuchilus et al. (2017)
Electronegativity of different substituted groups	Tan et al. (2016), Li et al. (2016)
pH of medium and type of solvent used for formation of polymeric solutions	Meng et al. (2015)
Surface morphology of polymeric films	Rossetti et al. (2017)
Synergistic antimicrobial effect of different reactive groups	Li et al. (2015), Tang et al. (2015), Tan et al. (2016), Li et al. (2016), Oyervides-Munoz et al. (2017), Ignatova et al. (2016), Logar et al. (2016), Mohamed et al. (2015)

Taking into account *hydrophilic–hydrophobic balance*, some researchers designed antimicrobials with polyampholyte or polyzwitterion character. Presence of hydrophobic *alkyl chains with variable lengths* between hydrophilic quaternary ammonium groups and polymer backbone could be tuned from synthesis conditions; the length of alkyl chain being thus a critical parameter. In this way, chemical structure of polymer, namely ratio between hydrophobic moiety and hydrophilic part, has a decisive role on antimicrobial activity. If hydrophobicity is enhanced by a long alkyl chain, penetration of quaternary ammonium groups through a hydrophobic biological membrane, mainly composed from proteins and phospholipids, is assured, and efficiency of antimicrobials with quaternary ammonium groups is improved (Meng et al. 2015; Bao et al. 2017). It seems that, usually, an octyl chain in structure of polymers is the best choice to design such polymeric antimicrobials containing quaternary ammonium moieties (Tuchilus et al. 2017; Qin et al. 2015). Since longer alkyl chains are more flexible, they can patch and mask the quaternary ammonium chains, so that electrostatic interactions will be limited and the antimicrobial potential of the substances will decrease (Lv et al. 2018).

Another issue concerns the correlation between self-aggregation state of quaternized macromolecules and their antimicrobial activity. Experiments revealed that some chemical agents were microbiologically active only in self-assembled form when minimum inhibitory concentration value was almost the same with that of critical micelle concentration; others were efficient at concentrations higher or lower than their critical micelle concentration. In addition, bacteriostatic or bactericidal character of a substance is dictated by relationship between minimum bactericidal concentration and minimum inhibitory concentration; for example, in case of quaternized dextrans, minumum inhibitory concentration recorded a value of 20 times greater than minimum bacterial concentration (Singh et al. 2008).

Electronegativity of different substituted groups with halogens in polymeric quaternary ammonium salts is a sensitive factor that influenced antifungal activities of halogenated derivatives of chitosan acetate (Tan et al. 2016) or of chitosan derivatives with halogeno-1,2,3-triazole (Li et al. 2016). It was observed that as electronegativity increased in the order trifluoromethyl > trichloromethyl > dichloromethyl > chloromethyl > bromomethyl, antifungal activity recorded same trend. Halogenated groups with stronger electronegativity have ability to draw more electrons from surrounding cationic amino groups of polymeric ammonium salts, and positive charge densities of cationic amino groups was consequently enhanced. Cationic amino groups possessing higher positive charge densities are more likely to interact with anionic components of fungal entities, such as mannan, glucan, proteins, and lipids, thereby blocking the proper transport of essential nutrients into cell.

pH of medium and type of solvent influence the polymer solubility, conformation of macromolecular chains and accessibility of cationic quaternary ammonium groups to anionic components of microorganisms. For example, chitosan, a biopolymer with intrinsec antimicrobial properties, become soluble in water if a small quantity of acid is added in solution such that glucosamine units are transformed into positively charged moieties. In addition, in order to increase solubility and antibacterial activity of this polysaccharide, introduction of substituting groups represented a feasible choice, especially in case of quaternary ammonium groups.

Compared with macromolecules in solutions, where antimicrobial activity depends especially on flexibility of macromolecular chains, in case of polymeric films containing quaternary ammonium moieties, surface morphology is related with position of biological active quaternary ammonium groups confined on film surface. On the other hand, *morphology, roughness and topography of surface* are in close relationship with antimicrobial activity. A surface with relatively smooth morphology and lower surface roughness value presents an increased contact area favoring microorganism adhesion (Rossetti et al. 2017).

In order to increase antimicrobial performance of materials, researchers chemically modify macromolecules such that equipped them not just with quaternary ammonium moieties, but also with other types of reactive antimicrobial groups: acyl thiourea, triazole, halogen, benzalchonium or pyridinium (Li et al. 2015; Tang et al. 2015; Tan et al. 2016; Li et al. 2016; Oyervides-Munoz et al. 2017). When they made physical mixture, beside quaternized polymer bearing quaternary ammonium cations, they used molecules with antimicrobial properties like silver, *k*-carrageenan or caffeic acid (Ignatova et al. 2016; Logar et al. 2016). In some cases, the intrinsic antimicrobial properties of polymers like chitosan were combined with the properties of quaternary ammonium cations (Mohamed et al. 2015). In this way, dual antimicrobial materials have a *synergistic antimicrobial effect* against a broad spectrum of microorganisms.

5.7 Conclusions

Quaternary ammonium groups are versatile chemical entities with antimicrobial properties that could be introduced in various type of polymers in order to design more efficient biocides. Incorporation of quaternary ammonium groups or moieties can be accomplished by two pathways or approaches: chemical and physical. Each of them has advantages and disadvantages. Antimicrobial agents bonded on matrix by physical forces are released in a controlled manner into environment until their concentration decreases by leaching of antimicrobial system. In return, chemical bonded antimicrobial agents, accomplished by binding biocide moieties to polymer chains, form a permanent bio-barrier and act as a biological obstacle for microorganisms that come in contact with polymeric matrix. Although, from economical point of view, a permanent biocidal material is preferred over physically bonded material, the latter possess a higher specific surface area available for more contacts with pathogenic entities. Even if polymeric quaternary ammonium salts have various advantages like chemical stability, no volatility, and generally do not penetrate mucosa, biocompatibility and cytotoxicity tests are required in order to assess potential toxic effects before introducing them into clinical use.

Currently, there are numerous roughly qualitative studies in which antimicrobial effects are generally observed. For the progress of pharmaceutical industry and responsible use of resources, the need for simulation studies of molecular dynamics regarding interactions between quaternary ammonium compounds and model molecules, which have chemical structures similar to each component of the microorganism, should be considered. Also, it is desirable and should insist on design of materials with dual-antimicrobial functional groups to prevent resistance of the most aggressive microorganisms to antimicrobial substances.

References

Bao Y, Guo J, Ma J, Li M, Li X (2017) Physicochemical and antimicrobial activities of cationic gemini surfactants with polyether siloxane linked group. J Mol Liq 242:8–15. https://doi.org/10.1016/j.molliq.2017.06.049

Campos DA, Ribeiro AC, Costa EM, Fernandes JC, Tavaria FK, Araruna FB, Eiras C, Eaton P, Leite JRSA, Pintado MM (2012) Study of antimicrobial activity and atomic force microscopy imaging of the action mechanism of cashew tree gum. Carbohyd Polym 90:270–274. https://doi.org/10.1016/j.carbpol.2012.05.034

Chen Y, Li J, Li Q, Shen Y, Ge Z, Zhang W, Chen S (2016) Enhanced water-solubility, antibacterial activity and biocompatibility upon introducing sulfobetaine and quaternary ammonium to chitosan. Carbohyd Polym 143:246–253. https://doi.org/10.1016/j.carbpol.2016.01.073

Cheng KC, Demirci A, Catchmark JM (2011) Pullulan: biosynthesis, production, and applications. Appl Microbiol Biotechnol 92:29–44. https://doi.org/10.1007/s00253-011-3477-y

Cui X, Qiao C, Wang S, Ding Y, Hao C, Li J (2015) Synthesis, surface properties, and antibacterial activity of polysiloxane quaternary ammonium salts containing epoxy group. Coll Polym Sci 293:1971–1981. https://doi.org/10.1007/s00396-015-3588-6

de Paula RCM, Healthy F, Budd PM (1998) Characterization of *Anacardiumoccidentale* exudate polysaccharide. Polym Int 45:27–35. https://doi.org/10.1002/(SICI)1097-0126(199801)45:1<27::AID-PI900>3.0.CO;2-9

Eweis M, Elkholy SS, Elsabee MZ (2006) Antifungal efficacy of chitosan and its thiourea derivatives upon the growth of some sugar-beet pathogens. Int J Biol Macromol 38:1–8. https://doi.org/10.1016/j.ijbiomac.2005.12.009

Fan L, Yang J, Wu H, Hu Z, Yi J, Tong J, Zhu X (2015) Preparation and characterization of quaternary ammonium chitosan hydrogel with significant antibacterial activity. Int J Biol Macromol 79:830–836. https://doi.org/10.1016/j.ijbiomac.2015.04.013

Francolini I, Vuotto C, Piozzi A, Donelli G (2017) Antifouling and antimicrobial biomaterials: an overview. APMIS 125:392–417. https://doi.org/10.1111/apm.12675

Gettings RL, White WC (1987) Progress in the application of a surface-bonded antimicrobial agent. BioProducts Division, Dow Corning Corporation, Midland, MI

Grigoras AG, Constantin M, Grigoras VC, Dunca SI, Ochiuz L (2013) Studies on physico-chemical and antibacterial properties of grafted pullulans solutions. React Funct Polym 73:1249–1254. https://doi.org/10.1016/j.reactfunctpolym.2013.06.009

He W, Zhang Y, Li J, Gao Y, Luo F, Tan H, Wang K, Fu Q (2016) A novel surface structure consisting of contact-active antibacterial upper-layer and antifouling sub-layer derived from gemini quaternary ammonium salt polyurethanes. Sci Rep-UK 6:32140. https://doi.org/10.1038/srep32140

https://emerypharma.com/biology/minimum-inhibitory-concentration/

Huang KS, Yang CH, Luang SL, Chen CY, Lu YY, Lin YS (2016) Recent advances in antimicrobial polymers: A mini-review. Int J Mol Sci 17:1578. https://doi.org/10.3390/ijms17091578

Huang M, Liu Z, Li A, Yang H (2017) Dual functionality of a graft starch flocculant: flocculation and antibacterial performance. J Environ Manag 196:63–71. https://doi.org/10.1016/j.jenvman.2017.02.078

Ignatova M, Manolova N, Rashkova I, Markova N (2016) Quaternized chitosan/κ-carrageenan/caffeic acid–coated poly(3-hydroxybutyrate) fibrous materials: preparation, antibacterial and antioxidant activity. Int J Pharm 513:528–537. https://doi.org/10.1016/j.ijpharm.2016.09.062

Jain A, Duvvuri LS, Farah S, Beyth N, Domb AJ, Khan W (2014) Antimicrobial polymers. Adv Healthc Mater 3:1969–1985. https://doi.org/10.1002/adhm.201400418

Jiao Y, Niu L, Ma S, Li J, Tay FR, Chen J (2017) Quaternary ammonium-based biomedical materials: state-of-the-art, toxicological aspects and antimicrobial resistance. Prog Polym Sci 71:53–90. https://doi.org/10.1016/j.progpolymsci.2017.03.001

Kenawy E-R, Worley SD, Broughton R (2007) The chemistry and applications of antimicrobial polymers: A state-of-the-art review. Biomacromolecules 8:1359–1384. https://doi.org/10.1021/bm061150q

Kenawy E-R, Ibrahim AS, Abo-Elghit EM, Al-Owais AA (2014) New trends in antimicrobial polymers: a state of the art review. Int J Chem Appl Biol Sci 1:95–105. https://doi.org/10.4103/2348-0734.146922

Lee SB, Koepsel RR, Morley SW, Matyjaszewski K, Sun Y, Russell AJ (2004) Permanent, nonleaching antibacterial surfaces. 1. Synthesis by atom transfer radical polymerization. Biomacromolecules 5:877–882. https://doi.org/10.1021/bm034352k

Lenoir S, Pagnoulle C, Galleni M, Compere P, Jerome R, Detrembleur C (2006) Polyolefin matrixes with permanent antibacterial activity: preparation, antibacterial activity, and action mode of the active species. Biomacromolecules 7:2291–2296. https://doi.org/10.1021/bm050850c

Li Z, Yang F, Yang R (2015) Synthesis and characterization of chitosan derivatives with dual-antibacterial functional groups. Int J Biol Macromol 75:378–387. https://doi.org/10.1016/j.ijbiomac.2015.01.056

Li Q, Tan W, Zhang C, Gu G, Guo Z (2016) Synthesis of water soluble chitosan derivatives with halogeno-1,2,3-triazole and their antifungal activity. Int J Biol Macromol 91:623–629. https://doi.org/10.1016/j.ijbiomac.2016.06.006

Lichter JA, Vliet KJV, Rubner MF (2009) Design of antibacterial surfaces and interfaces: polyelectrolyte multilayers as a multifunctional platform. Macromolecules 42:8573–8586. https://doi.org/10.1021/ma901356s

Liu G, Wu G, Jin C, Kong Z (2015) Preparation and antimicrobial activity of terpene-based polyurethane coatings with carbamate group-containing quaternary ammonium salts. Prog Org Coat 80:150–155. https://doi.org/10.1016/j.porgcoat.2014.12.005

Liu Z, Huang M, Li A, Yang H (2017) Flocculation and antimicrobial properties of a cationized starch. Water Res 119:57–66. https://doi.org/10.1016/j.watres.2017.04.043

Logar N, Klemenčič D, Tomšič B, Pavko Čuden A, Simončič B (2016) Tailoring of a dual-active antibacterial coating for polylactic acid fibres. Tekstilec 59:289–297. https://doi.org/10.14502/Tekstilec2016.59.289-297

Lv X, Liu C, Song S, Qiao Y, Hu Y, Li P, Li Z, Sun S (2018) Construction of a quaternary ammonium salt platform with different alkyl groups for antibacterial and biosensor applications. RSC Adv 8:2941–2949. https://doi.org/10.1039/C7RA11001D

Makvandi P, Jamaledin R, Jabbari M, Nikfarjam N, Borzacchiello A (2018) Antibacterial quaternary ammonium compounds in dental materials: a systematic review. Dent Mater 34:851–867. https://doi.org/10.1016/j.dental.2018.03.014

Maleki A, Shahmoradi B, Hayati B, Jebelli MA, Daraei H, Joo SW (2017) Synthesis of halogenated nanodendrimer as novel antimicrobial agents in water treatment. Desalin Water Treat 64:101–108. https://doi.org/10.5004/dwt.2017.20267

Meng J, Zhang X, Ni L, Tang Z, Zhang Y, Zhang Y, Zhang W (2015) Antibacterial cellulose membrane via one-step covalent immobilization of ammonium/amine groups. Desalination 359:156–166. https://doi.org/10.1016/j.desal.2014.12.032

Mohamed NA, El-Ghany NAA (2012) Preparation and antimicrobial activity of some carboxymethyl chitosan acyl thiourea derivatives. Int J Biol Macromol 50:1280–1285. https://doi.org/10.1016/j.ijbiomac.2012.03.011

Mohamed RR, Abu Elella MH, Saba MW (2015) Synthesis, characterization and applications of *N*-quaternized chitosan/poly(vinyl alcohol) hydrogels. Int J Biol Macromol 80:149–161. https://doi.org/10.1016/j.ijbiomac.2015.06.041

Munoz-Bonilla A, Fernandes-Garcia M (2012) Polymeric materials with antimicrobial activity. Prog Polym Sci 37:281–339. https://doi.org/10.1016/j.progpolymsci.2011.08.005

Oyervides-Munoz E, Pollet E, Ulrich G, de Jesús Sosa-Santillán G, Avérous L (2017) Original method for synthesis of chitosan-based antimicrobial agent by quaternary ammonium grafting. Carbohyd Polym 157:1922–1932. https://doi.org/10.1016/j.carbpol.2016.11.081

Pankey GA, Sabath LD (2004) Clinical relevance of bacteriostatic versus bactericidal mechanisms of action in the treatment of Gram-positive bacterial infections. Clin Infect Dis 38:864–870. https://doi.org/10.1086/381972

Peng N, Wang Y, Ye Q, Liang L, An Y, Li Q, Chang C (2016) Biocompatible cellulose-based superabsorbent hydrogels with antimicrobial activity. Carbohyd Polym 137:59–64. https://doi.org/10.1016/j.carbpol.2015.10.057

Qin X, Li Y, Zhou F, Ren L, Zhao Y, Yuan X (2015) Polydimethylsiloxane-polymethacrylate block copolymers tethering quaternary ammonium salt groups for antimicrobial coating. Appl Surf Sci 328:183–192. https://doi.org/10.1016/j.apsusc.2014.12.019

Quelemes PV, de Araújo AR, Plácido A, Delerue-Matos C, Maciel JS, Bessa LJ, Ombredane AS, Joanitti GA, Soares MJS, Eaton P, da Silva DA, Leite JRSA (2017) Quaternized cashew gum: An anti-staphylococcal and biocompatible cationic polymer for biotechnological applications. Carbohyd Polym 157:567–575. https://doi.org/10.1016/j.carbpol.2016.10.026

Rajkowska K, Kozirog A, Otlewska A, Piotrowska M, Nowicka-Krawczyk P, Brycky B, Kunicka-Styczynska A, Gutarowska (2016) Quaternary ammonium biocides as antimicrobial agents protecting historical wood and brick. Acta Biochim Pol 63:153–159. https://doi.org/10.18388/abp.2015_1134

Rossetti FF, Siegmann K, Köser J, Wegner I, Keskin I, Schlotterbeck G, Winkler M (2017) Antimicrobial polyethylene through melt compounding with quaternary ammonium salts. Int J Polym Sci, Article ID 2823604, 10 pages. https://doi.org/10.1155/2017/2823604

Santos MRE, Fonseca AC, Mendonça PV, Branco R, Serra AC, Morais PV, Coelho JFJ (2016) Recent developments in antimicrobial polymers: a review. Materials 9.:Article ID 599, 33 pages. https://doi.org/10.3390/ma9070599

Siedenbiedel F, Tiller JC (2012) Antimicrobial polymers in solution and on surfaces: overview and functional principles. Polymers 4:46–71. https://doi.org/10.3390/polym4010046

Singh RS, Saini GK, Kennedy JF (2008) Pullulan: Microbial sources, production and applications. Carbohyd Polym 73:515–531. https://doi.org/10.1016/j.carbpol.2008.01.003

Singh RS, Kaura N, Kennedy JF (2015) Pullulan and pullulan derivatives as promising biomolecules for drug and gene targeting. Carbohyd Polym 123:190–207. https://doi.org/10.1016/j.carbpol.2015.01.032

Song R, Zhong Z, Lin L (2016) Evaluation of chitosan quaternary ammonium salt-modified resin denture base material. Int J Biol Macromol 85:102–110. https://doi.org/10.1016/j.ijbiomac.2015.12.052

Staneva D, Vasileva-Tonkova E, Makki MSI, Sobahi TR, Abdel-Rahman RM, Asiri AM, Grabchev I (2015) Synthesis, photophysical and antimicrobial activity of new water soluble ammonium quaternary benzanthrone in solution and in polylactide film. J Photoch Photobio B 143:44–51. https://doi.org/10.1016/j.jphotobiol.2014.12.024

Tan W, Li Q, Dong F, Wei L, Guo Z (2016) Synthesis, characterization, and antifungal property of chitosan ammonium salts with halogens. Int J Biol Macromol 92:293–298. https://doi.org/10.1016/j.ijbiomac.2016.07.023

Tang Y, Xie L, Sai M, Xu N, Ding D (2015) Preparation and antibacterial activity of quaternized chitosan with iodine. Mat Sci Eng C-Mater 48:1–4. https://doi.org/10.1016/j.msec.2014.11.019

Tang R, Zhang Y, Zhang Y, Yu Z (2016) Synthesis and characterization of chitosan based dye containing quaternary ammonium group. Carbohyd Polym 139:191–196. https://doi.org/10.1016/j.carbpol.2015.12.047

Timofeeva L, Kleshcheva N (2011) Antimicrobial polymers: mechanism of action, factors of activity, and applications. Appl Microbiol Biot 89:475–492. https://doi.org/10.1007/s00253-010-2920-9

Tran PL, Huynh E, Hamood AN, de Souza A, Schultz G, Liesenfeld B, Mehta D, Webster D, Reid TW (2017) The ability of quaternary ammonium groups attached to a urethane bandage to inhibit bacterial attachment and biofilm formation in a mouse wound model. Int Wound J 14:79–84. https://doi.org/10.1111/iwj.12554

Tuchilus CG, Nichifor M, Mocanu G, Stanciu MC (2017) Antimicrobial activity of chemically modified dextran derivatives. Carbohyd Polym 161:181–186. https://doi.org/10.1016/j.carbpol.2017.01.006

Udabe E, Isik M, Sardon H, Irusta L, Salsamendi M, Sun Z, Zheng Z, Yan F, Mecerreyes D (2017) Antimicrobial polyurethane foams having cationic ammonium groups. Part of special issue: green and sustainable polyurethanes for advanced applications. J Appl Polym Sci., 7 pages. https://doi.org/10.1002/app.45473

Wang CH, Liu WS, Sun JF, Hou GG, Chen Q, Cong W, Zhao F (2016) Non-toxic *O*-quaternized chitosan materials with better water solubility and antimicrobial function. Int J Biol Macromol 84:418–427. https://doi.org/10.1016/j.ijbiomac.2015.12.047

Wiarachai O, Thongchul N, Kiatkamjornwong S, Hoven VP (2012) Surface-quaternized chitosan particles as an alternative and effective organic antibacterial material. Colloid Surf B 92:121–129. https://doi.org/10.1016/j.colsurfb.2011.11.034

Xue Y, Xiao H, Zhang Y (2015) Antimicrobial polymeric materials with quaternary ammonium and phosphonium salts. Int J Mol Sci 16:3626–3655. https://doi.org/10.3390/ijms16023626

Yao C, Li X, Neoh KG, Shi Z, Kang ET (2010) Antibacterial poly(D,L-lactide) (PDLLA) fibrous membranes modified with quaternary ammonium moieties. Chinese J Polym Sci 28:581–588. https://doi.org/10.1007/s10118-010-9094-x

Zhou F, Qin X, Li Y, Ren L, Zhao Y, Yuan X (2015) Fluorosilicone multi-block copolymers tethering quaternary ammonium salt groups for antimicrobial purpose. Appl Surf Sci 347:231–241. https://doi.org/10.1016/j.apsusc.2015.04.079

Chapter 6
Nanoparticles: Powerful Tool to Mitigate Antibiotic Resistance

Mitali Mishra, Shashank Patole, and Harapriya Mohapatra

Abstract The discovery of antibiotics has offered tremendous advantage for progress in medicine. It has ensured recuperation from deadly bacterial diseases and an increase in the longevity of human life. Bacteria, due to their versatile and quick adaptation towards a changing environment, inevitably emerged as winners in the struggle for survival. The bacteria have acquired resistance by means of genetic modifications, shared the resistance genes through horizontal gene transfer and evolved strategies to overcome lethal antimicrobials. This resulted in the emergence of resistance towards multiple antimicrobial agents. Concurrent with the emergence of resistance, better connectivity across the globe led to a rapid spread and dispersion of the resistance traits. Cumulatively, all the above, resulted in antimicrobial resistance emerging as the most significant human health crisis of the twenty-first century. Deaths attributed to antibiotic resistant infections have raised significantly worldwide, particularly in high and low-income nations. This crisis threatens to undo medical advances such as organ transplants and interventional surgery healing. Ongoing surveillance conducted by the World Health Organization on the occurrence of antibiotic resistant infections worldwide suggested approximately ten million deaths to occur by 2050. Such predicted death rates surpass those associated with other deadly diseases like cancer and diabetes. Several studies have highlighted the mechanisms behind such growing drug resistance, which unanimously urges us to look for alternatives to antibiotic and take action to tackle antibiotic resistant pathogens. The complexity of the problem is compounded with the bottlenecks in drug development and a lack of available new antimicrobials. Such a scenario has necessitated a search for alternatives to naturally occurring antimicrobials.

Nanoparticles/nanomaterials have emerged as promising alternatives with potential leads possessing enhanced antimicrobial activities. The nanoparticles are endowed with a wide spectrum of antimicrobial activity against multi drug resistant pathogens. Though in its primitive stage, the efficacy of nanomaterials can be

M. Mishra · S. Patole · H. Mohapatra (✉)
School of Biological Sciences, National Institute of Science Education and Research – Bhubaneswar, Jatni, Odisha, India

Homi Bhabha National Institute, Anushakti Nagar, Mumbai, Maharashtra, India
e-mail: hm@niser.ac.in

H. Panwar et al. (eds.), *Sustainable Agriculture Reviews 49*, Sustainable Agriculture Reviews 49, https://doi.org/10.1007/978-3-030-58259-3_6

enhanced with its physicochemical properties, antimicrobial efficacy and reduced cytotoxicity. Both inorganic (metallic and metal oxide nanoparticles) and organic nanoparticles have been extensively studied for their antimicrobial properties. Their ultra small size, easy penetration to the target cell and biocompatibility nature has only enhanced the popularity of nanoparticles to be used as an alternative antimicrobial agent. However, a lot of performance and quality assessment are essential before actual implementation of such nanoparticles in biomedicine.

The present chapter will focus on the development and diversity of metallic and non-metallic nanoparticles. Aspects of metallic nanoparticle synthesis, their mode of action along with use of non-metallic nanoparticles as drug delivery agent is also reviewed. The chapter finally concludes with discussion on limitations and future research potentials in the field.

Keywords Nanoparticles · Antibiotic resistance · Multi drug resistance · Silver nanoparticle · Bimetallic nanoparticle · Carbon nanoparticle · Fullerene · Graphene · Gold nanoparticle · Antibacterial activity

6.1 Introduction

Amongst significant developments in the history of medicine, discovery of the miracle molecule 'Penicillin' from the fungus *Penicillium notatum* by Alexander Fleming in 1928, was considered most relevant and decisive. Thereafter, by the mid-1940s, E. B. Chain and H. W. Florey were able to generate stable commercial formulations of Penicillin. In the year 1945, Fleming, Chain and Florey, were awarded the Nobel Prize in medicine for "the discovery of penicillin and its curative effect on various infectious diseases" (Lobanovska and Pilla 2017). Undoubtedly, over the past 70 years, antimicrobial therapy has enabled the treatment of a multitude of infectious diseases. It has contributed immensely to advances in medical interventions such as organ transplants. This, in turn has boosted the average life expectancy of individuals during the twentieth century.

However, within just 4 years of the discovery of commercial formulation of penicillin in 1943, there were reports of microbes developing resistance to this antibiotic by the production of a hydrolyzing enzyme 'penicillinase'. Resistance is the ability of a microorganism to escape or prevent the action of a drug that once successfully killed the same pathogen (Li and Webster 2018). Since then, the discovery of every new antimicrobial compound was challenged by superlative resistance mechanisms employed by pathogens. As a result of this, the antibiotic becomes ineffective against the infectious agent, resulting in treatment failure. This tug of war between pathogen and antimicrobial has eventually resulted in the development of multi drug resistant (MDR), extensive drug resistant (XDR) and pan drug resistant (PDR) pathogens (Magiorakos et al. 2012). The dissemination of antibiotic resistant genes among pathogens is associated with horizontal gene transfer, which is the exchange of plasmids bearing antibiotic resistance determinants and mutations. Integrons are another group of mobile genetic elements responsible for the transfer and insertion of resistance genes in gram negative pathogens (Davies and Davies 2010).

Overall the antimicrobial efficacy has been tremendously compromised due to evolution of drug resistance. The accumulation of multiple antimicrobial resistance mechanisms has resulted in evolution of bacteria that are immune towards multiple therapeutic drugs. Such 'superbugs' pose a threat towards the advancement of medical interventions and have globally emerged as a potential health threat. Moreover, antibiotic therapy options, being largely empirical, pose various side effects like toxicity, hypersensitivity, teratogenicity and/or mutagenicity (Hemeg 2017). In addition, the escalation of drug resistant pathogens and reduction in the potency of antibiotics is a major setback to public health with limited or no treatment options available in the future. Undoubtedly we are now in the "post-antibiotic era" and are exposed to a global health crisis (Ventola 2015). Considering the present situation, researchers have listed top six multi drug pathogens which are escalating rapidly worldwide resulting in higher mortality and morbidity in cases of antibiotic resistant infections. "ESKAPE", is the acronym for such group of opportunistic pathogens which includes *Enterococcus faecium, Staphylococcus aureus, Klebsiella pneumoniae, Acinetobacter baumannii, Pseudomonas aeruginosa*, and *Enterobacter* spp. The ESKAPE pathogens have rapidly developed resistance to primary, secondary and tertiary therapeutic agents and have posed a grave threat to healthcare practices globally over the last decade (Mulani et al. 2019; Boucher et al. 2009).

6.1.1 *Mechanisms of Antibiotic Resistance*

To mitigate the antimicrobial resistance problem, it is crucial to understand the tricks adopted by pathogens to escape the action of antimicrobials. This understanding is essential to develop counter strategies to combat resistant infections. Antimicrobial resistance mechanisms can broadly be classified into four categories *viz.* (1) modification and/or inactivation of drugs by various hydrolysing enzymes, (2) alteration of antibiotic target site, (3) limited membrane permeability thereby restricting the entry of antibiotic into the target cell, and, (4) active efflux pumps that expel antibiotics out of the cell (Li et al. 2015; Sherrard et al. 2014).

6.1.1.1 Drug Inactivation or Alteration

The first recognised and extensively studied antimicrobial resistance mechanism involves acquisition of genes encoding enzymes that alter or degrade the antibiotics, making them ineffective against their target, for instance β-lactamases and aminoglycoside modifying enzymes. β-lactamase enzymes are ancient, widely distributed in bacterial genera with activity on diverse substrates, and usually act by hydrolyzing the β-lactam rings (Santajit and Indrawattana 2016). Mutations in the genes encoding such enzymes produce extended spectra of resistance against β-lactams as well as cephalosporins. β-lactamase enzymes are classified into Ambler classes A, B, C and D (Bush and Jacoby 2010) based on their amino acid sequences. The ambler class A of serine β-lactamase enzymes include extended spectrum β-lactamases (ESBLs), mainly TEM, SHV, CTX-M and KPC (*Klebsiella pneumoniae* carbapenamase) types, which are prevalent in Enterobacteriaceae. Ambler class B includes metallo-β-lactamases such as IMP (active-on-imipenem), VIM (Verona integron-encoded) and NDM-1 (New Delhi metallo-β-lactamase), whereas the ambler class D include many oxacillin hydrolyzing enzymes (OXA) group of β-lactamases. The ambler class C includes AmpC β-lactamases, which are usually chromosomally encoded in many gram negative bacteria including *Citrobacter*, *Serratia* and *Enterobacter* spp. The presence of such chromosomal encoded genes result in low level resistance to the broad spectrum cephalosporin group of antibiotics due to their constitutive expression, however, expression of these enzymes is enhanced in the presence of antibiotics (Munita and Arias 2016).

Another important enzyme mediated antibiotic resistance mechanism is by shielding the target. An example of such mechanism is observed in resistance to fluoroquinolones facilitated by *qnr* (Quinolone resistance) genes. The *qnr* genes encode a family of DNA binding proteins that compete for the binding site in a gyrase-DNA complex. This lowers the ability of fluoroquinolones to bind and hence confer low levels of quinolone resistance (Strahilevitz et al. 2009).

6.1.1.2 Modification of Drug Binding Sites

Resistant pathogens avoid killing activity by antimicrobial agents by modifying their target sites. For example, penicillin binding proteins are enzymes usually anchored on the bacterial cytoplasmic membrane and offer resistance to β-lactam antibiotics. Mutation of such genes encoding for penicillin binding proteins result in low affinity for β-lactam antibiotics, and this in turn allows the pathogens to escape the antimicrobial action (Lambert 2005) and develop resistance.

6.1.1.3 Reduced Permeability of Antibiotics by Outer Membrane Proteins

The third most important drug resistance strategy involves limited membrane permeability that restricts the access of antibiotics through the intricate outer membrane and cell membrane barrier. This membrane mediated mechanism of antibiotic resistance is achieved through decreased membrane permeability by outer membrane proteins or porins, which are channel like proteins embedded in the cell membrane (Krishnamoorthy et al. 2017). These transport proteins form the primary mechanical barrier to antimicrobial therapy in gram negative pathogens by regulating the entry of hydrophilic antibiotics like β-lactams and fluoroquinolones, with porin modifications/mutations and downregulation of porin synthesis (Bolla et al. 2011).

6.1.1.4 Active Efflux Pumps Extruding Antibiotics

The rapid escalation of multi drug resistant pathogens is often characterized by the presence of active efflux pumps that expel antibiotics from the cytoplasm and periplasm, out of the cell (Piddock 2006). Both gram negative and gram positive pathogens harbour single component as well as multi component tripartite multi drug resistant efflux pumps from different families. Efflux mediated antibiotic resistance mechanisms were widely reported as a primary means of multi drug resistant phenotypes in many clinically significant pathogens owing to its substrate redundancy and over expression in stress conditions (Li et al. 2015) (Fig. 6.1).

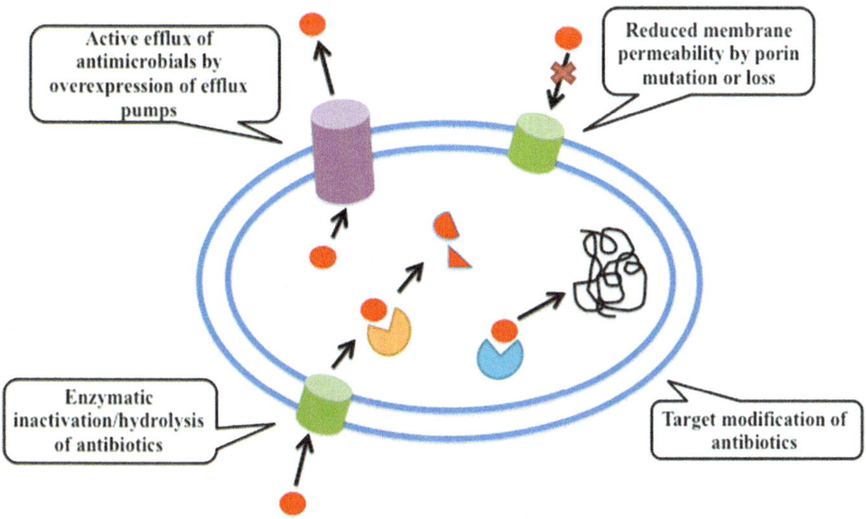

Fig. 6.1 A simplistic model depicting the broad categories of antibiotic resistance mechanisms employed by pathogens to avoid antimicrobial action. The figure summarizes the resistance strategies followed by bacteria mainly: antibiotic modifying/inactivating enzymes, change in target site of the antibiotic – both of this make the antibiotic non-functional/ineffective. Reduced outer membrane permeability by porins and active efflux of drugs by efflux pumps, both lower the effective concentration of the antibiotic inside the cell to be functional. All of these strategies in singular or in combination can exert resistance to the antimicrobial action in pathogens

6.1.2 *Current Status of Antibiotic Resistance*

Accurate prediction of worldwide healthcare associated infections caused by antimicrobial resistance is uncertain and often extrapolated, as it involves exclusive information obtained from regional/national level tertiary care hospitals, is not population centric and lacks data from countries with low or moderate income (Kraker et al. 2016). Nevertheless, significant efforts have been made by many international committees, namely, World Health Organization (WHO), Centre for Disease Control and prevention (CDC), European Centre for Disease Prevention and Control (ECDC), the Centre for Disease Dynamics, Economics and Policy (CDDEP), to contribute to our present knowledge of antimicrobial resistant infection statistics. As per the Centre for Disease Control and prevention (CDC) 2013 report on 'Antibiotic resistance threat' in the United States of America, every year two million people get affected and ~23,000 people die due to serious antimicrobial resistant infections (CDC 2013). Despite the availability of treatment options, infections due to drug resistant opportunistic and nosocomial pathogens account for 28–30% crude mortality rate in healthcare settings (WHO 2014). The present antibiotic resistance crisis has been largely attributed to overuse and misuse of antibiotics in clinics, veterinary, industry and agriculture settings, thus unknowingly aiding in the spread of resistant traits through diverse sources (Beceiro et al. 2013). Definitely, we have reached the 'post-antibiotic' era with mounting drug resistance due to the compromised efficacy of the available therapeutics, the recalcitrance of biofilms towards antibiotics, and development of resistance in bacteria to even the last-resort antibiotics, colistin (Aslam et al. 2018; Gupta et al. 2019). It was estimated that the mortality rates due to infections by antimicrobial resistant organisms could be approximately ten million by 2050 (O Neil 2014), which is even higher than other deadly diseases like cancer, diabetes, and is a matter of grave concern. Moreover, considering the amount of time, resources and precision required, developing new effective drugs to tackle this gigantic health issue seems practically impossible. This has necessitated the search for cost-effective and easily producible alternate treatment options, where nanoparticle based therapies have shown promising effects.

6.2 Nanoparticles: Boon in Post-antibiotic Era

Over the last decade, the utilization of nanotechnology in medicine has gained significant attention as a substitute to ameliorate the disastrous consequences of antibiotic resistance. Nanoparticles possess a surface area-to-volume ratio that is much larger than the bulk compounds originally used to synthesise them, which furnishes an abundance of functional sites for the compound to interact with the target. The nanoparticles are also less inclined to induce resistance in bacteria as compared to classical antibiotics (Natan and Banin 2017). Most of the work examining the therapeutic impact of nanoparticles has focused on capitalising on the pre-recognised antimicrobial properties of metal ions such as silver (Rai et al. 2009) and oxides of metals such as iron, titanium and zinc (Jiang et al. 2009).

Nanoparticles offer dual benefits; one, they combat antibiotic resistance and two, they offer the advantage of being used as drug carriers for antibiotics and natural compounds to increase their bioavailability. There are many important attributes of nanoparticles for which they have gained significant attention as a novel candidate to mitigate multi drug resistant pathogens:

1. Ultra small size coupled with greater surface area-to-volume ratio, which enables them to directly interact with the bacterial cell membrane without penetration, thus enhancing their antimicrobial property (Kim et al. 2007)
2. Wide spectrum antimicrobial activity against various gram positive and gram negative pathogens, with some nanoparticles exhibit antifungal and antiviral properties.
3. Increased drug solubility and stability in a chemical process (Huh and Kwon 2011).
4. Synthesis of nanoparticles is easy and reproducible in nature (Gholipourmalekabadi et al. 2017) and,
5. Biocompatibile with target drug and their regulated release, which can be modulated further by different stimuli, like light, pH and heat (Zhang et al. 2017).

Additionally, a combination of nanoparticles along with antibiotics makes them more effective in killing microorganisms due to increased target specificity (Wang and Hu 2017). Depending upon the type of materials used, nanoparticles can be broadly utilized for different applications including diagnosis using biosensors, cell and tissue imaging, food technology, textile industry, antimicrobial coatings, superconducters, optical devices, quantum lasers, energy and environment (Rudramurthy et al. 2016).

Another alternative that has been gaining greater attention is the use of nanoparticles as delivery vehicles to transport chemicals, antibiotics or other nanoparticles that have a proven antibacterial efficacy. Such nano encapsulated molecules can contain higher dose of antibiotics even in smaller volume and help in rapid absorption of the active drug material. Their ultra small size coupled with target specific property and less toxicity has helped the nanoparticles gain advantage over other delivery agents. There have been a plethora of nanomaterials that have been reported to be successful in the delivery of drugs and antibiotic compounds to treat infections, some of which include liposomes, dendrimers, solid lipid nanoparticles, nanotubes, polymeric micelles, and biodegradable polymer based nanoparticles (Huh and Kwon 2011; Gupta et al. 2017). Such antimicrobial compound nanoparticle composites have been associated with an increased solubility of the drug, a greater loading capacity for the drug, flexibility in the pathways of absorption, protection from oxidation, aggregation or metabolic degradation, and enabling sustained release of the drug/active-compound at the specific site (Gupta et al. 2017; Natan and Banin 2017). It is worth noting here that while these nanoparticles of organic origin themselves do not possess any antibacterial property like their metal counterparts; their properties have the potential and have already been applied to galvanize efforts to combat antibiotic resistance.

6.2.1 Characterization of Nanoparticles

Nanoparticles are particles of 1–100 nanometres in size and are generally composed of either organic matter, carbon, metal or metal oxides with unique physical and biochemical properties. Nanoparticles differ in their shape; could be spherical, cylindrical, tubular, spiral, conical etc. or irregular in size and structure depending on the matter from which it is synthesized. Certain nanoparticles have uniform surface structure, whereas others have surface variations (Ealias and Saravanakumar 2017).

Further, based upon the chemical composition of nanomolecules these can be further categorized as metallic nanoparticles, metal oxide nanoparticles, liposomes, dendrimers (highly branched, symmetric nano-sized complex); nano shells (dielectric core covered by a metal coat); quantum dots (tiny semiconductors bearing unique optical and electronic properties); polymeric nanospheres (spheres of micron size); nanobins; super paramagnetic iron oxide nanoparticles (SPIONs) that are very stable nanoparticles constituted of a magnetic core coated with either polysaccharides, or polymers/monomers, and ultra stable polymer coated nanocrystals.

6.2.2 Classification of Nanoparticles

While the classification and characterization of inorganic based nanomaterials, which consist of metal and metal oxide nanoparticles has been well studied and documented, the efficacy of nanomaterials derived from non-metallic compounds has been fairly understated in comparison. However, for easy understanding all the nanoparticles can broadly be categorized into three, namely, organic, inorganic and carbon nanoparticles (Kandi and Kandi 2015).

(A) **Organic nanoparticles**:

- Utilize non-covalent interactions for their assembly, such as dendrimers, liposomes, micelles, ferritins and polymer nanoparticles.
- Such nanomaterials are biodegradable, non-toxic in nature.
- Micelles that are fatty acid core enclosed within lipid monolayers, and liposomes made up of lipid bilayers; are sensitive to different stimuli like thermal and electromagnetic radiation such as heat and light.
- Applications in biomedical field include targeted drug delivery because they are highly efficient in injecting the nanomaterials into specific parts of the body.

(B) **Inorganic nanoparticles**:

- Include metal and metal oxide based nanoparticles, which are more advantageous due to their ability to sustain adverse conditions.
- Both the metallic and metal oxide nanoparticles have demonstrated excellent antimicrobial properties.
- *Metallic nanoparticles* – silver (Ag), copper (Cu), gold (Au), aluminium (Al), cobalt (Co), iron (Fe), cadmium (Cd), lead (Pb), and zinc (Zn) based nanoparticles. Metallic nanoparticles have distinctive features including nanoscale size range of 10–100 nm, greater surface area-to-volume ratio, surface charge density, pore size, structure, shape, colour, sensitivity and reactivity to different environmental stimuli.
- *Metal oxide nanoparticles* – They are synthesised in such a manner as to enhance the inherent properties of their respective metal based nanoparticles by increasing its reactivity and sensitivity. Examples include aluminium oxide (Al_2O_3), cerium oxide (CeO_2), iron oxide (Fe_2O_3), magnetite (Fe_3O_4), titanium oxide (TiO_2), silicon dioxide (SiO_2), zinc oxide (ZnO).

(C) **Carbon nanoparticles**:
These nanoparticles are composed essentially of carbon and can be categorized into graphene, fullerenes, carbon nanotubes (CNT), carbon black, carbon nanofibers and sometimes activated carbon.

(D) **Composite based nanomaterials**
Combinations of nanomaterials from either of the above mentioned three categories in combination with ceramic, metal, or polymer materials that are larger in dimension (Jeevanandam et al. 2018).

6.2.3 Synthesis of Nanoparticles

Synthesis of high throughput nanoparticles with good and regulated quality is highly desirable and has always been recommended for their successful applications in various fields. Commonly, there are two basic methods which are practiced to synthesize metallic nanoparticles that include -

1. **Top-down approach:** This is a destructive method where synthesis is initiated with the reduction of a bulk material to particles of nanometric scale. This is the most widely used approach utilized for synthesis of fine nanoparticles. Examples include mechanical milling, nanolithography, anodization, ion and plasma etching laser ablation, sputtering and thermal decomposition.
2. **Bottom-up approach:** This is a constructive method which involves the assembly of atoms to clusters to nanoparticles. Examples include self assembly of monomer/polymer molecules, spinning, sol–gel processing, chemical vapour deposition (CVD), laser pyrolysis and most importantly biosynthesis that are

eco-friendly, green synthesis approach for production of bio-degradable and non-toxic nanoparticles (Dhand et al. 2015).

In general, nanoparticles can be synthesized by different combinations of physical and chemical methods, but these methods are costly and potentially dangerous to the environment as they generate toxic by-products. Therefore, in recent years of nanotechnology advancement, biological methods of synthesis of nanoparticles, popularly known as 'green synthesis', have been widely adapted (Swamy et al. 2015), where biological entities are utilized as a substitute to toxic physicochemical methods, for the development of eco-friendly, cost-effective and non-toxic metallic and metal oxide nanoparticles (Graves et al. 2017).

In such cases of bio-assisted synthesis, three different approaches exist that utilize either living microorganisms (bacteria, fungi, viruses, actinomycetes etc.), or plant extracts/biomass or biomolecules (nucleic acids-DNA, membranes and diatoms) as a template, for the generation of nanoparticles (Zhang et al. 2016). Amongst these potential biological methods though, microbe assisted synthesis of nanoparticle is technically challenging perhaps owing to the need of highly aseptic conditions and their continuous maintenance throughout the production of nanoparticles (Sharma et al. 2015). As a result, use of plant extracts is more appropriate as compared to microorganisms due to the apparent improvement, low cell culture maintenance and other safety issues (Kuppusamy et al. 2016).

6.2.4 Inorganic Nanoparticles

Amongst various inorganic nanoparticles, metal and metal oxide based nanoparticles have been heavily documented for their antibacterial and antifungal activity, but development of resistance to nanomaterials in the microorganisms are less studied. Commonly used metals in inorganic nanoparticles include silver (Ag), gold (Au), zinc (Zn), copper (Cu), aluminium (Al), titanium (Ti), nickel (Ni), magnesium (Mg), iron (Fe), calcium (Ca) and silicon (Si). While certain metals such as zinc, silver, copper exhibit antimicrobial properties in their bulk form, metal oxides like iron oxide demonstrate antibacterial properties in nanoparticulate form. Compiling results from a greater number of studies, this book chapter will briefly focus on the different metallic nanoparticles, their efficacy and modes of action as antimicrobial agents.

6.2.4.1 Silver Nanoparticles

Silver nanoparticles are increasingly used in multiple applications including industry, healthcare products, medical device coatings, optical sensors, household, diagnostics, drug delivery, textile industry, food industry, wound dressings. Rationale behind such wide applications of silver nanoparticles are attributed to its unique physicochemical and biological properties, low side effects, easy availability and cost effective synthesis (Zhang et al. 2016; Bilal et al. 2017; Rai et al. 2012). The antimicrobial properties of Ag, Ag ions and Ag compounds have gathered much attention in the scientific field. The historical use of silver as an antimicrobial agent and antiseptic against numerous diseases has reinforced the development of silver nanoparticles as most promising nanoparticles in medicine (Franci et al. 2015). In addition to wide spectrum antimicrobial properties exhibited against both gram positive and gram negative pathogens, silver nanoparticles possess anti biofilm (Markowska et al. 2013), anti oxidant, anti inflammatory (Ravishankar and Jamuna Bai 2011) and anti tumor and anti angiogenic properties (Swamy et al. 2015); thus making silver nanoparticles as the most desirable metallic nanoparticle. In addition, silver nanoparticles have displayed minimal cytotoxicity and dose dependent killing activity at very less concentrations (Sanyasi et al. 2016).

Several reports have documented remarkably higher antibacterial activity of silver nanoparticles against many gram negative bacteria species (including *E. coli, K. pneumoniae, Enterobacter* spp., *Vibrio cholerae, Salmonella typhi, Acinetobacter baumannii* and *P. aeruginosa*) and gram positive bacteria (e.g. Methicillin resistant *Staphylococcus aureus*, *Staphylococcus epidermidis* and vancomycin resistant *Enterococcus faecium*) (Salomoni et al. 2017; Sanyasi et al. 2016; Losasso et al. 2014; Yuan et al. 2017). In addition, silver nanoparticles have also shown potential anti fungal activities against different fungal pathogens including *Candida albicans*, *Candida tropicalis*, *Aspergillus fumigatus*, *Cladosporium* spp., *Penicillium* spp. etc. (Zhang et al. 2016). Undoubtedly, the minimum bactericidal/inhibitory concentrations (MBCs/MICs) of silver nanoparticles would be strain specific but are far below the minimum inhibitory concentration of antibiotics tested for the organism.

Several studies have established the mechanism of microbicidal activity of silver nanoparticles and attributed to multiple factors. However, two major hypothetical modes of action of silver nanoparticles have been widely accepted. The first one attributes the microbicidal activity of silver nanoparticles to membrane destabilization and membrane perturbation (mainly pores). This is caused due to the release of Ag^+ ions upon interaction of silver nanoparticles with thiol groups present in sulfur containing membrane proteins and enzymes (Morones-Ramirez et al. 2013). The second hypothesis attributes the antimicrobial activity of silver nanoparticles to its larger surface area-to-volume ratio that increases membrane permeability. This increased membrane permeability (membrane damage) generates reactive oxygen species inside the cell, affecting DNA replication, cell division and metabolic process, ultimately leading to cell death (Dasgupta and Ramalingam 2016; AbdalDayem et al. 2017). Again, there are reports on interaction of silver nanoparticles with ribosomes and proteins that halt cellular, transcriptional and translational machineries affecting overall growth (Prabhu and Poulose 2012).

Besides working at cellular level, silver nanoparticles have also been implicated in inhibiting biofilm formation. Biofilm associated infections are essentially persistent infections and are difficult to treat due to poor penetration ability of antibiotics to the biofilm matrix, where silver nanoparticles have worked efficiently. Reports suggested that silver nanoparticles (with mean diameter of 50 nm) at an effective concentration of 100 nM completely prohibited biofilms formed by *P. aeruginosa* and *S. epidermidis*. (Kalishwaralal et al. 2010). Similar anti biofilm activities were also reported to reduce biofilm mediated infections with *Mycobacterium* spp., *Staphylococcus aureus* and *E. coli* (Markowska et al. 2013). Moreover, synergistic application of silver nanoparticles with antibiotics was observed to enhance the antimicrobial activities, suggesting that simultaneous use of antibiotics and silver nanoparticles may decrease the emergence of resistance in pathogens (Franci et al. 2015).

6.2.4.2 Gold Nanoparticles

The earliest recognized form of gold nanoparticles was colloidal gold, which was largely used for its healing activities. Gold nanoparticles have distinct physicochemical properties with a size range of 0.8–250 nm. They are inert, biologically compatible and can be prepared in different shapes and structures utilizing chemical and biological synthesis methods (Rai et al. 2016). The mode of action of gold nanoparticles include generation of pores in the bacterial cell membrane leading to cellular leakage, change in membrane potential, prevention of ATPase and inhibiting the subunit of ribosome for transfer RNA (tRNA) (Lima et al. 2013). Antimicrobial activities of gold nanoparticles largely depend on their surface area, shape, dispersion and surface capping. Gold nanoparticles, alone or in combination with antibiotics, have displayed antibacterial properties against multiple multi drug resistant pathogens such as *E. coli, E. cloacae* complex, *Salmonella typhimurium*, *P. aeruginosa*, Methicillin resistant *Staphylococcus aureus*, *S. epidermidis*, and even fungal pathogens including *Trichoderma viridae* (Rudramurthy et al. 2016).

6.2.4.3 Zinc Nanoparticles

Zinc nanomaterials are extensively used in biomedical applications such as drug delivery systems, bioimaging owing to their easy availability, low toxicity and unique electrical, optical and photocatalytic properties. Also zinc nanomaterials, particularly zinc oxide nanoparticles, display excellent antimicrobial activity against both gram positive (e.g. *B. subtilis*, *S. aureus*) and gram negative (*E. coli*, *Salmonella* spp., *Listeria monocytogenes*) pathogens (Ali et al. 2017). Antimicrobial mechanisms of zinc oxide nanoparticles was thought to be mediated by production of reactive oxygen species, such as hydrogen peroxide (H_2O_2), hydroxyl ions (OH^-) and superoxide molecules (Sharma et al. 2012). The hydrogen peroxide molecules react with the released Zn^{2+} ions causing damage to membrane proteins and lipids leading to diminished cell surface hydrophobicity. Further, the internalized nanoparticles interact with intracellular compartments, disturb metabolic pathways and subsequently inhibit bacterial growth (Lakshmi Prasanna and Vijayaraghavan 2015).

6.2.4.4 Aluminium Nanoparticles

Aluminium nanoparticles and its metallic oxide counterparts like aluminium oxide (Al_2O_3) are thermodynamically stable and have wide biomedical and industrial applications. In similar fashion to other metallic nanoparticles, the antimicrobial mechanisms employed by aluminium nanoparticles were attributed to cell membrane disruption and cell death *via* generation of reactive oxygen species (Ansari et al. 2014). Reports suggested growth inhibitory effect of aluminium nanoparticles towards several bacterial species including *B. subtilis, E. coli,* and *P. fluorescens* (Hemeg 2017) (Table 6.1).

6.2.4.5 Copper Nanoparticles

Historically, the element copper and its compounds were extensively used in the manufacture of weapons, ornaments and coins. Now, they have found broad applications because of their unique chemical stability, and physical properties involving heat resistance, spin dynamics, and superconductivity. Copper nanoparticles exert antimicrobial activity against both Gram positive (such as *Staphylococcus aureus* and *Bacillus subtilis*) as well as Gram negative pathogens (namely *E. coli, Klebsiella* spp. and *P. aeruginosa*) and fungal strains (Ramyadevi et al. 2012; Ahamed and Alhadlaq 2014; Kruk et al. 2015). The mechanism of their antimicrobial activity is attributed to a greater surface area-to-volume ratio, increasing adhesion of nanoparticles to bacterial cell walls of opposite electric charge. This adhesion facilitates penetration of copper nanoparticles to microbial membrane leading to generation of reactive oxygen species and subsequent oxidative stress induced damage to the pathogen. Though copper oxide nanoparticles were also shown to exhibit antibacterial effects but copper nanoparticles display greater activity in comparison, could be due to better electron transfer amongst the negatively charged bacteria and the metallic nanoparticles (Vimbela et al. 2017). Moreover, copper nanoparticles have stronger affinity towards amines and the carboxyl groups of the bacterial cell membrane, explaining their better antimicrobial efficacy. Very recently, efflux inhibitory properties of copper nanoparticles were also reported (Christena et al. 2015).

6.2.4.6 Bismuth Nanoparticles

Bismuth nanomaterials and its commonly found compounds such as bismuth oxide, bismuth sulfide and bismuth carbonate exhibit antimicrobial activity at relatively higher concentrations due to its poor water solubility. Generally, to enhance their efficacy at lower concentrations for an extended time point, their water solubility is increased upon addition of chelating agents like dimercaptoethanol. Bismuth nanoparticles which were synthesized using appropriate surface modifiers were utilized in the treatment of gastrointestinal disorders (Rudramurthy et al. 2016). Bismuth nanoparticles also are known to have potential antibacterial, antifungal as

Table 6.1 Overview of different mechanisms of antimicrobial actions of metal and metal oxide nanoparticles

Type of metallic nanoparticles	Mode of action	Target organisms	References
Silver nanoparticles	Disturb the electron transport chain machinery	Vancomycin resistant *Enterococcus faecalis*, methicillin resistant *Staphylococcus aureus*, *Staphylococcus epidermidis*, *Pseudomonas fluorescens*, *Pseudomonas aeruginosa*, *Klebsiella pneumoniae*, *Escherichia coli*, *Bacillus subtilis*, *Acinetobacter baumannii*, *Mycobacterium smegmatis*, *Vibrio fluvialis*	Zhang et al. (2016), Wan et al. (2016), Franci et al. (2015), and Yuan et al. (2017)
	Cell membrane damage and reactive oxygen species generation		
	Prevent cell wall synthesis, protein and nucleic acid synthesis and cascade of intracellular reaction		
	Evasion of multi drug efflux pumps		
	Penetration in the bacterial cell wall and biofilms		
	Combination with antibiotics		
	Anti inflammatory and antioxidant properties		
	Also anti fungal and anti viral agent		
Gold nanoparticles	Disruption of bacterial cell wall.	Methicillin resistant *Staphylococcus aureus*, *E. coli*, *Enterobacter aerogenes*, *E. cloacae*, *Klebsiella pneumoniae*, *Salmonella typhimurium*, *P. aeruginosa*, *A. baumannii*, *S. epidermidis*, *S. haemolyticus*, *Proteus species*	Lima et al. (2013), Roshmi et al. (2015), Rai et al. (2016), and Li et al. (2014)
	DNA damage and inhibit the transcription process.		
	Anti inflammatory properties as it limit the enzymatic activity of liposomes in macrophages.		
	Penetration through biofilms and interaction with intracellular components		
Magnesium oxide nanoparticle	Generation of reactive oxygen species, lipid peroxidation and electrostatic interactions in cell membranes and cell damage due to alkaline effect.	*S. aureus*, *E. coli*, *Bacillus megaterium*, *Bacillus subtilis*	Stankic et al. (2016)

(continued)

Table 6.1 (continued)

Type of metallic nanoparticles	Mode of action	Target organisms	References
Titanium dioxide nanoparticle	Formation of reactive oxygen species, and targeted DNA damage, photocatalytic properties	*S. aureus*, *E. coli* and also anti fungal in nature	Lai et al. (2015)
Zinc oxide nanoparticles	Primarily by reactive oxygen species production. Released Zn^{2+} ions damage cell membrane proteins and interfere the metabolic pathways inhibiting growth.	*E. coli*, *K. pneumoniae*, *Salmonella* sp., *Listeria monocytogenes*, *S. aureus*, *B. subtilis*	Yu et al. (2014) and Lakshmi Prasanna and Vijayaraghavan (2015)
Copper/ copper oxide nanoparticles	Penetration of the cell wall. Disrupt biochemical processes, Inhibition of biofilm formation, efflux inhibition.	*P. aeruginosa*, *E. coli*, *B. subtilis*, *S. aureus*.	Chen et al. (2014) and Kruk et al. (2015)
Iron oxide nanoparticles	Reactive oxygen species mediated oxidative stress. Interference with electron transfer system	*S. aureus*, *P. aeruginosa*, *E. coli*, *S. epidermidis*	Behera et al. (2012)
Aluminium nanoparticles	Disruption of cell walls, reactive oxygen species generation.	*E. coli*, *S. aureus*	Ansari et al. (2014)
Bismuth nanoparticles	Interfere the Krebs cycle and disturb amino acid and nucleotide metabolism.	Multiple antibiotic resistant *Helicobacter pylori*	Baptista et al. (2018)
Silver-gold bimetallic nanoparticles	Disruption of bacterial cell wall, inactivate the proteins and enzymes for adenosine-triphosphate (ATP) production.	*E. coli*, *S. aureus*, *E. faecalis*, *P. aeruginosa*	Ramasamy et al. (2017) and Sharma et al. (2019)

well as antiviral activity primarily through alternations in the Kreb's cycle, disruption of amino acid and nucleotide metabolism (Baptista et al. 2018). However their toxicity aspects still remains to be investigated in detail.

6.2.4.7 Titanium Nanoparticles

Titanium nanomaterials are successfully employed in dentistry and orthopaedic implants and prosthetics, because of its non-toxicity, biocompatibility and good optical and mechanical properties. Titanium dioxide nanoparticles are also heavily used in pharmaceuticals, food industry, cosmetics, due to significant antibacterial activity towards *E. coli*, *S. epidermidis*, *S. aureus* and fungal pathogens like *Aspergillus niger*. Titanium dioxide nanoparticles exhibit photocatalytic activity that results in antimicrobial effects. In the presence of light, titanium dioxide nanoparticles generate hydroxyl ions (OH^-) that ruptures the cell membrane resulting in cell death of the microorganism (Slavin et al. 2017). Similar to other metallic and metal oxide nanoparticles, titanium dioxide nanoparticles exhibit an antimicrobial response primarily by the generation of reactive oxygen species that act on phospholipids on the bacterial surface, resulting in alteration of membrane permeability and site specific DNA damage (Vimbela et al. 2017; Ranjan and Ramalingam 2016).

6.2.4.8 Magnesium Nanoparticles

Inorganic metal oxides like magnesium oxide nanoparticles, similar to zinc oxide nanoparticles, are utilized in biomedical applications. Their antimicrobial properties coupled with other physicochemical parameters such as biocompatibility, biodegradable in nature and high abundance; make these metals preferable for such applications (Rudramurthy et al. 2016). Moreover, the antimicrobial activity doesn't rely on the photoactivation and magnesium oxide nanoparticles also exhibit anti inflammatory and antioxidant properties. Mechanisms behind antimicrobial actions of magnesium oxide nanoparticles were attributed to multiple factors, which include generation of reactive oxygen species, lipid peroxidation and electrostatic interactions between bacterial cell membrane and the nanoparticles, resulting in cell death (Vimbela et al. 2017). It is also believed that upon contact with the bacterial cell surface, the high pH of magnesium oxide nanoparticles results in an alkaline effect that damages the cell (Rudramurthy et al. 2016). Nonetheless, reports suggest potential antimicrobial activity of magnesium oxide nanoparticles against Gram positive such as *S. aureus*, *B. subtilis*, *Bacillus megaterium* as well as Gram negative bacterial species; including *E. coli*, *P. aeruginosa* (Stankic et al. 2016).

6.2.4.9 Iron Containing Nanoparticles

Iron oxide nanoparticles have broad spectrum applications in food industry, as biosensors, as antimicrobial agents, targeted drug delivery vehicles, in magnetic resonance imaging, in cell sorting and as anti cancer agents. The antimicrobial mechanism of these iron containing nanoparticles is mainly contributed by generation of reactive oxygen species, resulting in oxidative stress induced cell death (Wang and Hu 2017). It is believed that upon interaction with microbial cells, these nanoparticles penetrate the membrane and disturb the functioning of electron transfer, as well as damage macromolecules like DNA and proteins (Behera et al. 2012). Several studies on the antimicrobial properties of ferrosoferric oxide (Fe_3O_4) nanoparticles revealed its notable growth inhibitory activities against multi drug resistant bacteria such as *S. epidermidis*, *Staphylococcus saprophyticus*, Methicillin resistant *Staphylococcus aureus*, *E. coli*, *P. vulgaris* and *Xanthomonas*.

6.2.4.10 Bimetallic Nanoparticles

With the ongoing development of metallic and metal oxide nanoparticles, the recent focus on bimetallic nanoparticles has enhanced to further improvise the efficiency and sensitivity of metallic nanoparticles. One such important example is gold-silver bimetallic nanoparticles to enhance the drug action with required dose to minimize the cytotoxicity. Though individually both silver nanoparticles and gold nanoparticles possess excellent antimicrobial properties; in combination they form bimetallic nanoparticles with significantly enhanced antimicrobial activity (Arvizo et al. 2010; Singh et al. 2016). Such bimetallic gold-silver nanoparticles overcome the limitation of silver nanoparticles to function in conjunction with biomolecules and drugs. In addition, these bimetallic nanoparticles also possess improved characteristics such as better optical, electronic and catalytic properties (Santos et al. 2012). Further, compared to silver nanoparticles, gold nanoparticles are well known as better delivery vectors for pharmacologic compounds. Therefore, gold-silver bimetallic nanoparticles are highly effective with superb antimicrobial activity of silver coupled with improved stability and ease in functioning supported by gold (Doria et al. 2010; Santos et al. 2012).

6.2.5 Mechanism of Action of Metallic Nanoparticles

Metallic nanoparticles utilize pleiotropic ways to disrupt the normal functioning of multi drug resistant pathogens and successfully eliminate microbes from the sites of infection (Sharma et al. 2012; Wang and Hu 2017). The molecular mechanism behind antimicrobial actions of metallic nanoparticles has been extensively investigated and has been summarized below in Fig. 6.2.

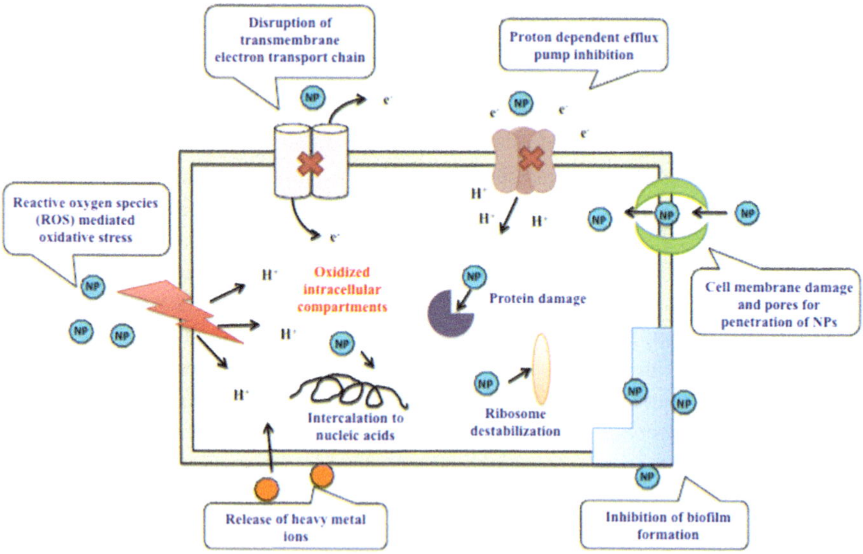

Fig. 6.2 Probable modes of antimicrobial action of metallic nanoparticles against multi drug resistant bacterial pathogens. The figure summarizes different mechanisms employed by metallic nanoparticles (labelled as NPs in the figure) to tackle multi drug resistant bacterial pathogens, such as: reactive oxygen species (ROS) dependent oxidative stress, efflux pump inhibition, release of heavy metal ions that damages cellular proteins and nucleic acids, disruption of biofilms, ribosome destabilization, interference in electron transport chain and destabilization of bacterial membrane integrity by causing pores for nanoparticle to penetrate host cell

6.2.5.1 Generation of Reactive Oxygen Species

One of the principal strategy employed by maximum metallic nanoparticles is the generation of reactive oxygen species- hydroxyl radicals, superoxide ions, hydrogen peroxide, which subsequently induce lipid peroxidation, compromise membrane permeability and affects bacterial replication as well as translational process leading to cell death (Seil and Webster 2012). For instance, silver nanoparticles generate hydroxyl radicals (OH^-) and zinc oxide nanoparticles produce hydrogen peroxide (H_2O_2), that damage their target organisms *via* reactive oxygen species mediated oxidative stress. Moreover, release of heavy metal ions such as Cu^{2+} from copper nanoparticles, were also responsible for formation of reactive oxygen species.

6.2.5.2 Release of Heavy Metal Ions

Microorganisms have different sensitivities towards heavy metal ions. The significantly enhanced antibacterial activity of silver nanoparticles and zinc oxide nanoparticles have been due to interaction of released metal ions (Ag^+ and Zn^{2+}) with the bacterial cell wall that disrupt the membrane integrity. It is suggested that Ag^+ has a strong affinity towards the sulfhydryl groups of bacterial membrane proteins and enzymes in many Gram negative and Gram positive pathogens, making them dysfunctional (Hemeg 2017). In similar fashion, in case of the Gram positive pathogen *Bacillus subtilis*, Cu^{2+} interacts with amines and carboxyl groups of the microbial surface, resulting in membrane disruption (Ahamed et al. 2014).

6.2.5.3 Affecting Bacterial Membrane Permeability

Metallic nanoparticles, particularly silver nanoparticles and zinc oxide nanoparticles, adhere to the bacterial cell surface, alter membrane permeability and interfere with the transmembrane electron transport system. Positively charged metal ions, e.g. Ag^+, released from silver nanoparticles interact with the negatively charged lipopolysaccharide in the bacterial membrane, dissipate the electrochemical proton gradient across the membrane, resulting in cell lysis. Similar loss of membrane potential and inhibition of respiratory chain was also reported as a probable mode of antimicrobial action for other metallic and metal oxide nanoparticles including gold, copper and nickel oxide nanoparticles (Baptista et al. 2018).

6.2.5.4 Adsorption of Nanoparticles to Bacterial Cell and Its Penetration

In bacteria, the cell membrane behaves as the primary defensive barriers, which protect the organisms against external environment. Gram negative bacterial cell wall is composed of lipoproteins, phospholipids and lipopolysaccharides, whereas the cell wall of Gram positive bacteria is made up of a thin layer of peptidoglycans (Kumar et al. 2018). Upon electrostatic interaction between the metallic nanoparticles and its target microbial cells, altered membrane permeability and production of reactive oxygen species, the metallic nanoparticles can then internalize through generated pores or perturbations in the cell envelope. This eventually results in a fall in cytoplasmic pH, which raises the membrane potential. The adhesion of silver nanoparticles and zinc oxide nanoparticles to bacterial cell envelope cause damage to membrane lipids and proteins (Wang and Hu 2017). Aluminium oxide nanoparticles cause oxidative damage to membrane and enter cytoplasm. Both silver and gold nanoparticles have been reported to exert toxicity by penetrating inside the cell and denaturing the 30S ribosomal subunit, thereby impeding protein translation (Hemeg 2017).

6.2.5.5 Affecting Nucleic Acid Replication

Inhibition of the cellular DNA replication machinery and DNA degradation has been well documented with copper nanoparticles. Moreover, titanium oxide nanoparticles in *E. coli* were shown to downregulate the gene expression of precursor molecules to nucleic acid synthesis (Slavin et al. 2017). Bismuth nanoparticles in combination with X-ray treatment emit electrons, with the formation of free radicals that damage bacterial DNA (Rudramurthy et al. 2016). It was also reported that Ag^{+} ions released from silver nanoparticles intercalate with DNA, inhibiting DNA replication and thereby cell division.

6.2.5.6 Disruption of Bacterial Biofilms

One important cause of persistent drug resistant infections is bacterial biofilms, because they evade antibiotic actions and escape innate immune activity. During bacterial biofilm maturation, the extracellular polymeric substance generated, prevents penetration of the antibiotics to target sites. Several reports have suggested metallic nanoparticles like silver nanoparticles to inhibit the microbial biofilm formation (Mu et al. 2016) by interacting with extracellular polymeric substance molecules and by hampering quorum sensing of *E. coli* and *S. aureus*. Magnetic nanoparticles such as super paramagnetic iron oxide nanoparticles coated with silver or gold exhibit the greatest activity against bacterial biofilms (Baptista et al. 2018).

6.2.5.7 Efflux Inhibitory Properties of Nanoparticles

While relatively new, this mechanistic approach of metallic nanoparticles' antimicrobial action against drug resistant pathogens was supported by many studies. This is a very good way to tackle the emerging drug resistant bacteria by utilizing nanoparticles as efflux pump inhibitors, which block the activity of efflux pumps and enhance the concentration of the antibiotic inside the cell for it to be effective in killing pathogens (Sun et al. 2014). For instance, copper nanoparticles were known to exhibit significant efflux inhibitory properties against multi drug resistant *P. aerugionsa* and *S. aureus* (Christena et al. 2015). Similar reports of efflux inhibitory activities of silver nanoparticles and bimetallic gold-silver nanoparticles against AcrAB-TolC type resistance nodulation division (RND) efflux pumps was recently demonstrated in multi drug resistant *Enterobacter cloacae* isolates (Mishra et al. 2018).

6.2.6 *Antimicrobial Efficacy of Carbon Nanoparticles*

Carbon nanoparticles or nanostructures, have become increasingly popular owing to a profusion of properties that they afford. These include mechanical strength, photo luminescence, thermal and electrical conductivity, in addition to a high surface area and improved structural stability (Al-Jumaili et al. 2017). They also have been found to exhibit bactericidal effect (Kang et al. 2008). The antibacterial activity of carbon based nanoparticles is a function of their size and surface area; greater the surface area and smaller the size of the nanoparticle, higher is the antimicrobial activity associated with it (Rudramurthy et al. 2016). However, the exact mode of action against bacterial cells has been hard to predict. The efficacy of carbon nanoparticles has been demonstrated against bacteria, with most of the work done either using non-resistant, non-clinical type strains or by demonstrating activity against resistant strains *in vitro* (Lyon et al. 2006; Kang et al. 2007), but the explanation for their potency is currently at best speculative.

6.2.6.1 Fullerenes

Fullerenes and their derivatives are known to possess potent antibacterial activity against microorganisms by virtue of their intrinsic molecular architecture. They are generally closed-cage nanoparticles with conjugate double bonds maintaining π-electrons in the molecule. Upon illumination by photons, the fullerene is energized to an excited state, from the ground state. The excited state is very short lived, and rapidly decays to a longer lasting triplet state which, in the presence of molecular oxygen tends to form reactive oxygen species, including singlet oxygen ($^1O_2$) and the superoxide anion (O_2^-). These unstable chemical species are intensely lethal in high concentrations, leading to the peroxidation of lipids, protein and nucleic acids in eukaryotes (Al-Jumaili et al. 2017). The surface of fullerenes is highly hydrophobic. It has the potential to interact with membrane lipids in the bacterial outer membrane, resulting in cleavage of DNA and disruption of the cell membrane (Grinholc et al. 2015). Fullerenes have been seen to negatively affect the growth of Gram positive bacteria as well as yeasts that colonize and infect the skin (Aoshima et al. 2009). However, antibacterial activity of fullerenes has been observed to be higher in Gram positive bacteria rather than their Gram negative counter parts (Markovic and Trajkovic 2008). It has been postulated that a high concentration of fullerenes increase oxygen uptake, with a concomitant increase in its conversion to hydrogen peroxide that in turn interferes with the cellular respiratory chain (Mashino et al. 2003). A polyhydroxylated derivative of fullerene, fullerol, has been gaining attention as an antimicrobial agent for exhibiting activity against a host of microorganisms with the advantage of being less toxic than fullerene to the host (Aoshima et al. 2009).

6.2.6.2 Carbon Nanotubes

Carbon nanotubes were first reported to possess antibacterial properties against *E. coli* (Kang et al. 2008). The small cross section of single walled carbon nanotubes allowed partitioning of and penetration into the bacterial cell membrane. With a larger surface area, they induce a greater amount of oxidative stress responses in conjunction with the resultant membrane stress response. These were seen to negatively impact cell morphology, metabolism and envelope integrity, precipitating in cell death. The more complex variants of these nanoparticles, i.e., multi walled carbon nanotubes, also exhibit antibacterial action, where particles longer than 50 μm are seen to wrap around the bacterial cell and induce osmotic lysis (Chen et al. 2013). Single walled carbon nanotubes have been demonstrated to have antibacterial activity against *Salmonella enterica*, *E. coli*, and *Enterococcus faecium* (Dong et al. 2012). Like fullerenes, carbon nanotubes also possess the ability to generate reactive oxygen species in response to stimulation by ultraviolet radiation, with both single- and multi- walled nanotubes producing far greater reactive species than fullerenes (Chae et al. 2011).

6.2.6.3 Graphene

Graphene is a family that comprises of many nanomaterial formulations, not restricted to pristine graphene, but also include graphite, graphene oxide and its reduced form, multi layered graphene, and graphene nanosheets. Graphene oxide has been seen to exhibit the most antibacterial activity, followed by reduced graphene oxide and graphite, when tested against *Pseudomonas aeruginosa*. Though the exact mode of action is not known, simulations have pointed towards graphene sheets penetrating the cell membrane through slow diffusion. While small sheets leave the phospholipid order intact, larger sheets tend to disrupt the distribution and density of phospholipids within the layer (Dallavalle et al. 2015). The main mechanism of antibacterial action, however, has been proposed to be by generation of reactive oxygen species, an overproduction of which confers oxidative stress upon the cell (Krishnamoorthy et al. 2012). Graphene oxide was seen to be adept at inactivating *S. aureus* better than *E. coli* (Akhavan et al. 2011) in-vitro. A unique antibacterial mechanism of graphene has been reported using aggregated graphene sheets. These structures have the property to entrap bacterial cells, physically isolating them from nutrients in their vicinity and inducing a proliferative slowdown, akin to bacteriostatic action (Akhavan et al. 2011).

6.2.7 Organic Nanomaterials and Their Biomedical Applications

6.2.7.1 Improving the Bioavailability of Drug Molecules

Roxithromycin, a semisynthetic derivative of erythromycin, has a low bioavailability of 50% (absolute oral bioavailability) due to its hydrophobic nature. To exploit its effectiveness as an antimicrobial agent used against multi drug resistant Gram positive bacteria, nanoparticles were prepared using roxithromycin and Poly-(lactic-co-glycolic acid) (PLGA) and showed a greater antibacterial activity against multi drug resistant strains of *E. coli* and *S. aureus* (Masood et al. 2016). A report by Marslin et al. (2015) delineates the synthesis and potency of a multi-faceted composite nanoparticle that not only increases the effective concentration of the active drug molecule over sustained time duration, but also helps prevent the development of antibiotic resistance. A copolymer synthesized using polyethylene glycol and polylactic-co-glycolic acid (abbreviated as mPEG-PLGA), acted as a carrier for the fluoroquinolone ofloxacin, which was encapsulated within the nanoparticle. This formulation was demonstrated to increase uptake of the drug, thus exhibiting increased antimicrobial activity against the bacterial cells, as compared to the free drug. This enhanced antimicrobial activity was attributed to the binding of polyethylene glycol to DNA thereby releasing the fluoroquinolone in the direct vicinity of its target molecules (DNA gyrase and topoisomerase). In contrast to fluoroquinolones, polyethylene glycol did not induce mutations and thus prevented evolution of antibiotic resistance in the bacterium *Bacillus subtilis*. Further, efficacy of polyethylene glycol to enhance the antimicrobial resistance could also be attributed to its efflux pump inhibitory property as resistance to fluoroquinolones in clinical cases of *B. subtilis* is mostly mediated by the efflux pump *bmr* (Ahmed et al. 1995).

6.2.7.2 Enhancing the Efficacy of Existing Metal Nanoparticles

Silver nanoparticles are known to bind with high avidity to negative side groups of biomolecules that are present in bacterial cells, an act which alters the structure of the bound molecule, rendering it non-functional. Silver has also been reported to affect various intracellular molecules or molecular complexes, thereby interfering with membrane transport, cell wall synthesis, electron transport, protein folding and function, translation, and nucleic acid synthesis. Bacterial growth is consequently inhibited or the bacteria are killed (Kalhapure et al. 2015). There however has been an increasing reportage of adverse responses by these same nanoparticles *in vitro* as well as *in vivo* (Vazquez-Muñoz et al. 2017). The application of silver, therefore, has been directed towards and found more success in complexes with antimicrobial drugs encapsulated within lipid nanoparticles. Kalhapure et al. (2015) demonstrated the efficacy of clotrimazole-silver complexes encapsulated within solid-lipid nanoparticles against methicillin resistant *Staphylococcus aureus*. Entrapment within the lipid compartment allowed release of the drug-silver complex in a controlled manner, in sufficient quantities to inhibit the growth of bacteria. It has also been postulated that the silver molecules released supplement the antibacterial activity of the drug-silver complex release from the nanoparticle. The use of carbon nanoparticles has been extended to incorporate silver ions in complexes with N-heterocyclic carbene. When encapsulated within L-tyrosine phosphate micelles, these have been shown to augment the antimicrobial activity of silver *in vitro* without causing toxicity to human fibroblast cells. The most striking feature of these nanoparticles, however, is their ability to overcome the inherent resistance of bacteria through sustained dosing over a period of time. Vancomycin resistant *Enterococcus faecium* were found to resist single doses of the silver-carbene complexes, but was killed by half the concentration of the microbicidal dose of the nanoparticle upon consecutive dosing for 24 h (Leid et al. 2011).

6.2.7.3 Re-introducing Toxic Antimicrobials into Therapeutic Use

Certain antimicrobial compounds have remained unsuitable for therapeutic use owing to their toxicity and the deleterious effects on the human host system. These are of special interest in tackling antimicrobial resistance, given the lack of resistance available against them owing to their insubstantial use in the past. Nanoparticles have provided a way to reintroduce the compounds into mainstream treatment by alleviating the ill effects that they cause without diminishing their antimicrobial potency.

Chloramphenicol inhibits protein chain elongation in the bacterial ribosome, and has been established as a broad spectrum bacteriostatic drug. The hydrophobic nature of chloramphenicol prevents penetration and transport by the vascular system. Coupled with its propensity to cause bone marrow toxicity, the use of chloramphenicol in therapeutic regimens has been stringently controlled. Kalita et al. (2015) devised a work around wherein they synthesized nanoparticles that are a composite of poly (ε-caprolactone) and pluronic with chloramphenicol encapsulated within. While the former is frequently used in subcutaneous drug delivery systems, pluronic is a surfactant polyol that solubilizes water insoluble compounds. They observed the nanoparticles to inculcate 98.3% of the chloramphenicol within themselves and release 81% of it in a sustained manner over a time period of 36 days. The pluronic encapsulated chloramphenicol retain their size and encapsulation efficiency when stored for 6 months at 4° and 25 °C respectively. But more importantly, a significant enhanced antimicrobial activity was observed against methicillin resistant *Staphylococcus aureus* strains, with a reduction in hemolytic activity and cytotoxicity as compared to the free drug.

There has been increasing reports of botanical extracts and their effect on bacteria, with multiple reports on the effectiveness of various natural products against mounting challenge of multi drug resistance in bacteria. While this shows promise, in reality, a large number of natural extracts and botanical compounds that show antimicrobial activity *in vitro* suffer from weak solubility in aqueous solvents, poor stability resulting in rapid degradation and low bioavailability *in vivo*. One such example is the molecule 'curcumin', the active ingredient of turmeric. Krausz et al. (2015) created composite nanoparticles using silane, organized to form a porous lattice structured within which curcumin was accommodated. The formulation was seen to not only inhibit the growth of methicillin resistant *Staphylococcus aureus in vitro* but also reduce the bacterial load in burn wounds infected by methicillin resistant *Staphylococcus aureus* in a murine model.

6.3 Potential Limitations of Metallic Nanoparticles

The mechanisms of metallic nanoparticles against its target biological entities are being gradually explored. However, the major challenge routinely faced in nanotechnology research is to regulate the size and shape of monodispersed nanoparticles without affecting its activity and retaining stability during synthesis. Furthermore, the critical parameter of any nanoparticles is its size which defines its permeation ability, for which they are known as a substitute to antibiotics or drug delivery agents. Since it was noticed that most of these metallic nanoparticles penetrate cell envelope, they are likely to even disseminate by blood vessels to different regions of the human body including the lymphatic vascular system and nerve cells (Khan et al. 2017). Therefore, metallic nanoparticles due to their selective aggregation in different cells and tissues of the body, or other sub-cellular structures possess potential health threats. It is also pertinent to mention here that the potential risks attached with metallic nanoparticles vary significantly with the type of nanoparticles.

Consequently, researchers have also investigated the defence mechanism employed by bacterial pathogens against antibacterial action of metallic and metal oxide nanoparticles that resulted in the developing resistance towards nanoparticles. Firstly, the larger metallic nanoparticles, i.e., greater than 10–20 nm in size, can be limited by production of extracellular flagellin matrix that agglomerate these metallic nanoparticles and thus prevents its antibacterial action. Secondly, certain bacterial species produce pigments like pyocyanin which is capable of inactivating ions released by the metallic nanoparticles (Martinez et al. 2019). Even it was also observed that certain microorganisms were able to modulate their electrical surface charge in order to avoid the nanoparticle action with different charge surface. Besides, efflux pumps which has recently gained attention in providing resistance to bacterial cells against metallic nanoparticles, there are other methods like mutations, bio-precipitation, enzyme detoxification, biofilm formation, pigment production etc. which could possibly contribute to development of resistance against antimicrobial nature of nanoparticles (Martinez et al. 2019). It is noteworthy that excessive use of metallic and metal oxide nanoparticles has also facilitated co-selection and co-expression of antibiotic resistance genes, which could be a potential limitation for usage of nanoparticles in medicine.

One of the most significant hurdles to the large scale deployment of organic nanoparticles, or any nanomaterials *per se*, in therapeutic regimens against bacteria is their biological toxicity. Metallic nanoparticles can easily prevent themselves from the immune defense mechanism of the host body, because of their small size, and disseminate through epithelial and endothelial cells into the blood, eventually spread to other parts of the body *via* lymphatic circulation (Leucuta 2014). The generation of reactive oxygen species by nanoparticles are primary cause to subsequent inflammation and toxicity, triggering apoptosis followed by the activation of signalling pathways, leading to the progression of several critical health disorders. For example, in case of pulmonary diseases, experimental evidences have identified a strong relationship between pulmonary inflammation and detrimental effects of ultrafine particles (Hoet et al. 2004). It was also noticed in human as well as animal studies, that nanomaterials get translocated from extrapulmonary sites (such as the liver, heart and brain) to the systemic circulation. Therefore, the severity of the toxic effect of nanoparticles depends, to some extent, on their route of introduction into the biological system.

Several nanoparticles have reportedly exhibited toxicity in multiple organs, including hepatotoxicity and nephrotoxicity, which is caused primarily due to oxidative stress generated by the interaction of free radicals of the nanoparticles with cell components (De Jong and Borm 2008). Reports also indicated that intravenous injection of nanoparticles leads to its accumulation in the liver, lung, colon, spleen, bone marrow, and lymphatic system (Hagens et al. 2007). Again, inhalation of nanoparticles was observed to induce cytotoxicity in different parts of the body like lungs, liver, even heart and spleen through systemic circulation (Poma and Di Giorgio 2008; Leucuta 2014).

The biocompatibility of nanoparticles, that is the ability of the nanomaterial to function inside host body in a certain way so that the host responds in a particular way, is another crucial parameter usually validated through cell culture based *in vitro* assays. As earlier mentioned that depending upon its usage as an antimicrobial agent, nanoparticles can permeate through inhalation, skin contact, ingestion, and even oral and intravenous injections. Hence, for better estimating the host response to nanoparticles, in the context of metabolism, associated toxicity and clearance from host; *in vivo* models must be utilized (Beyth et al. 2015). Carbon nanoparticles particularly face the acute problems of a high production cost, considerable batch-to-batch variation in the properties of nanomaterials synthesized and poor yield (Al-Jumaili et al. 2017).

6.4 Future Research Directions

Different methods and studies have been proposed to evaluate the safety and environmental impacts of metallic and non-metallic nanoparticles. Various *in vivo* and *in vitro* studies have given us insights on the specific strategy employed by nanoparticles; by which its surface can be modified limiting its adverse effects and making them safer and less toxic – thus being more appropriate for use (De Matteis 2017). Future applications of nanoparticles would be greatly dependent on their toxicology profile, for which, optimization of the *in vitro* methodologies based on good laboratory practiceas well as the generation of reliable and flexible databases is extremely necessary. Together, these studies will provide valuable information on the accurate dosage for a particular metallic nanoparticle to be effective to pathogens, while considered safe and appropriate for medical use. Since, the effect of nanoparticles on biological systems is less explored, so the deleterious effects and limitations of nanoparticles should be carefully investigated.

As mentioned previously, nanomaterials possess great potential to be used as an alternative to antimicrobial therapeutics, though several challenges still remain unsettled for its actual implementation in the clinics. One of the major problems include standardizing the accurate dose and appropriate routes of administration of the nanoparticles, that will be the decisive factor for interactions of nano antibiotics with their respective target cells/tissues and organs (Sandhiya et al. 2009). However, effective administration of nanoparticles in the hospitals will further require to adapt and practice a set of predesigned approaches to evaluate their mechanism of action. In addition to the rapid development of nanomedicines, it's commercialization and effective biomedical applications needs to be carefully validated. Appropriate guidelines for eco-friendly synthesis of the nanoparticles, their physicochemical characterization, biocompatibility check and optimization of nanotoxicology assays and protocols for easy comparison of datasets originating from *in vitro* and *in vivo* studies; should be strictly followed to understand their metabolism in host (Duncan and Gaspar 2011; Beyth et al. 2015; Rai et al. 2016). For this, several assessment criteria and reference standards have been designed and some are still under development (Halamoda-Kenzaoui et al. 2019). However, literatures suggested critical gaps in determining the quality and safety measures of the nanomaterials that further necessitates the correct assessment of all of its features along with drug load and release aspects of the nanomaterial when used as a carrier/vehicle before its actual applications and commercialization.

Ultimately, the larger community still needs to figure out the environmental and socio-economical impact of translation of such nanomaterials to the health centres. It would be rightful to state that, there are still plenty of real life issues and challenges that persist in the field of health sciences, which needs to be quickly managed before our humankind actually gets benefitted from the advantageous effects of nanomaterials.

6.5 Conclusion

Taking into consideration the valuable therapeutic potential and wide range of applications, it is becoming extremely important to gain knowledge regarding modes of action underlying antimicrobial activity of the metallic nanomaterials on multi drug resistant pathogens. Simultaneous development of beneficial aspects of nanoparticles and reducing toxic side effects, would significantly help the medical researchers to mitigate this escalating antimicrobial resistance problem. Undoubtedly, metallic nanoparticles could be utilized as a powerful tool against such multi drug resistant infectious agents in this post antibiotic era, if taken care with judicious applications.

References

AbdalDayem A, Hossain M, Lee S, Kim K, Saha S, Yang GM, Choi H, Cho SG (2017) The role of reactive oxygen species (ROS) in the biological activities of metallic nanoparticles. Int J Mol Sci:1–21. https://doi.org/10.3390/ijms18010120

Ahamed M, Alhadlaq HA, Majeed Khan MA, Karuppiah P, Al-Dhabi NA (2014) Synthesis, characterization, and antimicrobial activity of copper oxide nanoparticles. J Nanomater 10:4. https://doi.org/10.1155/2014/637858

Ahmed M, Lyass L, Markham PN, Taylor SS, Vázquez-Laslop N, Neyfakh AA (1995) Two highly similar multidrug transporters of Bacillus subtilis whose expression is differentially regulated. J Bacteriol 177:3904 LP–3903910. https://doi.org/10.1128/jb.177.14.3904-3910.1995

Akhavan O, Ghaderi E, Esfandiar A (2011) Wrapping Bacteria by graphene nanosheets for isolation from environment, reactivation by sonication, and inactivation by near-infrared irradiation. J Phys Chem B 115:6279–6288. https://doi.org/10.1021/jp200686k

Ali SS, Morsy R, El-Zawawy NA, Fareed MF, Bedaiwy MY (2017) Synthesized zinc peroxide nanoparticles (ZnO2-NPs): a novel antimicrobial, anti-elastase, anti-keratinase, and anti-inflammatory approach toward polymicrobial burn wounds. Int J Nanomedicine 12:6059–6073. https://doi.org/10.2147/IJN.S141201

Al-Jumaili A, Alancherry S, Bazaka K, Jacob M (2017) Review on the antimicrobial properties of carbon nanostructures. Materials (Basel) 10:1066. https://doi.org/10.3390/ma10091066

Ansari MA, Khan HM, Khan AA, Ahmad MK, Mahdi AA, Pal R, Cameotra SS (2014) Interaction of silver nanoparticles with *Escherichia coli* and their cell envelope biomolecules. J Basic Microbiol 54:905–915. https://doi.org/10.1002/jobm.201300457

Aoshima H, Kokubo K, Shirakawa S, Ito M, Yamana S, Oshima T (2009) Antimicrobial activity of fullerenes and their hydroxylated derivatives. Biocontrol Sci 14:69–72. https://doi.org/10.4265/bio.14.69

Arvizo RR, Miranda OR, Thompson MA et al (2010) Effect of nanoparticle surface charge at the plasma membrane and beyond. Nano Lett 10:2543–2548. https://doi.org/10.1021/nl101140t

Aslam B, Wang W, Arshad MI et al (2018) Antibiotic resistance: a rundown of a global crisis. Infect Drug Resist 11:1645–1658. https://doi.org/10.2147/IDR.S173867

Baptista PV, McCusker MP, Carvalho A et al (2018) Nano-strategies to fight multidrug resistant bacteria-“A Battle of the Titans”. Front Microbiol 9:1–26. https://doi.org/10.3389/fmicb.2018.01441

Beceiro A, Tomás M, Bou G (2013) Antimicrobial resistance and virulence: a successful or deleterious association in the bacterial world? Clin Microbiol Rev 26:185–230. https://doi.org/10.1128/CMR.00059-12

Behera SS, Patra JK, Pramanik K, Panda N, Thatoi H (2012) Characterization and evaluation of antibacterial activities of chemically synthesized Iron oxide nanoparticles. World J Nano Sci Eng 02:196–200. https://doi.org/10.4236/wjnse.2012.24026

Beyth N, Houri-Haddad Y, Domb A et al (2015) Alternative antimicrobial approach: nano-antimicrobial materials. Evid Based Complement Altern Med 2015:1–16. https://doi.org/10.1155/2015/246012

Bilal M, Rasheed T, Iqbal HMN et al (2017) Silver nanoparticles: biosynthesis and antimicrobial potentialities. Int J Pharmacol 13:832–845

Bolla JM, Alibert-Franco S, Handzlik J et al (2011) Strategies for bypassing the membrane barrier in multidrug resistant gram-negative bacteria. FEBS Lett 585:1682–1690. https://doi.org/10.1016/j.febslet.2011.04.054

Boucher HW, Talbot GH, Bradley JS et al (2009) Bad bugs, no drugs: no ESKAPE! An update from the infectious diseases society of America. Clin Infect Dis. https://doi.org/10.1086/595011

Bush K, Jacoby GA (2010) Updated functional classification of β-lactamases. Antimicrob Agents Chemother 54:969–976. https://doi.org/10.1128/AAC.01009-09

Centers for Disease Control and Prevention (2013) Antibiotic resistance threats. Cent Dis Control Prev:22–50. CS239559-B

Chae S-R, Watanabe Y, Wiesner MR (2011) Comparative photochemical reactivity of spherical and tubular fullerene nanoparticles in water under ultraviolet (UV) irradiation. Water Res 45:308–314. https://doi.org/10.1016/j.watres.2010.07.067

Chen H, Wang B, Gao D, Guan M, Zheng L, Ouyang H, Chai Z, Zhao Y, Feng W (2013) Broad-spectrum antibacterial activity of carbon nanotubes to human gut bacteria. Small 9:2735–2746. https://doi.org/10.1002/smll.201202792

Chen F, Ehlerding EB, Cai W (2014) Theranostic nanoparticles. J Nucl Med 55:1919–1922. https://doi.org/10.2967/jnumed.114.146019

Christena LR, Mangalagowri V, Pradheeba P et al (2015) Copper nanoparticles as an efflux pump inhibitor to tackle drug resistant bacteria. RSC Adv 5:12899–12909. https://doi.org/10.1039/C4RA15382K

Dallavalle M, Calvaresi M, Bottoni A, Melle-Franco M, Zerbetto F (2015) Graphene can wreak havoc with cell membranes. ACS Appl Mater Interfaces 7:4406–4414. https://doi.org/10.1021/am508938u

Dasgupta N, Ramalingam C (2016) Silver nanoparticle antimicrobial activity explained by membrane rupture and reactive oxygen generation. Environ Chem Lett 14:477–485. https://doi.org/10.1007/s10311-016-0583-1

Davies J, Davies D (2010) Origins and evolution of antibiotic resistance. Microbiol Mol Biol Rev 74:417–433. https://doi.org/10.1128/mmbr.00016-10

De Jong WH, Borm PJ (2008) Drug delivery and nanoparticles: applications and hazards. Int J Nanomedicine 3:133–149

De Matteis V (2017) Exposure to inorganic nanoparticles: routes of entry, immune response, biodistribution and in vitro/in vivo toxicity evaluation. Toxics 5:29. https://doi.org/10.3390/toxics5040029

Dhand C, Dwivedi N, Loh XJ, Ying AN, Verma NK, Beuerman RW, Lakshminarayanan R, Ramakrishna S (2015) Methods and strategies for the synthesis of diverse nanoparticles and their applications: a comprehensive overview. RSC Adv 5:105003–105037. https://doi.org/10.1039/C5RA19388E

Dong L, Henderson A, Field C (2012) Antimicrobial activity of single-walled carbon nanotubes suspended in different surfactants. J Nanotechnol 2012. https://doi.org/10.1155/2012/928924

Doria G, Larguinho M, Dias JT et al (2010) Gold-silver-alloy nanoprobes for one-pot multiplex DNA detection. Nanotechnology 21. https://doi.org/10.1088/0957-4484/21/25/255101

Duncan R, Gaspar R (2011) Nanomedicine (s) under the microscope. Mol Pharm 8:2101–2141. https://doi.org/10.1021/mp200394t

Ealias AM, Saravanakumar MP (2017) A review on the classification, characterisation, synthesis of nanoparticles and their application. IOP Conf Ser Mater Sci Eng 263. https://doi.org/10.1088/1757-899X/263/3/032019

Franci G, Falanga A, Galdiero S et al (2015) Silver nanoparticles as potential antibacterial agents. Molecules 20:8856–8874. https://doi.org/10.3390/molecules20058856

Gholipourmalekabadi M, Mobaraki M, Ghaffari M, Zarebkohan A, Omrani VF, Urbanska AM, Seifalian A (2017) Targeted drug delivery based on gold nanoparticle derivatives. Curr Pharm Des 23:2918–2929. https://doi.org/10.2174/1381612823666170419105413

Graves J, Thomas M, Ewunkem J (2017) Antimicrobial nanomaterials: why evolution matters. Nano 7:283. https://doi.org/10.3390/nano7100283

Grinholc M, Nakonieczna J, Fila G, Taraszkiewicz A, Kawiak A, Szewczyk G, Sarna T, Lilge L, Bielawski KP (2015) Antimicrobial photodynamic therapy with fulleropyrrolidine: photoinactivation mechanism of *Staphylococcus aureus*, in vitro and in vivo studies. Appl Microbiol Biotechnol 99:4031–4043. https://doi.org/10.1007/s00253-015-6539-8

Gupta M, Sharma V, Chauhan NS (2017) Nanotechnology for oral delivery of anticancer drugs: an insight potential. Nanostruct Oral Med:467–510. https://doi.org/10.1016/B978-0-323-47720-8.00017-1

Gupta R, Ahad MZ, Udupa A, Varma M, Mukhopadhyay C, Ke V (2019) Blood stream infections by carbapenem resistant bacteria: critical perspectives from Indian tertiary care hospital. Int J Infect Dis 79:40. https://doi.org/10.1016/j.ijid.2018.11.111

Hagens WI, Oomen AG, de Jong WH, Cassee FR, Sips AJ (2007) What do we (need to) know about the kinetic properties of nanoparticles in the body? Reg Toxicol Pharmacol 49:217–229. https://doi.org/10.1016/j.yrtph.2007.07.006

Halamoda-Kenzaoui B, Holzwarth U, Roebben G, Bogni A, Bremer-Hoffmann S (2019) Mapping of the available standards against the regulatory needs for nanomedicines. Wiley Interdiscip Rev Nanomed Nanobiotechnol 11(1):e1531

Hemeg HA (2017) Nanomaterials for alternative antibacterial therapy. Int J Nanomedicine 12:8211–8225. https://doi.org/10.2147/IJN.S132163

Hoet PHM, Brüske-Hohlfeld I, Salata OV (2004) Nanoparticles – known and unknown health risks. J Nanobiotechnol 2:1–15. https://doi.org/10.1186/1477-3155-2-12

Huh AJ, Kwon YJ (2011) "Nanoantibiotics": a new paradigm for treating infectious diseases using nanomaterials in the antibiotics resistant era. J Control Release 156:128–145. https://doi.org/10.1016/J.JCONREL.2011.07.002

Jeevanandam J, Barhoum A, Chan YS, Dufresne A, Danquah MK (2018) Review on nanoparticles and nanostructured materials: history, sources, toxicity and regulations. Beilstein J Nanotechnol 9:1050–1074. https://doi.org/10.3762/bjnano.9.98

Jiang W, Mashayekhi H, Xing B (2009) Bacterial toxicity comparison between nano- and micro-scaled oxide particles. Environ Pollut 157:1619–1625. https://doi.org/10.1016/J.ENVPOL.2008.12.025

Kalhapure RS, Sonawane SJ, Sikwal DR, Jadhav M, Rambharose S, Mocktar C, Govender T (2015) Solid lipid nanoparticles of clotrimazole silver complex: an efficient nano antibacterial against *Staphylococcus aureus* and MRSA. Colloid Surf B. https://doi.org/10.1016/j.colsurfb.2015.10.003

Kalishwaralal K, BarathManiKanth S, Pandian SR, Deepak V, Gurunathan S (2010) Silver nanoparticles impede the biofilm formation by *Pseudomonas aeruginosa* and *Staphylococcus epidermidis*. Colloids Surf B Biointerfaces 79:340–344. https://doi.org/10.1016/j.colsurfb.2010.04.014

Kalita S, Devi B, Kandimalla R, Sharma KK, Sharma A, Kalita K, Ch Kataki A, Kotoky J (2015) Chloramphenicol encapsulated in poly(epsilon- caprolactone)-pluronic composite: nanoparticles for treatment of MRSA-infected burn wounds. Int J Nanomedicine 10:2971. https://doi.org/10.2147/IJN.S75023

Kandi V, Kandi S (2015) Antimicrobial properties of nanomolecules: potential candidates as antibiotics in the era of multi-drug resistance. Epidemiol Health 37:e2015020. https://doi.org/10.4178/epih/e2015020

Kang S, Pinault M, Pfefferle LD, Elimelech M (2007) Single-walled carbon nanotubes exhibit strong antimicrobial activity. Langmuir 23:8670–8673. https://doi.org/10.1021/la701067r

Kang S, Herzberg M, Rodrigues DF, Elimelech M (2008) Antibacterial effects of carbon nanotubes: size does matter! Langmuir 24:6409–6413. https://doi.org/10.1021/la800951v

Khan I, Saeed K, Khan I (2017) Nanoparticles: properties, applications and toxicities. Arab J Chem. https://doi.org/10.1016/j.arabjc.2017.05.011

Kim JS, Kuk E, Yu KN et al (2007) Antimicrobial effects of silver nanoparticles. Nanomed Nanotechnol Biol Med 3:95–101. https://doi.org/10.1016/j.nano.2006.12.001

Kraker MEA, Stewardson AJ, Harbarth S (2016) Will 10 million people die a year due to antimicrobial resistance by 2050? PLoS Med 13:e1002184. https://doi.org/10.1371/journal.pmed.1002184

Krausz AE, Adler BL, Cabral V, Navati M, Doerner J, Charafeddine RA, Chandra D, Liang H, Gunther L, Clendaniel A, Harper S, Friedman JM, Nosanchuk JD, Friedman AJ (2015) Curcumin-encapsulated nanoparticles as innovative antimicrobial and wound healing agent. Nanomedicine 11:195–206. https://doi.org/10.1016/j.nano.2014.09.004

Krishnamoorthy K, Veerapandian M, Zhang L-H, Yun K, Kim SJ (2012) Antibacterial efficiency of graphene Nanosheets against pathogenic bacteria via lipid peroxidation. J Phys Chem C 116:17280–17287. https://doi.org/10.1021/jp3047054

Krishnamoorthy G, Leus IV, Weeks JW et al (2017) Synergy between active efflux and outer membrane diffusion defines rules of antibiotic permeation into gram-negative Bacteria. MBio 8:1–16. https://doi.org/10.1128/mbio.01172-17

Kruk T, Szczepanowicz K, Stefańska J, Socha RP, Warszyński P (2015) Synthesis and antimicrobial activity of monodisperse copper nanoparticles. Colloids Surf B 128:17–22. https://doi.org/10.1016/j.colsurfb.2015.02.009

Kumar M, Curtis A, Hoskins C (2018) Application of nanoparticle technologies in the combat against anti-microbial resistance. Pharmaceutics 10:1–17. https://doi.org/10.3390/pharmaceutics10010011

Kuppusamy P, Yusoff MM, Maniam GP, Govindan N (2016) Biosynthesis of metallic nanoparticles using plant derivatives and their new avenues in pharmacological applications– an updated report. Saudi Pharm J 24:473–484. https://doi.org/10.1016/j.jsps.2014.11.013

Lai HZ, Chen WY, Wu CY, Chen YC (2015) Potent antibacterial nanoparticles for pathogenic bacteria. ACS Appl Mater Interfaces 7:2046–2054. https://doi.org/10.1021/am507919m

Lakshmi Prasanna V, Vijayaraghavan R (2015) Insight into the mechanism of antibacterial activity of ZnO: surface defects mediated reactive oxygen species even in the dark. Langmuir 31:9155–9162. https://doi.org/10.1021/acs.langmuir.5b02266

Lambert PA (2005) Bacterial resistance to antibiotics: modified target sites. Adv Drug Deliv Rev 57:1471–1485. https://doi.org/10.1016/j.addr.2005.04.003

Leid JG, Ditto AJ, Knapp A, Shah PN, Wright BD, Blust R, Christensen L, Clemons CB, Wilber JP, Young GW, Kang AG, Panzner MJ, Cannon CL, Yun YH, Youngs WJ, Seckinger NM, Cope EK (2011) In vitro antimicrobial studies of silver carbene complexes: activity of free and nanoparticle carbene formulations against clinical isolates of pathogenic bacteria. J Antimicrob Chemother 67:138–148. https://doi.org/10.1093/jac/dkr408

Leucuta SE (2014) Subcellular drug targeting, pharmacokinetics and bioavailability. J Drug Target 22:95–115. https://doi.org/10.3109/1061186X.2013.848453

Li B, Webster TJ (2018) Bacteria antibiotic resistance: new challenges and opportunities for implant-associated orthopedic infections. J Orthop Res 36:22–32. https://doi.org/10.1002/jor.23656

Li X, Robinson SM, Gupta A, Saha K, Jiang Z, Moyano DF, Sahar A, Riley MA, Rotello VM (2014) Functional gold nanoparticles as potent antimicrobial agents against multi-drug-resistant bacteria. ACS Nano 8:10682–10686. https://doi.org/10.1021/nn5042625

Li XZ, Plésiat P, Nikaido H (2015) The challenge of efflux-mediated antibiotic resistance in gram-negative bacteria. Clin Microbiol Rev. https://doi.org/10.1128/CMR.00117-14

Lima E, Guerra R, Lara V, Guzmán A (2013) Gold nanoparticles as efficient antimicrobial agents for *Escherichia coli* and *Salmonella typhi*. Chem Cent J 7:1–7. https://doi.org/10.1186/1752-153X-7-11

Lobanovska M, Pilla G (2017) Penicillin's discovery and antibiotic resistance: lessons for the future? Yale J Biol Med 90:135–145

Losasso C, Belluco S, Cibin V, Zavagnin P, Mičetić I, Gallocchio F, Zanella M, Bregoli L, Biancotto G, Ricci A (2014) Antibacterial activity of silver nanoparticles: sensitivity of different *Salmonella*serovars. Front Microbiol 5:1–9. https://doi.org/10.3389/fmicb.2014.00227

Lyon DY, Adams LK, Falkner JC, Alvarez PJJ (2006) Antibacterial activity of fullerene water suspensions: effects of preparation method and particle size. Environ Sci Technol 40(14):4360–4366. https://doi.org/10.1021/es0603655

Magiorakos AP, Srinivasan A, Carey RB et al (2012) Multidrug-resistant, extensively drug-resistant and pandrug-resistant bacteria: an international expert proposal for interim standard definitions for acquired resistance. Clin Microbiol Infect. https://doi.org/10.1111/j.1469-0691.2011.03570.x

Markovic Z, Trajkovic V (2008) Biomedical potential of the reactive oxygen species generation and quenching by fullerenes (C60). Biomaterials 29:3561–3573. https://doi.org/10.1016/J.BIOMATERIALS.2008.05.005

Markowska K, Grudniak AM, Wolska KI (2013) Silver nanoparticles as an alternative strategy against bacterial biofilms. Acta Biochim Pol 60:523–530

Marslin G, Revina AM, Khandelwal VKM, Balakumar K, Sheeba CJ, Franklin G (2015) PEGylated ofloxacin nanoparticles render strong antibacterial activity against many clinically important human pathogens. Colloids Surf B 132:62–70. https://doi.org/10.1016/J.COLSURFB.2015.04.050

Mashino T, Usui N, Okuda K, Hirota T, Mochizuki M (2003) Respiratory chain inhibition by fullerene derivatives: hydrogen peroxide production caused by fullerene derivatives and a respiratory chain system. Bioorg Med Chem 11:1433–1438. https://doi.org/10.1016/S0968-0896(02)00610-7

Masood F, Yasin T, Bukhari H, Mujahid M (2016) Characterization and application of Roxithromycin loaded cyclodextrin based nanoparticles for treatment of multidrug resistant Bacteria. Mater Sci Eng C 61:1–7. https://doi.org/10.1016/j.msec.2015.11.076

Mishra M, Kumar S, Majhi RK, Goswami L, Goswami C, Mohapatra H (2018) Antibacterial efficacy of polysaccharide capped silver nanoparticles is not compromised by AcrAB-TolC efflux pump. Front Microbiol 9. https://doi.org/10.3389/fmicb.2018.00823

Morones-Ramirez JR, Winkler JA, Spina CS, Collins JJ (2013) Silver enhances antibiotic activity against gram-negative bacteria. Sci Transl Med 19. https://doi.org/10.1038/mp.2011.182

Mu H, Tang J, Liu Q et al (2016) Potent antibacterial nanoparticles against biofilm and intracellular bacteria. Sci Rep 6:1–9. https://doi.org/10.1038/srep18877

Mulani MS, Kamble EE, Kumkar SN et al (2019) Emerging strategies to combat ESKAPE pathogens in the era of antimicrobial resistance: a review. Front Microbiol 10. https://doi.org/10.3389/fmicb.2019.00539

Munita JM, Arias CA (2016) Mechanisms of antibiotic resistance. Microbiol Spectr 4:1–37. https://doi.org/10.1128/microbiolspec.VMBF-0016-2015

Natan M, Banin E (2017) From nano to micro: using nanotechnology to combat microorganisms and their multidrug resistance. FEMS Microbiol Rev 41:302–322. https://doi.org/10.1093/femsre/fux003

Niño-Martínez N, Salas Orozco MF, Martínez-Castañón GA, Torres Méndez F, Ruiz F (2019) Molecular mechanisms of bacterial resistance to metal and metal oxide nanoparticles. Int J Mol Sci 20(11):2808

O'Neill J (2014) Review on antimicrobial resistance. Antimicrobial resistance: tackling a crisis for the health and wealth of nations, 2014, 4 (December). https://doi.org/10.1038/510015a

Piddock LJV (2006) Clinically relevant chromosomally encoded multidrug resistance efflux pumps in bacteria. Clin Microbiol Rev 19:382–402. https://doi.org/10.1128/CMR.19.2.382

Poma A, Di Giorgio ML (2008) Toxicogenomics to improve comprehension of the mechanisms underlying responses of in vitro and in vivo systems to nanomaterials: a review. Curr Genomics 9:571–585. https://doi.org/10.2174/138920208786847962

Prabhu S, Poulose EK (2012) Silver nanoparticles: mechanism of antimicrobial action, synthesis, medical applications, and toxicity effects. Intnano Lett 2:1–10. https://doi.org/10.1186/2228-5326-2-32

Rai M, Yadav A, Gade A (2009) Silver nanoparticles as a new generation of antimicrobials. Biotechnol Adv 27:76–83. https://doi.org/10.1016/J.BIOTECHADV.2008.09.002

Rai MK, Deshmukh SD, Ingle AP, Gade AK (2012) Silver nanoparticles: the powerful nanoweapon against multidrug-resistant bacteria. J Appl Microbiol 112:841–852. https://doi.org/10.1111/j.1365-2672.2012.05253.x

Rai M, Deshmukh SD, Ingle AP, Gupta IR, Galdiero M, Galdiero S (2016) Metal nanoparticles: the protective nanoshield against virus infection. Crit Rev Microbiol 42:46–56. https://doi.org/10.3109/1040841X.2013.879849

Ramasamy M, Lee JH, Lee J (2017) Development of gold nanoparticles coated with silica containing the antibiofilm drug cinnamaldehyde and their effects on pathogenic bacteria. Int J Nanomedicine 12:2813–2828. https://doi.org/10.2147/IJN.S132784

Ramyadevi J, Jeyasubramanian K, Marikani A, Rajakumar G, Rahuman AA (2012) Synthesis and antimicrobial activity of copper nanoparticles. Mater Lett 71:114–116. https://doi.org/10.1016/j.matlet.2011.12.055

Ranjan S, Ramalingam C (2016) Titanium dioxide nanoparticles induce bacterial membrane rupture by reactive oxygen species generation. Environ Chem Lett 14:487–494. https://doi.org/10.1007/s10311-016-0586-y

Ravishankar Rai V, Jamuna Bai A (2011) Nanoparticles and their potential application as antimicrobials (A Méndez-Vilas A, eds). Formatex, Mysore

Roshmi T, Soumya KR, Jyothis M, Radhakrishnan EK (2015) Effect of biofabricated gold nanoparticle-based antibiotic conjugates on minimum inhibitory concentration of bacterial isolates of clinical origin. Gold Bull 48:63–71. https://doi.org/10.1007/s13404-015-0162-4

Rudramurthy GR, Swamy MK, Sinniah UR, Ghasemzadeh A (2016) Nanoparticles: alternatives against drug-resistant pathogenic microbes. Molecules 21:1–30. https://doi.org/10.3390/molecules21070836

Salomoni R, Léo P, Montemor AF, Rinaldi BG, Rodrigues MF (2017) Antibacterial effect of silver nanoparticles in *Pseudomonas aeruginosa*. Nanotechnol Sci Appl 10:115–121. https://doi.org/10.2147/NSA.S133415

Sandhiya S, Dkhar SA, Surendiran A (2009) Emerging trends of nanomedicine–an overview. Fundam Clin Pharmacol 23:263–269. https://doi.org/10.1111/j.1472-8206.2009.00692.x

Santajit S, Indrawattana N (2016) Mechanisms of antimicrobial resistance in ESKAPE pathogens. Biomed Res Int 2016:1–8. https://doi.org/10.1155/2016/2475067

Santos MM, Queiroz MJ, Baptista PV (2012) Enhancement of antibiotic effect via gold:silver-alloy nanoparticles. J Nanopart Res 14. https://doi.org/10.1007/s11051-012-0859-8

Sanyasi S, Majhi RK, Kumar S, Mishra M, Ghosh A, Suar M, Satyam PV, Mohapatra H, Goswami C, Goswami L (2016) Polysaccharide-capped silver nanoparticles inhibit biofilm formation and eliminate multi-drug-resistant bacteria by disrupting bacterial cytoskeleton with reduced cytotoxicity towards mammalian cells. Sci Rep 6:24929. https://doi.org/10.1038/srep24929

Seil JT, Webster TJ (2012) Antimicrobial applications of nanotechnology: methods and literature the need for novel antibiotics. Int J Nanomedicine 7:2767–2781. https://doi.org/10.2147/IJN.S24805

Sharma A, Kumar Arya D, Dua M, Chhatwal GS, Johri AK (2012) Nano-technology for targeted drug delivery to combat antibiotic resistance. Expert Opin Drug Deliv 9:1325–1332. https://doi.org/10.1517/17425247.2012.717927

Sharma D, Kanchi S, Bisetty K (2015) Biogenic synthesis of nanoparticles: a review. Arab J Chem. https://doi.org/10.1016/j.arabjc.2015.11.002

Sharma G, Kumar A, Sharma S, Naushad M, Dwivedi RP, ALOthman ZA, Mola GT (2019) Novel development of nanoparticles to bimetallic nanoparticles and their composites: a review. J King Saud Univ Sci 31(2):257–269

Sherrard LJ, Tunney MM, Elborn JS (2014) Antimicrobial resistance in the respiratory microbiota of people with cystic fibrosis. Lancet 384:703–713. https://doi.org/10.1016/S0140-6736(14)61137-5

Singh R, Nawale L, Arkile M et al (2016) Phytogenic silver, gold, and bimetallic nanoparticles as novel antitubercular agents. Int J Nanomedicine 11:1889–1897. https://doi.org/10.2147/IJN.S102488

Slavin YN, Asnis J, Häfeli UO, Bach H (2017) Metal nanoparticles: understanding the mechanisms behind antibacterial activity. J Nanobiotechnol 15:1–20. https://doi.org/10.1186/s12951-017-0308-z

Stankic S, Suman S, Haque F, Vidic J (2016) Pure and multi metal oxide nanoparticles: synthesis, antibacterial and cytotoxic properties. J Nanobiotechnol 14:1–20. https://doi.org/10.1186/s12951-016-0225-6

Strahilevitz J, Jacoby GA, Hooper DC, Robicsek A (2009) Plasmid-mediated quinolone resistance: a multifaceted threat. Clin Microbiol Rev 22:664–689. https://doi.org/10.1128/CMR.00016-09

Sun J, Deng Z, Yan A (2014) Bacterial multidrug efflux pumps: mechanisms, physiology and pharmacological exploitations. Biochem Biophys Res Commun. https://doi.org/10.1016/j.bbrc.2014.05.090

Swamy M, Sudipta KM, Jayanta K, Balasubramanya S (2015) The green synthesis, characterization, and evaluation of the biological activities of silver nanoparticles synthesized from Leptadenia reticulata leaf extract. Appl Nanosci 5:73–81. https://doi.org/10.1007/s13204-014-0293-6

Vazquez-Muñoz R, Borrego B, Juárez-Moreno K, García-García M, Mota Morales JD, Bogdanchikova N, Huerta-Saquero A (2017) Toxicity of silver nanoparticles in biological systems: does the complexity of biological systems matter? Toxicol Lett 276:11–20. https://doi.org/10.1016/J.Tox.Lett.2017.05.007

Ventola CL (2015) The antibiotic resistance crisis part 1: causes and threats. P T J 40(4):277–283

Vimbela GV, Ngo SM, Fraze C et al (2017) Antibacterial properties and toxicity from metallic nanomaterials. Int J Nanomedicine 12:3941–3965. https://doi.org/10.2147/IJN.S134526

Wan G, Ruan L, Yin Y, Yang T, Ge M, Cheng X (2016) Effects of silver nanoparticles in combination with antibiotics on the resistant bacteria *Acinetobacter baumannii*. Int J Nanomedicine 11:3789–3800. https://doi.org/10.2147/IJN.S104166

Wang L, Hu C (2017) The antimicrobial activity of nanoparticles: present situation and prospects for the future. Int J Nanomedicine 12:1227–1249. https://doi.org/10.2147/IJN.S121956

WHO (2014) Antimicrobial resistance global report on surveillance 2014. World Heal Organization, Geneva

Yu L, Zhang Y, Zhang B, Liu J (2014) Enhanced antibacterial activity of silver nanoparticles/halloysite nanotubes/graphene nanocomposites with sandwich-like structure. Sci Rep 4:4551. https://doi.org/10.1038/srep04551

Yuan YG, Peng QL, Gurunathan S (2017) Effects of silver nanoparticles on multiple drug-resistant strains of *Staphylococcus aureus* and *Pseudomonas aeruginosa* from mastitis-infected goats: an alternative approach for antimicrobial therapy. Int J Mol Sci 18. https://doi.org/10.3390/ijms18030569

Zhang X, Liu Z, Shen W, Gurunathan S (2016) Silver nanoparticle: synthesis, characterization, properties, applications, and therapeutic approaches. https://doi.org/10.3390/ijms17091534

Zhang J, Tang H, Liu Z, Chen B (2017) Effects of major parameters of nanoparticles on their physical and chemical properties and recent application of nanodrug delivery system in targeted chemotherapy. Int J Nanomedicine 12:8483–8493. https://doi.org/10.2147/IJN.S148359

Chapter 7
Antimicrobial Peptides and Peptidomimetics for the Control of Antimicrobial Resistance

Richard Weeks, Ammar Algburi, and Michael Chikindas

Abstract Bacterial resistance to conventional antibiotics is a growing issue, and the development of novel antimicrobial compounds has not been able to keep pace with the emergence of multi drug resistant pathogens. Antimicrobial peptides are source of inspiration for the development of next generation antimicrobial drugs; however, there are key limitations to the use of natural antimicrobial peptides, owing in large part to common pharmacological features that preclude their use outside of topical applications. The development of novel antimicrobial peptides and peptidomimetics via strategic chemical alterations is a means of improving on the functionality of natural antimicrobial peptides while tuning their pharmacological properties and in some instances, imparting novel mechanisms of action and functions outside of bactericidal activity as well.

Herein we first review natural antimicrobial peptides, their current use as clinical agents, and the ways in which they are typically classified. An overview of the key physicochemical properties of antimicrobial peptides and the ways in which they relate to each other and the impact they have on pharmacological properties is then presented together with a discussion of key limitations relating to bioavailability, toxicity, resistance development, and production and synthesis. Lastly, an overview of several approaches for the improvement and development of novel peptides and

R. Weeks
Health Promoting Naturals Laboratory, School of Environmental and Biological Sciences, Rutgers State University, New Brunswick, NJ, USA

A. Algburi
Health Promoting Naturals Laboratory, School of Environmental and Biological Sciences, Rutgers State University, New Brunswick, NJ, USA

Department of Biotechnology, Science College, Diyala University, Baqubah, Iraq

M. Chikindas (✉)
Health Promoting Naturals Laboratory, School of Environmental and Biological Sciences, Rutgers State University, New Brunswick, NJ, USA

Don State Technical University, Rostov-on-Don, Russia
e-mail: tchikind@sebs.rutgers.edu

H. Panwar et al. (eds.), *Sustainable Agriculture Reviews 49*, Sustainable Agriculture Reviews 49, https://doi.org/10.1007/978-3-030-58259-3_7

peptidomimetics via chemical modifications and strategic alterations are given. Together, these sections should contain a means for the understanding of antimicrobial peptides and the ways in which they are able to target resistant pathogens, and provides a framework for the development of fine-tuned synthetic antimicrobial peptides and peptidomimetics (see Fig. 7.1).

Keywords Antimicrobial peptides · Cationic amphiphiles · Peptidomimetics · Structure-activity relationships · Biofilms · Synergy · Physicochemical properties

7.1 Introduction

Antimicrobial resistance is a growing problem worldwide, with at least two million people in the USA contracting some form of antibiotic resistant infection each year, resulting in approximately 23,000 deaths (CDC 2013). Globally, infections due to antimicrobial resistant bacteria are responsible for 700,000 deaths each year, with more extreme predictions estimating an increase of up to ten million deaths annually by 2050 (O'Neil 2014). The associated cost of antimicrobial resistance is

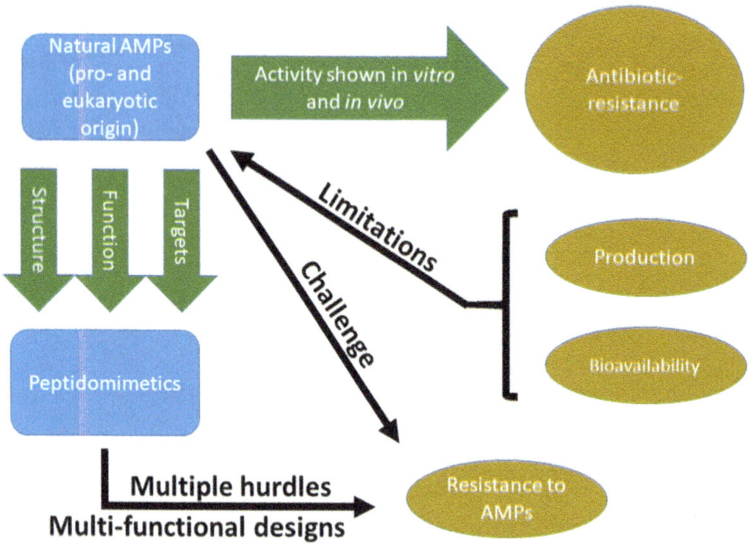

Fig. 7.1 Towards the development of novel antibiotics based on antimicrobial peptides (AMPs), their key properties, and how they may be strategically modified in the development of next generation peptidomimetics. Inspiration should be taken from naturally occurring antimicrobials, with structural changes made to alter peptide function and provide target specificity. Critical challenges and key limitations that are typically associated with natural AMPs must also be taken into consideration, as the interplay between both the positive and negative aspects of these compounds, relating primarily to structure, is complex

also growing, with an estimated annual cost of $5–20 billion in the United States alone (Pendleton et al. 2013). A large proportion of US hospital infections are attributed to a group of multi drug resistant bacteria known as the ESKAPE pathogens (*Enterococcus faecium, Staphylococcus aureus, Klebsiella pneumoniae, Acinetobacter baumannii, Pseudomonas aeruginosa* and *Enterobacter* spp.), in reference to the particular genera and their ability to 'escape' the biocidal action of most antibiotics and other antimicrobial drugs used by western medicine (Pendleton et al. 2013). The increasing threat posed by antimicrobial resistance is driven by several factors, including but not limited to: (1) the over-prescription and misuse of current generation antibiotics, leading to increased incidence of resistance development; (2) a lack of industry interest and research into novel antimicrobial compounds; and (3) insufficient resources and regulation for surveillance and response measures against antimicrobial resistant pathogens and outbreaks. Resistance to even the last-resort antibiotics colistin and carbapenems, typically used in the treatment of particularly difficult Gram negative infections, is no longer uncommon. For example, a mobilized colistin resistance gene (*mcr-1*) was found in bacteria isolated from pigs in China in November 2015, and has now been found in *Escherichia coli* and *K. pneumoniae* isolates worldwide. Since its discovery, at least eight additional mcr variants have been described (Dalmolin et al. 2018). Similarly, carbapenem resistance genes are also spreading, with particularly rapid and alarming rates of resistance development in *Pseudomonas spp.* and *Acinetobacter spp.* (Righi et al. 2017) (Fig. 7.1).

In a 2014 report delivered to the President of the United States of America, three areas of focus regarding the emergence and prevention of antimicrobial resistance were outlined: "(1) improving our surveillance of the rise of antibiotic resistant bacteria to enable effective response, (2) increasing the longevity of current antibiotics. (3) increasing the rate at which new antibiotics, as well as other interventions, are discovered and developed" (PCAST 2014). The first two are not within the scope of this review, though they are essential to a comprehensive understanding of the growing threat of antimicrobial resistance, and as such, a thorough review on surveillance and antimicrobial resistance stewardship efforts involving current antibiotics are provided by Marwick et al. (2017), Tacconelli et al. (2018), and Gregory (2018).

In the search for new antibiotics, great attention is now being focused on antimicrobial peptides, a group of compounds that had been somewhat overlooked and understudied until relatively recently. Antimicrobial peptides are a diverse group of evolutionarily conserved molecules that have been expressed in nearly all living organisms for millions of years, yet have maintained their protective role and remain potent antimicrobials (Wang 2015). This persistence is just one aspect that underscores antimicrobial peptides' potential use as antibiotics, as they have other promising characteristics as well. Many display a broad spectrum of activity and may be effective against Gram positive and Gram negative bacteria, fungi, parasites, or even viruses and cancer cells (for review see Chikindas et al. 2018). There is also limited potential for the development of antimicrobial resistance, largely related to their unique, membrane targeting activity. Some antimicrobial peptides show synergy with non-peptide antibiotics, allowing for a multi-hurdle approach to treatment that can greatly reduce the risk of developed resistance (Al-Gburi et al. 2015). While promising, naturally occurring antimicrobial peptides have critical limitations that are preventing their widespread use, including: (1) impaired bioavailability, (2) toxicity (particularly in antimicrobial peptides of eukaryotic origin), (3) high cost and difficulty of production, (4) limited and contradictory pharmacological data, and (5) reduced activity under certain physiological conditions (Semreen et al. 2018). Alternatives to naturally occurring antimicrobial peptides are currently being developed to address the above concerns, while maintaining or improving upon their positive characteristics, and in some instances even imparting entirely novel activities or functions. One such alternative, peptidomimetics, have essential elements that are able to mimic natural antimicrobial peptides, thus imparting the same targets, activities, or mechanisms. At the same time, peptidomimetics' non-peptide structures are thought to circumvent certain critical limitations such as stability against proteolysis and poor bioavailability, though there are *in vivo* studies indicating otherwise (van Staden et al. 2012; Campione et al. 2013), while some *in vitro* observations do not necessarily translate to an *in vivo* environment.

The design of novel antimicrobial peptides and peptidomimetics hinges on the development of structure-activity relationships by which the role of key physicochemical properties and specific structural elements may be analyzed and minimal active sequences and fundamental pharmacophore properties identified. The first step in this process is the selection or discovery of an initial lead compound and its thorough characterization, followed by structure-activity relationship guided modifications, resulting in libraries of finely-tuned drug candidates that may then be tested against pathogens of interest. The number of rounds of modification and characterization is indefinite, as numerous variables must be taken into account, and the interplay between different modifications can often lead to unexpected results. Once promising candidates are identified, they may be produced either biologically or through entirely synthetic processes, with difficulty of synthesis and cost as somewhat challenging factors. Additional factors must also be taken into account at this stage, such as drug formulation and delivery strategies, but these aspects are more related to clinical application and product design, and as such, are not within the scope of this chapter.

7.1.1 Antimicrobial Peptides

Antimicrobial peptides have been considered as a potential source of novel antibiotics for the past several decades, with several key eukaryotic antimicrobial peptides discoveries in the 1980s (cecropins, human α-defensins and histatins, magainins, etc.) sparking a renewed interest in both innate immunity research and antimicrobial peptides. Thousands of antimicrobial peptides have since been identified, with 3110 unique antimicrobial peptides cataloged in the Antimicrobial Peptide Database (APD) as of August 5, 2019, and 19,899 entries in the Data Repository of Antimicrobial Peptides (DRAMP). Approximately 25% of those entries are natural or synthetic antimicrobial peptides, while the rest consist of patent antimicrobial peptides (DRAMP 2019; Fan et al. 2016). Regardless of origin, antimicrobial peptides are ubiquitous in nature and are produced by nearly all living organisms. They often target a broad range of organisms, including bacteria, parasites, viruses, fungi, and animals. Antimicrobial peptides are also referred to as "host defense peptides", as they play an essential role as the first line of defense against infectious or competitive agents. In higher-level organisms, antimicrobial peptides may have several other functions outside of direct antimicrobial activity, including immunomodulatory effects and cell-signaling functions, and as such can also be referred to as "innate immune peptides" (Wang 2017a, b). Antimicrobial peptides, while diverse, share common features, with structural variations allowing for the observed range of functions, activities, and targets. Antimicrobial peptides are most often short oligopeptides, with sequences ranging from 2 to 100 amino acids, with the majority of antimicrobial peptides under 50 amino acids in length. The hydrophobicity of an antimicrobial peptide, defined as the ratio of hydrophobic amino acids to total amino acid content, is also important for antimicrobial peptide functionality, with the majority of antimicrobial peptides having a ratio between 30% and 60% (Wang 2017a, b). Net charge is another defining characteristic, with antimicrobial peptides classified as either cationic, neutral, or anionic depending on both amino acid content and additional chemical modifications. The vast majority are positively charged, with approximately 12% of antimicrobial peptides in the Antimicrobial Peptide Database being neutral or negatively charged. Hydrophobic content, net charge, and amphipathicity play a major role in determining how antimicrobial peptides interact with cellular membranes, influencing both antimicrobial potency and selectivity, as well as toxicity and hemolytic activity observed in mammalian cells (Bobone and Stella 2019).

7.1.2 Antimicrobial Peptides as Clinical Agents

To date, antimicrobial peptides have seen limited clinical use, and very few have made it past the initial stages of discovery and *in vitro* characterization of antimicrobial potential. This is due, in large part, to discrepancies between demonstrated *in vitro* efficacy and actual performance *in vivo*. While antimicrobial peptides may display broad spectrum antibacterial activity coupled with limited risk of antimicrobial resistance development, many suffer from different critical defects, as described above. Despite these hurdles, several antimicrobial peptides have made their way through the drug development pipeline, and are U.S. Food and Drug Administration approved for use in humans. A large portion of those antimicrobial peptides are produced by *Bacillus* ssp., and examples include bacitracin, polymyxin, gramicidin, and tyrothricin (Sumi et al. 2014). Tyrothricin was first discovered by René Dubos in the 1930s and is a mixture of tyrocidines and gramicidins produced by the soil bacteria originally reported as *Bacillus brevis* (Lang and Staiger 2016; Wenzel et al. 2018). As with many antimicrobial peptides, tyrothricin has hemolytic properties and as such is only used as a topical agent (DRUGBANK 2017). Tyrocidine A and gramicidin S are broad spectrum cyclopeptides that belong to the same antibiotic class as tyrothricin, and are also limited to topical applications (i.e. superficial skin and throat infections) due to hemolytic activity. Bacitracin (Neosporin™) is another mixture of cyclic polypeptides that is combined with the aminoglycoside antibiotic neomycin and another important antimicrobial peptide, polymyxin. Bacitracin is available as an over-the-counter drug, and is also used to treat eye and skin infections, but must be used with caution due to high renal toxicity (DRUGBANK 2019a, b). Polymyxin is one of the few U.S. Food and Drug Administration approved antimicrobial peptides for systemic use and oral administration, and is used as last resort against multi drug resistant bacterial infections, primarily against Gram negative pathogens or when other first line antibiotics are either ineffective or contraindicated (Kaur et al. 2015). Daptomycin is a cyclic antimicrobial lipopeptide used against systemic infections caused by Gram positive pathogens, with particular use against multi drug resistant pathogens due to its distinct membrane targeting mechanism of action. Vancomycin is a glycopeptide originally isolated from *Streptomyces orientalis* that is able to inhibit cell wall assembly in Gram positive bacteria, and is ineffective against Gram negative bacilli, mycobacteria, and fungi (Shen et al. 1982; DRUGBANK 2019a, b). Vancomycin can be administered through various methods, and is used for the treatment of severe infections caused by susceptible strains of methicillin resistant (β-lactam-resistant) staphylococci. Additionally, an FDA-approved oral liquid treatment is used for the treatment of *Clostridium difficile* associated diarrhea and enterocolitis caused by *Staphylococcus aureus*, including methicillin-resistant strains (U.S. Food and Drug Administration 2018). As with the other approved antimicrobial peptides, vancomycin can be toxic at higher doses, especially in the kidneys and inner ear.

There are currently 76 peptide drugs in development catalogued in the Data Repository of Antimicrobial Peptides (that are in various stages of development, with the vast majority focused on topical applications and skin infections due to Gram positive bacteria (DRAMP 2019)). The focus on topical administration is in large part due to the toxicity issues mentioned above as well as generally high susceptibilities to proteolytic degradation *in vivo*. A recent review of antimicrobial peptides and peptidomimetics undergoing clinical tries is provided by Greber and Dawgul (2017) and Molchanova et al. (2017).

7.1.3 Antimicrobial Peptide Classification

Antimicrobial peptides can be grouped using a variety of category based approaches, and while engineered synthetic peptides and peptidomimetics may not necessarily fit into some of these classifications, they are still useful in understanding antimicrobial peptides and the ways in which they are related. As such, classification should be considered when selecting natural antimicrobial peptides and lead compounds, which through structure-activity studies may serve as the starting point for the development of novel antimicrobial peptides and peptidomimetics.

Classification by source kingdom or domain is common and was the first means of organization used by the Antimicrobial Peptide Database (Wang et al. 2009). Examples exist for each kingdom, but the vast majority of known antimicrobial peptides (~77%) are from animal origins, as that is where the majority of research has been focused until more recently. Plants and bacteria are the next most common sources of antimicrobial peptides in the Antimicrobial Peptide Database, and represent approximately 12% and 10% of the Antimicrobial Peptide Database, respectively. More detailed classification of antimicrobial peptides based on source kingdom is complicated, with each having its own methods of organization, most often based on shared structural features, sequence similarity, or source organism. The classification of animal antimicrobial peptides is complex, as many examples have been found in vastly different organism, where they may serve very different purposes. For example, antimicrobial peptides derived from insect and other venoms are quite toxic and serve a dual purpose in both predation and defense, whereas human and other vertebrate antimicrobial peptides often serve a primary purpose of host defense in the exposed tissues in the respiratory and gastrointestinal tracts, but may also act upon the adaptive immune system (Gao and Zhu 2018). For reviews on animal antimicrobial peptides of particular interest, please see Shabir et al. (2018) and Semreen et al. (2018) for fish and marine antimicrobial peptides and Yi et al. (2014) for a review of insect antimicrobial peptides. For major antimicrobial peptides from amphibians see Conlon (2008) and Amiche et al. (2008), and for mammalian and human antimicrobial peptides see Dutta and Das (2016) and Wang (2014), respectively. Bacterial ribosomally synthesized antimicrobial peptides are known as bacteriocins, and represent a fast growing source of novel antimicrobial peptides. Bacteriocins are of particular interest in the search for novel antimicrobial peptides, as they may be produced in broadly different environmental conditions (halophiles, extremophiles, etc.), and may have unknown or unexpected activities that may be exploited in drug design (Coker 2016; Chikindas et al. 2018). Plant antimicrobial peptides are also well researched and are currently separated into nine different groups based on sequence similarity and cysteine motifs. A review of plant antimicrobial peptides can be found in Tam et al. (2015), and Salas et al. (2015).

One of the most important methods of grouping antimicrobial peptides is by three-dimensional structure, as an understanding of structure-activity relationships is necessary for the rational design of peptides and peptidomimetics. Structural determination has mainly been achieved using nuclear magnetic resonance or circular dichroism spectroscopy and crystallographic analysis, though spectroscopic methods are far more common due to the small size of most antimicrobial peptides and the resistance of membrane targeting antimicrobial peptides to crystallization (Wang 2017a, b; Yang et al. 2017). It is important that the structure of antimicrobial peptides is determined in a variety of conditions, as many factors can affect peptide structure in solution. Additionally, membrane active antimicrobial peptides often undergo structural changes upon membrane interaction, which are critical to the antimicrobial activity of these compounds. A variety of model membranes are commonly used, such as dodecylphosphocholine or phosphatidylglycol micelles, with electron microscopy of bacterial antimicrobial peptide interactions often used to confirm activity and the mechanism of activity. Non-membrane targeting antimicrobial peptides often form large complexes with their targets, for example, proline rich antimicrobial peptides are known to bind ribosomes and inhibit protein synthesis, but the large size of the proline rich antimicrobial peptide ribosome complex necessitated the use of x-ray crystallography as opposed to nuclear magnetic resonance spectroscopy (Roy et al. 2015; Seerfeldt et al. 2015).

The first proposed 3D-strucutre based classes included α-helical, β-sheet, and glycine, proline, tryptophan/arginine or histidine rich peptides (Boman 2003). An overlapping classification for folded antimicrobial peptides has also been proposed, separating them into β-sheet, α-helix, extended, and looped structures. A comprehensive classification scheme based on 3D structure was recently put forth by Wang (2017a), where antimicrobial peptides are again grouped into four families: α-helical, β-sheet, mixed αβ structures, and non-αβ structures.

The majority of α-helical antimicrobial peptides are membrane targeting cationic amphiphiles, though some examples do exist with intracellular and non-membrane based mechanisms. Antimicrobial peptides may have multiple α-helices, such is the case with caenopore-5 from *Caernorhabditis elegans* and its five amphipathic helices (Wang 2017b), though they are often short, containing a single helix that may associate to form complexes upon membrane contact, as exemplified by alamethicin and magainin-2 (Li and Salditt 2006). A large portion of α-helical cationic amphiphiles have a disordered structure in aqueous solutions, only adopting helical structures upon membrane binding. Some α-helical antimicrobial peptides like caenopore-5 are able to maintain helical structures in an aqueous environment due to the presence of disulfide bonds or other covalent modifications, a fact that may be exploited in the design of more stable peptide drugs (Wang 2017b).

β-sheet peptides must contain a minimum of two β-strands, and are often stabilized by one or more disulfide bonds. S-S bonds are often essential both in maintaining folded structures and in some membrane interactions. One important example of a linear β-sheet antimicrobial peptide is thanatin, isolated from the spined soldier bug, which contains a single disulfide bond that drives a specific-interaction with Gram negative *E. coli*, but has no impact on non-specific binding to the Gram positive *Micrococcus luteus* (Imamura et al. 2008). Interestingly, thanatin is thought to kill bacteria by cell agglutination and interactions with lipopolysaccharides, but may have intracellular targets as well that disrupt the bacterial respiratory pathway (Jackson and Miller-White 2018; Sinha et al. 2017). Other β-sheet antimicrobial peptides such as θ-defensins are non-linear, existing as a closed loop due to a peptide bond between the N- and C- terminus, with the overall structure stabilized by an additional three disulfide bonds. The flexible loop regions outside of the β-strands are often used in the stabilization of bioactive epitopes by peptide grafting, which will be discussed further on when considering design strategies and specific alterations (Conibear et al. 2016). Other β-sheet peptides include lasso peptides, which are typified by an N-terminal macrocyclic ring composed of 7–9 amino acids and a C-terminal tail that may thread through the ring. Lassos may or may not contain disulfide bonds, and the ring structure provides enhanced stability against chemical, thermal and proteolytic degradation (Martin-Gmez and Tulla-Puche 2018). This makes them particularly attractive candidates for drug discovery, and the advantages imparted by macrocyclic rings have been studied in de novo peptides generation as well (Vinogradov et al. 2019).

As the name implies, αβ antimicrobial peptides contain a mixture of both α-helices and β-sheets, and they are represented across all kingdoms. A major class of αβ antimicrobial peptides are defensins, which are cysteine-rich antimicrobial peptides found in both plants and animals, that are structurally and functionally diverse, with different ratios of α/β features, and distinct folding patterns. Defensins are separated into three families, α-, β-, and θ-defensins, based on the arrangement of their disulfide bridges (Mishra et al. 2018). Many act through membrane permeation followed by the production of reactive oxygen species within the cell (Islam et al. 2017), with mitochondrial membrane collapse also occurring in some instances (Souza et al. 2018). Plant and insect defensin are able to target fungal membranes due to sphingolipid recognition (Parisi et al. 2019). Human defensins are more effective against bacterial membranes, with human neutrophils peptides-1 to -3, which integrate into bacterial membranes throughout phagocytosis, disturbing ion stabilities, leading to lysis and cell death (Oyinloye et al. 2015). Other human defensins have broad spectrum activity and include α-defensins and β-defensins, with α-defensins being expressed mainly by myeloid cells, and β-defensins expressed in epithelial cells (Ouellette 2015).

Antimicrobial peptides belonging to the αβ family have no discernable α or β features, and their function and structure are instead characterized by an abundance of certain amino acids. Two major examples of αβ peptide groups are the tryptophan rich and proline rich. Both kill microorganisms by targeting intracellular pathways, with some tryptophan rich peptides such as indolicidin acting via membrane lysis mechanisms (Subbalakshmi and Sitaram 1998). Tryptophan rich peptides are able to adopt amphipathic structures due to the way in which the indole ring interacts with both bacterial membranes and amino acids within the peptide, driven by hydrogen bonding potential and other properties including dipole and quadrupole moments, with a combination of hydrophobic and hydrophilic attributes making it ideal from membrane insertion (Vogel et al. 2002). A minimum length of six amino acids is required for high antimicrobial activity in Tryptophan rich peptides, with examples ranging from 5 to 11 residues in length (Strøm et al. 2003; Shagaghi et al. 2016). The positioning of tryptophan residues relative to other amino acids has a direct effect on antimicrobial activity, while the number of residues is less important (Mishra et al. 2018). Proline rich antimicrobial peptides are intracellular acting peptides, with both ribosomes and the heat shock protein DnaK currently identified as major proline rich peptide targets (Kragol et al. 2001). Structural analysis has shown the binding of the proline rich antimicrobial peptide oncocin to the ribosome, where it is able to block both the peptidyl transferase center and the peptide-exit tunnel, thereby inhibiting protein synthesis (Seefeldt et al. 2015; Roy et al. 2015). Other proline rich antimicrobial peptides have low sequence homology, but are structurally similar, with a certain degree of proline content (~30%) and proline-arginine-proline motifs being common features (Li et al. 2014).

Another useful way of grouping antimicrobial peptides is by peptide chain bonding patterns, with various chain connections generating different conserved topologies that have a large influence on antimicrobial peptide activity and stability (Wang 2015). These categories are linear, sidechain-linked, sidechain-backbone linked, and backbone-linked circular antimicrobial peptides. Interestingly, each class possesses overlapping and highly conserved amino acid sequences, a fact that can be exploited in the prediction based design of peptidomimetics (Wang 2017b).

There are several other means of identifying and grouping antimicrobial peptides, including but not limited to: synthesis (gene-encoded and non-gene-encoded), chemical modifications, and mechanism of action. Means of biological synthesis is not necessarily relevant in designing antimicrobial peptides and peptidomimetics, especially in the case of fully synthetic peptidomimetics with little to no peptide character, though it is useful when considering biotechnological methods of production. Both antimicrobial targets and mechanisms of action are dependent on peptide structure and key physicochemical properties, as briefly mention above, though more detailed examination of known mechanisms of action will be described further on. Structural modifications are of particular relevance to antimicrobial peptides and peptidomimetics, as they represent a direct way of altering antimicrobial peptides with the goal of reducing toxicity, imparting resistance to proteolysis, or increasing antimicrobial activity, specificity, and imparting novel functions.

7.2 Mechanisms of Action

Before discussing the various antibacterial mechanisms of action of both antimicrobial peptides and peptidomimetics, it is important to note that many have multiple functions that are often concentration dependent. An additional concern that is difficult to account for is how antimicrobial peptide function may be influenced or induced *in vivo*, resulting in changes to activity that may not be obvious or easily predicted through *in vitro* studies. As such, the summary given below may be considered a general overview of the subject (summarized in Fig. 7.2), with a focus on the mechanism itself, and does not cover every possible function of each antimicrobial peptide that is used as an example. For a review of the multifunctionality of antimicrobial peptides with a focus on bacteriocins, see Chikindas et al. (2018).

Antimicrobial peptides can be divided into two groups when considering their potential use against pathogens: antimicrobial peptides that have a direct killing effect, and those with indirect effects such as antibiofilm, toxin neutralization, or immunomodulatory activities. Antimicrobial peptides with a direct killing effect can be further categorized into membrane targeting and non-membrane targeting or intracellular targeting mechanisms. In both instances, interaction with the cell membrane is a critical step and is necessary for the bactericidal effects of antimicrobial

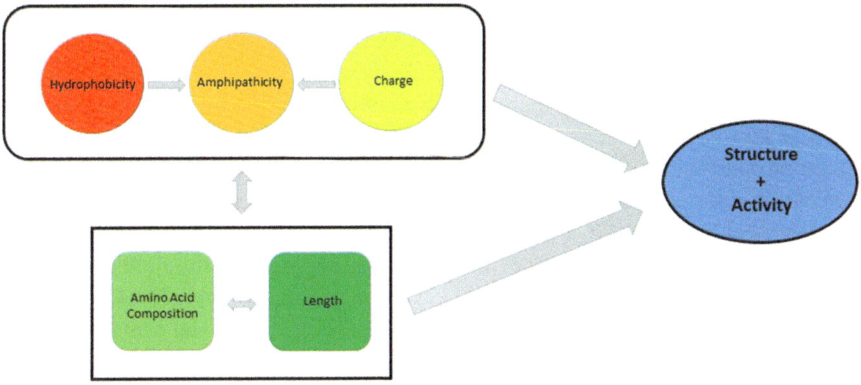

Fig. 7.2 Overview of the most common mechanisms of action of antimicrobial peptides, divided into direct effects that result in cell death, and other effects that may indirectly influence the antimicrobial activity of peptides and peptidomimetics in other ways

peptides. In terms of target selectivity, antimicrobial peptides can be either non-selective, effecting both mammalian and bacterial cells, or they may display varying degrees of selectivity, and may be active against Gram positive or Gram negative bacteria, fungi, viruses, and parasites, or some combination of the above targets, without damaging eukaryotic cells at similar concentrations (Segev-Zarko et al. 2017). The physicochemical properties of an antimicrobial peptide such as net charge, charge distribution, and hydrophobicity greatly influence antimicrobial peptide membrane interactions, and often determine the potential targets an antimicrobial peptide is able interact with and the strength of that interaction, due to the inherent differences between the membranes of bacterial, fungal, and mammalian cells. Examples of non-selective antimicrobial peptides include the bee and wasp venom derived peptides melittin and mastoparan (Moreno and Giralt 2015), and mosquito derived cecropin (Kaushal et al. 2016; Zheng et al. 2017; Agrawal et al. 2019). Cell selectivity is achieved either through receptor-mediated mechanisms or through a combination of biophysical properties that makes interaction with the targeted cell membrane more favorable than interactions with eukaryotic cells. Examples of reported receptor-mediated antimicrobial peptides include some bacteriocins such as nisin (Shin et al. 2015), class IIa (Kjos et al. 2009), and IId bacteriocins (Diep et al. 2007), and antimicrobial peptides of eukaryotic origin such as magainin (Arnusch et al. 2012). These antimicrobial peptides contain both receptor binding domains and pore-forming domains, allowing for receptor mediated attachment to the cell surface, followed by pore formation and eventual cell death. Receptor mediated antimicrobial peptides may not be the best choice in considering drug development with the goal of combating or preventing the development of antibiotic resistance, as they suffer from a flaw common to many antibiotics. They act on or through a singular target that through mutations, may be changed in such a way that the interactions between the receptor binding domain and its target are no longer possible. The majority of known membrane targeting antimicrobial peptides belong to the second group, and their activity is a direct consequence of their physicochemical properties. The most common membrane lytic antimicrobial peptides are cationic amphiphiles, containing both hydrophobic and positively charged regions that are essential for their selective antimicrobial activity against bacterial cells. It should be mentioned that anionic antimicrobial peptides such as subtilosin A are presently receiving some deserved attention and are reported as being active against foodborne pathogens (Van Kuijk et al. 2011), also in synergistic action with conventional antibiotics (Cavera et al. 2015), and against enveloped viruses such as herpes simplex virus (Quintana et al. 2014). The degree of hydrophobicity and the distribution of charged amino acids are key properties that play a critical role in cell specificity and antimicrobial activity, as well as in the observed toxicity towards mammalian cells.

7.2.1 Membrane Lytic Antimicrobial Peptides

There are several different models for the killing action of membrane lytic cationic amphiphiles, and a key stage in each is the attraction of antimicrobial peptides to the cell surface and binding to the targeted cell. The positive charge of the antimicrobial peptide allows it to come into initial contact with bacterial membranes, which contain a large fraction of negatively charged lipids, such as lipopolysaccharides in Gram negative species and lipoteichoic acid in Gram positive species (Sani and Separovic 2016). Additionally, the outer leaflets of bacterial membranes contain a high number of anionic phospholipids such as phosphatidylglycerol. As such, the bacterial membrane maintains a high electrical potential gradient, attracting the positively charged antimicrobial peptides. While mammalian cell membranes also contain negatively charged components like sialic acid, their distribution across the plasma membrane is different than in bacteria. In addition, the cell membrane is primarily composed of zwitterionic phospholipids, discouraging the binding of the positively charge cationic amphiphiles (Sani and Separovic 2016). Once initial contact with the bacterial membrane is established, cationic amphiphiles may act through a variety of possible mechanisms to disrupt the cell membrane, leading to pore formation, cell lysis, and eventual cell death. Popular models for pore formation include carpet/detergent-like, membrane thinning, aggregate, toroidal pore, and barrel stave interactions (Bozelli et al. 2017). The majority of antimicrobial peptides exhibit a distinct secondary structure upon contacting the membrane, a feature considered essential for their membrane lytic effects in bacteria (Takahashi et al. 2010). In the barrel stave model, peptides insert into the lipid bilayer, and are able to form a stable state perpendicular to the membrane, leading to the recruitment of additional peptide molecules, resulting in the formation of a barrel like pore (Yamamoto et al. 2019). The carpet or detergent like model begins with the same initial interaction of peptide monomers and oligomers with the membrane surface. Hydrophobic portions are attracted to the membrane surface, while hydrophilic regions face outwards. Cationic amphiphiles continue to accumulate on the surface until a critical threshold concentration is reached, leading to membrane permeation (Chung and Khanum 2017). Other membrane interaction models, while mechanistically different, lead to the same end result, and will not be discussed in depth.

7.2.2 *Intracellular Targets*

Some antimicrobial peptides have been found to exhibit a killing effect only after crossing the bacterial outer and inner membranes and interacting with various intercellular targets, leading to inhibition of protein synthesis, transcription and replication, cell wall synthesis and outer membrane biogenesis, inhibition of cytokinesis, and various other less documented membrane independent mechanisms (Scocchi et al. 2017). The exact means by which antimicrobial peptides with intracellular targets enter the cell remains unclear, with two possible mechanisms currently proposed: bacterial protein mediated and spontaneous translocation. Proline rich antimicrobial peptides have shown to cross the membrane via protein mediated transportation. Many act using the inner membrane protein SBmA to penetrate the membrane, as observed in *E. coli* and other Gram negative bacteria (Scocchi et al. 2011). Some proline rich antimicrobial peptides seem to need the SbmA uptake system to function, while others may act through multiple potential bacterial transports, making resistance development more difficult for those antimicrobial peptides. Examples include oncocin and Bac7(1-35), which may be able to use the recently identified *yjiL-mdtM* gene cluster (Krizsan et al. 2014). Spontaneous translocation is similar in concept to the pore-forming models used for membrane lytic cationic amphiphiles, though pore formation is only transient and occurs at lower concentrations than needed for cell lysis, thereby preserving membrane integrity during passage (Ulmschneider 2017).

Upon entering the cell, antimicrobial peptides may have single or multiple targets. Inhibition of protein synthesis and molecular chaperones has been demonstrated for various non-lytic peptides, both *in vivo* and *in vitro*. Well-documented examples include oncocin, Bac7, and pyrrhocoricin which have all been observed binding to DnaK and the bacterial ribosome, with apidaecin and pyrrhocoricin binding to GroEL as well (Scocchiet al. 2017). The exact mechanisms and specificities for many antimicrobial peptides remain unclear, with targets ranging from DNA as seen with buforin II leading to inhibition transcription and replication (Uyterhoeven et al. 2008), or lipid II binding by nisin or copsin, which can lead to the inhibition of cell wall synthesis and bacterial membrane biogenesis (Essig et al. 2014; ‘t Hart et al. 2016).

7.2.3 Non-killing Actions

Some antimicrobial peptides are able to exert indirect pressure on pathogens through a variety of methods outside of direct bactericidal or bacteriostatic mechanisms. Examples include antibiofilm effects, either through inhibition of surface attachment or biofilm formation, or through biofilm dispersion and degradation. Antimicrobial peptide-host interactions are another potential area of interest, with some antimicrobial peptides having immunomodulatory, wound healing, angiogenic or anti-inflammatory effects. Antimicrobial peptides may also exert similar effects through interactions with bacterial secondary metabolites and endotoxins such as lipopolysaccharides, lipoteichoic acid, anthrax lethal toxin, shiga toxin, etc. (Kim et al. 2005; Nell et al. 2006; Yamada et al. 2006; Golec 2007).

Biofilms are structured microbial communities that form on surfaces or at interphase and reside in an extracellular matrix composed of extracellular polymeric substances, primarily polysaccharides and proteins, with other molecules such as DNA and lipids found in smaller amounts. Biofilm formation is a key factor in many infectious diseases, providing increased protection against antibiotics and the innate immune response, thus creating a safe haven for pathogens, resulting in increased persistence and infection recurrence. In fact, is has been show that biofilms may be 1000 times more tolerant to conventional antibiotics than their planktonic counterparts (Olsen 2015). Infection persistence and recurrence are often due to so-called "persister-cells", a subpopulation of bacteria within the biofilm matrix that remain in a dormant and drug tolerant state, further increasing the likelihood of resistance development (Gerdes and Semsey 2016; Wood 2017). Many antimicrobial peptides and peptidomimetics have been shown to have biofilm killing, prevention, or dispersion effects. A natural human derived cathelicidin antimicrobial peptide LL-37 and related peptidomimetic NA-CATH:ATRA1-ATRA1 have been shown to inhibit biofilm production by *S. aureus* biofilms at sub-antimicrobial concentrations (Dean et al. 2011). Another series of LL-37 based peptidomimetics was recently developed by de Brej et al. (2018) with the lead compound from the series, SAAP-148, able to kill antibiotic resistant pathogens on *ex vivo* human skin cells and biofilms, without the development of resistance, even after long term exposure. Other antimicrobial peptides have shown anti biofilm activity when used on medical devices against *S. aureus* and *P. aeruginosa,* and include lactoferrin, conjugated lactoferrin, melamine and citropin 1.1. These antimicrobial peptides also showed synergy with the traditional antibiotics rifampicin and minocycline (Yoshinari et al. 2010). Other peptidomimetic compounds have also shown anti biofilm activity, a series of recently designed lipopeptidomimetic cationic amphiphiles has demonstrated activity against both planktonic and biofilm embedded methicillin resistant *S. aureus* (Joshi et al. 2018).

7.3 Key Physicochemical Properties

As shown above, antimicrobial peptides are structurally and functionally diverse, and it is often difficult to identify commonalities that exist between all known examples. There is also tremendous interplay between the various physicochemical properties of antimicrobial peptides and peptidomimetics, driven by various factors including amino acid sequence; chemical or post-translational alterations; covalent modifications, salt bridges, and other means of stabilization (Avan et al. 2014). As such, it is often difficult to isolate the effect of individual features and to determine the degree of influence they may have on an individual peptides function, and it is more difficult still to apply any knowledge gained towards the design of *de novo* peptide and peptidomimetic antimicrobials. Nevertheless, research efforts continue to examine these key properties and how they may be fine tuned for rational design. It is important to note that the properties discussed below are not necessarily applicable to all engineered antimicrobial peptides and peptidomimetics, but are instead most commonly associated with membrane lytic cationic amphiphiles, which have seen the greater part of research and design efforts in the field. Thus, we present the following information as a general starting point in understanding the interplay between these features (as shown in Fig. 7.3), which can in turn be used as a set of "guiding principles" during the step wise engineering of novel peptide and peptidomimetic antimicrobials against the ESKAPE pathogens and other emerging multi drug resistant species.

7.3.1 Length

The length of the peptide chain is an important structural aspect of antimicrobial peptides, with minimal optimal lengths required for maintaining the activity of the pharmacophore or other functionally active sequences (e.g. protein binding, lipopolysaccharide binding, surface tethering regions, etc.) (Hilpert et al. 2009), which can vary greatly between different antimicrobial peptides. This makes the impact of length on the activity of different antimicrobial peptides difficult to compare, as there likely is no universally optimal peptide length, and length-activity relationships should instead be determined for each antimicrobial peptide of interest, and only used when designing antimicrobial peptides and peptidomimetics based on the data gained from studying that example. Length is particularly important in the case of membrane targeting amphiphiles, as at least 7–8 amino acids are necessary to form an amphipathic structure with both hydrophilic and hydrophobic regions on opposite sides of the polypeptide (Bahar and Ren 2013). Additionally, a certain length is required for an antimicrobial peptide to properly anchor to and transverse the bacterial lipid membrane, with at least 22 amino acids and eight amino acids needed for α-helical and β-sheet antimicrobial peptides to properly function under the barrel-stave model, for example (Westerhoff et al. 1989). One way of examining

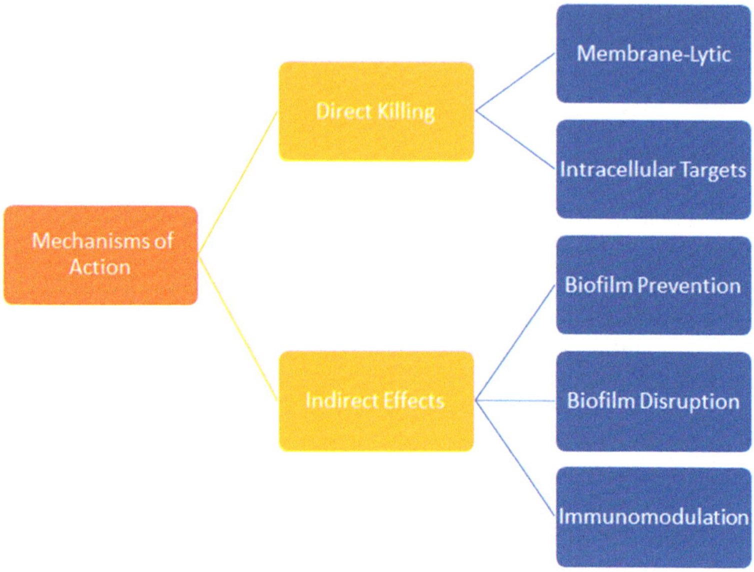

Fig. 7.3 Key physicochemical properties of natural antimicrobial peptides and how they interact to determine the structure and by consequence, the function of a typical antimicrobial peptide. Both charge and hydrophobicity are critical in determining the amphipathicity of an antimicrobial peptide, which is a key characteristic driving the membranolytic action of many peptides. These features are primarily a consequence of amino acid sequence, length, and various chemical modifications, and the interplay between all these features is what determines the structure and resulting functionality of a given antimicrobial peptide

length effects is through the generation of novel peptides libraries with the use of different and often repeating amino-acid sequence-motif based building blocks. For example, Deslouches et al. (2005) developed a series of 12-residue lytic base unit peptides composed of arginine and valine, and found an increase in antimicrobial activity against *P. aeruginosa* and *S. aureus* when increasing the length from 12-mer to 24-mer, with increase in length beyond that having little impact on antimicrobial activity. A similar length effect was also observed in a series of α-peptide/β-peptoid chimeras, with an increase in length from 8 to 12 to 16 residues showing increased activity against *E. coli*, *L. monocytogenes*, and *S. aureus* isolates (Hein-Kristensen et al. 2011). More recently, Gagnon et al. (2017) generated a series of α-helical peptides using a repeating KIAGKIA (~ two turns of the helix) sequence, which were designed so that other features such as the polar sector size, hydrophobic moment, mean hydrophobicity, and charge density (charge per amino acid) were nearly unchanged for the series. This allowed length effects to be effectively isolated, and they were able to establish a relationship between membrane thickness and peptide length, with only helices that are long enough to span the membrane resulting in leakage. The length of the peptide chain can also have an impact on cytotoxicity, with a truncated form of melittin exhibiting markedly less toxicity to rat and human erythrocytes as compared to the natural form (Subbalakshmi et al.

1999). Other reports have also demonstrated a relationship between toxicity and length, with longer peptide chains showing increased toxicity towards mammalian cells (Javadpour et al. 1996). Increased length has also been shown to have an effect on antibacterial activity as shown in a series of $(RW)_{(n)}$ repeat peptides, where increased chain length resulted in both increased toxicity and antimicrobial activity (Liu et al. 2007). From just these few studies, representing a small fraction of the literature in which length-activity relationships have been examined, it is easy to see the importance of peptide length in antimicrobial design, but they also draw attention to the importance of amino acid sequences and motifs and the consequences impact they may have on antimicrobial peptide characteristics.

7.3.2 Amino Acid Sequence

As with length, there is tremendous variety in amino acid composition between different antimicrobial peptides. Amino acids may exert their effect individually, or in concert with other amino acids or as part of a functional sequence motif. In peptidomimetic and *de novo* antimicrobial peptide it is also important to consider the impact of unnatural and chemically modified amino acids, whose impact and use will be discussed further on. The different structure-based and bonding-pattern-based antimicrobial peptide classes have different amino acid ratios and certain residues are dominant in each (Mishra and Wang 2012). The α-helical antimicrobial peptides tend to have Leucine as the primary hydrophobic residue, while lysine is the dominant charged amino acid. In the case of β-stranded antimicrobial peptides, the polypeptide fold is an important structural feature that relies on cysteine for disulfide bond stabilization, while arginine is favored over lysine for providing positive charge. In αβ structures, a high proportion of cysteine is used as the major hydrophobic component required for peptide folding, while both arginine and lysine are used equally. As mentioned above non-αβ peptides most often favor the used of specific amino acids that are necessary for their observed effects, with tryptophan, proline, and arginine all playing a major role. As mentioned earlier, peptides may be classified based on chain binding patterns, each with its own distinct sequence signature: Linear antimicrobial peptides tend to favor leucine, alanine, glycine, and lysine; sidechain linked favor cysteine, glycine, and lysine; sidechain-backbone linked favor valine, alanine, and glycine; and backbone linked cyclic antimicrobial peptides favor cysteine and glycine (Wang et al. 2016).

Amino acid composition also plays a major role in various antimicrobial peptide functions, with different amino acid compositions common among peptides with similar targets and antibacterial mechanisms. For example, clear differences exist between antimicrobial peptides with Gram positive and Gram negative selectivity, with antimicrobial peptides active against Gram positive bacteria containing relatively similar amounts of leucine and cysteine, while antimicrobial peptides that only target Gram negative species have higher numbers of leucine and lower cysteine content by comparison (Mishra and Wang 2012).

Lysine and arginine are both commonly found in peptide sequences due to their positive charge, which enables electrostatic interactions between antimicrobial peptides and the negatively charged bacterial membrane. While both are widely used, the differences in their side chain chemistry give them markedly different properties. The guanidinium group of arginine allows for a greater potential for multiple interactions to occur, primarily due to the more dispersed charge as compared to lysine. Arginine also has the ability to interact with the aromatic system in tryptophan via cation-π interactions (Aliste et al. 2003). Numerous studies have been carried out to elucidate the effects of the two amino acids on antimicrobial peptide activity. These studies often utilize amino acid substitution and the generation of novel peptides sequences based on arginine or lysine heavy repeating motifs. Most arginine and lysine often are used in a repeating series with hydrophobic residues to develop cationic amphiphiles, and they are also sometimes used as a positive chain at the end of a peptide to encourage antimicrobial peptide membrane interactions (Duval et al. 2009). Lysine → arginine substitution is often shown to increase the antimicrobial activity of many natural antimicrobial peptides due to the more favorable interactions of guanidinium moiety of arginine with membranes (Li et al. 2013; Arias et al. 2018). This was demonstrated recently with two mutants of the antimicrobial peptide KR-12, one in which lysine residues were replaced with arginine (R-KR12) and another with arginine residues mutated to lysine (K-KR12) (Rice and Wereszczynski 2017). It was shown that the lysine → arginine mutants interacted weakly with a model membrane, and that the arginine → lysine mutants formed significantly more hydrogen bonds with the bilayer. The use of arginine over lysine is also commonly associated with enhanced antimicrobial activity. In a study, comparing 8-mer to 18-mer WK and WR peptides, the 8-mer and 10-mer arginine containing peptides showed increased activity over the analogous lysine containing peptides (Deslouches et al. 2016). Length again played a role in antimicrobial activity and cytotoxity, with optimal activity occurring with the 12-mer peptides, which also showed negligible hemolytic and cytotoxic effects.

Cysteine plays a major role in the structure of natural antimicrobial peptides, particularly in β and αβ structures, where the formation of disulfide bonds via the oxidation of the thiol group of cysteine are necessary for proper folding and resulting antimicrobial activity. The formation of disulfide bonds provides the additional benefit of increased protection to proteolysis as well (Tanabe et al. 2007). The role of disulfide bonds in determining antimicrobial activity is complex, and the formation, location, and reduction of disulfide bonds can have very different impacts depending on the antimicrobial peptide in question. For example, protegrin-1 contains two internal disulfide bridges that are integral to its structure and antibacterial activity, as their removal via cysteine replacement can be correlated to a loss of bactericidal activity (Harwig et al. 1996). In contrast, human β-defensin 1 (HBD-1) shows minimal antimicrobial activity as compared to other human defensins, however, disulfide bond reduction has been shown to induce increased antimicrobial activity (Schroeder et al. 2011). This highlights the potential role of disulfide bond reduction and free cysteine residues in the antimicrobial action of similar defensins when expressed in reducing environments, i.e., the gastrointestinal tract. Indeed, proteolytic degradation of reduced HBD-1 leads to the development of peptide fragments with antimicrobial activity, with similar active antimicrobial fragments having been generated from HD-5 and HD-6 as well (Wendler et al. 2019; Ehmann et al. 2019). Interestingly, reduction of disulfide bridges in HBD-3 does not appear to influence its anti-bacterial activities, but does impact chemotactic activity (Klüver et al. 2005; Zhang 2017). Taken together, these studies highlight the complex relationship between cysteine residues, disulfide bridges, and antimicrobial peptide function.

7.3.3 Charge

The effects of charge on an antimicrobial peptide's activity is primarily a consequence of amino acid composition and the number and position of charged residues within the peptide structure. The majority of antimicrobial peptides are net positive, with charges ranging from +2 to +13, primarily due to large proportions of lysine and arginine residues, with histidine occurring far less often in natural antimicrobial peptides (Mishra and Wang 2012). Cationicity is a major determining factor in antimicrobial peptide membrane interactions, and numerous studies have shown correlations between charge and antimicrobial activity, toxicity, and selectivity. In a series of α-helical cationic amphiphiles, using a previously designed α-helical cationic amphiphile L-V13K (Chen et al. 2005), Jiang et al. showed improved antimicrobial activity with increased charge up to +8, while a decrease in activity against *P. aeruginosa* was observed when the charge was < +4 (Jiang et al. 2008). Similarly, increasing the charge of magainin 2 from +3 to +5 improves antimicrobial activity against bacteria, but further increases to charge resulted in increased hemolytic activity and a loss of antimicrobial activity (Dathe et al. 2001). While a net positive-charge of antimicrobial peptides is important in determining antimicrobial peptide membrane interactions, especially in the case of negatively charged bacterial membranes, it is not the sole determining factor in those interactions. In addition to overall charge, charge distribution also seems to play a major role in peptide membrane interactions (Mihajlovic and Lazaridis 2012). Charge does not necessarily come from amino acid sequence alone, as different charged moieties may be added via post-translation modification or thought chemical alterations and the addition of unnatural moieties in peptidomimetics. While cationic amphiphiles are dominant among known antimicrobial peptides, there are outliers that are either net neutral or anionic that nonetheless demonstrates antimicrobial activity, such as dermcidin, which may act through ion channel formation stabilized by a zinc ion bridge between negatively charged histidine residues and negatively charged membrane features (Becucci et al. 2014).

7.3.4 Hydrophobicity

Hydrophobicity is another feature that plays a major role in determining the degree of antimicrobial activity and the range of target cells for membrane targeting antimicrobial peptides (Kustanovich et al. 2002; Zelezetsky et al. 2005). While examples exist for antimicrobial peptides with a hydrophobicity ranging from 0% to 100%, the majority of antimicrobial peptides fall between 50% and 78% (Wang 2017a). Hydrophobicity has a direct effect on antimicrobial peptide-membrane interactions, influencing the ability to penetrate a lipid bilayer and the range and degree of interactions with different membrane compositions (Pasupuleti et al. 2012). In addition, increasing hydrophobicity has a well-documented correlation to decreased antibacterial specificity and increased toxicity to mammalian cells (Chen et al. 2007; Yin et al. 2012). Returning to the example of V681, Chen et al. (2007) found that strong hemolytic activity and decreased antimicrobial activity of the peptide series was linked to increased hydrophobicity. Decreased specificity and hemolytic activity might be explained by the more hydrophobic peptides ability to penetrate further into the hydrophobic core an erythrocyte membrane, while decreased antimicrobial activity could be explained by increased self-association of the peptides in solution, negatively impacting peptide-membrane interactions. This is supported by a series of cationic amphiphiles, in which increased hemolytic activity and decreased antimicrobial activity were also linked to increased self-aggregation. Indeed, Yin et al. showed a correlation between hydrophobicity and cell selectivity, with more hydrophobic peptides based on alanine to leucine substitutions showing increased hemolytic activity and destruction of mammalian model membranes (Yin et al. 2012). Interestingly, all peptides of the series displayed similar antimicrobial activity against *P. aeruginosa* strain PAO1, demonstrating once again that observations in one antimicrobial peptide series may not necessarily translate to other antimicrobial peptides, and that the relationship between physicochemical properties and observed activities is complex.

7.3.5 Amphipathicity

Amphipathicity in antimicrobial peptides refers to the relative abundance and distribution of hydrophobic and hydrophilic domains, and is often considered a defining and necessary feature for the activity of many antimicrobial peptides. Indeed, as discussed above, most known examples are positively charged, ranging from +1 to +7 and have approximately 50% hydrophobic amino acids (Wang 2017a). The interplay between charged groups and hydrophobic residues is complex, with the degree and positioning of positive charge playing a large role in membrane recognition and attachment, with hydrophobicity being essential for proper membrane insertion, disruption, or transversal. Amphipathicity is not simply a product of the rations of hydrophobic and charged residues present in the primary sequence, but is highly linked to the 2D or 3D structure of a given antimicrobial peptide. For example, amphipathicity can occur in a variety of forms, such as facial amphipathicity, as exemplified by α-helical cationic amphiphiles, in which one side of the helix is composed primarily of hydrophobic residues, while the opposite side is cationic (Li et al. 2017). A key descriptor of amphipathicity in α-helical cationic amphiphiles is the hydrophobic moment (defined as vector sum of individual amino acid hydrophobicity that is standardized to an idealized helix model) which is often used together with helical wheel projections in discussing the influence of facial amphipathicity on membrane interactions (Eisenberg et al. 1982; Vishnepolsky and Pirtskhalave 2014). Another form of amphipathicity that is often used in the design of very short cationic amphiphile mimics is bola-like amphipathicity, with two cationic moieties positioned on either side of a hydrocarbon chain (Moretti et al. 2019).

As with the other features described above, amphipathicity is known to have impacts on antimicrobial activity and toxicity, though a clear relationship is difficult to determine, as the degree of amphipathicity has sometimes shown disparate and contradictory effects when comparing different antimicrobial peptides. For example, many studies have shown that disruption of amphipathicity in α helical antimicrobial peptides can increase antimicrobial activity and reduce hemolytic activity (Kumar et al. 2018). However, contradictory results were found in the study of melittin related peptides, with increased amphipathicity leading to increased hemolysis instead (Zhang et al. 2016). Furthermore, other peptides studies have demonstrated a correlation between increased amphipathicity and both increased antimicrobial and hemolytic activity (Chen et al. 2005; Fernandez-Vidall et al. 2007).

7.3.6 Interplay Between the Physicochemical Properties of Antimicrobial Peptides and Peptidomimetics

The studies on length, amino acid sequence, charge, hydrophobicity, and amphipathicity described above highlight the complex and interconnected relationship between each of these properties. It is prudent to consider correlations between physicochemical characteristics and the pharmacological properties of antimicrobial peptides as general guiding principles, and to not mechanistically follow them when approaching antimicrobial peptide design. It is likely essential that any rationally designed antimicrobial peptide be probed for structure activity relationships on an individual basis, with each subsequent series of modifications leading to the selection of the next generation of lead compounds, repeated as needed until a comprehensive library of compounds with structure-activity relationship data have been generated, with finely tuned lead compounds then being selected for more advanced studies. Changes to any one of these properties will likely impact others, and can have unexpected and inconsistent effects when not carefully considered, especially when moving from *in vitro* to *in vivo* and clinical studies.

7.4 Limitations and Challenges

While antimicrobial peptides have displayed great promise as alternatives to traditional antibiotics, there are still several factors that have so far limited their use as clinical agents. These factors are in part, a consequence of the features described above, with the complex interplay between physicochemical properties (i.e. charge, hydrophobicity, amphipathicity) often resulting in undesirable pharmacological features that may preclude their use *in vivo*; relating to the absorption, distribution, metabolism, elimination, and toxicity (ADMET) of an antimicrobial peptide. Indeed, the majority of naturally occurring peptides have an oral bioavailability no greater than 1% (Di 2015). There are other factors to consider that are not directly related to ADMET, and those include production and synthesis considerations as well as bacterial resistance to antimicrobial peptides. A brief overview of some of these issues is presented below, followed by a review of modification and design strategies for the development of improved antimicrobial proteins and peptidomimetics aimed at addressing these key limitations.

7.4.1 Solubility and Proteolytic Degradation

In order for an antimicrobial peptide to exhibit its desired effect, it is necessary for it to be able to effectively reach and then act upon or pass through the membranes of bacterial targets. The solubility of antimicrobial peptides under physiological condition has a large impact on activity, and many naturally occurring antimicrobial peptides have issues related to auto-aggregation and exhibit poor solubility in an aqueous environment (Fosgerau and Hoffman 2015). Peptide solubility may be affected by numerous other factors, such as solvent composition and the presence of ions, salts, proteins, etc. (Schein 1990; Mohammad et al. 2015). The inherent insolubility of some peptides *in vivo* may be addressed through several different methods, including structural alterations, often through modifications to hydrophobic regions, achieved through amino-acid substitutions or the N-methylation of specific residues. For example, a chimeric antimicrobial peptide made from cecropin and melittin was found to naturally associate into dimers, reducing bioavailability *in vivo*. It was then found that by changing the amino acid composition of the nonpolar face of the compound via the substitution of a charged lysine residue prevented dimerization, leading to reduced hemolytic activity and improved incorporation into lipid membranes (Chen et al. 2005). It is important to note that the aggregation of antimicrobial peptides is not always negative, as exemplified by self-assembled small cationic amphiphiles and peptidomimetics that form supramolecular nanostructures such as nanovesicles or hydrogels. These structures, which may be necessary for antimicrobial activity, may lead to improvements in biocompatibility, stability, and the solubility of peptide drugs (Liu et al. 2009; Zhang et al. 2017; Eskandari et al. 2017; Moretti et al. 2019). Other factors that may affect antimicrobial peptide solubility are charge distribution and the isoelectric point of the peptide, with changes made in relation to the pH of the desired formulation of the final product (Rollema et al. 1995; Yin et al. 2012). It is also possible to circumvent the inherent insolubility of certain peptide compounds without direct modifications to peptide structure; examples include the use of drug delivery systems (Nordström and Malmsten 2017) and surface immobilization techniques (Costa et al. 2011).

Natural antimicrobial peptides, are subject to proteolytic degradation by proteases such as chymotrypsin, greatly limiting their oral availability. Additionally, antimicrobial peptides may also be digested by proteases expressed by targeted pathogens, as in the case of LL-37 degradation by *S. aureus*, *P. aeruginosa, P. mirabilis,* and *E. faecalis* enzymes (Schmidtchen et al. 2002). This has been one of the driving factors behind the pharmaceutical industries' focus on topical applications, as systemic applications may be hindered by the action of proteases, which greatly reduce the half-life of a peptide drug *in vivo*. There are many methods for the stabilization of peptide structures, including covalent modifications such as the addition of disulfide/diselenide bonds or backbone-based cyclization, and the use of unnatural amino acids and chemical alterations (Sieprawska-Lupa et al. 2004; Meng and Kumar 2007; Carmona et al. 2013). In addition to protection against proteolytic degradation, such alterations have potential to alter antimicrobial peptide function in other ways, and may result in reduced activity, which can be corrected through further chemical alterations to restore the original active structure. Overall, the less peptide character a peptidomimetic antimicrobial contains, the more stable it will be against proteolytic degradation (Gentilucci et al. 2010).

7.4.2 Toxicity

Toxicity towards eukaryotic cells is a common feature of many naturally occurring peptides, and is often directly tied to the direct action of antimicrobial peptides, most often studied *in vitro,* resulting in membrane level cytotoxity and hemolysis. Toxicity to the host is often more complicated and toxic effects may occur through complex pathways leading to systemic toxicity, as exemplified by polymyxin B, which is demonstrably safe against eukaryotic cells *in vitro*, but can result in extensive nephrotoxicity and neurotoxicty *in vivo* (Falagas and Kasiakou 2006; Roberts et al. 2015). Cytoxicity in eukaryotic *vs* bacterial cells is largely a consequence of the differences between eukaryotic and bacterial membranes, and the degree to which antimicrobial peptides are able to associate with them. A desirable property in antimicrobial peptide design is cell selectivity, i.e., bactericidal activity at concentrations that cause little to no damage to the cells of the host (Bonbone and Stella 2019). As demonstrated above, cytotoxicity and selectivity rely on a complex interplay between factors such as charge or charge distribution, hydrophobicity, and amphipathicity, and alterations to these properties can have sizeable impact. Other alterations to reduce toxicity can include the substitution or addition of polar residues to the hydrophobic side of an α-helical cationic amphiphile, resulting in imperfect amphipathicity, or through the addition of helix-breaking residues, such as proline, glycine, D-amino acids, or peptoids (Bonbone and Stella 2019). It has also been shown that certain amino acids (cysteine, histidine, asparagine, and proline) are more commonly found in toxic peptides, and are preferred in certain positions, a fact that is exploited in the *in silico* prediction of toxicity using tools such as ToxinPred (Gupta et al. 2013). Other strategies to reduce cytotoxicity include peptide grafting (Sahariah et al. 2015), i.e. the use of antimicrobial peptide prodrugs that are released by proteolysis in the host (Pereira et al. 2015), or formulation and delivery-based systems (Ragioto et al. 2014).

It should be noted that while cytotoxicity towards eukaryotic cells is generally undesirable in regards to antimicrobial peptides when they are to be used against pathogens, there are instances where selective toxicity towards certain eukaryotic cell types may be desirable. This is exemplified by antimicrobial peptides that have both antimicrobial and anticancer activities. The principles behind antimicrobial peptides actions against cancer cells are similar to their antibacterial activity in that they are also based on differences in the membrane composition of a normal versus a typical cancer cell. While cancer cells are heterogenous as a whole, they share some common modifications that make them susceptible to membranolytic antimicrobial peptides. These changes include the presence of negatively charged phosphatidylserine on the surface of the cell membrane, as well as other changes that result in an increased transmembrane potential, surface area, and membrane fluidity (Felício et al. 2017). For a review on antimicrobial peptides with potential anticancer applications, please see Felício et al. (2017) and Deslouches and Di (2017).

7.4.3 Difficulty of Production and Manufacturing Cost

There are several options when considering the large scale production of antimicrobial peptides, such as chemical synthesis, the use of bacterial expression systems, cell free expression systems, and even transgenic plants. Techniques such as solid phase synthesis are commonly used when designing novel peptides, but become prohibitively costly when scaled up for production, with synthesis and production costs that are approximately 10–100 fold higher than traditional small molecule drugs (Di 2015). Production costs can be minimized by concentrating on the development of short antimicrobial peptides and peptidomimetics, and in the case of peptidomimetics, focusing on the use of readily available, inexpensive, or generally recognized as safe (GRAS) building blocks (Moretti et al. 2019). Indeed, ~ 85% of peptide drugs are synthetically produced, with the rest produced largely using recombinant technology (Di 2015). Examples of recombinant technologies that may be used in antimicrobial peptide production include the use of transgenic plants. This is commonly associated with *Nicotinia tabacum* or *Nicotinia benthamiana* and the use of *Agrobacterium tumefaciens* with plasmids that encode viral

RNAs replicons in a process known as magnifection. Magnifection can reduce the cost of production, as it is a rapid and efficient system, with potential yields of up to 5 g of peptide per kilogram of fresh tobacco leaves (da Cunha et al. 2017). Prokaryotic expression systems are also a viable option for antimicrobial peptide production, with examples including the hybrid peptide cecropin A-LL37 produced by recombinant *E. coli* and plectasin from *Bacillus subtilis*, where the authors were able to achieve peptide yields of 17.5 mg/L and 35.8 mg/L, respectively (Wei et al. 2018; Chen et al. 2015). A review of current methods for biosynthetic antimicrobial peptide production is provided by da Cunha et al. (2017), and further information on solid phase peptide synthesis can be found in Münzker et al. (2017).

7.4.4 Resistance to Antimicrobial Peptides

Antimicrobial peptides are considered as promising alternatives to current antibiotics due to their low propensity for resistance development, attributed in part to the non-specific membrane targeting mechanism of many cationic amphiphiles, the speed at which they are able to kill target cells, and the high energy cost associated with many forms of resistance (Li et al. 2017). Bacterial resistance to antimicrobial peptides is not unusual though, and numerous examples exists for both intrinsic and acquired resistance to antimicrobial peptides. Intrinsic resistance takes the form of evolutionarily driven changes in bacteria that have developed over time in response to regular and sustained exposure to antimicrobial peptides in the natural environment (da Cunha et al. 2017). Intrinsic resistance may be either passive or inducible. Passive resistance is often driven by reduced interaction between antimicrobial peptides and the bacterial membrane as result of more positively charged lipid A molecules, a feature common to several species such as *Proteus mirabilis*, *Morganella morganii*, *Providencia rettgeri,* etc. (Basu et al. 1986; Olaitan et al. 2014; Maria-Neto et al. 2015). There are also other means by which bacteria may gain a degree of resistance to the action of antimicrobial peptides that are not directly related to exposure, such as the protection conferred by bacterial biofilms (Rabin et al. 2015). Induced resistance is an inherent response mechanism in many species, triggered by changing environmental conditions, leading to the transient expression of genes with a wide range of effects. Examples include modifications of membrane composition and intracellular targets or the activation of proteolytic enzymes and efflux pumps (Andersson et al. 2016).

Acquired resistance is a primary concern with the use of antibiotics as a whole, and is the main driver behind the rapid development of resistance to conventional antibiotics. It has long been thought that bacterial resistance to antimicrobial peptides is both unlikely to develop and difficult to acquire. This is due in part to the high energy cost associated with changes to membrane composition and other inducible mechanisms, but detrimental effects can be associated with acquired resistance and the expression of resistance genes as well (Lofton et al. 2013). An example is found in the colistin resistance gene *mcr-1*, the expression of which is associated with decreased cellular growth and viability, degradation of membrane components and intracellular structures, resulting in decreased overall fitness of species expressing *mcr-1* (Yang et al. 2017). Studies on acquired resistance are few, however several examples have been reported, with examples including resistance to LL-37, lactoferrin B, and some defensins in *S. aureus* linked to *hemB* (Gläser et al. 2014), and resistance to colistin and polymyxin B in *A. baumannii* through *lpxA*, *lpxD* or *lpxC* (Moffat et al. 2010).

As with all drug resistance, the rate at which resistance to antimicrobial peptides may develop and spread is driven by a combination of many factors, such as mutation supply rate, mutant fitness, selection strength, etc., which are reviewed in detail by Andersson et al. (2016). An additional concern with acquired antimicrobial peptide resistance is that the resistance to one antimicrobial peptide may provide resistance to other antimicrobial peptides with similar mechanisms, and could even undermine the effect of naturally occurring human defense peptides, weakening the immune response. This has been demonstrated with antimicrobial peptide resistant *S. aureus* and human defensins and cathelicidins (Kubicek-Sutherland et al. 2017). Several therapeutic strategies have been proposed for the mitigation of resistance development, including multiple hurdle approaches, which consider the application of antimicrobial peptides with multiple mechanism of action, or "cocktail treatments" of multiple antimicrobial peptides and/or other antibiotics, with additive effects and synergy reducing the concentrations needed for bactericidal action, greatly decreasing the potential for resistance. In regards to multiple mechanisms or combination treatments, the use of biofilm preventing/penetrating and anti-infective and wound healing peptides can reduce the potential for infection recurrence and decrease overall treatment times, respectively (Nuri et al. 2015).

7.5 Chemical Modifications and Peptidomimetics

While antimicrobial peptides have several promising characteristics, there are several hurdles to their clinical implementation, and many have failed to display any advantages over existing treatment options (Costa et al. 2019). Modified and synthetic antimicrobial peptides and peptidomimetics represent a growing class of engineered compounds that are effective antimicrobial agents against multi drug resistant pathogens, with design strategies involving chemical modifications that are implemented to reduce, eliminate, or circumvent the limitations described above. Chemical and structural modifications are often inspired by post-translation modifications in naturally occurring antimicrobial peptides. Some antimicrobial peptides require post-translation modifications to properly function, often occurring when they are first produced, but they may also be initiated under specific conditions, with examples including the increased activity of some human defensins upon disulfide bond reduction, or the activation of PEGylated antimicrobial peptide prodrugs *via* proteolytic cleavage (Böttger et al. 2016; Zhu et al. 2017). Common modifications that have shown potential for the improvement of therapeutic peptides and peptidomimetics include amidation (Bradbury and Smyth 1991; Mura et al. 2016), disulfide bond addition and other covalent modifications (Robinson et al. 2005; Ma et al. 2016; Dolle et al. 2019), glycosylation (Moradi et al. 2016; Bednarska et al. 2017), addition of D-amino acids (Genchi 2017), and proteolytic cleavage (Shinnar et al. 2003).

Peptidomimetics are small protein like molecules that take inspiration from naturally occurring antimicrobial peptides, and are designed to mimic their structure with the goal of increased activity against targeted pathogens while also improving upon key pharmacological properties. Major classes of peptidomimetics include small synthetic antimicrobial peptidomimetics (Ghosh and Haldar 2015), ultrashort peptidomimetics (Ahn et al. 2017), peptoids, β^3 -peptides, α/β^3 -peptides, peptide/peptoid hybrids, AApeptides, and oligoacyllysines (Molchanova et al. 2017).

This section will focus on the principles behind the design of peptidomimetics and antimicrobial peptides in a step-wise manner, starting with the selection of a natural antimicrobial peptide as a scaffold for antimicrobial peptide development and the identification of active peptide fragments and sequences, followed by a short review of common chemical modifications used to improve selectivity, resistance to degradation, etc. A schematic representation of peptidomimetic building blocks and chemical alteration strategies is given in Fig. 7.4.

7.5.1 Peptide Truncation and Antimicrobial Fragment Prediction

Most naturally occurring peptides are between 20 and 50 amino acids in length, which can make their synthesis both costly and difficult. However, not all naturally occurring peptides need the entirety of their sequence to function, and efforts have been made to reduce antimicrobial peptides in size and to identify essential elements and minimally active sequences in naturally occurring peptides and proteins. Structure–activity relationships have shown the importance of the different physicochemical properties of antimicrobial peptides, but comprehensive rules for the prediction of peptide function remain just out of reach. Similarly, it is difficult to predict the effect truncation may have on a given peptide sequence, as mechanistically relevant sections may be found at any point in the peptide sequence. As such, *in silico* prediction packages such as those provided by the Data Repository of Antimicrobial Peptides or Antimicrobial Peptide Database can be utilized to determine potential antimicrobial fragments within a larger peptide or protein (Liu et al. 2017; Egan et al. 2018), while other *in silico* methods may be used to predict antimicrobial peptides from relevant genomes (Amaral et al. 2012) driving down the cost of discovery and development by limiting the number and range of potential antimicrobial peptides that will undergo further *in vitro* and *in vivo* testing. A good example of a natural peptide that has been developed in this fashion is the human cathelicidin LL-37, a linear antimicrobial peptide with broad spectrum activity, and one of the

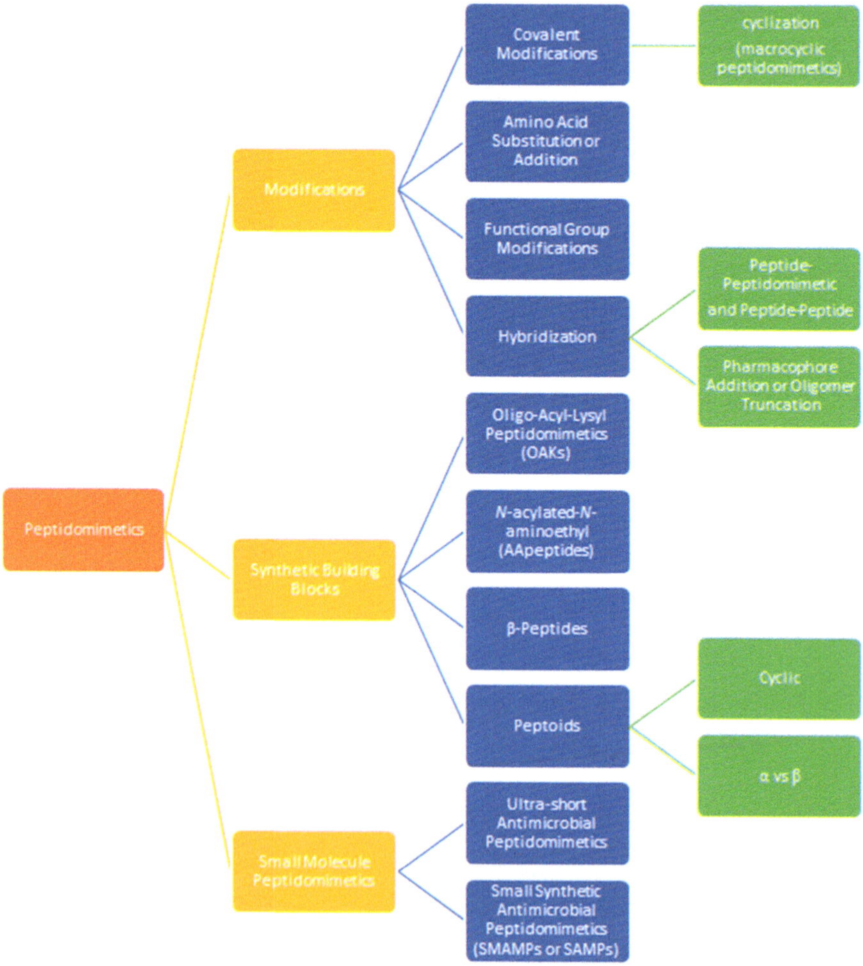

Fig. 7.4 Taxonomy of key design elements and principles that may be used in the development of novel synthetic antimicrobial peptides and peptidomimetics. Examples are given for several different means of modifying an existing peptide, and several major classes of peptidomimetic "building blocks" are presented as well

most extensively studied host-defense peptides. Determination of the 3D structure led to the identification of the key antimicrobial region in the middle of the peptide sequence, as confirmed by several research groups (Li et al. 2006). The resulting peptide was termed FK-16, and a new peptide termed GF-17, was obtained by addition of a glycine to the N-terminus of FK-16. Many derivatives have since been developed, primarily through library screening with structure based design, with a range of peptides having been developed showing a wide range of activities against a variety of targets (Kiattiburut et al. 2018). Other examples of peptide truncation resulting in small synthetic antimicrobial peptides include histone derived antimicrobial fragments (Gao and Elmore 2019), with examples including H2A derived sphistin and its even shorter analogs, Sph_{12-38}, Sph_{20-38} and Sph_{30-38}, with Sph_{12-38} having the greatest antimicrobial activity, potentially through membrane disruption but with the added ability to target genomic DNA as well (Ma et al. 2017). Peptide truncation is also studied in more developed peptidomimetics such as with P_5, a cecropin A-magainin 2 hybrid analog peptide with antimicrobial activity against Gram negative and Gram positive bacteria, and the study of several truncated analogs with good potential for use as novel antibiotics (Kwon et al. 2019). Such studies outline the need for the continuous study and implementation of structure activity relationships for each successive generation of derived antimicrobial peptides, driving the development of even more effective antimicrobial peptides with each series of potential modifications.

7.5.2 Unnatural Amino Acids and Side Chain Modifications

A common strategy to modify and improve upon the properties of antimicrobial peptides involves the substitution of naturally occurring L-amino with D-amino acids or other unnatural analogs (Molhoek et al. 2011). In the case of the LL-37 derived peptide GF-17, several such modifications were made in an effort to reduce the susceptibility of GF-17 to proteolytic degradation by chymotrypsin (Wang et al. 2014). Several different peptides were generated with different numbers and positions of D-amino acid substitutions, resulting in a new protease resistant template GF-17d3, that was found to have reduced antimicrobial activity due to its unusual amphipathic structure containing hydrophobic defects. Altering the aromatic structure of two AA residues *via* the replacement of two phenylalanines with biphenylalanine resulted in a new non-αβ compound, 17BIPHE2, with activity against the ESKAPE pathogens and potential biofilm prevention and immunomodulatory activity as well (Wang et al. 2014). Other studies have shown the utility of D-amino acids in improving stability, and they are commonly incorporated in a wide range of structures to reduce proteolytic degradation (Khara et al. 2016). The range of unnatural amino acids that may be included in antimicrobial peptide design go far beyond simple D-amino acid substitutions, and the sheer number of possible non-canonical amino acids that may be incorporated allows for near limitless chemical diversification of antimicrobial peptides and peptidomimetics. Examples include a series of synthetic peptides utilizing tetrahydroisoquinolinecarboxylic acid and octahydroindolecarboxylic acid dipeptide units that have shown promise against the ESKAPE pathogens (Hicks et al. 2013), and the use of ornithine and norleucine in a series of Cbf-14 (derived from cathelicidin-BF) analogs, generating antimicrobial peptides with improved antimicrobial activity and decreased toxicity (Kang et al. 2017).

Another common modification is the addition of lipid moieties, a strategy used by bacteria to give an advantage over antimicrobial peptides produced by closely related strains (Mojsoska et al. 2015). Lipopeptides are formed by the conjugation of a peptide to either a lipid tail or similarly lipophilic compounds (Cochrane and

Vederas 2016) and the addition of acyl chains of various lengths is a key way in which the hydrophobicity, and consequentially, the activity of a peptide may be modified. Indeed, adding aliphatic chains to the N-terminus of an antimicrobial peptide can result in improved antimicrobial properties (Shalev et al. 2006). Natural lipopeptides typically contain a cyclic peptide head group attached to a single lipid chain (Hamley 2015), with cyclization enhancing the *in vivo* stability as compared to linear analogs. Synthetic lipopeptides and lipopeptidomimetics are structurally diverse, as the addition of lipid moieties is often combined with numerous other chemical alterations, generating a plethora of unique and interesting compounds. LTX-109 is a synthetic antimicrobial peptide that is in clinical trials that has both lipid and aromatic modifications (Nilsson et al. 2015), and other short lipopeptidomimetics have shown promise against planktonic and biofilm associated methicillin resistant *S. aureus* (Joshi et al. 2018). Another heavily modified synthetic lipopeptide, (dBacK-(cap)) was derived from the cyclic peptide bactenecin, combining a variety of chemical alterations, including amino acid substitution, incorporation of d-amino acids, and lipidation (Sim et al. 2019). The resulting dBacK-(cap) compound has potent antibacterial activity against Gram positive and Gram negative species, with rapid killing kinetics and potent membrane permeabilization as well.

7.5.3 Covalent and Backbone Modifications

Covalent modifications are commonly used to impart stability upon antimicrobial peptides, and they can impact other key antimicrobial peptide characteristics as well. Cyclization of peptides may be achieved through disulfide or diselenide bonds (Li and Brimble 2019) or other backbone based covalent modifications, such as hydrocarbon stapling or macrocyclization which may be achieved through a variety of methods (Barrett et al. 2004; Yoo et al. 2010; Ibrahim et al. 2015). The addition of disulfide bonds or other covalent modifications generally provide increased stability against proteolysis, but can have unforeseen impacts on antimicrobial activity and toxicity (Bahar and Ren 2013). The cyclization of peptoids has been demonstrated to increase antimicrobial activity without significantly impacting hemolytic activity (Huang et al. 2012). Covalent modifications can also be used for the surface immobilization of antimicrobial peptides, a strategy that is being applied to medical devices and implants, where the immobilized antimicrobial peptides impart anti-infective and wound healing properties (Nie et al. 2016).

Backbone modifications can impart resistance to proteolysis, but may also lead to changes to the electrostatic properties and structure of a peptidomimetic chain, and can have varying effects on key pharmacological properties. The inherent flexibility of natural peptides can make it easy for interactions with proteolytic enzymes to occur, and the reduced flexibility of conformationally restricted peptidomimetics has the added benefit of potentially increased affinity towards bacterial membranes and surface proteins (Avan et al. 2014). There are a large number of possible backbone modifications that can be made, and a thorough review of common modifications and resulting peptidomimetics is given by Avan et al. (2014) and Mojsoska et al. (2015). Peptoids are one of the major groups of peptidomimetic compounds, in which the side-chain is shifted to the α-amino group, resulting in an alkylated peptide bond that imparts resistance towards degradation, which can increase bioavailability and membrane permeabilization in some instances. β-peptidomimetics are a result of increased carbon numbers along the peptide chain, with no changes to side chain chemistry, that have shown great potential in the development of ultra short peptide mimics against methicillin resistant *S. aureus* and methicillin resistant *Staphylococcus epidermidis* (Hansen et al. 2010). While backbone modifications is generally a good strategy for increasing stability, the conformational changes may result in decreased activity, and other modifications are added to restore or improve upon the original activity, resulting in heavily modified peptidomimetics.

7.5.4 Chimeric Antimicrobial Peptides and Peptidomimetics

An emerging strategy for the development of antimicrobial peptides with novel function is the creation of chimeric or hybrid peptides, in which functional elements from two or more peptides are combined to impart novel or improved function on the newly created hybrids. The potential diversity of chimeric peptides is quite large, as such, only a few examples will be presented.

Commonly, chimeras are produced from the combinations of different regions from naturally occurring antimicrobial peptides. Hybrids constructed from the natural antimicrobial peptides PG-1, bovine lactoferricin and cecropin A were found to be active anti-infectious agents (Liu et al. 2013). Other α-helical hybrid peptides developed from PRW4, fowlicidin-2, protegrin-3 and tritrpticin sequences were able to effectively neutralize endotoxins and reduce cytotoxicity as well (Ma et al. 2015). Other forms of hybridization combine peptide and peptidomimetic features, as demonstrated by α-peptide/β-peptoid chimeras, which combine both peptide and non-peptide characteristics, and are generally stable toward proteolysis, non-hemolytic, and may possess increased or comparable antibacterial activity to their natural analogs (Olsen et al. 2007).

An interesting example of peptide hybridization involved the combination of antimicrobial peptides with different mechanisms of action, with regions from two membrane translocation peptides, buforin II and DesHDAP1 being combined with the membrane permeabilizing antimicrobial peptides magainin 2 and parasin (Wade et al. 2019). They found the permeabilizing mechanism to be dominant, with hybrid peptide found to be more effective than combinations of the original peptides, and also found that the ordering of the two peptide sequences had a bearing on activity. Similarly, conjugation to active regions of membrane translocating peptides have been considered for either the delivery of antibiotics that have lost the ability to cross the bacterial membrane due to developed resistance, or for the delivery of antisense DNA analogs to inhibit transcription (Kauffman et al. 2018).

Another interesting example of chimeric peptides with a novel mechanism of action are those that are now being designed for use in photodynamic therapy. Photodynamic antimicrobial therapy involves the use of visible light and a non-toxic photosensitizer, which upon exposure to certain wavelengths causes the production of reactive oxygen species, effectively killing bacterial cells. Examples include a recently developed membrane binding chimeric peptide PpIX-[PEG_8-$(KLAKLAK)_2]_2$ that successfully combined the photosensitizer protoporphyrin IX (PpIX) with an antimicrobial peptide $(KLAKLAK)_2$ (KLA), which was effective against *S. aureus* and *E. coli* (Zhang et al. 2019). Other studies have combined PpIX, PEG and Cholesterol segments (Chol-PEG-PpIX) to effectively photoinactivate both Gram negative and Gram positive bacteria (Jia et al. 2017).

7.6 Concluding Remarks

Antimicrobial peptides are a promising source of inspiration for the creation of novel antimicrobial peptide and peptidomimetic antibiotics. While naturally occurring antimicrobial peptides have several promising characteristics that make them ideal candidates for drug development, they also have some limitations. Both the negative and positive aspects of antimicrobial peptides are a consequence of the complex interplay between certain key physicochemical properties and the structure and resulting activity of a given peptide antimicrobial. The relationship between the physicochemical properties of an antimicrobial peptide is complex, and different structural changes may have impacts on certain antimicrobial peptides that cannot easily be translated to other examples. However, knowledge of the general trends seen for hydrophobicity, charge, amphipathicity, etc., is useful in making informed chemical alterations with the goal of determining structure activity relationships that may then be applied during each stage of development for synthetic peptides and peptidomimetics. Numerous chemical alterations are commonly used in the development of peptidomimetics that may alter side chain or backbone chemistry that may improve the stability and functionality of the compounds as drug candidates, but may also lead to decreased activity and other negative outcomes. As such, the design of new antimicrobial peptides and peptidomimetics is now at a stage in which lead compounds are identified, informed chemical modifications are made, structure activity relationships developed, and new lead compounds identified. This process can be both costly and lengthy, and several generations of lead compounds are often necessary before meaningful progress is made. However, as the body of data on structure function relationships for diverse groups of compounds continues to grow, we may yet reach a point where universal design strategies might be employed, with the development of a "unified algorithm", in which all the associated variables are present and the weighted value of each has accounted for, such that an output is given showing the effects any one change may have on relevant physicochemical and pharmacological properties. Such a systematic development strategy is not out of reach, and advances in machine learning and database design are now driving the rapid identification and creation of potential antimicrobial sequences, with the ability to estimate potential toxicity as well.

Acknowledgement MLC was supported in part by the Ministry of Science and Higher Education of the Russian Federation (Project Number 075-15-2019-1880).

References

't Hart P, Oppedijk SF, Breukink E, Martin NI (2016) New insights into nisin's antibacterial mechanism revealed by binding studies with synthetic lipid II analogues. Biochemistry 55:232–237. https://doi.org/10.1021/acs.biochem.5b01173

Agrawal A, Rangarajan N, Weisshaar JC (2019) Resistance of early stationary phase E. coli to membrane permeabilization by the antimicrobial peptide cecropin A. Biochim Biophys Acta Biomembr 1861:182990. https://doi.org/10.1016/j.bbamem.2019.05.012

Ahn M, Gunasekaran P, Rajasekaran G, Kim EY, Lee SJ, Bang G, Cho K, Hyun JK, Lee HJ, Jeon YH, Kim NH, Ryu EK, Shin SY, Bang JK (2017) Pyrazole derived ultra-short antimicrobial peptidomimetics with potent anti-biofilm activity. Eur J Med Chem 125:551–564. https://doi.org/10.1016/j.ejmech.2016.09.071

Al-Gburi A, Volski A, Chikindas ML (2015) Natural antimicrobials subtilosin and lauramide arginine ethyl ester (LAE) synergize with conventional antibiotics clindamycin and metronidazole against biofilms of *Gardnerella vaginalis* but not against biofilms of healthy vaginal lactobacilli. Pathog Dis 73:ftv018. https://doi.org/10.1093/femspd/ftv018

Aliste MP, MacCallum JL, Tieleman DP (2003) Molecular dynamics simulations of pentapeptides at interfaces: salt bridge and cation-pi interactions. Biochemistry 42:8976–8987. https://doi.org/10.1021/bi027001j

Amaral AC, Silva ON, Mundim NCCR, de Carvalho MJA, Migliolo L, Leite JRSA, Prates MV, Bocca AL, Franco OL, Felipe MSS (2012) Predicting antimicrobial peptides from eukaryotic genomes: *in silico* strategies to develop antibiotics. Peptides 37:301–308. https://doi.org/10.1016/j.peptides.2012.07.021

Amiche M, Ladram A, Nicolas P (2008) A consistent nomenclature of antimicrobial peptides isolated from frogs of the subfamily phyllomedusinae. Peptides 29:2074–2082. https://doi.org/10.1016/j.peptides.2008.06.017

Andersson DI, Hughes D, Kubicek-Sutherland JZ (2016) Mechanisms and consequences of bacterial resistance to antimicrobial peptides. Drug Resist Updat 26:43–57. https://doi.org/10.1016/j.drup.2016.04.002

APD (2019) Antimicrobial peptide database. http://aps.unmc.edu/AP/main.php. Accessed 15th June 2019

Arias M, Piga KB, Hyndman ME, Vogel HJ (2018) Improving the activity of Trp-rich antimicrobial peptides by Arg/Lys substitutions and changing the length of cationic residues. Biomol Ther 8:19. https://doi.org/10.3390/biom8020019

Arnusch CJ, Pieters RJ, Breukink E (2012) Enhanced membrane pore formation through high-affinity targeted antimicrobial peptides. PLoS One 7:e39768. https://doi.org/10.1371/journal.pone.0039768

Avan I, Hall C, Katritzky A (2014) Peptidomimetics via modifications of amino acids and peptide bonds. Chem Soc Rev 43:3575–3594. https://doi.org/10.1039/c3cs60384a

Bahar AA, Ren D (2013) Antimicrobial peptides. Pharmaceuticals (Basel) 6:1543–1575. https://doi.org/10.3390/ph6121543

Barrett AG, Hennessy AJ, Vézouët RL, Procopiou PA, Seale PW, Stefaniak S, Upton RJ, White AJP, Williams DJ (2004) Synthesis of diverse macrocyclic peptidomimetics utilizing ring-closing metathesis and solid-phase synthesis. J Organomet Chem 69:1028–1037. https://doi.org/10.1021/jo0352629

Basu S, Radziejewska-Lebrecht J, Mayer H (1986) Lipopolysaccharide of Providencia rettgeri. Chemical studies and taxonomical implications. Arch Microbiol 144(3):213–218. https://doi.org/10.1007/BF00410949

Becucci L, Valensin D, Innocenti M, Guidelli R (2014) Dermcidin, an anionic antimicrobial peptide: influence of lipid charge, pH and Zn2+ on its interaction with a biomimetic membrane. Soft Matter 10:616–626. https://doi.org/10.1039/c3sm52400k

Bednarska NG, Wren BW, Willcocks SJ (2017) The importance of the glycosylation of antimicrobial peptides: natural and synthetic approaches. Drug Discov Today 22:919–926. https://doi.org/10.1016/j.drudis.2017.02.001

Bobone S, Stella L (2019) Selectivity of antimicrobial peptides: a complex interplay of multiple equilibria. Adv Exp Med Biol 1117:175–214. https://doi.org/10.1007/978-981-13-3588-4_11

Boman HG (2003) Antibacterial peptides: basic facts and emerging concepts. J Intern Med 254:197–215. https://doi.org/10.1046/j.1365-2796.2003.01228.x

Böttger R, Knappe D, Hoffmann R (2016) Readily adaptable release kinetics of prodrugs using protease-dependent reversible PEGylation. J Control Release 230:88–94. https://doi.org/10.1016/j.jconrel.2016.04.010

Bozelli JC, Schreier S, Epand RM (2017) Microbial membranes and the action of antimicrobial peptides. In: Wang, G (ed). Antimicrobial peptides: discovery, design, and novel therapeutic strategies. CABI, Oxfordshire, pp 135–213

Bradbury AF, Smyth DG (1991) Peptide amidation. Trends Biochem Sci 16:112–115. https://doi.org/10.1016/0968-0004(91)90044-V

Campion A, Casey PG, Field D, Cotter PD, Hill C, Ross RP (2013) *In vivo* activity of nisin A and nisin V against *Listeria monocytogenes* in mice. BMC Microbiol 13:23. https://doi.org/10.1186/1471-2180-13-23

Carmona G, Rodriguez A, Juarez D, Corzo G, Villegas E (2013) Improved protease stability of the antimicrobial peptide Pin2 substituted with D-amino acids. Protein J 32:456–466. https://doi.org/10.1007/s10930-013-9505-2

Cavera VL, Volski A, Chikindas ML (2015) The natural antimicrobial subtilosin a synergizes with lauramide arginine ethyl ester (LAE), ε-poly-l-lysine (Polylysine), clindamycin phosphate and metronidazole, against the vaginal pathogen *Gardnerella vaginalis*. Probiotics Antimicrob Proteins 7:164–171. https://doi.org/10.1007/s12602-014-9183-1

CDC (2013) Antibiotic resistance threats in the United States. CDC, Atlanta

Chen Y, Mant CT, Farmer SW, Hancock RE, Vasil ML, Hodges RS (2005) Rational design of alpha-helical antimicrobial peptides with enhanced activities and specificity/therapeutic index. J Biol Chem 280:12316–12329. https://doi.org/10.1074/jbc.M413406200

Chen Y, Guarnieri MT, Vasil AI, Vasil ML, Mant CT, Hodges RS (2007) Role of peptide hydrophobicity in the mechanism of action of alpha-helical antimicrobial peptides. Antimicrob Agents Chemother 51:1398–1406. https://doi.org/10.1128/AAC.00925-06

Chen X, Shi JW, Chen R, Wen YA, Shi Y, Zhu Z, Guo SW, Li L (2015) Molecular chaperones (TrxA, SUMO, Intein, and GST) mediating expression, purification, and antimicrobial activity assays of plectasin in Escherichia coli. Biotechnol Appl Biochem 62:606–614. https://doi.org/10.1002/bab.1303

Chikindas ML, Weeks RM, Drider D, Chistyakov VA, Dicks LMT (2018) Functions and emerging applications of bacteriocins. Curr Opin Biotechnol 49:23–28. https://doi.org/10.1016/j.copbio.2017.07.011

Chung PY, Khanum R (2017) Antimicrobial peptides as potential anti-biofilm agents against multidrug-resistant bacteria. J Microbiol Immunol Infect 50:405–410. https://doi.org/10.1016/j.jmii.2016.12.005

Cochrane SA, Vederas JC (2016) Lipopeptides from *Bacillus* and *Paenibacillus* spp.: a gold mine of antibiotic candidates. Med Res Rev 36:4–31. https://doi.org/10.1002/med.21321

Coker JA (2016) Extremophiles and biotechnology: current uses and prospects. F1000Res 5:396. https://doi.org/10.12688/f1000research.7432.1

Conibear A, Chaousis S, Durek T, Johan Rosengren K, Craik D, Schroeder C (2016) Approaches to the stabilization of bioactive epitopes by grafting and peptide cyclization. Pept Sci 106:89–100. https://doi.org/10.1002/bip.22767s

Conlon JM (2008) Reflcctions on a systemic nomenclature for antimicrobial peptides from the skins of frogs of the family *Ranidae*. Peptides 29:1815–1819. https://doi.org/10.1016/j.peptides.2008.05.029

Costa F, Carvalho IF, Montelaro RC, Gomes P, Martins MC (2011) Covalent immobilization of antimicrobial peptides (antimicrobial peptides) onto biomaterial surfaces. Acta Biomater 7:1431–1440. https://doi.org/10.1016/j.actbio.2010.11.005

Costa F, Teixeira C, Gomes P, Martins MCL (2019) Clinical application of antimicrobial peptides. In: Matsuzaki K (ed) Antimicrobial peptides: basics for clinical application, Advances in experimental medicine and biology 1117. Springer, Singapore, pp 281–298. https://doi.org/10.1007/978-981-13-3588-4_15

da Cunha NB, Cobacho NB, Viana JF, Lima LA, Sampaio KB, Dohms SS, Ferreira ACR, de la Fuente-Núñez C, Costa FF, Franco OL, Dias SC (2017) The next generation of antimicrobial peptides (antimicrobial peptides) as molecular therapeutic tools for the treatment of diseases with social and economic impacts. Drug Discov Today 22:234–248. https://doi.org/10.1016/j.drudis.2016.10.017

Dalmolin TV, de Lima-Morales D, Barth AL (2018) Plasmid-mediated colistin resistance: what do we know? J Inf Secur 1:16–22. https://doi.org/10.3390/microorganisms7020055

Dathe M, Nikolenko H, Meyer J, Beyermann M, Bienert M (2001) Optimization of the antimicrobial activity of magainin peptides by modification of charge. FEBS Lett 501:146–150. https://doi.org/10.1016/s0014-5793(01)02648-5

de Breij A, Riool M, Cordfunke RA, Malanovic N, de Boer L, Koning R, Ravensbergen E, Franken M, van der Heijde T, Boekema BK, Kwakman PHS, Kamp N, El Ghalbzouri A, Lohner K, Zaat SAJ, Drijfhout JW, Nibbering PH (2018) The antimicrobial peptide SAAP-148 combats drug-resistant bacteria and biofilms. Sci Transl Med 10:eaan4044. https://doi.org/10.1126/scitranslmed.aan4044

Dean SN, Bishop BM, van Hoek ML (2011) Natural and synthetic cathelicidin peptides with antimicrobial and anti-biofilm activity against *Staphylococcus aureus*. BMC Microbiol 11:114. https://doi.org/10.1186/1471-2180-11-114

Deslouches B, Phadke SM, Lazarevic V, Cascio M, Islam K, Montelaro RC, Mietzner TA (2005) *De novo* generation of cationic antimicrobial peptides: influence of length and tryptophan substitution on antimicrobial activity. Antimicrob Agents Chemother 49:316–322. https://doi.org/10.1128/AAC.49.1.316-322.2005

Deslouches B, Hasek ML, Craigo JK, Steckbeck JD, Montelaro RC (2016) Comparative functional properties of engineered cationic antimicrobial peptides consisting exclusively of tryptophan and either lysine or arginine. J Med Microbiol 65:554–565. https://doi.org/10.1099/jmm.0.000258

Di L (2015) Strategic approaches to optimizing peptide ADME properties. AAPS J 17:134–143. https://doi.org/10.1208/s12248-014-9687-3

Diep DB, Skaugen M, Salehian Z, Holo H, Nes IF (2007) Common mechanisms of target cell recognition and immunity for class II bacteriocins. Proc Natl Acad Sci U S A. 104(7):2384–2389. https://doi.org/10.1073/pnas.0608775104

Dolle A, Nagati VB, Hunashal Y, Krishnamurthy K, Pasupulati AK, Raghothama S, Gowd KH (2019) Disulfide engineering on temporin-SHf: stabilizing the bioactive conformation of an ultra-short antimicrobial peptide. Chem Biol Drug Des 94:1634–1646. https://doi.org/10.1111/cbdd.13525

DRAMP (2019) DRAMP database. http://dramp.cpu-bioinfor.org/browse/ClinicalTrialsData.php. Accessed 15th June 2019

DRUGBANK (2017) Tyrothricin. DRUGBANK. https://www.drugbank.ca/drugs/DB13503. Accessed 15th June 2019

DRUGBANK (2019a) Bacitracin. DRUGBANK. http://www.drugbank.ca/drugs/DB00626. Accessed 15th June 2019

DRUGBANK (2019b) Vancomycin. DRUGBANK. https://www.drugbank.ca/drugs/DB00512#label-reference. Accessed 15th June 2019

Dutta P, Das S (2016) Mammalian antimicrobial peptides: promising therapeutic targets against infection and chronic inflammation. Curr Top Med Chem 16:99–129. https://doi.org/10.2174/1568026615666150703121819

Duval E, Zatylny C, Laurencin M, Baudy-Floc'h M, Henry J (2009) KKKKPLFGLFFGLF: a cationic peptide designed to exert antibacterial activity. Peptides 30:1608–1612. https://doi.org/10.1016/j.peptides.2009.06.022

Egan K, Field D, Ross RP, Cotter PD, Hill C (2018) *In silico* prediction and exploration of potential bacteriocin gene clusters within the bacterial genus *Geobacillus*. Front Microbiol 9:2116. https://doi.org/10.3389/fmicb.2018.02116

Ehmann D, Wendler J, Koeninger L, Larsen IS, Klag T, Berger J, Marette A, Schaller M, Stange EF, Malek NP, Jensen BAH, Wehkamp J (2019) Paneth cell α-defensins HD-5 and HD-6 display differential degradation into active antimicrobial fragments. PNAS 116:3746–3751. https://doi.org/10.1073/pnas.1817376116

Eisenberg D, Weiss RM, Terwilliger TC (1982) The helical hydrophobic moment: a measure of the amphiphilicity of a helix. Nature 299:371–374. https://doi.org/10.1038/299371a0

Eskandari S, Guerin T, Toth I, Stephenson RJ (2017) Recent advances in self-assembled peptides: implications for targeted drug delivery and vaccine engineering. Adv Drug Deliv Rev 110–111:169–187. https://doi.org/10.1016/j.addr.2016.06.013

Essig A, Hofmann D, Münch D, Gayathri S, Künzler M, Kallio PT, Sahl HG, Wider G, Schneider T, Aebi M (2014) Copsin, a novel peptide-based fungal antibiotic interfering with the peptidoglycan synthesis. J Biol Chem 289:34953–34964. https://doi.org/10.1074/jbc.M114.599878

Falagas ME, Kasiakou SK (2006) Toxicity of polymyxins: a systematic review of the evidence from old and recent studies. Crit Care 10:R27. https://doi.org/10.1186/cc3995

Fan L, Sun J, Zhou M, Zhou M, Zhou J, Lau X, Zheng H, Xu H (2016) DRAMP: a comprehensive data repository of antimicrobial peptides. Sci Rep 6:24482. https://doi.org/10.1038/srep24482

Felício MR, Silva ON, Gonçalves S, Santos NC, Franco OL (2017) Peptides with dual antimicrobial and anticancer activities. Front Chem 5:5. https://doi.org/10.3389/fchem.2017.00005

Fernandez-Vidall M, Jayasinghe S, Ladokhin AS, White SH (2007) Folding amphipathic helices into membranes: amphiphilicity trumps hydrophobicity. J Mol Biol 370:459–470

Fosgerau K, Hoffmann T (2015) Peptide therapeutics: current status and future directions. Drug Discov Today 20:122–128. https://doi.org/10.1016/j.drudis.2014.10.003

Gagnon MC, Strandber E, Grau-Campistany A, Wadhwani P, Reichert J, Burck J, Rabanal F, Auguer M, Paqui JF, Ulrich AS (2017) Influence of the length and charge on the activity of α-helical amphipathic antimicrobial peptides. Biochemistry 56:1680–1695. https://doi.org/10.1021/acs.biochem.6b01071

Gao K, Elmore DE (2019) Can molecular dynamics simulations predict the effect of truncating histone-derived antimicrobial peptides? Biophys J 116:84a. https://doi.org/10.1016/j.bpj.2018.11.497

Gao B, Zhu S (2018) Mesobuthus Venom-derived antimicrobial peptides possess intrinsic multifunctionality and differential potential as drugs. Front Microbiol 9:320. https://doi.org/10.3389/fmicb.2018.00320

Genchi G (2017) An overview on d-amino acids. Amino Acids 49:1521–1533. https://doi.org/10.1007/s00726-017-2459-2465

Gentilucci L, De Marco R, Cerisoli L (2010) Chemical modifications designed to improve peptide stability: incorporation of non-natural amino acids, pseudo-peptide bonds, and cyclization. Curr Pharm Des 16:3185–3203. https://doi.org/10.2174/138161210793292555

Gerdes K, Semsey S (2016) Microbiology: pumping persisters. Nature 534:41–42. https://doi.org/10.1038/nature18442

Ghosh C, Haldar J (2015) Membrane-active small molecules: designs inspired by antimicrobial peptides. Chem Med Chem 10:1606–1624. https://doi.org/10.1002/cmdc.201500299

Gläser R, Becker K, von Eiff C, Meyer-Hoffert U, Harder J (2014) Decreased susceptibility of *Staphylococcus aureus* small-colony variants toward human antimicrobial peptides. J Invest Dermatol 134:2347–2350. https://doi.org/10.1038/jid.2014.176

Golec M (2007) Cathelicidin LL-37: LPS-neutralizing, pleiotropic peptide. Ann Agric Environ Med 14:1–4

Greber KE, Dawgul M (2017) Antimicrobial peptides under clinical trials. Curr Top Med Chem 17:620–628. https://doi.org/10.2174/1568026616666160713143331

Gregory J (2018) A review of the opportunities and shortcomings of antibiotic stewardship. US Pharm 43:HS-7–HS-12

Gupta S, Kapoor P, Chaudhary K, Gautam A, Kumar R, Open Source Drug Discovery Consortium, Raghava GP (2013) *In silico* approach for predicting toxicity of peptides and proteins. PLoS One 8:e73957. https://doi.org/10.1371/journal.pone.0073957

Hamley IW (2015) Lipopeptides: from self-assembly to bioactivity. Chem Commun (Camb) 51:8574–8583. https://doi.org/10.1039/c5cc01535a

Hansen T, Alst T, Havelkova M, Strøm MB (2010) Antimicrobial activity of small β-peptidomimetics based on the pharmacophore model of short cationic antimicrobial peptides. J Med Chem 53:595–606. https://doi.org/10.1021/jm901052r

Harwig SS, Waring A, Yang HJ, Cho Y, Tan L, Lehrer RI (1996) Intramolecular disulfide bonds enhance the antimicrobial and lytic activities of protegrins at physiological sodium chloride concentrations. Eur J Biochem 240:352–357. https://doi.org/10.1111/j.1432-1033.1996.0352h.x

Hein-Kristensen L, Knapp KM, Franzyk H, Gram L (2011) Bacterial membrane activity of α-peptide/β-peptoid chimeras: influence of amino acid composition and chain length on the activity against different bacterial strains. BMC Microbiol 11:144. https://doi.org/10.1186/1471-2180-11-144

Hicks RP, Abercrombie JJ, Wong RK, Leung KP (2013) Antimicrobial peptides containing unnatural amino acid exhibit potent bactericidal activity against ESKAPE pathogens. Bioorg Med Chem 21:205–214. https://doi.org/10.1016/j.bmc.2012.10.039

Hilpert K, Elliott M, Jenssen H, Kindrachuk J, Fjell CD, Körner J, Winkler DF, Weaver LL, Henklein P, Ulrich AS, Chiang SH, Farmer SW, Pante N, Volkmer R, Hancock RE (2009) Screening and characterization of surface-tethered cationic peptides for antimicrobial activity. Chem Biol 16:58–69. https://doi.org/10.1016/j.chembiol.2008.11.006

Huang ML, Shin SB, Benson MA, Torres VJ, Kirshenbaum K (2012) A comparison of linear and cyclic peptoid oligomers as potent antimicrobial agents. Chem Med Chem 7:114–122. https://doi.org/10.1002/cmdc.201100358

Ibrahim MA, Panda SS, Oliferenko AA, Oliferenko PV, Girgis AS, Elagawany M, Küçükbay FZ, Panda CS, Pillai GG, Samir A, Tämm K, Halla CD, Katritzkya AR (2015) Macrocyclic peptidomimetics with antimicrobial activity: synthesis, bioassay, and molecular modeling studies. Org Biomol Chem 13:9492–9503. https://doi.org/10.1039/C5OB01400J

Imamura T, Yamamoto N, Tamura A, Murabayashi S, Hashimoto S, Shimada H, Taguchi S (2008) NMR based structure-activity relationships of an antimicrobial peptide, thanatin, engineered by site-specific chemical modification: activity improvement and spectrum alteration. Biochem Biophys Res Commun 369:609–615. https://doi.org/10.1016/j.bbrc.2008.02.057

Islam KT, Velivelli SLS, Berg RH, Oakley B, Shah DM (2017) A novel bi-domain plant defensin MtDef5 with potent broad-spectrum antifungal activity binds to multiple phospholipids and forms oligomers. Sci Rep 7:16157. https://doi.org/10.1038/s41598-017-16508-w

Jackson KE, Miller-White T (2018) The intracellular target of the antimicrobial peptide thanatin. J Immunol 200(1 Suppl):170.17

Javadpour MM, Juban MM, Lo WC, Bishop SM, Alberty JB, Cowell SM, Becker CL, McLaughlin ML (1996) *De novo* antimicrobial peptides with low mammalian cell toxicity. J Med Chem 39:3107–3113. https://doi.org/10.1021/jm9509410

Jia HR, Zhu YX, Chen Z, Wu FG (2017) Cholesterol-assisted bacterial cell surface engineering for photodynamic inactivation of Gram-positive and Gram-negative bacteria. ACS Appl Mater Interfaces 9:15943–11595. https://doi.org/10.1021/acsami.7b02562

Jiang Z, Vasil A, Hale J, Hancock R, Vasil M, Hodges R, Jiang Z (2008) Effects of net charge and the number of positively charged residues on the biological activity of amphipathic alpha-helical cationic antimicrobial peptides. Biopolymers 90:369–383. https://doi.org/10.1002/bip.20911

Joshi S, Mumtaz S, Singh J, Pasha S, Mukhopadhyay K (2018) Novel miniature membrane active lipopeptidomimetics against planktonic and biofilm embedded methicillin-resistant *Staphylococcus aureus*. Sci Rep 18:1021. https://doi.org/10.1038/s41598-017-17234-z

Kang W, Liu H, Ma L, Wang M, Wei S, Sun P, Jiang M, Guo M, Zhou C, Dou J (2017) Effective antimicrobial activity of a peptide mutant Cbf-14-2 against penicillin-resistant bacteria based on its unnatural amino acids. Eur J Pharm Sci 105:169–177. https://doi.org/10.1016/j.ejps.2017.05.030

Kauffman WB, Guha S, Wimley WC (2018) Synthetic molecular evolution of hybrid cell penetrating peptides. Nat Commun 9:2568. https://doi.org/10.1038/s41467-018-04874-6

Kaur K, Sign I, Kaur P, Kaur R (2015) Food and Drug Administration (FDA) approved peptide drugs. AJRBPS 3:75–88

Kaushal A, Gupta K, Shah R, van Hoek ML (2016) Antimicrobial activity of mosquito cecropin peptides against *Francisella*. Dev Comp Immunol 63:171–180. https://doi.org/10.1016/j.dci.2016.05.018

Khara JS, Priestman M, Uhía I, Hamilton MS, Krishnan N, Wang Y, Yang YY, Langford PR, Newton SM, Robertson BD, Ee PL (2016) Unnatural amino acid analogues of membrane-active helical peptides with anti-mycobacterial activity and improved stability. J Antimicrob Chemother 71:2181–2191. https://doi.org/10.1093/jac/dkw107

Kiattiburut W, Zhi R, Lee SG, Foo AC, Hickling DR, Keillor JW, Goto NK, Li W, Conlan W, Angel JB, Wang G, Tanphaichitr N (2018) Antimicrobial peptide LL-37 and its truncated forms, GI-20 and GF-17, exert spermicidal effects and microbicidal activity against *Neisseria gonorrhoeae*. Hum Reprod 33:2175–2183. https://doi.org/10.1093/humrep/dey315

Kim C, Gajendran N, Mittrücker HW, Weiwad M, Song YH, Hurwitz R, Wilmanns M, Fischer G, Kaufmann SH (2005) Human α-defensins neutralize anthrax lethal toxin and protect against its fatal consequences. Proc Natl Acad Sci U S A 102:4830–4835. https://doi.org/10.1073/pnas.0500508102

Kjos M, Nes IF, Dzung BD (2009) Class II one-peptide bacteriocins target a phylogenetically defined subgroup of mannose phosphotransferase systems on sensitive cells. Microbiology 155:2949–2961. https://doi.org/10.1099/mic.0.030015-0

Klüver E, Schulz-Maronde S, Scheid S, Meyer B, Forssmann WG, Adermann K (2005) Structure–activity relation of human β-defensin 3: influence of disulfide bonds and cysteine substitution on antimicrobial activity and cytotoxicity. Biochemistry 44:9804–9816. https://doi.org/10.1021/bi050272k

Kragol G, Lovas S, Varadi G, Condie BA, Hoffmann R, Otvos L (2001) The antibacterial peptide pyrrhocoricin inhibits the ATPase actions of DnaK and prevents chaperone-assisted protein folding. Biochemistry 40:3016–3026. https://doi.org/10.1021/bi002656a

Krizsan A, Volke D, Weinert S, Sträter N, Knappe D, Hoffmann R (2014) Insect derived proline-rich antimicrobial peptides kill bacteria by inhibit bacterial protein translation at the 70S ribosome. Angew Chem Int Ed Eng 53:12236–12239. https://doi.org/10.1002/anie.201407145

Kubicek-Sutherland JZ, Lofton H, Vestergaard M, Hjort K, Ingmer H, Andersson DI (2017) Antimicrobial peptide exposure selects for *Staphylococcus aureus* resistance to human defence peptides. J Antimicrob Chemother 72:115–127. https://doi.org/10.1093/jac/dkw381

Kumar P, Kizhakkedathu JN, Straus SK (2018) Antimicrobial peptides: diversity, mechanism of action and strategies to improve the activity and biocompatibility *in vivo*. Biomol Ther 8:4. https://doi.org/10.3390/biom8010004

Kustanovich I, Shalev DE, Mikhlin M, Gaidukov L, Mor A (2002) Structural requirements for potent versus selective cytotoxicity for antimicrobial dermaseptin s4 derivatives. J Biol Chem 277:16941–16951. https://doi.org/10.1074/jbc.M111071200

Kwon JY, Kim MK, Mereuta L, Seo CH, Luchian T, Park Y (2019) Mechanism of action of antimicrobial peptide P5 truncations against *Pseudomonas aeruginosa* and *Staphylococcus aureus*. AMB Express 9:122. https://doi.org/10.1186/s13568-019-0843-0

Lang C, Staiger C (2016) Tyrothricin – an underrated agent for the treatment of bacterial skin infections and superficial wounds? Pharmazie 71:299–305. https://doi.org/10.1691/ph.2016.6038

Li F, Brimble M (2019) Using chemical synthesis to optimize antimicrobial peptides in the Fight against antimicrobial resistance. Pure Appl Chem 91:181–198(18). https://doi.org/10.1515/pac-2018-0704

Li C, Salditt T (2006) Structure of magainin and alamethicin in model membranes studied by x-ray reflectivity. Biophys J 91:3285–3300. https://doi.org/10.1529/biophysj.106.090118

Li X, Li Y, Han H, Miller DW, Wang G (2006) Solution structures of human LL-37 fragments and NMR-based identification of a minimal membrane-targeting antimicrobial and anticancer region. J Am Chem Soc 128:5776–5785. https://doi.org/10.1021/ja0584875

Li L, Vorobyov I, Allen TW (2013) The different interactions of lysine and arginine side chains with lipid membranes. J Phys Chem B 117(40):11906–11920. https://doi.org/10.1021/jp405418y

Li W, Tailhades J, O'Brien-Simpson NM, Separovic F, Otvos L, Hossain MA, Wade JD (2014) Proline-rich antimicrobial peptides: potential therapeutics against antibiotic-resistant bacteria. Amino Acids 46:2287–2294. https://doi.org/10.1007/s00726-014-1820-1

Li J, Koh JJ, Liu S, Lakshminarayanan R, Verma CS, Beuerman RW (2017) Membrane active antimicrobial peptides: translating mechanistic insights to design. Front Neurosci 11:73. https://doi.org/10.3389/fnins.2017.0007

Liu ZG, Brady A, Young A, Rasimick B, Chen K, Zhou CH, Kallenbach NR (2007) Length effects in antimicrobial peptides of the (rw)(n) series. Antimicrob Agents Chemother 51:597–603. https://doi.org/10.1128/AAC.00828-06

Liu L, Xu K, Wang H, Tan PK, Fan W, Venkatraman SS, Li L, Yang YY (2009) Self-assembled cationic peptide nanoparticles as an efficient antimicrobial agent. Nat Nanotechnol 4:457. https://doi.org/10.1038/nnano.2009.153

Liu YF, Xia X, Xu L, Wang YZ (2013) Design of hybrid β-hairpin peptides with enhanced cell specificity and potent anti-inflammatory activity. Biomaterials 34:237–250. https://doi.org/10.1016/j.biomaterials.2012.09.032

Liu S, Fan L, Sun J, Lao X, Zheng H (2017) Computational resources and tools for antimicrobial peptides. J Pept Sci 23:4–12. https://doi.org/10.1002/psc.2947

Lofton H, Pränting M, Thulin E, Andersson DI (2013) Mechanisms and fitness costs of resistance to antimicrobial peptides LL-37, CNY100HL and wheat germ histones. PLoS One 8:e68875. https://doi.org/10.1371/journal.pone.0068875

Ma Z, Wei D, Yan P, Zhu X, Shan A, Bi Z (2015) Characterization of cell selectivity, physiological stability and endotoxin neutralization capabilities of α-helix-based peptide amphiphiles. Biomaterials 52:517–530. https://doi.org/10.1016/j.biomaterials.2015.02.063

Ma B, Niu C, Zhou Y, Xue X, Meng J, Luo X, Hou Z (2016) The disulfide bond of the peptide thanatin is dispensible for its antimicrobial activity *in vivo* and *in vitro*. Antimicrob Agents Chemother 60:4283. https://doi.org/10.1128/AAC.00041-16

Ma XW, Hou L, Chen B, Fan DQ, Chen YC, Yang Y, Wang KJ (2017) A truncated Sph12-38 with potent antimicrobial activity showing resistance against bacterial challenge in *Oryzias melastigma*. Fish Shellfish Immunol 67:561–570. https://doi.org/10.1016/j.fsi.2017.06.013

Maria-Neto S, de Almeida KC, Macedo ML, Franco OL (2015) Understanding bacterial resistance to antimicrobial peptides: from the surface to deep inside. Biochim Biophys Acta 1848:3078–3088. https://doi.org/10.1016/j.bbamem.2015.02.017

Martin-Gmez H, Tulla-Puche J (2018) Lasso peptides: chemical approaches and structural elucidation. Org Biomol Chem 16:5065–5080. https://doi.org/10.1039/c8ob01304g

Marwick C, Guthrie B, Davey P (2017) Hospital antimicrobial stewardship: the way forward. Lancet Infect Dis 17:1119–1120. https://doi.org/10.1016/S1473-3099(17)30566-2

Meng H, Kumar K (2007) Antimicrobial activity and protease stability of peptides containing fluorinated amino acids. J Am Chem Soc 129:15615–15622. https://doi.org/10.1021/ja075373f

Mihajlovic M, Lazaridis T (2012) Charge distribution and imperfect amphipathicity affect pore formation by antimicrobial peptides. Biochim Biophys Acta 1818:1274–1283. https://doi.org/10.1016/j.bbamem.2012.01.016

Mishra B, Wang G (2012) The importance of amino acid composition in natural antimicrobial peptides: an evolutional, structural, and functional perspective. Front Immunol 3:221. https://doi.org/10.3389/fimmu.2012.00221

Mishra AK, Choi J, Moon E, Baek KH (2018) Tryptophan-rich and proline-rich antimicrobial peptides. Molecules 23:815. https://doi.org/10.3390/molecules23040815

Moffatt JH, Harper M, Harrison P, Hale JDF, Vinogradov E, Seemann T, Henry R, Crane B, St. Michael F, Cox AD, Adler B, Nation RL, Li J, Boyce JD (2010) Colistin resistance in *Acinetobacter baumannii* is mediated by complete loss of lipopolysaccharide production. Antimicrob Agents Chemother 54:4971–4977. https://doi.org/10.1128/AAC.00834-10

Mohammad H, Thangamani S, Seleem MN (2015) Antimicrobial peptides and peptidomimetics - potent therapeutic allies for staphylococcal infections. Curr Pharm Des 21(16):2073–2088. https://doi.org/10.2174/1381612821666150310102702

Mojsoska B, Jenssen H, Mojsoska B (2015) Peptides and peptidomimetics for antimicrobial drug design. Pharmaceuticals 8:366–415. https://doi.org/10.3390/ph8030366

Molchanova N, Hansen PR, Franzyk H (2017) Advances in development of antimicrobial peptidomimetics as potential drugs. Molecules 22:1430. https://doi.org/10.3390/molecules22091430

Molhoek EM, van Dijk A, Veldhuizen EJ, Haagsman HP, Bikker FJ (2011) Improved proteolytic stability of chicken cathelicidin-2 derived peptides by D-amino acid substitutions and cyclization. Peptides 32:875–880. https://doi.org/10.1016/j.peptides.2011.02.017

Moradi SV, Hussein WM, Varamini P, Simerska P, Toth I (2016) Glycosylation, an effective synthetic strategy to improve the bioavailability of therapeutic peptides. Chem Sci 7:2492–2500. https://doi.org/10.1039/c5sc04392a

Moreno M, Giralt E (2015) Three valuable peptides from bee and wasp venoms for therapeutic and biotechnological use: melittin, apamin and mastoparan. Toxins 7:1126–1150. https://doi.org/10.3390/toxins7041126

Moretti A, Weeks RM, Chikindas M, Uhrich KE (2019) Cationic amphiphiles with specificity against Gram-positive and Gram-negative bacteria: chemical composition and architecture combat bacterial membranes. Langmuir 35:5557–5567. https://doi.org/10.1021/acs.langmuir.9b00110

Münzker L, Oddo A, Hansen PR (2017) Chemical synthesis of antimicrobial peptides. In: Hansen P (ed) Antimicrobial peptides, Methods in molecular biology 1548. Humana Press, New York, pp 35–49. https://doi.org/10.1007/978-1-4939-6737-7_3

Mura M, Wang J, Zhou Y, Pinna M, Zvelindovsky AV, Dennison SR, Phoenix DA (2016) The effect of amidation on the behaviour of antimicrobial peptides. Eur Biophys J 45:195–207. https://doi.org/10.1007/s00249-015-1094-x

Nell MJ, Tjabringa GS, Wafelman AR, Verrijk R, Hiemstra PS, Drijfhout JW, Grote JJ (2006) Development of novel LL-37 derived antimicrobial peptides with LPS and LTA neutralizing and antimicrobial activities for therapeutic application. Peptides 27:649–660. https://doi.org/10.1016/j.peptides.2005.09.016

Nie BE, Ao H, Chen C, Xie K, Zhou J, Long T, Tang T, Yue B (2016) Covalent immobilization of KR-12 peptide onto a titanium surface for decreasing infection and promoting osteogenic differentiation. RSC Adv 6:46733–46743. https://doi.org/10.1039/C6RA06778F

Nilsson AC, Janson H, Wold H, Fugelli A, Andersson K, Håkangård C, Olsen P, Olsen WM (2015) LTX-109 is a novel agent for nasal decolonization of methicillin-resistant and-sensitive

Staphylococcus aureus. Antimicrob Agents Chemother 59:145–151. https://doi.org/10.1128/AAC.03513-14

Nordström R, Malmsten M (2017) Delivery systems for antimicrobial peptides. Adv Colloid Interf Sci 242:17–34. https://doi.org/10.1016/j.cis.2017.01.005

Nuri R, Shprung T, Shai Y (2015) Defensive remodeling: how bacterial surface properties and biofilm formation promote resistance to antimicrobial peptides. Biochim Biophys Acta 1848:3089–3100. https://doi.org/10.1016/j.bbamem.2015.05.022

O'Neill J (2014) Review on antimicrobial resistance: tackling a crisis for the health and wealth of nations. Review on Antimicrobial Resistance, London

Olaitan AO, Morand S, Rolain JM (2014) Mechanisms of polymyxin resistance: acquired and intrinsic resistance in bacteria. Front Microbiol 5:643. https://doi.org/10.3389/fmicb.2014.00643

Olsen I (2015) Biofilm-specific antibiotic tolerance and resistance. Eur J Clin Microbiol Infect Dis 34:877–886. https://doi.org/10.1007/s10096-015-2323-z

Olsen CA, Bonke G, Vedel L, Adsersen A, Witt M, Franzyk H, Jaroszewski JW (2007) α-peptide/β-peptoid chimeras. Org Lett 9:1549–1552. https://doi.org/10.1021/ol070316c

Ouellette AJ (2015) Defensins in enteric mucosal immunity. Mucosal Immunol (Fourth Ed) 1:271–285. https://doi.org/10.1016/B978-0-12-415847-4.00016-1

Oyinloye BE, Adenowo AF, Kappo AP (2015) Reactive oxygen species, apoptosis, antimicrobial peptides and human inflammatory diseases. Pharmaceuticals (Basel) 8:151–175. https://doi.org/10.3390/ph8020151

Parisi K, Shafee T, Quimbar P, van Der Weerden N, Bleackley M, Anderson M, Parisi K (2019) The evolution, function and mechanisms of action for plant defensins. Semin Cell Dev Biol 88:107–118. https://doi.org/10.1016/j.semcdb.2018.02.004

Pasupuleti M, Schmidtchen A, Malmsten M (2012) Antimicrobial peptides: key components of the innate immune system. Crit Rev Biotechnol 32:143–171. https://doi.org/10.3109/07388551.2011.594423

PCAST (2014) Report to the president on combating antibiotic resistance. President's Council of Advisors on Science and Technology, Washington, DC

Pendleton JN, Gorman SP, Gilmore BF (2013) Clinical relevance of the ESKAPE pathogens. Expert Rev Anti-Infect Ther 11:297–308. https://doi.org/10.1586/eri.13.12

Pereira MP, Shi J, Kelley SO (2015) Peptide targeting of an antibiotic prodrug toward phagosome-entrapped mycobacteria. ACS Infect Dis 1:586–592. https://doi.org/10.1021/acsinfecdis.5b00099

Quintana VM, Torres NI, Wachsman MB, Sinko PJ, Castilla V, Chikindas M (2014) Antiherpes simplex virus type 2 activity of the antimicrobial peptide subtilosin. J Appl Microbiol 117:1253–1259. https://doi.org/10.1111/jam.12618

Rabin N, Zheng Y, Opoku-Temeng C, Du Y, Bonsu E, Sintim HO (2015) Biofilm formation mechanisms and targets for developing antibiofilm agents. Future Med Chem 7:493–512. https://doi.org/10.4155/fmc.15.6

Ragioto DA, Carrasco LD, Carmona-Ribeiro AM (2014) Novel gramicidin formulations in cationic lipid as broadspectrum microbicidal agents. Int J Nanomedicine 9:3183–3192. https://doi.org/10.2147/IJN.S65289

Rice A, Wereszczynski J (2017) Probing the disparate effects of arginine and lysine residues on antimicrobial peptide/bilayer association. Biochim Biophys Acta Biomembr 1859:1941–1950. https://doi.org/10.1016/j.bbamem.2017.06.002

Righi E, Peri AM, Harris PNA, Walian AM, Liborio M, Lane SW, Paterson DL (2017) Global prevalence of carbapenem resistance in neutropenic patients and association with mortality and carbapenem use: systematic review and meta-analysis. J Antimicrob Chemother 72:668–677. https://doi.org/10.1093/jac/dkw459

Roberts KD, Azad MA, Wang J, et al (2015) Antimicrobial activity and toxicity of the major lipopeptide components of polymyxin B and colistin: Last-line antibiotics against multidrug-resistant Gram-negative bacteria. ACS Infect Dis 1(11):568–575. https://doi.org/10.1021/acsinfecdis.5b00085

Robinson JA, Shankaramma SC, Jetter P, Kienzl U, Schwendener RA, Vrijbloed JW, Obrecht D (2005) Properties and structure–activity studies of cyclic β-hairpin peptidomimetics based on the cationic antimicrobial peptide protegrin I. Bioorg Med Chem 13:2055–2064. https://doi.org/10.1016/j.bmc.2005.01.009

Rollema HS, Kuipers OP, Both P, De Vos WM, Siezen RJ (1995) Improvement of solubility and stability of the antimicrobial peptide nisin by protein engineering. Appl Environ Microbiol 61:2873–2878

Roy RN, Lomakin IB, Gagnon MG, Steitz TA (2015) The mechanism of inhibition of protein synthesis by the proline rich peptide oncocin. Nat Struct Mol Biol 22:466–469. https://doi.org/10.1038/nsmb.3031

Sahariah P, Sørensen KK, Hjálmarsdóttir MÁ, Sigurjónsson ÓE, Jensen KJ, Másson M, Thygesen MB (2015) Antimicrobial peptide shows enhanced activity and reduced toxicity upon grafting to chitosan polymers. Chem Commun (Camb) 51:11611–11614. https://doi.org/10.1039/c5cc04010h

Salas CE, Badillo-Corona JA, Ramirez-Sotelo G, Oliver-Salvador C (2015) Biologically active and antimicrobial peptides from plants. Biomed Res Int 2015:1–11. https://doi.org/10.1155/2015/102129

Sani MA, Separovic F (2016) How membrane-active peptides get into lipid membranes. Acc Chem Res 49:1130–1138. https://doi.org/10.1111/jam.12618

Schein CH (1990) Solubility as a function of protein structure and solvent components. Nat Biotechnol 8:308–317. https://doi.org/10.1038/nbt0490-308

Schmidtchen A, Frick IM, Andersson E, Tapper H, Björck L (2002) Proteinases of common pathogenic bacteria degrade and inactivate the antibacterial peptide LL-37. Mol Microbiol 46:157–168. https://doi.org/10.1046/j.1365-2958.2002.03146.x

Schroeder BO, Wu Z, Nuding S, Groscurth S, Marcinowski M, Beisner J, Buchner J, Schaller M, Stange EF, Wehkamp J (2011) Reduction of disulphide bonds unmasks potent antimicrobial activity of human β-defensin 1. Nature 469:419–423. https://doi.org/10.1038/nature09674

Scocchi M, Tossi A, Gennaro R (2011) Proline rich antimicrobial peptides: converging to a non-membrane lytic mechanism of action. Cell Mol Life Sci 68:2317–2330. https://doi.org/10.1007/s00018-011-0721-7

Scocchi M, Mardirossian M, Runti G, Benincasa M (2017) Non-membranolytic mechanisms of action of antimicrobial peptides – novel therapeutic opportunities? In: Wang G (ed) Antimicrobial peptides: discovery, design, and novel therapeutic strategies. CABI, Oxfordshire, pp 149–160

Seefeldt AC, Nguyen F, Antunes S, Pérébaskine N, Graf M, Arenz S, Inampudi KK, Douat C, Guichard G, Wilson DN, Innis CA (2015) The proline rich antimicrobial peptide Onc112 inhibits translation by blocking and destabilizing the initiation complex. Nat Struct Mol Biol 22:470–475. https://doi.org/10.1038/nsmb.3034

Segev-Zarko L, Mangoni ML, Shai Y (2017) Antimicrobial peptides: multiple mechanism against a variety of targets. In: Wang G (ed) Antimicrobial peptides: discovery, design, and novel therapeutic strategies. CABI, Oxfordshire, pp 119–127

Semreen M, El-Garmal M, Abdin S, Alkhazraji H, Kamal L, Hammad S, El-Awady F, Waleed D, Kourbaj L (2018) Recent updates of marine antimicrobial peptides. Saudi Pharm J 26:396–409. https://doi.org/10.1016/j.jsps.2018.01.001

Shabir U, Ali S, Magray AR, Ganai BA, Firdous P, Hassan T, Nazir R (2018) Fish antimicrobial peptides (AMP's) as essential and promising molecular therapeutic agents: a review. Microb Pathog 114:50–56. https://doi.org/10.1016/j.micpath.2017.11.039

Shagaghi N, Palombo EA, Clayton AHA, Bhave M (2016) Archetypal tryptophan-rich antimicrobial peptides: properties and applications. World J Microbiol Biotechnol 32:31. https://doi.org/10.1007/s11274-015-1986-z

Shalev DE, Rotem S, Fish A, Mor A (2006) Consequences of n-acylation on structure and membrane binding properties of dermaseptin derivative k4-s4-(1–13). J Biol Chem 281:9432–9438. https://doi.org/10.1074/jbc.M513051200

Shen LP, Pictet RL, Rutter WJ (1982) Human somatostatin I sequence of the cDNA. Proc Natl Acad Sci U S A 79:4575–4579. https://doi.org/10.1073/pnas.79.15.4575

Shin JM, Gwak JW, Kamarajan P, Fenno JC, Rickard AH, Kapila YL (2015) Biomedical applications of nisin. J Appl Microbiol 120:1449–1465. https://doi.org/10.1111/jam.13033

Shinnar AE, Butler KL, Park HJ (2003) Cathelicidin family of antimicrobial peptides: proteolytic processing and protease resistance. Bioorg Chem 31:425–443. https://doi.org/10.1016/s0045-2068(03)00080-4

Sieprawska-Lupa M, Mydel P, Krawczyk K, Wójcik K, Puklo M, Lupa B, Suder P, Silberring J, Reed M, Pohl J, Shafer W, McAleese F, Foster T, Travis J, Potempa J (2004) Degradation of human antimicrobial peptide LL-37 by *Staphylococcus aureus*-derived proteinases. Antimicrob Agents Chemother 48:4673–4679. https://doi.org/10.1128/AAC.48.12.4673-4679.2004

Sim JY, Kim S, Lee J, Lim H, Kim HH, Park ZY, Kim JI (2019) A significantly enhanced antibacterial spectrum of D-enantiomeric lipopeptide bactenecin. Biochem Biophys Res Commun 514:497–502. https://doi.org/10.1016/j.bbrc.2019.04.153

Sinha S, Zheng L, Mu Y, Ng WJ, Bhattacharjya S (2017) Structure and interactions of a host defense antimicrobial peptide thanatin in lipopolysaccharide micelles reveal mechanism of bacterial cell agglutination. Sci Rep 7:17795. https://doi.org/10.1038/s41598-017-18102-6

Souza GS, de Carvalho LP, de Melo EJT, Gomes VM, Carvalho AO (2018) The toxic effect of Vu-Defr, a defensin from *Vigna unguiculata* seeds, on *Leishmania amazonensis* is associated with reactive oxygen species production, mitochondrial dysfunction, and plasma membrane perturbation. Can J Microbiol 64:455–464. https://doi.org/10.1139/cjm-2018-0095

Strøm MB, Haug BE, Skar ML, Stensen W, Stiberg T, Svendsen JS (2003) The pharmacophore of short cationic antibacterial peptides. J Med Chem 46:1567–1570. https://doi.org/10.1021/jm0340039

Subbalakshmi C, Sitaram N (1998) Mechanism of antimicrobial action of indolicidin. FEMS Microbiol Lett 160:91–96. https://doi.org/10.1111/j.1574-6968.1998.tb12896.x

Subbalakshmi C, Nagaraj R, Sitaram N (1999) Biological activities of c-terminal 15-residue synthetic fragment of melittin: design of an analog with improved antibacterial activity. FEBS Lett 448:62–66. https://doi.org/10.1016/S0014-5793(99)00328-2

Sumi CD, Yang BW, Yeo IC, Hahm YT (2014) Antimicrobial peptides of the genus *Bacillus*: a new era for antibiotics. Can J Microbiol 61:93–103. https://doi.org/10.1139/cjm-2014-0613

Tacconelli E, Sifakis F, Harbarth S, Schrijver R, an Mourik M, Voss A, Sharland M, Rajendran NB, Rodriguez-Bano J, EPI-Net COMBACTE-MAGNET Group (2018) Surveillance for control of antimicrobial resistance. Lancet Infect Dis 28:e-99–e-106. https://doi.org/10.1016/S1473-3099(17)30485-1

Takahashi D, Shukla SK, Prakash O, Zhang G (2010) Structural determinants of host defense peptides for antimicrobial activity and target cell selectivity. Biochimie 92:1236–1241. https://doi.org/10.1016/j.biochi.2010.02.023

Tam J, Wang S, Wong KH, Tan WL (2015) Antimicrobial peptides from plants. Pharmaceuticals 8:711–757. https://doi.org/10.3390/ph8040711

Tanabe H, Ayabe T, Maemoto A, Ishikawa C, Inaba Y, Sato R, Moriichi K, Okamoto K, Watari J, Kono T, Ashida T, Kohgo Y (2007) Denatured human alpha-defensin attenuates the bactericidal activity and the stability against enzymatic digestion. Biochem Biophys Res Commun 358:349–355. https://doi.org/10.1016/j.bbrc.2007.04.132

Ulmschneider JP (2017) Charged antimicrobial peptides can translocate across membranes without forming channel-like pores. Biophys J 113:73–81. https://doi.org/10.1016/j.bpj.2017.04.056

U.S. Food and Drug Administration (2018) Center for Drug Evaluation and Research. Firvanq NDA 208910 Approval Letter, Reference ID: 4213175, Approval Date January 22, 2018. From: https://www.accessdata.fda.gov/drugsatfda_docs/nda/2018/208910Orig1s000Approv.pdf

Uyterhoeven ET, Butler CH, Ko D, Elmore DE (2008) Investigating the nucleic acid interactions and antimicrobial mechanism of buforin II. FEBS Lett 582:1715–1718. https://doi.org/10.1016/j.febslet.2008.04.036

Van Kuijk S, Noll KS, Chikindas ML (2011) The species-specific mode of action of the antimicrobial peptide subtilosin against *Listeria monocytogenes* Scott A. J Appl Microbiol 54:52–58. https://doi.org/10.1111/j.1472-765X.2011.03170.x

van Staden AD, Brand AM, Dicks LMT (2012) Nisin F-loaded brushite bone cement prevented the growth of *Staphylococcus aureus in vivo*. J Appl Microbiol 112:831–840. https://doi.org/10.1111/j.1365-2672.2012.05241.x

Vinogradov A, Yin Y, Suga H (2019) Macrocyclic peptides as drug candidates: recent progress and remaining challenges. J Am Chem Soc 141:4167–4181. https://doi.org/10.1021/jacs.8b13178

Vishnepolsky B, Pirtskhalava M (2014) Prediction of linear cationic antimicrobial peptides based on characteristics responsible for their interaction with the membranes. J Chem Inf Model 54:1512–1523. https://doi.org/10.1021/ci4007003

Vogel HJ, Schibli DJ, Jing W, Lohmeier-Vogel EM, Epand RF, Epand RM (2002) Towards a structure-function analysis of bovine lactoferricin and related tryptophan- and arginine-containing peptides. Biochem Cell Biol 80:49–63. https://doi.org/10.1139/o01-213

Wade HM, Darling LE, Elmore DE (2019) Hybrids made from antimicrobial peptides with different mechanisms of action show enhanced membrane permeabilization. Biochim Biophys Acta Biomembr 1861:182980. https://doi.org/10.1016/j.bbamem.2019.05.002

Wang G (2014) Human antimicrobial peptides and proteins. Pharmaceuticals (Basel) 7:545–594. https://doi.org/10.3390/ph7050545

Wang G (2015) Improved methods for classification, prediction, and design of antimicrobial peptides. Methods Mol Biol 1268:43–66. https://doi.org/10.1007/978-1-4939-2285-7_3

Wang G (2017a) Discovery classification and functional diversity of antimicrobial peptides. In: Wang G (ed) Antimicrobial peptides: discovery, design, and novel therapeutic strategies. CABI, Oxfordshire, pp 1–14

Wang G (2017b) Structural insight into the mechanisms of action and antimicrobial and structure-based design. In: Wang G (ed) Antimicrobial peptides: discovery, design, and novel therapeutic strategies. CABI, Oxfordshire, pp 169–180

Wang G, Li X, Wang Z (2009) APD2: the updated antimicrobial peptide database and its application in peptide design. Nucleic Acids Res 37:D933–D937. https://doi.org/10.1093/nar/gkn823

Wang G, Hanke ML, Mishra B, Lushnikova T, Heim CE, Chittezham Thomas V, Bayles KW, Kielian T (2014) Transformation of human cathelicidin LL-37 into selective, stable, and potent antimicrobial compounds. ACS Chem Biol 9:1997–2002. https://doi.org/10.1021/cb500475y

Wang G, Li X, Wang Z (2016) APD3: the antimicrobial peptide database and its application. Nucleic Acids Res 44:D1087–D1093. https://doi.org/10.1093/nar/gkv1278

Wei XB, Wu RJ, Zhang LL, Ahmad B, Si DY, Zhang RJ (2018) Expression, purification, and characterization of a novel hybrid peptide with potent antibacterial activity. Molecules 23:1491. https://doi.org/10.3390/molecules23061491

Wendler J, Schroeder BO, Ehmann D, Koeninger L, Mailänder-Sánchez D, Lemberg C, Wanner S, Schaller M, Stange EF, Malek NP, Weidenmaier C, LeibundGut-Landmann S, Wehkamp J (2019) Proteolytic degradation of reduced human beta defensin 1 generates a novel antibiotic octapeptide. Sci Rep 9:3640. https://doi.org/10.1038/s41598-019-40216-2

Wenzel M, Rautenback M, Vosloo JA, Siersma T, Aisenbrey CHM, Zaitseva E, Laubscher W, Rensburg W, Behrends J, Bechinger B, Hamoen L (2018) The multifaceted antibacterial mechanisms of the pioneering peptide antibiotics Tyrocidine and Gramicidin S. Am Soc Microbiol 9:e00802–e00818. https://doi.org/10.1128/mBio.00802-18

Westerhoff HV, Juretic D, Hendler RW, Zasloff M (1989) Magainins and the disruption of membrane-linked free-energy transduction. Proc Natl Acad Sci U S A 86:6597–6601. https://doi.org/10.1073/pnas.86.17.6597

Wood TK (2017) Strategies for combating persister cell and biofilm infections. Microb Biotechnol 10:1054–1056. https://doi.org/10.1111/1751-7915.12774

Yamada Y, Miura Y, Sakaki A, Yoshida T, Kobayashi K (2006) Design of multifunctional peptides expressing both antimicrobial activity and Shiga toxin neutralization activity. Bioorg Med Chem 14:77–82. https://doi.org/10.1016/j.bmc.2005.07.052

Yamamoto T, Umegawa Y, Yamagami M, Suzuki T, Tsuchikawa H, Hanashima S, Matsumori N, Murata M (2019) The perpendicular orientation of amphotericin b methyl ester in hydrated lipid bilayers supports the barrel-stave model. Biochemistry 58:2282–2291. https://doi.org/10.1021/acs.biochem.9b00180

Yang Q, Li M, Spiller OB, Andrey DO, Hinchliffe P, Li H, MacLean C, Niumsup P, Powell L, Pritchard M, Papkou A, Shen Y, Portal E, Sands K, Spencer J, Tansawai U, Thomas D, Wang S, Wang Y, Shen J, Walsh T (2017) Balancing mcr-1 expression and bacterial survival is a delicate equilibrium between essential cellular defence mechanisms. Nat Commun 8:2054. https://doi.org/10.1038/s41467-017-02149-0

Yi HY, Chowdhury M, Huang YD, Yu XQ (2014) Insect antimicrobial peptides and their applications. Appl Microbiol Biotechnol 98:5807–5822. https://doi.org/10.1007/s00253-014-5792-6

Yin LM, Edwards MA, Li J, Yip CM, Deber CM (2012) Roles of hydrophobicity and charge distribution of cationic antimicrobial peptides in peptide-membrane interactions. J Biol Chem 287:7738–7745. https://doi.org/10.1074/jbc.M111.303602

Yoo B, Shin SBY, Huang ML, Kirshenbaum K (2010) Peptoid macrocycles: making the rounds with peptidomimetic oligomers. Chemistry 16:5528–5537. https://doi.org/10.1002/chem.200903549

Yoshinari M, Kato T, Matsuzaka K, Hayakawa T, Shiba K (2010) Prevention of biofilm formation on titanium surfaces modified with conjugated molecules comprised of antimicrobial and titanium-binding peptides. Biofouling 26:103–110. https://doi.org/10.1080/08927010903216572

Zelezetsky I, Pacor S, Pag U, Papo N, Shai Y, Sahl HG, Tossi A (2005) Controlled alteration of the shape and conformational stability of alpha-helical cell-lytic peptides: effect on mode of action and cell specificity. Biochem J 390:177–188. https://doi.org/10.1042/BJ20042138

Zhang L (2017) Different dynamics and pathway of disulfide bonds reduction of two human defensins, a molecular dynamics simulation study. Proteins 85:665–681. https://doi.org/10.1002/prot.25247

Zhang SK, Song JW, Gong F, Li SB, Chang HY, Xie HM, Gao HW, Tan YX, Ji SP (2016) Design of an α-helical antimicrobial peptide with improved cell-selective and potent anti-biofilm activity. Sci Rep 6:27394. https://doi.org/10.1038/srep27394

Zhang Y, Algburi A, Wang N, Kholodovych V, Oh DO, Chikindas M, Uhrich KE (2017) Self-assembled cationic amphiphiles as antimicrobial peptides mimics: role of hydrophobicity, linkage type, and assembly state. Nanomedicine 13:343–352. https://doi.org/10.1016/j.nano.2016.07.018

Zhang AN, Wu W, Zhang C, Wang QY, Zhuang ZN, Cheng H, Zhang XZ (2019) A versatile bacterial membrane-binding chimeric peptide with enhanced photodynamic antimicrobial activity. J Mater Chem B 7:1087–1095. https://doi.org/10.1039/C8TB03094D

Zheng Z, Tharmalingam N, Liu Q, Jayamani E, Kim W, Fuchs BB, Zhang R, Vilcinskas A, Mylonakis E (2017) Synergistic efficacy of aedes aegypti antimicrobial peptide cecropin a2 and tetracycline against *Pseudomonas aeruginosa*. Antimicrob Agents Chemother 61:e00686–e00617. https://doi.org/10.1128/AAC.00686-17

Zhu C, Schneider EK, Wang J, Kempe K, Wilson P, Velkov T, Li J, Davis TP, Whittaker MR, Haddleton DM (2017) A traceless reversible polymeric colistin prodrug to combat multidrug-resistant (MDR) Gram-negative bacteria. J Control Release 259:83–91. https://doi.org/10.1016/j.jconrel.2017.02.005

Chapter 8
Exploiting the Achilles' Heel of Iron Dependence in Antibiotic Resistant Bacteria with New Antimicrobial Iron Withdrawal Agents

Bruce E. Holbein, M. Trisha C. Ang, David S. Allan, Wangxue Chen, and Christian Lehmann

> *It is quite probable that spatial and temporal fluctuations of iron availability in a single host organism do occur and that these are sufficient to permit microbial growth in one portion and microbial death in another part of the same tissue.*
>
> *E.D. Weinberg (1978)*

Abstract Pathogenic microorganisms including bacteria and fungi have irreplaceable needs for iron as critically needed for the activities of a wide array of essential enzymes that are vital for energy production, metabolism, nucleic acid synthesis and cellular defense. Various virulence-associated iron acquisition mechanisms are deployed by microbes as iron availability in vertebrate hosts is quite limited and

B. E. Holbein (✉)
Chelation Partners Inc., The Labs at Innovacorp, Life Sciences Research Institute, Halifax, NS, Canada

Department of Microbiology and Immunology, Dalhousie University, Halifax, NS, Canada; https://www.chelationpartners.com/

M. T. C. Ang · D. S. Allan
Chelation Partners Inc., The Labs at Innovacorp, Life Sciences Research Institute, Halifax, NS, Canada

W. Chen
Human Health Therapeutics Research Center, National Research Council Canada, Ottawa, ON, Canada

C. Lehmann
Department of Microbiology and Immunology, Dalhousie University, Halifax, NS, Canada

Department of Anesthesia, Pain Management and Perioperative Medicine, Dalhousie University, Halifax, NS, Canada

H. Panwar et al. (eds.), *Sustainable Agriculture Reviews 49*, Sustainable Agriculture Reviews 49, https://doi.org/10.1007/978-3-030-58259-3_8

host innate defense mechanisms seek to further withdraw iron availability during infection. Antibiotic resistant microbes appear unaltered in their iron requirement, but iron withdrawal can enhance microbial sensitivity to various antibiotics and suppress outgrowth of antibiotic-exposed resistant survivors. Thus, iron dependence of antibiotic resistant microbes represents an Achilles' heel that can be exploited as the basis of alternative therapeutic approaches to address infection. Three major therapeutic approaches can potentially exploit this susceptibility of antibiotic resistant microbes. Gallium, a non-functional iron analogue metal can be used to thwart microbes as it can substitute and effectively displace functional iron, resulting in loss of iron dependent enzymes critical for microbial growth. A second approach utilizes synthetic copies of microbial iron acquisition siderophores chemically linked to antibiotics resulting in Trojan-horse carriers that are imported into microbial cells utilizing their own siderophore uptake systems to thereby deliver antibiotics to their cytoplasmic targets. Thirdly, new generation iron chelators that have been purpose-designed as antimicrobials offer advantages over conventional hematologically used chelators for selective iron withdrawal from antibiotic sensitive or resistant pathogens. Importantly, these chelators also function to bolster innate iron withdrawal defenses of the infected host. To date, the 3-hydroxypyridin-4-one containing chelators appear to have the most promise. DIBI (developmental name) is an example of these new agents and it is a low molecular weight, water-soluble copolymer with strong antimicrobial activity yet it exhibits a very low toxicity profile for animals.

Keywords Iron dependence · Iron acquisition · Iron withdrawal · Virulence · Antibiotic resistance · Iron chelators

8.1 Introduction

Antibiotic resistance of microbial pathogens has become a massive and growing global problem. Morbidity and mortality are rapidly increasing as effective antibiotic choices dwindle (Friedman et al. 2016; Barrasa-Villar et al. 2017). Health care burdens are escalating (Naylor et al. 2018) with some antibiotic resistant infections becoming essentially untreatable (Ventola 2015; Frieria et al. 2017). Relatively few new antibiotics are being introduced or are on the development horizon given the dwindling choices of new classes of antibiotics that could attack yet-to-be exploited targets (Culyba et al. 2015). There are also relative economic disincentives for big pharma companies to develop new antibiotics, from potentially reduced financial returns due to freshly acquired microbial resistance to a new agent early after its expensive development and introduction (Mullard 2014; Culyba et al. 2015).

In perspective, our antibiotic resistance problem is not all that surprising given most antibiotics are, or are derived from, natural microbial products (Katz and Baltz 2016; Movassaghi and van der Donk 2018). Antibiotics also tend to target one or only a few related microbial target(s) (Luepke et al. 2017). The positive selection pressure from antibiotic use thus readily favours survival-selection and growth of antibiotic resistant clones (Bengtsson-Palme et al. 2018).

New alternative approaches to conventional antibiotics are urgently needed to address antibiotic resistance and various possibilities are being considered. However, the top-tier ranked alternative approaches as recently reviewed (Czaplewski et al. 2016) including the use of bacteriophage and bacterial lysins have yet to yield useful new therapeutics despite over 10 years of active investigation. One new alternative approach is to target pathogens based on their heightened requirement for a growth essential trace metal during infection. Palmer and Skaar (Palmer and Skaar 2016) have recently reviewed the potential of requirements for key essential metals (e.g., Fe, Cu, Mn, and Zn) as alternative targets. The basis for this approach is to utilize metal sequestering therapeutics which withdraw and withhold the essential metal supply from microbes during infection but without causing undue effects to the infected host. Iron requirements of pathogens stand out as the top metal candidate as almost all bacterial and fungal pathogens have irreplaceable requirements for iron (Weinberg 2009; Ganz 2018) for their growth and survival.

The broad strengths of exploiting the iron needs of microbes are based on several key aspects. The needs for iron by major pathogens are evident during infection (Weinberg 2009; Palmer and Skaar 2016; Ganz 2018). Also, vertebrate hosts already possess innate iron withdrawal defense mechanisms that attempt to limit infection (Ganz and Nemeth 2015, Nairz et al. 2018). There are also multiple, essential iron dependent targets in microbes (Palmer and Skaar 2016; Ganz 2018), so iron withdrawal would have broad based effects on a given microbe. Given this breadth of iron dependent microbial targets, pathogens would also have a greatly reduced capacity to overcome an iron withdrawal therapeutic or become resistant to such agents.

Various iron chelators now in clinical use for other medical needs have been investigated for their antimicrobial potential with mixed results. There is also some skepticism among toxicologists and clinicians as to potential host toxicity using iron chelators to suppress iron availability during infection (Czaplewski et al. 2016). Such concerns appear to stem largely from the known toxicity issues of conventional chelators as currently used to treat chronic iron metabolism disorders, especially abnormal iron overload hematological disorders such as Thalassemia. These iron overload disorders already feature iron toxicity as excess tissue iron is itself toxic (Hershko 2010; Mobarra et al. 2016). It is also important to note that hematological chelators were not developed for anti-infective activity and can be accessed for iron by some microbes as will be discussed later in this chapter. For utility as anti-infectives, new iron chelators need to preferentially target and withdraw microbial accessible iron and not interfere with longer term host iron homeostasis. In this regard, new generation iron chelators and in particular those utilizing hydroxypyridinone metal binding groups have been purpose-designed as anti-infectives. Of these, hydroxypyridinone functionalized polymers have demonstrated particular promise.

Here, we review the problem of antibiotic resistance of microbial pathogens in the context of their iron acquisition and host iron withdrawal defenses. Our focus is primarily on extracellular bacterial pathogens as these predominate medically, i.e., both obligate extracellular pathogens and those that set up an initial phase of extracellular infection prior to later lodging intracellularly. Of relevance to antibiotic resistance is the evidence that microbial iron needs are quite separate from antibiotic resistance mechanisms and that effective iron withdrawal from microbes can enhance antibiotic activity including for antibiotic resistant isolates.

These features provide foundations for the alternate therapeutic approach of denying microbes iron as a promising strategy for addressing antibiotic resistant infection. Advantageously, three distinct therapeutic approaches can exploit the iron dependence of antibiotic resistant microbes. First, gallium, a non-functional iron analogue metal can be used to thwart microbes as it can substitute for and effectively displace functional iron, resulting in loss of iron dependent enzymes critical for microbial growth. A second approach utilizes synthetic copies of microbial iron acquisition siderophores, chemically linked to antibiotics resulting in Trojan-horse carriers of antibiotics. These are carried into microbes utilizing their own iron acquisition uptake systems but to then deliver antibiotics inside the microbial cell. Thirdly, new generation iron chelators that have been purpose-designed as antimicrobials offer advantages over conventional hematologically used chelators for selective iron withdrawal from antibiotic sensitive and resistant pathogens. Importantly, these chelators also appear to function through bolstering innate iron withdrawal defenses of the infected host that already operate during infection. Given this additional benefit new generation antimicrobial iron chelators hold the highest promise.

8.2 Iron Is Essential for Pathogenic Microorganisms

8.2.1 Microbial Iron Acquisition Virulence mechanisms

Iron is one of the most important micronutrients required for microbes for growth and survival. Iron is also essential for expression of many key virulence determinants. Under normal physiological conditions, iron availability is extremely limited within the human body and also with other vertebrate species, iron being sequestered in proteins such as haemoglobin, lactoferrin, transferrin and other iron binding proteins (Caza and Kronstad 2013; Johnstone and Nolan 2015; Sheldon and Heinrichs 2015; Sheldon et al. 2016; Thompson et al. 2015).

On the other hand, bacterial and fungal pathogens have developed sophisticated and often redundant mechanisms to counter these host defenses and capture iron from various sources with high efficiency. In this regard, microbes not only need a mechanism to acquire iron from the host, but also need to out-compete other microbes for the same scarce iron source and supply. These host and microbe inter-relationships are shown diagrammatically in Fig. 8.1.

Bacteria have evolved various strategies and mechanisms to obtain their needed iron from the host (Bairwa et al. 2017; Bilitewski et al. 2017; Caza and Kronstad 2013; Foley and Simeonov 2012; Sheldon and Heinrichs 2015; Sheldon et al. 2016; Thompson et al. 2015). These include: (1) siderophore production and transport, (2) iron acquisition from heme, (3) iron acquisition from host iron sequestering proteins such as lactoferrin and transferrin and (4) reduction of ferric to ferrous iron

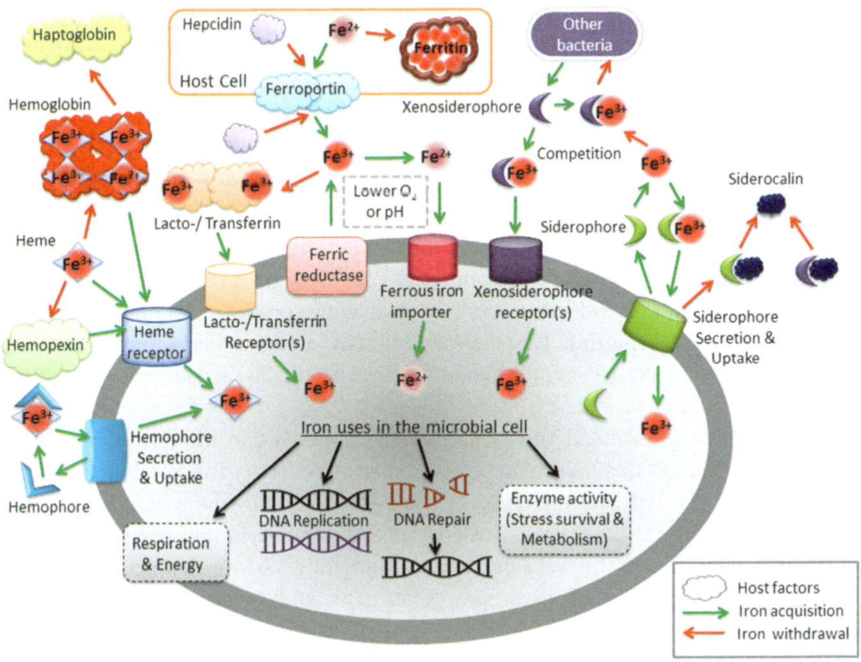

Fig. 8.1 The interface of microbial iron acquisition and host iron withdrawal during infection Gram (−) and Gram (+) bacteria and fungi have developed multiple often redundant systems to acquire growth essential iron from the host environment, including siderophores, hemes, heme proteins, and transferrin/lactoferrin. These systems predominantly acquire iron in the extracellular compartments of the infected host for delivery into the microbe for internal needs related to energy production, replication and defense. At the same time the host deploys various defense mechanisms triggered during infection, to withdraw and reduce availability of iron in the extracellular compartments. An innate nutritional immune response regulated by hepcidin occurs and it lowers the concentration of extracellular iron carried systemically on transferrin through promoting intracellular iron storage in ferritin. Siderocalins attempt to neutralize microbial siderophores and hemopexin binds and removes free heme as released from damaged host cells to be taken up by the liver and spleen. These various microbial iron acquisition and host iron withdrawal mechanisms largely determine the course of infection and provide various avenues for medical intervention to exploit or bolster these

(Kelson et al. 2013, Sheldon et al. 2016). These various microbial strategies are depicted in Fig. 8.1 and reviewed below.

8.2.1.1 Iron Acquisition by Siderophore Systems

In the mammalian host, extracellular iron is usually present as Fe (III) and complexed with transport proteins such as transferrin and lactoferrin. Many bacteria and fungi can access ferric iron, Fe (III) for growth through producing siderophores to compete, acquire, and transport iron (Foley and Simeonov 2012; Sheldon and Heinrichs 2015; Sheldon et al. 2016). Siderophores are typically low molecular weight (<1500 Da) iron chelating molecules with extremely high affinity for iron i.e., dissociation constants for iron ranging from 10^{-20} to 10^{-52} M (Foley and Simeonov 2012). They are secreted into the extracellular milieu to capture Fe (III) from their environment (soil, water, or the vertebrate body) being capable of stripping Fe (III) from host sequestering proteins (Chitambar 2016; Thompson et al. 2015).

To date, >500 different siderophores have been identified and characterized structurally (Kelson et al. 2013). Although structurally diverse, most siderophores have some common features, including their metal binding donor atoms which are typically oxygen and nitrogen (Kelson et al. 2013). A bacterial species will often produce its own unique siderophore(s). Some bacteria produce just one siderophore while others secrete multiple types, allowing them to effectively sequester iron and to better colonize varied environments (Kelson et al. 2013; Bairwa et al. 2017; Sheldon and Heinrichs 2015).

Based on their chemical functionality, siderophores can be divided into three general chemical classes: hydroxamates, catecholates and hydroxycarbonates (Caza and Kronstad 2013; Bilitewski et al. 2017; Foley and Simeonov 2012). Table 8.1 summarizes these different chemical classes and provides some key example siderophores as produced by various bacteria and fungi. More detailed reviews on siderophores can be found elsewhere (Ellermann and Arthur 2017; Holden and Bachman 2015; Johnstone and Nolan 2015; Wilson et al. 2016). The chemistry of these siderophores is discussed in more detail later in this chapter. The overall generalized system of siderophore production, secretion, iron capture and uptake are depicted in Fig. 8.1.

Siderophores typically chelate Fe (III) with high-affinity and therefore often outcompete the iron sequestering molecules of the host (Ellermann and Arthur 2017; Wilson et al. 2016). After binding ferric ion, ferri-siderophores are retrieved from the extracellular environment by their cognate receptors either on the outer membrane of Gram negative bacteria or on cell wall associated receptors of Gram positive bacteria. These receptors facilitate translocation of the iron complex into the periplasmic space (Bairwa et al. 2017; Caza and Kronstad 2013; Foley and Simeonov 2012; Holden and Bachman 2015; Johnstone and Nolan 2015; Khan et al. 2018; Sheldon and Heinrichs 2015; Wilson et al. 2016). The specific Gram negative bacterial surface receptors (such as FepA, IroN, and PfeA from *Escherichia coli*,

Table 8.1 Chemical classes of microbial siderophores and examples produced by pathogens

Chemical class	Example	Microbial pathogen[a]
Hydroxamate	Ferrichrome	*Ustilago sphaerogena*
	Deferoxamine, clinically used as Desferal®	*Streptomyces pilosus, S. coelicolor*
	Alcaligin	*Bordetella sp.*
	Fusarinine C	*Fusarium roseum*
	Ornibactin	*Burkholderia cepacia*
	Rhodotorulic acid	*Rhodotorula pilimanae*
Phenolate/ Catecholate	Enterobactin	*Escherichia coli, other Enteric bacteria*
	Acinetobactin	*Acinetobacter baumannii*
	Salmochelin	*Salmonella sp.*
	Bacillibactin	*Bacillus subtilis, B. anthracis*
	Vibriobactin	*Vibrio cholera*
	Petrobactin	*B. anthracis*
	Corynebactin	*B. subtilis*
	Cepaciachelin	*B. cepacia*
Carboxylate	Staphyloferrin A	*Staphylococcus*
	Rhizoferrin	*R. microspores*
Mixed class	Azotobactin	*Azotobacter vinelandii*
	Pyoverdine	*Pseudomonas aeruginosa*
	Yersiniabactin	*Yersinia pestis*
	Acinetoferrin	*Acinetobacter spp.*
	Rhizobactin	*Rhizobium meliloti*
	Aerobactin	*E. coli, Shigella sp.*
	Mycobactins	*Mycobacterium spp.*

[a]Examples of human, animal and plant microbial pathogens. Based on (Foley and Simeonov 2012; Kelson et al. 2013) and https://en.wikipedia.org/wiki/Siderophore

Salmonella enterica and *Pseudomonas aeruginosa*, respectively) are all members of the well known TonB dependent transporter family and are usually regulated by the ferric uptake regulator protein, Fur (Caza and Kronstad 2013).

Periplasmic ferri-siderophore binding proteins then shuttle the molecules to specific cell membrane associated ABC transporters, which hydrolyse ATP to drive transport of the iron bearing cargo into the bacterial cytosol (Foley and Simeonov 2012). Once the molecule reaches the intracellular space, its iron can be released by physical degradation of the siderophore or through the chemical reduction of Fe (III) to Fe (II) using ferri-siderophore reductases or esterases (Caza and Kronstad 2013; Foley and Simeonov 2012; Kelson et al. 2013; Zhou et al. 2012).

Given the importance of iron, microbial pathogens often deploy multiple iron acquisition systems or siderophores to ensure iron acquisition from the infected host (Bairwa et al. 2017; Caza and Kronstad 2013; Sheldon and Heinrichs 2015; Sheldon et al. 2016). While different microbial receptors are often selective for a particular ferri-siderophore complexes, some bacteria possess broader receptor/uptake systems for various siderophores secreted by other bacteria (i.e., xenosiderophores) to achieve what has been termed iron piracy (Caza and Kronstad 2013). In addition, some bacteria release siderophores to deprive microbial competitors of iron availability in the community, for example in the soil.

Some microbes such as *Listeria monocytogenes* and *Candida albicans* do not produce siderophores; instead utilizing heterogeneous xenosiderophores produced by other microbes (Caza and Kronstad 2013). Yet other microbial pathogens such as *P. aeruginosa* although producing its own siderophores, can also use xenosiderophores to better compete for iron (Caza and Kronstad 2013).

8.2.1.2 Heme Acquisition and Utilization

Most iron in the mammalian body is bound to biological molecules such as haemoglobin within a porphyrin ring as ferriprotoporphyrin IX (heme) and this is not directly accessible by microbes (Kelson et al. 2013). Heme is the main iron component and constitutes >70% of the total iron in mammalian hosts. Heme is a general component of intracellular proteins. It is accessible as an iron source by intracellular pathogens or by extracellular pathogens that produce cytotoxins (such as cytolysins or hemolysins) that lyse host cells (e.g., red blood cells) to release hemeproteins. Implicitly lysin production would require bacterial multiplication and thus iron for initial infection growth that would likely be dependent on non-heme host iron supplies. In severe sepsis, free heme levels in plasma can also be elevated (Larsen et al. 2010) and therefore under these conditions additional extracellular heme would presumably become available to extracellular pathogens.

Bacteria have developed strategies to obtain heme iron from the host during infection by targeting heme, hemoglobin, or complexes containing these molecules (e.g., haptoglobin-hemoglobin, hemopexin-heme). These strategies are depicted in Fig. 8.1 and require access to host heme sources. Thus, a number of pathogenic bacteria and fungi secrete a variety of exotoxins (hemolysins), rhamnolipids, and surfactants to lyse host cells so they can then capture either the released hemoglobin or heme (Bilitewski et al. 2017; Bairwa et al. 2017; Sheldon and Heinrichs 2015; Foley and Simeonov 2012). In this regard, hemolysins are well characterized in Gram negative bacteria, such as pathogenic *E. coli* (Caza and Kronstad 2013; Sheldon and Heinrichs 2015).

Bacteria can utilize two main strategies to scavenge and transport iron from heme and heme containing proteins: (1) direct contact between the bacterium and the exogenous heme sources, and/or (2) production of extracellular hemophores (heme chelating proteins, analogous to siderophores), which bind heme with high affinity and return it to specific bacterial receptors (Chitambar 2016; Kelson et al. 2013). The direct heme uptake system (for example, Phu system in *P. aeruginosa* and Isd system in *S. aureus*) generally extracts heme from hemoglobin or hemoglobin-haptoglobin complexes directly and transfers it to an ATPase transporter complex (Bilitewski et al. 2017). This is achieved by recognition and binding to a specific receptor. These surface receptors can directly bind heme and process its transport, but they are also usually able to bind heme-containing proteins like hemoglobin, haptoglobin-hemoglobin, hemopexin-heme, and myoglobin (Wandersman and Delepelaire 2004). For these, heme is extracted from the complexes and transported into the periplasm in a TonB dependent manner (Caza and Kronstad 2013; Sheldon and Heinrichs 2015; Sheldon et al. 2016). Once in the periplasm, heme is bound to a heme transport protein and delivered to an ABC transporter on the inner membrane. Heme is then transported into the cytoplasm in an ATP dependent fashion with subsequent degradation and iron release by bacterial heme oxygenases (Anzaldi and Skaar 2010; Caza and Kronstad 2013). Multiple heme acquisition systems (i.e., different surface receptors and ABC transporters) are generally present in the Gram positive bacteria as reviewed in detail elsewhere (Sheldon and Heinrichs 2015).

Hemophores are surface exposed or secreted bacterial proteins such as HasA from *Serratia marcescens* with the ability to bind free heme and/or extract heme from heme containing proteins in the extracellular environment (Sheldon and Heinrichs 2015; Caza and Kronstad 2013, Sheldon et al. 2016). HasA interacts with and transfers heme to the specific outer membrane hemophore receptor HasR (Anzaldi and Skaar 2010, Bilitewski et al. 2017). HasR can uptake heme from hemoglobin alone, but the process is 100 times more efficient with the participation of HasA (Caza and Kronstad 2013). The HasA system is negatively regulated by iron and Fur and positively regulated by a sigma and anti-sigma (HasI and HasS) signaling cascade triggered by heme loaded hemophore-HasR complexes (Caza and Kronstad 2013, Sheldon and Heinrichs 2015, Sheldon et al. 2016).

After binding, heme is extracted from hemoproteins and transferred to the periplasm in a TonB dependent mechanism and shuttled to ABC transporters that pump heme into the cytosol (Caza and Kronstad 2013, Sheldon and Heinrichs 2015). Once internalized, heme is either degraded to release free iron or used intact as a cofactor in catalases, cytochromes and other bacterial hemoproteins (Foley and Simeonov 2012). It has been suggested that *S. aureus* and some strains of *A. baumannii* may have more active iron acquisition systems using heme-based than siderophore-based iron sources (Kelson et al. 2013, de Leseleuc et al. 2014).

8.2.1.3 Transferrin, Lactoferrin and Ferritin

Various bacterial pathogens can utilize non-heme, iron-containing proteins such as transferrin, lactoferrin, and ferritins as sources of iron (Caza and Kronstad 2013; Chitamber 2010). Acquisition from transferrin and lactoferrin is typically through receptors for these proteins (Chitambar 2016) as depicted in Fig. 8.1. The uptake of ferric iron from transferrin and lactoferrin is facilitated by TbpAB and LbpAB system, respectively (Caza and Kronstad 2013). The TbpAB system consists of two transferrin binding proteins expressed from a biscistronic operon that is regulated by Fur. The TbpAB system consists of the TonB dependent protein TbpA and the lipoprotein TbpB that acts as a co-receptor. TbpA binds apo and holo-transferrin with similar affinities, whereas TbpB binds preferentially to iron containing transferrin. TbpA is a TonB dependent protein and catalyzes a conformational change that leads to iron release and dissociation of apo-transferrin with the help of the TonB complex. The released iron is then transported into the cytosol through the periplasmic ferric binding protein FbpA (Caza and Kronstad 2013; Noinaj et al. 2012a, b). The lactoferrin uptake system LbpAB is overall, very similar to TbpAB in that LbpA is a TonB dependent outer membrane protein and LbpB is a lipoprotein that serves as a co-receptor for LbpA (Caza and Kronstad 2013).

In addition, bacteria elaborate cell surface ferric reductases to reduce free ferric iron to ferrous iron which can then be taken up and utilized by the bacterial cell. Ferrous iron ions are believed to diffuse freely through the outer membrane of Gram negative bacteria, with subsequent transport through the inner membrane by the ABC transporter FeoABC (Caza and Kronstad 2013), which is under control of *fnr* (for anaerobes) and *fur* regulatory elements (Caza and Kronstad 2013).

8.2.1.4 Fungal Iron Acquisition

Most of our current knowledge and understanding of iron acquisition in fungi is derived from the studies of *Saccharomyces cerevisiae* and from the three pathogenic species: *Aspergillus fumigatus*, *Candida albicans* and *Cryptococcus neoformans* (Caza and Kronstad 2013; Bairwa et al. 2017). These have been reviewed in detail recently (Bairwa et al. 2017; Caza and Kronstad 2013).

In common with bacterial pathogens, pathogenic fungi have also evolved a number of mechanisms to acquire iron from different sources in the mammalian host with many of these mechanisms sharing functional similarities with bacterial pathogens. Caza and Kronstad (2013) have comprehensively compared the shared and different iron acquisition mechanisms between pathogenic bacteria and fungi. The similarities include: (1) both pathogenic bacteria and fungi possess multiple mechanisms for exploiting the potential iron sources in vertebrate hosts; (2) the mechanisms that mediate iron acquisition from heme and heme containing proteins are far less known in fungi in that the key components such as the hemophore system that perform analogous functions in fungal pathogens are just now being identified and characterized; (3) siderophore mediated iron acquisition, in particular the biosynthesis of siderophores, is well studied in fungi although more studies on siderophore transport in fungal pathogens are needed; (4) reductive iron uptake systems are additional similarities between bacteria and fungi for the uptake of ferrous iron. There are, however, clear differences with accessing iron containing host proteins, such as transferrin, lactoferrin and ferritin, between bacterial and fungal pathogens (Bairwa et al. 2017; Caza and Kronstad 2013).

8.2.2 Irreplaceable Iron Need Is an Achilles' Heel of Microbes

The evidence reviewed above demonstrates that the need for iron is widely shared among pathogenic microbes. Thus, with iron being irreplaceable this critical requirement represents a key Achilles' heel. Iron withdrawal strategies to restrict supply of essential iron to microbes would have broad microbial physiological effects, ranging from impairment in energy production to DNA synthesis to cellular defense. Later in this chapter, we will show that antibiotic resistant microbes retain their iron dependence. This therefore opens a new avenue to address these pathogens by iron withdrawal. Importantly, as reviewed below, iron withdrawal is already attempted by the host as part of innate immunity (termed nutritional immunity) and thus bolstering this natural defense mechanism has appeal.

8.3 Role of Iron in Host Defenses to Microbial Infection

Iron plays Janus-faced roles in the host defense and immune response to infection: on one side iron deprivation is a useful defense system to limit microbial growth. On the other side, the host's ability to kill microbial invaders depends at least partly on the generation of enough Reactive Oxygen Species (ROS) through the Haber-Weiss and Fenton reactions and thus, key reactive iron pools also play a role in this defense mechanism.

Under normal conditions (physiological iron levels) efficient host defense will result in transiently decreased systemic iron levels. However, in chronic infection this can lead to iron deficiency anemia (Cartwright et al. 1946). On the contrary, under conditions with pre-existing excess iron overload (e.g. hemochromatosis) an increased incidence of infections is observed (Schaible and Kaufmann 2004).

Later in this chapter, we will further differentiate the relative needs for key host iron pools and illustrate why new antimicrobial iron chelators, to be effective, should not inappropriately affect host intracellular iron pools or disrupt host iron homeostasis, i.e., over a prolonged period. Such novel chelators should, however, help restrict extracellular iron pools to withdraw sufficient amounts of microbe sought iron, i.e., as in play for most pathogenic microbes in the early stages of infection. The rationale for this is that most microbial pathogens are either exclusively extracellular or likely require an initial phase of extracellular growth before entering host cells to take up intracellular residence. The key aspects of iron related host defenses as related to iron withdrawal from invading microbes are also shown in Fig. 8.1 and further discussed below.

8.3.1 Innate Iron Sequestration Immunity

Invasion by microbes triggers an inflammatory host response via different pathways. For example, lipopolysaccharide (LPS; synonym: endotoxin) from Gram negative bacteria binds to Toll-like receptor 4 (TLR4). TLR4 activation causes translocation of nuclear factor-kB (NF-kB) into the nucleus of innate immune cells and transcription, translation and cellular release of inflammatory mediators such as tumor necrosis factor-alpha (TNF-α) and interleukin 6 (IL-6). IL-6 is known to increase synthesis of hepcidin in the liver (Johnson and Wessling-Resnick 2012). Hepcidin is the main regulator of host iron homeostasis: increased hepcidin levels cause cellular internalization and lysosomal degradation of ferroportin, a transporter protein responsible for iron release to extracellular compartments. The overall response from these pathways decreases extracellular iron availability, initially for microbes and then ultimately the host (Barton and Acton 2019). It is important to appreciate that most microbes do not store excess iron for future needs and generally come from iron limited environments. Thus, when microbes find the opportunity to initiate an infection on/in a vertebrate host they predictably require immediate access to iron, i.e., to grow and evade host defense clearance mechanisms.

8.3.2 Hypoferremic Response to Infection

Hepcidin release during the innate immune response to microbes reduces systemic iron levels by internalization or "hiding" of iron in various cells (e.g., intestinal epithelial cells, immune cells). The resulting extracellular iron levels in the blood stream are therefore lowered, which is described as the "hypoferremic response". Other factors involved in modulation of extracellular iron availability are for example lactoferrin and lipocalin (siderocalin). Constitutively high levels of lactoferrin are found in most mucosal surface secretions, including tears, saliva, bile, and breast milk (Ward et al. 2002). Pro-inflammatory cytokines such as TNF-α also induce the release of lactoferrin from neutrophilic granules at the site of infection (Afeltra et al. 1997). Accordingly, the addition of exogenous lactoferrin has been shown to reduce pulmonary *M. tuberculosis* burden in a mouse model of iron overload (Schaible et al. 2002) and growth of *S. aureus* in the mammary system of cows with mastitis (Lacasse et al. 2008). The capacity of lactoferrin to sequester iron also has been implicated in the ability of patients with cystic fibrosis to control opportunistic *P. aeruginosa* infection and biofilm formation in the respiratory tract (Britigan et al. 1993).

8.3.3 Iron Dysregulation in Sepsis

Sepsis is defined as life-threatening organ dysfunction caused by a dysregulated host response to infection (Singer et al. 2016). It is considered as "worst case" of an infection, where the body's overwhelming immune response leads to tissue damage, organ failure, and death. Sepsis has been named as the most expensive in-patient cost in American hospitals with an average of over $18,000 per hospital stay. With over 1.5 million sepsis hospital stays per year, sepsis costs total $27 billion each year in the USA alone (Paoli et al. 2018). At present, there is no FDA approved therapeutic for sepsis available. Therefore, it might be useful to study the role of iron in sepsis as a potential treatment target.

Clinical findings have confirmed that the known physiological mechanisms of iron restriction in infection also have implications for sepsis as critically ill sepsis patients have low systemic iron levels as a consequence of the host defense to infection (Tacke et al. 2016). Animal experiments showed beneficial effects of iron chelation in sepsis with reduced hyper-inflammation and improved survival (Lehmann et al. 2014). The beneficial effects of iron chelation in experimental sepsis studies are most likely due to the Janus-faced roles of iron in infection: iron deprivation reduces bacterial growth including for antibiotic resistant bacteria (Parquet et al. 2019) and reduced iron availability also attenuates the overproduction of ROS known to occur in sepsis as the main cause of organ dysfunction and organ failure in sepsis (Lehmann et al. 2014). Clinical trials with iron chelators to treat sepsis have not yet been carried out but these may prove worthwhile.

8.3.4 Reactive Oxygen Species (ROS) Related Defense Mechanisms

ROS also display Janus-faced roles in the host defense to microbes. As described above, ROS are important for bacterial killing but under some circumstances such as in sepsis, overproduction of ROS can be harmful to host tissue. The pathophysiological response to infection suggests that the body prioritizes iron restriction in order to reduce bacterial growth over providing ample iron for ROS generation. Some antibiotics, such as metronidazole, are known to have antioxidant properties, in line with its inferiority of ROS-induced bacterial killing over primary reduction of bacterial proliferation (Pélissier et al. 2007). Studies by our group and others have demonstrated the impact of iron chelation on ROS production in experimental infection (Heli et al. 2011). Furthermore, we have also shown that iron deprivation (and thus potentially reduced ROS production) did not have a detrimental impact on suppression of bacterial growth and animal survival in *in vivo* infection experiments (Aali et al. 2019; Thorburn et al. 2017; Islam et al. 2016).

It should also be noted that antimicrobial ROS activity is primarily intracellular such as in phagocytes. Thus, appropriate iron withdrawal of extracellular iron pools by therapeutics that do not readily permeate host cells and immediately affect host intracellular iron pools, should not affect host defensive ROS activity. Longer term iron withdrawal might conceivably modulate excess inappropriate ROS production.

8.4 Exploiting Microbial Iron Needs

As discussed above, bacteria and fungi possess several, often redundant, iron acquisition systems which allow them to adapt to different iron sources available in their environment. Since pathogenic microbes are highly dependent on iron acquisition for their virulence and colonization during infection, these systems are attractive targets for the rational development of antimicrobial therapeutics or vaccination strategies.

The biosynthesis of siderophores and their uptake systems are most frequently targeted. There are several approaches to this targeting strategy, including siderophore inhibitors or siderophore-antibiotic conjugates (Trojan horses) (Budzikiewicz 2001; Ellermann and Arthur 2017; Foley and Simeonov 2012; Ghosh et al. 2017; Johnstone and Nolan 2015; Mollmann et al. 2009; Wandersman and Delepelaire 2004; Wilson et al. 2016). However, some pathogens, such as *S. aureus* and certain *A. baumannii* clinical strains, can rely on heme utilization and inhibition of the access to heme proteins could also be a valuable therapeutic target (Anzaldi and Skaar 2010; Bilitewski et al. 2017, Kelson et al. 2013; Zhou et al. 2012; de Leseleuc et al. 2014). Over the last several decades, a number of approaches and platforms have been developed and evaluated for their potential to exploit the essential nature of these pathways of bacterial virulence to provide compounds that may prove suitable for development into new antibacterial agents (Foley and Simeonov 2012). The main approaches taken are described below.

8.4.1 Gallium a Non-functional Iron Mimic

Iron (III) can be displaced by gallium (III) (Ga) in most iron complexes but gallium does not have the essential redox properties of iron (III) and thus Ga-substituted complexes are non-functional. Gallium (III) salts, such as gallium nitrate, gallium maltolate, or gallium citrate, or gallium organo-complexes have been investigated as anti-infectives (Banin et al. 2008; Chitambar 2016, 2017; Kelson et al. 2013; Rangel-Vega et al. 2015; Stojiljkovic et al. 1999). Gallium and its complexes may block bacterial iron acquisition through several mechanisms: a) displacing iron from siderophores, b) uptake by microorganisms as a Ga siderophore, such as Ga-pyochelin in *P. aeruginosa* infection, c) disturbing the regulation of iron acquisition systems by repressing bacterial siderophore transcriptional regulators (such as pvdS of *P. aeruginosa*) and d) interfering with the biofilm formation (Chitambar 2016; Kelson et al. 2013; Lessa et al. 2012, Thompson et al. 2015).

Gallium has several unique properties and advantages as a potential antimicrobial agent. It has been used in diagnostic imaging and in cancer chemotherapy for decades. Gallium compounds such as gallium nitrate have well characterized pharmokinetics in human patients and are anticipated to have an excellent bio-distribution profile in the host (Kelson et al. 2013). Although gallium maltolate is the most common compound used in preclinical evaluation for its antimicrobial potential, many other forms of gallium salts and gallium complexes have been developed over the years with several licensed and others in clinical trials (Banin et al. 2008; Chitambar 2016, 2017; Kelson et al. 2013; Rangel-Vega et al. 2015; Stojiljkovic et al. 1999; Thompson et al. 2015). In addition, the indication that some gallium compounds are orally bioavailable (Kelson et al. 2013) provides another advantage for gallium as an alternative to antibiotics.

Gallium has been investigated as an antimicrobial agent with a large panel of pathogenic bacteria, fungi and parasites and has demonstrated encouraging results for many of those pathogens as evident by its effect on reducing tissue and blood bacterial burdens, disruption of biofilm formation, and improvement of infection associated inflammation and tissue healing (Chitambar 2017; Kelson et al. 2013; Lessa et al. 2012; Rangel-Vega et al. 2015; Thompson et al. 2015; Goss et al. 2018). Gallium citrate, for example, shows activity against a range of Gram negative bacteria with a minimum inhibitory concentration ranging from 1 to 5 μg/mL (Bilitewski et al. 2017). Phase 1/2a clinical trials with an intravenous gallium nitrate-citrate formulation and gallium citrate (Panaecin), respectively, have shown promising results for *P. aeruginosa* lung infections in patients with cystic fibrosis (Bilitewski et al. 2017). Other gallium complexes based on siderophore and heme structures have also exhibited clinically relevant levels of potency (0.008–4 mg/mL range) and the selectivity for microbial targets (Kelson et al. 2013; Banin et al. 2008; Chitambar 2016, 2017; Rangel-Vega et al. 2015; Stojiljkovic et al. 1999; Thompson et al. 2015).

In addition to gallium salts, several gallium organic complexes have been investigated for their anti-microbial potential. Such complexes could also improve the therapeutic efficacies and reduce the toxicity associated with gallium salts. For example, pharmaceutically active organic ligands have been assessed as useful carriers of gallium for their uptake by bacteria and their additive or synergistic antimicrobial effects (Lessa et al. 2012). It has been shown that non-iron metalloporphyrins, such as gallium-protophorphyrin-IX, have potent antibacterial activity against both Gram negative and Gram positive bacteria by exploiting the bacterial heme uptake systems (Stojiljkovic et al. 1999; de Leseleuc et al. 2014). Alternatively, conjugating gallium to siderophores, such as deferoxamine mesylate has been shown to improve the efficacies of gentamicin in a rabbit model of *P. aeruginosa* corneal infection (Banin et al. 2008). Synergism of Ga (III) and antibiotics holds promise as a last resort therapy for infections sustained by pandrug-resistant bacteria (Minandri et al. 2014).

Despite these promising results, there are several challenges to the use of gallium as an alternative to antibiotics. First, not all bacterial strains are susceptible to gallium. For example, some *A. baumannii* strains can circumvent gallium nitrate activity with a heme receptor (de Leseleuc et al. 2014). In addition, there is the toxicity concern when high or prolonged doses of gallium are used since the toxicity of gallium and its compounds have yet to be fully studied (Chitambar 2016, 2017). Gallium would presumably also displace host iron and since there are no excretion mechanisms available for iron, gallium administered parenterally could accumulate in the body. Clearly, further elucidation of the uptake and metabolism mechanisms of iron and gallium in bacteria will help define and optimize the use of gallium complexes *in vivo*. Moreover, further evaluation of gallium based drugs particularly as related to potential host toxicity issues and their effects on innate host iron withdrawal defense mechanisms is needed to establish whether these have a significant place in the treatment of infections in humans.

8.4.2 Trojan Horse Antibiotic-Siderophore Conjugates

Antibiotic-siderophore conjugates utilize a siderophore structure as a bait to deliver an antibiotic cargo into the periplasm or cytosol of microbial cells through the cell surface siderophore specific receptors; akin to a "Trojan horse". This can be achieved by conjugating a specific siderophore to an antibiotic molecule via linkage chemistry. These conjugates depend on siderophore transporters within the target bacterial cells for active transport of the conjugate into the cytosol where subsequent chemical cleavage can release the free active antibiotic to then kill the pathogen (Budzikiewicz 2001; Mollmann et al. 2009). A range of natural and synthetic Trojan horse antibiotic conjugates have been identified, synthesized and evaluated for their safety and efficacies *in vitro* and in animal models over the past 50 years with generally mixed results. None of these has reached late stage clinical trials (Budzikiewicz 2001; Mollmann et al. 2009; Ghosh et al. 2017; Ji et al. 2012).

Two major classes of siderophore-conjugated antibiotics are documented in the literature, as categorized by the producing bacterium and particular siderophore moiety and as previously reviewed (Johnstone and Nolan 2015). The sideromycins (including the salimycins, albomycins, and ferrimycins) are naturally produced by Gram positive soil actinomycetes (Bilitewski et al. 2017; Budzikiewicz 2001; Foley and Simeonov 2012). Because of their potential attractiveness, rationally designed synthetic antibiotic-siderophore conjugates comprising different classes of antibiotics and relevant or specific siderophores of the desired target pathogen have been constructed with some being evaluated for efficacy *in vivo* (Budzikiewicz 2001; Ghosh et al. 2018; Ji et al. 2012; Mohammadi et al. 2011; Zheng and Nolan 2014) and with the siderophore-lactam conjugates being the most commonly investigated.

Despite the availability of substantial chemical synthesis and characterization data, there are relatively few studies on *in vivo* efficacy and very little safety data on antibiotic siderophore conjugates. It has been shown that the tetra-acetylated form of a synthetic bis-catechol conjugate (HKI-9924154) was recognized by outer membrane siderophore receptors of targeted Gram negative bacteria and it was effective against *P. aeruginosa, E. coli, S. maltophilia,* and *Klebsiella pneumoniae* (Mollmann et al. 2009). In addition, the promising activities of tricatechol–ampicillin conjugates against select strains of *P. aeruginosa* (Ji et al. 2012) and enterobactin (tricatechol)-β-lactam conjugates against pathogenic strains of *E. coli* (Zheng and Nolan 2014) have been recently reported. More recently, a conjugate of daptomycin and a fimsbactin mimic showed outstanding *in vitro* and *in vivo* activities against *A. baumannii* (Ghosh et al. 2017). Furthermore, covalent attachment of daptomycin, an antibiotic typically active for only Gram positive bacteria, with siderophore mimetics that are recognized by Gram negative bacteria, provided conjugates that were active against virulent strains of antibiotic resistant *A. baumannii*, including carbapenemase and cephalosporinase producers (Ghosh et al. 2018). These two resistance associated enzymes inactivate carbapenem and cephalosporin class antibiotics, respectively and this type of resistance mechanism is discussed later in this chapter.

The factors contributing to the antimicrobial efficacies of antibiotic siderophore conjugates have also been studied. For example, the enterobactin-ciprofloxacin conjugate (Ent-Cipro) can be activated through an esterase catalysed hydrolysis of the conjugate (Neumann et al. 2018). Ent-Cipro provides antibacterial activity comparable to unmodified ciprofloxacin against the uropathogenic *E. coli* UTI89 and CFT073, highlighting the potential for targeting endogenous pathogen associated microbial enzymes for narrow spectrum antibacterial delivery. Furthermore, those authors also synthesized and evaluated Ent-Cipro that contains a self immolative disulfide linkage (Ent-SS-Cipro) (Neumann and Nolan 2018). This linkage was designed to be cleaved after uptake in the reducing environment of the bacterial cytoplasm for the release of the active antibiotic. However, *in vitro* antimicrobial assays showed that Ent-SS-Cipro exhibits activity against only some but not all *E. coli* isolates, suggesting that a disulfide linker may not be generally applicable for this strategy (Neumann and Nolan 2018).

The antibiotic siderophore conjugate strategy has potential advantages in the case of Gram negative pathogens, where the permeability of the outer membrane is a significant barrier for many antibiotics and other anti-infectives (Foley and Simeonov 2012). In addition to potentially increasing the efficacies of antibiotics, this approach has the potential to convert effective Gram positive exclusive antibiotics to also work against Gram negative bacteria. In addition, the large substituents of the conjugate seem to reduce β-lactamase activity (a microbial resistance enzyme that inactivates β-lactam class antibiotics, a resistance mechanism discussed later in this chapter). The use of a bacterial species specific siderophore such as pyoverdin for *P. aeruginosa* (Budzikiewicz 2001) as a transport vehicle has the additional advantage of possibly avoiding collateral damage to other normal host microbiota (Budzikiewicz 2001; Foley and Simeonov 2012).

Despite the above advantages and some promising *in vitro* and *in vivo* activity, selection of the appropriate siderophore will remain challenging due to: (1) the rapid emergence of potential resistance due to the presence of multiple siderophore receptors by many bacteria; (2) the existence of bacterial "cheaters" which take siderophores from other bacteria rather than their own, a common feature in polymicrobial infections and (3) the potential down-regulation of the siderophore receptors on the cell surface of bacterial targets (Budzikiewicz 2001; Foley and Simeonov 2012). In addition, a recent report of an *in vivo* failure of sideromycin treatment implies efflux pumping as a potential resistance mechanism to siderophore-antibiotic conjugates; possibly this resistance might be overcome by the use of efflux inhibitors (Johnstone and Nolan 2015; Thompson et al. 2015; Tomaras et al. 2013; Tomaras et al. 2015; Budzikiewicz 2001). Efflux pumping as an antibiotic resistance mechanism is discussed later in this chapter.

8.4.3 Synthetic Chelators to Intercept and Deny Iron

Iron sequestration or competition for iron has been explored for many years as a potential alternative to antibiotics. To counter iron dependent bacterial processes, natural or synthetic iron chelators with high iron binding affinity have been investigated with the objective of outcompeting native bacterial siderophores and other bacterial iron acquisition mechanisms (Bairwa et al. 2017; Bilitewski et al. 2017; Johnstone and Nolan 2015; Khan et al. 2018; Roosenberg et al. 2000; Thompson et al. 2012; Zhou et al. 2012; Ang et al. 2018).

For iron chelators to compete effectively with bacterial siderophores they should bind iron more tightly and possess a sufficiently different structure to those of bacterial siderophores, thereby minimising interaction with the outer membrane iron siderophore receptors (Bairwa et al. 2017; Khan et al. 2018; Roosenberg et al. 2000; Thompson et al. 2012; Ang et al. 2018). It has been suggested that hexadentate iron binding molecules will have greater potential in this role than corresponding bidentate and tridentate ligands, while hydroxypyridinone containing ligands are less likely to be recognised as siderophores by bacterial receptors (Roosenberg et al. 2000; Thompson et al. 2012; Zhou et al. 2012; Ang et al. 2018).

New synthetic chelators providing competition with siderophores represent a promising alternative to antibiotics for combating antimicrobial resistance. Natural siderophores such as deferoxamine, a siderophore from *Streptomyces pilosus* and synthetic molecules such as deferiprone and deferasirox have been approved and used clinically for treatment of iron overload in Thalassemia patients (Foley and Simeonov 2012). These chelators are reasonably well tolerated in iron overloaded patients but there have been some issues as to toxicity. These clinical chelators have been tested for their antimicrobial activity against several genera of human pathogens including *Pseudomonas*, *Acinetobacter* and *Staphylococcus* (Foley and Simeonov 2012; Parquet et al. 2018; Ang et al. 2018) but with mixed to poor results (see below). Investigations on the potential antimicrobial activity of other iron chelators such as 8-hydroxyquinoline and related compounds, the hexadentate chelator *N,N′*-ethylenebis[2-(2-hydroxyphenyl)-glycine, EDTA and DTPA have also yielded mixed results (Zhou et al. 2012). Yet other synthetic iron chelator ligands, such as polyaminocarboxylates and organophosphonates are also known for their bacteriostatic properties (Bilitewski et al. 2017). The chemical and microbiological bases for the variable results obtained with these various chelators are further addressed below.

8.4.4 Hematologically Useful Iron Chelators Are Often Utilizable by Microbes

Iron (III) is the most stable oxidation state of iron in aerobic aqueous media and behaves as a hard Lewis acid. As a hard Lewis acid, iron (III) will bind strongly to hard donor atoms, such as negatively charged oxygen and amine nitrogen atoms. Microbes have taken advantage of this characteristic and produce siderophores that have catechol, hydroxamic acid, and α-hydroxycarboxylic acid functional groups (Fig. 8.2, left), all rich in these useful donor moieties. Siderophores must selectively bind iron tightly in order to solubilize the metal ion and prevent its hydrolysis, as well as effectively compete with other chelators in the host system. The functional groups form five membered chelate rings upon binding that is effective for iron complexes due to the size of the metal and the bite angles formed in chelation (Fig. 8.2, right). As such, microbes have evolved to produce siderophores that are selective for iron, even among other metal ions that are generally present at higher concentrations.

Clinically relevant hematological chelators, deferoxamine (DFO), deferiprone (DFP) and deferasirox (DEF) have chemical structures that also contain oxygen and nitrogen donor atoms, i.e., characteristic to those of siderophores (Fig. 8.3). As a measure of coordinative strength and a useful parameter under biologically relevant conditions and to compare iron affinity among chelators over the conventional stability constant, is the pFe^{3+} value (Raymond et al. 1984). The pFe^{3+} is defined as the negative logarithm of the concentration of the free iron (III) in solution when in the presence of a chelator. For clinically relevant conditions, pFe^{3+} values are typically calculated for total [ligand] = 1 μM and total [iron] = 10 μM at pH 7.4. Unlike the stability constant, log K or log β_3, the pFe^{3+} value considers ligand protonation, denticities, and difference in metal ligand stoichiometries. Among the hematological chelators, deferoxamine has the strongest binding affinity ($pFe^{3+} = 26$), followed by deferasirox ($pFe^{3+} = 22.5$) and then deferiprone ($pFe^{3+} = 19.4$) (Heinz et al. 1999).

The iron binding affinity hierarchy of these chelators has precedence by the "iron-shuttle" hypothesis with the dual treatment using both deferoxamine and deferiprone for β-thalassemia (Link et al. 2001; Giardina and Grady 2001). It has been described that iron is bound to a "shuttle"- oral agent, such as deferiprone, that mobilizes tissue iron which is then exchanged in the bloodstream with a "sink" such as deferoxamine, that is then excreted with iron through the kidneys allowing the deferiprone iron shuttle to be reused again (Giardina and Grady 2001). As a

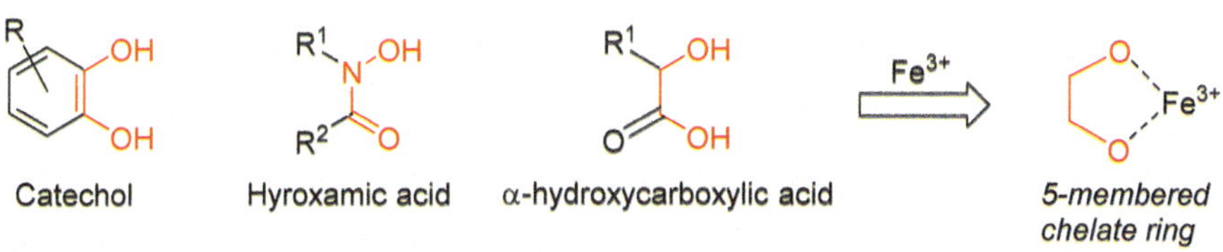

Fig. 8.2 Common siderophore functional groups that can form 5-membered chelate rings

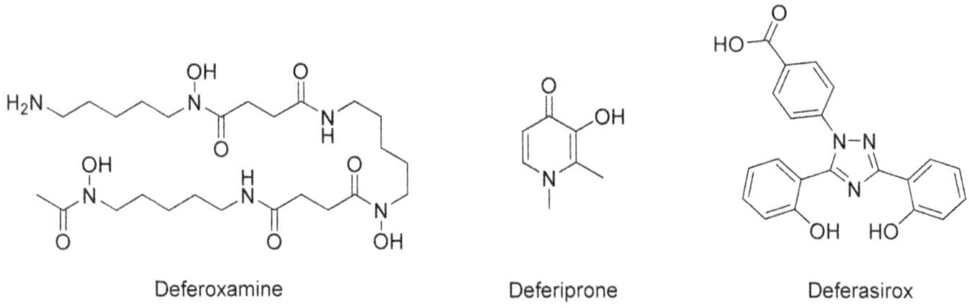

Fig. 8.3 Hematological chelators Deferoxamine (DFO), Deferiprone (DFP) and Deferasirox (DEF)

testament to its higher binding affinity, deferoxamine can remove the chelated iron from the 3:1 deferiprone: iron complex (Liu and Hider 2002).

The above three clinically used chelators are effective for the treatment of iron overload diseases and while they exhibit some antimicrobial activity alone, it does not preclude them from being sources of iron for a number of microorganisms. Kontoghiorghes et al. examined how the chelators can affect iron uptake by microbial pathogens in patients that are treated for iron overload diseases (Kontoghiorghes et al. 2010). The addition of chelators can inhibit or promote microbial growth and proliferation, especially in an iron deprived condition. Specific to this case, the iron load of the patient, the length of the treatment and the minimum therapeutic dose that can be safely used has to be considered.

The antimicrobial activity of deferoxamine is compromised by the molecule itself being a microbial siderophore and influences the growth of various microbes. Its xenosiderophore activity has been demonstrated for many pathogenic bacteria (Chan et al. 2009; Thompson et al. 2012; Lesic et al. 2002; Banin et al. 2005; Holbein and Mira de Orduña 2010; Ang et al. 2018). Microbes that are challenged with deferoxamine likely harbor a receptor capable of capturing the molecule when complexed to iron. Consistent with this is that prolonged administration of deferoxamine to humans with β-thalassemia increases their susceptibility to infection (Kontoghiorghes et al. 2010).

Deferoxamine, deferiprone and deferasirox have differing antimicrobial activities. Lesic et al. compared the antimicrobial activity of deferiprone to deferoxamine and evaluated the potential of deferiprone to promote the growth of pathogenic *Yersinia enterocolitica* (Lesic et al. 2002). It was found that while deferoxamine promoted the growth of *Y. enterocolitica*, deferiprone at the same concentration did not. There are several reported and unreported cases that deferoxamine facilitates the growth of *Yersinia enterocolitca* infections in thalassemia patients and in some cases with a fatal outcome (Robins-Browne and Prpic 1983; Robins-Browne and Prpic 1985). In contrast to deferoxamine, deferiprone does not promote *Y. enterocolitica* septicemia in the mouse experimental model. The growth of other bacterial organisms isolated from infected Thalassemic patients was studied in the presence of iron chelators. Chan et al. evaluated the growth *in vitro* of two pathogenic organisms *Klebsiella pneumoniae* and *Aeromonas hydrophila* derived from Thalassemic patients using the three iron chelators (Chi-Fung Chan et al. 2009). Deferoxamine induced proliferation of *K. pneumoniae*, while deferiprone and deferasirox did not. However, all three chelators studied did not affect the growth of *A. hydrophila*. The authors attributed this null effect to the highly specific ligand exchange process of *A. hydrophila* (Stintzi et al. 2000). Stintzi et al. studied the iron uptake mechanism of *A. hydrophila* where the exchange of iron at the membrane surface from an iron bound siderophore to an iron free siderophore bound to a receptor, while hypothesizing that this acquisition process would likely be widespread in Gram negative bacteria (Stintzi et al. 2000).

Pseudomonas aeruginosa is an example pathogen that has a broad iron uptake capability and it produces two known siderophores, pyoverdine and pyochelin, while also using a range of heterologous siderophore molecules including deferoxamine. Thompson et al (Thompson et al. 2012) evaluated the *in vitro* antimicrobial activities of several FDA-approved iron chelators (deferasirox, deferoxamine and deferiprone (also called ApoL1) as well as novel chelators (Apo6619 and VK28 dihydrochloride) against a panel of healthcare associated bacterial pathogens (*A. baumannii, S. aureus, P. aeruginosa, K. pneumoniae,* and *E. coli*). When tested in cation-adjusted Mueller-Hinton broth, deferoxamine showed no effect on bacterial growth (Minimum Inhibitory Concentration (MIC)>512 μg/ml for all bacteria tested). In contrast, VK28 inhibited the growth of all strains of *A. baumannii*, *E. coli*, and *S. aureus* tested. Deferiprone (ApoL1) inhibited the growth of all strains of *E. coli* and *A. baumannii*, some strains of *P. aeruginosa* and *K. pneumoniae*, but had no effect on *S. aureus*. When RPMI medium was used for the assay, the MICs were reduced by 4- to 64-fold for VK28 and by 2- to 4-fold for deferiprone and Apo6619 (Thompson et al. 2012). Further studies in a time-kill assay showed that VK28, ApoL1 and Apo6619 inhibited the growth of *S. aureus* at 1x and 2x the Minimum Inhibitory Concentration (MIC) and demonstrated a bacteriostatic effect on *E. coli* at 2X the MIC, suggesting the promise of those new iron chelators as alternatives to antibiotics. Unfortunately, the effect of those iron chelators on recent clinical isolates or in animal models were not evaluated (Thompson et al. 2012). In addition to the chelating iron, some iron chelators have also demonstrated additive or synergistic effects to enhance the activity of known antibiotics up to 50-fold (Foley and Simeonov 2012; Luo et al. 2014). Ang et al. (2018) has demonstrated that the effective concentrations required for antimicrobial activity of deferiprone and deferoxamine are not useful in comparison to a novel chelator, DIBI which was >1000X more inhibitory.

Deferoxamine also promotes the growth of fungi. The antimicrobial activity of deferoxamine, deferiprone and ciclopirox ranged from none for deferoxamine to modest for the others against *A. fumigatus in vitro* (Zarember et al. 2009). The same observation of iron uptake from deferoxamine was found for *Rhizopus microspores* (de Locht et al. 1994) and *C. albicans* (Holbein and Mira de Orduña 2010).

8.4.5 Problem of Weak Antimicrobial Activity of Low Molecular Weight Chelators

The use of low molecular weight iron chelators as anti-infective alternatives to antibiotics, including those now used clinically for hematological disorders has so far generated only mixed success (Thompson et al. 2012; Bilitewski et al. 2017; Johnstone and Nolan 2015; Khan et al. 2018; Zhou et al. 2012; Ang et al. 2018). We have proposed that these limitations in antimicrobial activities of these various chelators are related to their small molecule nature (i.e., Mw<1500 Da). For antimicrobial activity of a synthetic iron chelator, it is essential to ensure that the iron complex formed by the chelators cannot be taken up, accessed or otherwise utilized by a pathogen, as this would lead to access to the chelated iron and thus microbial growth.

Siderophores are essential for microorganisms to survive in their natural iron limited environment. In the infected host, they represent virulence factors of pathogenic bacteria and fungi. A variety of artificial siderophores have been synthesized and studied to learn more about their specific interactions with microbial iron transport systems and their potential as alternatives to antibiotics to outcompete with the native siderophores (Roosenberg et al. 2000; Roosenberg and Miller 2000). For example, Mohammodi et al. synthesized and characterized a highly effective iron chelator that mimics the enterobactin structure (Mohammadi et al. 2011) which dramatically improved the iron binding affinity and iron selectivity of the final siderophore mimetic hydrogel. Since the chemical coordinating groups commonly found in natural siderophores are likely to be recognised by microbial transporters, these chemical groups might be avoided in the design of new synthetic antimicrobial iron chelators (Foley and Simeonov 2012).

8.4.6 Requirements of New Microbial Specific Iron Withdrawal Agents

Based on our understanding of microbial iron acquisition mechanisms, microbial utilization of host iron pools and the mixed results obtained to date when hematologically useful chelators have been trialed as antimicrobials, some key requirements for new iron withdrawal therapeutics emerge. Key requirements for new purpose directed antimicrobial iron chelators in contrast to current hematologically useful chelators (deferoxamine, deferiprone, deferasirox) are summarized in Table 8.2. We believe that the key aspects for useful antimicrobial activity are molecular size being >1500 Da (i.e., above the lowest size freely accessible for bacterial uptake) and chemical composition, i.e., not similar to bacterial siderophores in terms of iron chelating component groups. An overarching requirement is that a new antimicrobial chelator should have low toxicity to the infected host, i.e. high microbial toxicity but low host toxicity. These various attributes are further discussed below in relation to recently advanced novel chelators.

Table 8.2 Desired properties for novel antimicrobial iron chelators as compared to conventional hematological chelators

Chelator property	Hematological chelator	Antimicrobial chelator	Significance
Molecular weight	<1500 Da	≥1500 Da	Hematologicals access intracellular host iron Antimicrobials should primarily access extracellular iron pools
Antimicrobial activity spectrum	Narrow	Broad	Hematologicals not broadly effective and support growth for some microbes
Antimicrobial activity	Poor with high to very high Minimum Inhibitory Concentrations (MICs)	High with very low MICs, ideally similar effective concentration range as for antibiotics	Hematologicals are weak anti-infectives with high MICs
Host toxicity	Varied cytotoxicity issues related to reactive iron depending on chelator loading	Low with iron fully coordinated and less reactive	Fully coordinated iron is less-reactive as to cytotoxicity
Water solubility	Soluble to limited solubility	High solubility	Water solubility improves utility for topical and systemic administration

8.5 Novel Purpose Designed Antimicrobial Iron Sequestering Agents

8.5.1 Hydroxypyridinone, a Preferred Iron Ligand

Among the hematological chelators that contain various iron binding groups and have potential as antimicrobial agents, the hydroxypyridinone group is driven forward. Hydroxypyridinones combine the characteristics of both hydroxamate and catecholate groups. While catecholate ligands, such as enterobactin and analogues, have higher stability constants for iron (III) than hydroxypyridinones, under acidic conditions they are limited by their weak acid nature and require the loss of six protons to bind iron (III). Hydroxypyridinones are monoprotic acids and require the loss of three protons to form a neutral tris-coordinated iron (III) complex. The structure of the chelate thus differs significantly from siderophores and may not be readily recognized by bacteria.

There are three classes of hydroxypyridinones; 1-hydroxypyridin-2-ones; 3-hydroxypyridin-2-ones and 3-hydroxypyridin-4-ones (Fig. 8.4). Of the three classes of hydroxypyridinone ligands, 3-hydroxypyridin-4-one class possesses the highest affinity for iron (III) with an association constant of 10^{37}. This is due to the higher pK_a value that is attributed to the 4-oxo group when compared to the 2-oxo

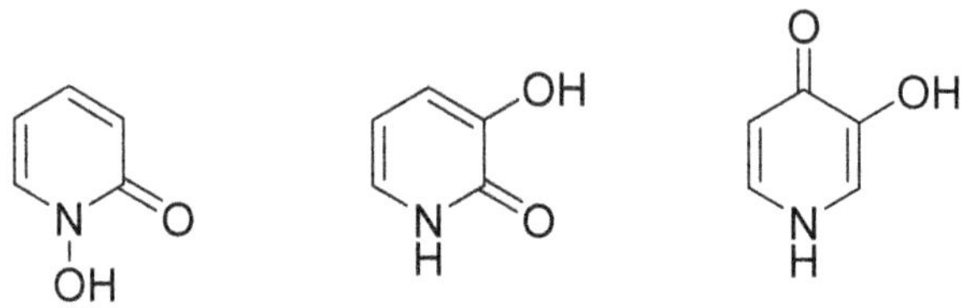

Fig. 8.4 Three classes of hydroxypyridinones: 1-hydroxypyridin-2-one (left), 3-hydroxypyridin-2-one (middle), 3-hydroxypyridin-4-one (right)

congeners. While catechol derivatives possess higher formation constant values than that of 3-hydroxypyridin-4-one for iron (III), their corresponding pFe^{3+} values are lower, due to the higher affinity for protons by the catechol derivatives. The oxygen atoms of the hydroxypyridinone binds to iron in a 3:1 fashion and it forms five membered chelate rings upon coordination and the chelate is stable over a wide physiological pH range. Deprotonation of the hydroxypyridinone produces a zwitterionic aromatic resonance form. The electron pair of the nitrogen atom delocalizes on the carbonyl oxygen and the electron pair is shared between the two vicinal oxygen atoms.

Because of their high affinity for iron (III), 3-hydroxypyridin-4-ones have been considered for several therapeutic applications (Liu and Hider 2002). Deferiprone, also known as ferriprox or L1, is a clinically used iron chelator that contains a 3-hydroxypyridin-4-one group and is widely used for the treatment of iron overload associated with β-thalassemia (Balfour and Foster 1999). The compound is characterized by two protonation constants ($logK_1 = 9.64$ and $logK_2 = 3.56$), the first is related to the hydroxy group and the second is related to the keto group (Nurchi et al. 2008). At pH 7.4, deferiprone is found in its neutral form and the iron (III) complex carries no net charge and can thus penetrate membranes easily to remove potentially toxic iron from tissues (Liu and Hider 2002). The low molecular weight of deferiprone allows its efficient absorption into the intestinal tract and penetration into cells. In addition, it can remove iron (III) from ferritin and transferrin (Dobbin et al. 1993).

The low molecular weight of deferiprone increases its oral bioavailability in comparison to hexadentate chelators, such as deferoxamine, however it has limited clinical efficacy. The two main disadvantages of deferiprone are its rapid metabolism (Singh et al. 1992) and reversible agranulocytosis, as induced in approximately 1% of patients receiving the drug (Ceci et al. 2002). The metabolism of deferiprone is from its susceptibility to glucuronidation of the 3-hydroxyl group that inactivates its iron chelating capability. As such, the deferiprone dose necessary to maintain an iron negative balance is 75–100 mg/kg/day (Balfour and Foster 1999) and adverse side effects have been observed (Olivieri et al. 2019). Further support of this are indicated by recovery studies that reported >85% of the administered dose in man is recovered in the urine as the non-chelating 3-*O*-glucuronide conjugate (Singh et al. 1992).

Chemically modifying hydroxypyridinone groups changes their hydrophilic/lipophilic characteristics without changing the iron binding affinity (Dobbin et al. 1993). To illustrate this, increasing the length of the alkyl substituent at the 1-position of the pyridinone ring increases the lipophilicity of the molecule and minimizes the inhibition of non-heme iron containing enzymes such as lipoxygenase, that are affected by hydrophobic chelators. Brain barrier penetration of 3-hydroxypyridin-4-ones is strongly dependent on lipophilicity (Habgood et al. 1999), where branched alkyl substituents at the 1-position penetrate more slowly than simple 1-alkyl substituents.

Hexadentate chelators that contain three 3-hydroxypyridin-4-one groups on a molecular scaffold can act as siderophore analogues as shown in Fig. 8.5 (Qiu et al. 2011; Xu et al. 2011; Zhou et al. 2015b; Streater et al. 1990). Incorporating the hydroxypyridinone group increases the potential of not being recognized by bacteria as a source of iron. By affixing three 3-hydroxypyridin-4-one moieties increases the iron (III) binding affinity while still maintaining a stronger acid nature than catechols, such as enterobactin, where three protons are released instead of six. Having a higher iron (III) binding affinity reduces the likelihood of "loosely" bound iron that could have the opportunity to redox cycle between the two most stable oxidation states of iron (II) and iron (III) thus generating toxic oxygen derived free radicals such as hydroxyl, that would cause oxidative tissue damage.

The denticity nature of the iron coordination complex influences the dissociation constant. The dissociation of iron for a tris-bidentate octahedral metal complex is dependent on $[\text{ligand}]^3$, where with a hexadentate ligand–metal complex dissociation of iron is dependent on [ligand]. Hence, the sensitivity of concentration dilution for iron-complex dissociation follows the order hexadentate $<$ tridentate $<$ bidentate ligands. As a result, the majority of natural siderophores are hexadentate compounds that can scavenge iron (III) efficiently at low metal concentrations (Hider and Konga 2010).

While there have been several hexadentate chelators designed and synthesized for potential antimicrobial agents, their activity appears limited by their poor water solubility and molecular weight. Two early examples of hexadentate chelators reported by Qui et al. (**Q1** and **Q2**, Fig. 8.5) were evaluated against Gram positive and Gram negative bacteria in comparison to the antimicrobial activity of diethylenetriamine pentaacetic acid (DTPA) (Qiu et al. 2011). It was found among these three chelators that **Q1** gave the highest antimicrobial activity followed by DTPA and **Q2**. The authors ascribed **Q1** to having the highest activity due to its higher affinity for iron (III) ($\log K = 30.7$, $pFe^{3+} = 30.5$) than DTPA ($\log K = 28.6$) (Sohnle et al. 2001). The low inhibitory effect of **Q2** was explained by its poor water solubility and because of its molecular weight was above the 500-600 molecular weight cut-off point (Hancock and Nikaido 1978).

Molecular weight was also considered a factor in influencing the antimicrobial activity of compounds **X1** and **X2** (Fig. 8.5) (Xie et al. 2013). In most cases, **X1** and **X2** outcompeted DTPA against the Gram positive and Gram negative bacteria studied where this was attributed to the hexadentate chelators having a higher affinity for iron (III) and would not have the ability to cross bilayer membranes by

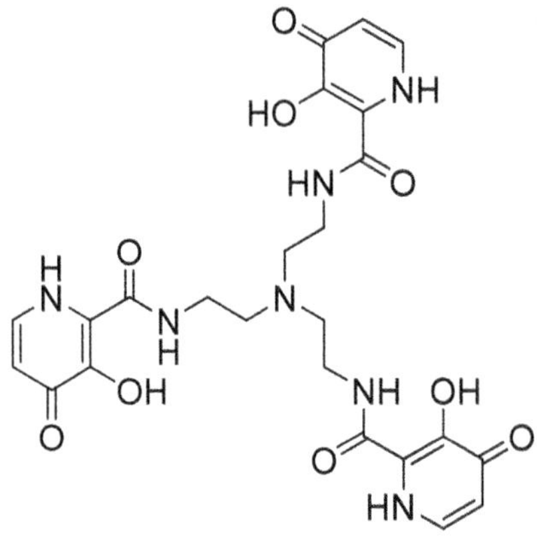

Q1

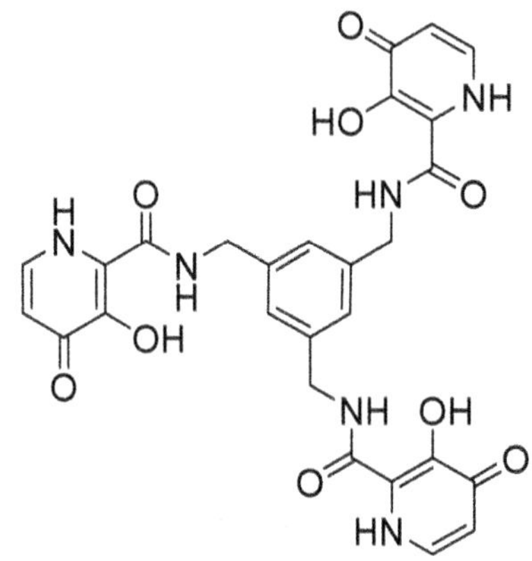

Q2

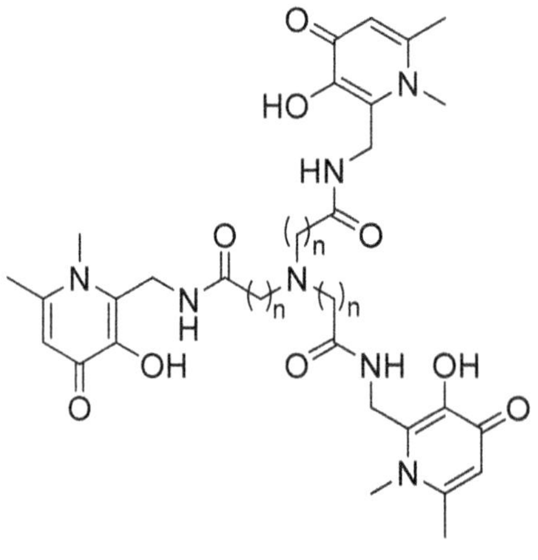

n = 1, **X1**
= 2, **X2**

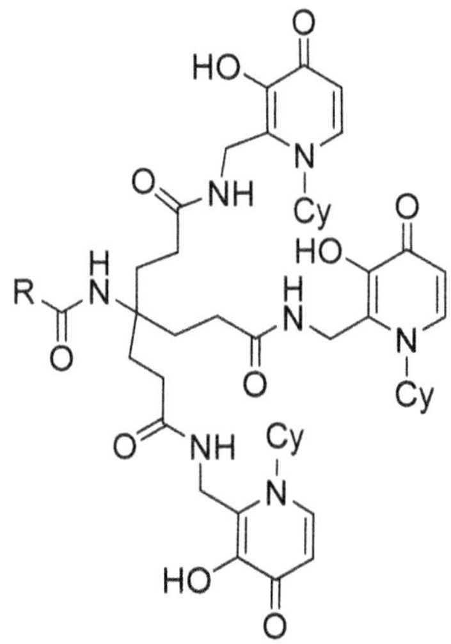

R = CH_3, **Z1**
= n-C_3H_7, **Z2**

Fig. 8.5 Representative hexadentate 3-hydroxypyridin-4-one chelators that exhibit antimicrobial activity

non-facilitated diffusion. The authors hypothesized that **X1** and **X2** would likely gain access to the periplasmic space of the Gram negative bacteria and restrict iron from them. As an extension to these structures, derivatives were synthesized that are highly hydrophilic and their antimicrobial activity was evaluated in comparison to DTPA (Xie et al. 2013). The antimicrobial activities of hydrophilic derivatives that contained various substituents at the nitrogen center were strongest against the Gram negative bacteria than the Gram positive bacteria studied. Like **X1** and **X2** their activity was regarded as having ready access to the periplasmic space of Gram negative bacteria and removal of iron(III) from the immediate area surrounding Gram positive bacteria while having a higher affinity for iron (III) than DTPA (Xie et al. 2013).

Hexadentate chelators have been developed that exhibit moderate antimicrobial activity against methicillin resistant *Staphylococcus aureus* (MRSA) and Gram negative bacteria *P. aeruginosa* (Zhou et al. 2015b). Overall, it was found that the *Pseudomonas* strains were more sensitive to all the test chelators studied than were the MRSA strains. Compounds **Z1** and **Z2** that have a hexyl group substituted at the 1-position of the pyridinone ring, were the most hydrophobic and possessed the strongest inhibitory activity against MRSA and *P. aeruginosa* compared to the other compounds tested.

The design of a rhodamine-labelled hexadentate chelators that contain 3-hydroxypyridin-4-one moieties balances the hydrophilic/lipophilic character to combat growth of *Mycobacterium avium* (Moniz et al. 2013). The hexadentate chelator that contains rhodamine B isothiocyanate (Fig. 8.6) exhibited the strongest inhibitory activity at concentrations as low as 1 μM. The authors described that the rhodamine B labelled chelator strongly interacts with lipid phases and previous confocal microscopic studies showed that the rhodamine counterpart remains largely membrane bound (Nunes et al. 2010). They speculated that the fluorescent chelators are targeting the phagosomal compartment of macrophages where this bacterium grows, and that the fluorophore can anchor into the phagosomal membrane to tether the chelator and compete against mycobacterial siderophores.

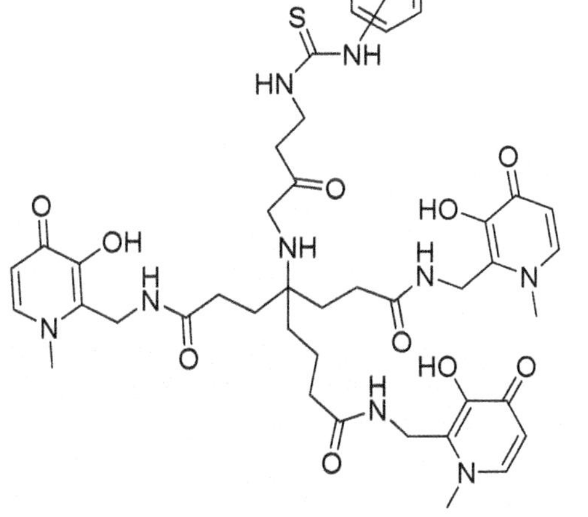

Fig. 8.6 Representative Rhodamine B labelled hexadentate 3-hydroxypyridin-4-one chelator

There is limited literature that investigates 1-hydroxypyridin-2-ones for antimicrobial activity, as these chelators have a lower iron affinity than their 3-hydroxypyridin-4-one isomers. Workman et al. used these pyridinones in their hexadentate chelators with a triaza macrocycle backbone (Workman et al. 2016). The lower pK_a values of these hydroxypyridinones make them charged molecules at physiological pH making them less likely to penetrate the host. This could potentially lead to safety benefits to treat systemic infections. The authors demonstrated the utility of these hexadentate chelators as bacteriostatic however with limited activity. Minimum inhibitory concentration values obtained for the four tested Gram negative bacteria were higher than the tested Gram positive bacteria. The most resistant strains were *P. aeruginosa*, *K. pneumoniae*, and *E. coli.*

The hexadentate hydroxypyridinone chelators exhibit moderate antimicrobial activity and have a high affinity for iron (III). Their molecular size lowers the probability of cell permeation and toxicity than their bidentate conjugates; however, their iron capacity is the same as their bidentate counterparts.

8.5.2 Polymeric Iron Chelators

As illustrated in the previous section, molecular weight is a critical factor for the rate of drug absorption, uptake by microbes and can influence drug toxicity. There is no clear "cut-off" value for the transcellular route but the reported polyethylene glycol (PEG) permeability, penetration falls off rapidly with molecular weights greater than 500 Da (Maxton et al. 1986). A low molecular weight chelator combined with an overall neutral charge upon the complexation of iron (III) enables permeation through cells. Using deferiprone as an example, the iron (III) complex has a zero charge at neutral pH that allows excretion of this complex. However, this iron complexation is highly concentration dependent and at relatively low concentrations (<5 μM) the iron-deferiprone complex will redistribute iron to competing ligands (Yokel et al. 1995). This leads to a high drug dose requirement with associated toxicity and hence its useful partnering with the kinetically more stable deferoxamine for treatment of iron overload conditions. The hexadentate chelators offer a stronger iron (III) binding affinity, although due to their similar iron capacity to a bidentate chelator, this translates to a similar concentration dependency for effectiveness.

The antimicrobial activity of dendritic chelators containing hexadentate 3-hydroxypyridin-4-one head-groups were evaluated and compared to that of deferiprone (Zhou et al. 2014; Zhou et al. 2018). The **Zh1** dendrimer investigated (Fig. 8.7) showed the strongest inhibitory effects on two strains of *P. aeruginosa* and was more efficient than that of deferiprone. However, none of the dendrimer chelators were able to completely inhibit the growth of *E. coli* at up to 500 μg/mL. The chelators were more effective against the *P. aeruginosa* strains with **Zh1** completely inhibiting growth. With respect to the Gram positive bacteria, *S. aureus* and *Bacillus subtilis*, the chelators were found to be less effective than deferiprone. Upon testing

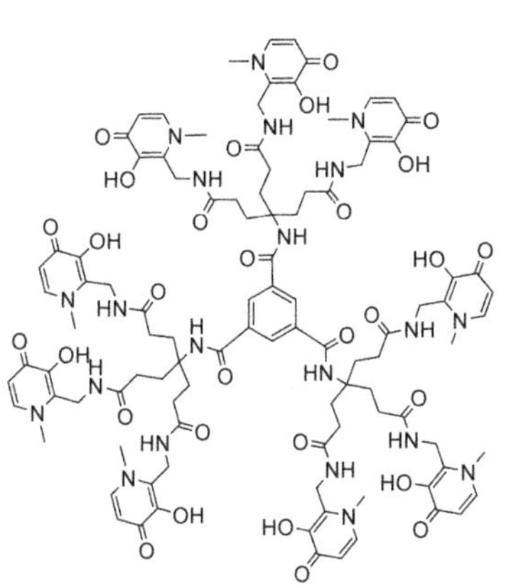

Zh1

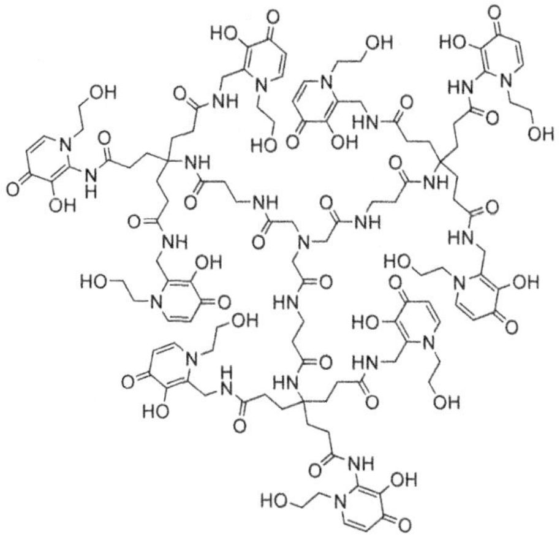

Zh2

Fig. 8.7 Representative dendrimers (**Zh1** and **Zh2**) that contains a hexadentate 3-hydroxypyridin-4-one head-group

norfloxacin in combination with **Zh1** there was a dramatic enhancement in the inhibition of *E. coli* and *S. aureus* than with either agent alone. Norfloxacin is a fluoroquinoline antimicrobial agent that can bind metal ions at the carbonyl and carboxyl groups of its pyridinone ring, a region that also interacts with DNA gyrase, essential for DNA replication. The authors described that iron (III) complexation of **Zh1** would indirectly increase the interaction of DNA gyrase with norfloxacin. A more recent example, (**Zh2**, Fig. 8.7) showed enhanced antimicrobial activity against *E. coli* than the previous dendrimer and among the suite of dendrimers reported (Zhou et al. 2018) with a bactericidal rate reaching 99.7% at a markedly lower concentration of 100 μg/mL than the early example dendrimer. At the same concentration, **Zh2** exhibited superior activity against the Gram positive bacteria *S. aureus* and *B. subtilis* in comparison to deferiprone, something that was not achieved with the early dendrimer, **Zh1**. The authors predicted the activity to scavenging iron around the bacteria and differences in activity could be attributed to their differences in water solubility.

Cross-linked polymers have been developed and tested as antibiotics and adjuvants for potential use in wound dressing materials (El-Gendy et al. 2015). Polyallylamine was simultaneously cross-linked by *N,N′*-methylenebis (acrylamide) and conjugated with 2,3-dihydroxybenzoic acid (DHBA) molecules that serve as iron-chelation sites. The "iron affinity index" was used as a measure for the iron affinity of the cross-linked particles, due to the heterogeneous nature of the polymeric material, in comparison to a reference iron chelator, in this case, EDTA. For all the samples tested, they were at least 10^3 times stronger than EDTA. It is noted that upon increasing the content of DHBA from 5% to 30% the affinity indexes of the polymers decreased. This decrease was attributed to the increase of hydrophobicity of the material that may have hindered the iron (III) access or coordination and reducing the apparent iron affinity indexes. Following the incubation of the polymer samples with iron (III) solution for one week, the highest iron capacity plateaued at around 20 mg of iron (III) per gram of polymer. The antimicrobial activity of a chosen cross-linked derivative was examined against *P. aeruginosa* and in combination with the antibiotics ciprofloxacin or gentamicin. Treating the growth media with the cross-linked polymer reduced the iron to undetectable levels and led to stopping growth and eventual death of the bacteria.

To afford larger scaffolds and more flexibility in the structure, a hexadentate 3-hydroxypyridin-4-one monomer was co-polymerized with 2-hydroethyl acrylate (HEA) using azobisisobutyronitrile (AIBN) as the initiator (Zhou et al. 2015a). The hexadentate chelator possessed a high affinity for iron (III) ($logK_1$ = 33.6 and pFe^{3+} = 30.4). The bulky monomer rendered the polymerization difficult where the weight recovery of the co-polymers decreased with increasing percentage of hexadentate chelator. This in turn affected the iron binding capacity and the highest achieved was a co-polymer synthesized with an initial monomer mole ratio of 9% and iron capacity of 370 μmol of iron per gram of polymer. In addition, the calculated pFe^{3+} values of the hexadentate monomer and co-polymer were similar, 29.7 and 29.8 respectively, indicating either species had similar affinity for iron (III). Similarly, it was observed that the hexadentate hydroxypyridinone head-group and the formed dendrimer shared a similar affinity for iron (III) (Zhou et al. 2006). The co-polymer chosen for further investigation contained a mole ratio of monomer at 5% (200 μmol of iron per gram of polymer capacity) and an average molecular weight of about 180 kDa (measured by GPC). The iron affinity of monomer and chosen co-polymer were similar and had similar antimicrobial potency against five bacterial strains. The authors described the polymer as a potential material to be incorporated into wound dressing materials and less likely to access systemic circulation.

Poly (glycidyl methacrylate) (PGMA) polymers were synthesized *via* Reversible Addition-Fragmentation Chain Transfer (RAFT) polymerization and conjugated with amine-containing 3-hydroxypyridin-4-ones to create polymeric iron chelators with controlled molecular weights (Li et al. 2016). Glycerol monomethacrylate was polymerized in anhydrous toluene at 62 °C using AIBN as an azo initiator and a dithiobenzoate-based RAFT agent to produce well defined RAFT PGMA epoxy functional groups. Bidentate hydroxypyridinone ligands were then used as nucleophiles to ring-open the epoxide groups for post polymerization modification. Among the five hydroxypyridinone conjugative groups, only two of those containing a pegylated chain, produced two water soluble polymers (Fig. 8.8). The other hydroxypyridinone conjugative groups produced water insoluble polymers or those soluble in aqueous DMSO solutions. The authors described the insolubility to the removal of the hydrogen bonding capability when transforming a primary amine to a secondary amine that dramatically decreased the solubility of the macromolecular chelators. It was determined for one series of polymers that the highest number of chelating units per polymer chain was 106 and M_n = 15 200. The highest metal capacity achieved for one of the water soluble polymers (M_n = 50 100), was calculated to be 843 μmol/g. The same polymer exhibited the highest potency

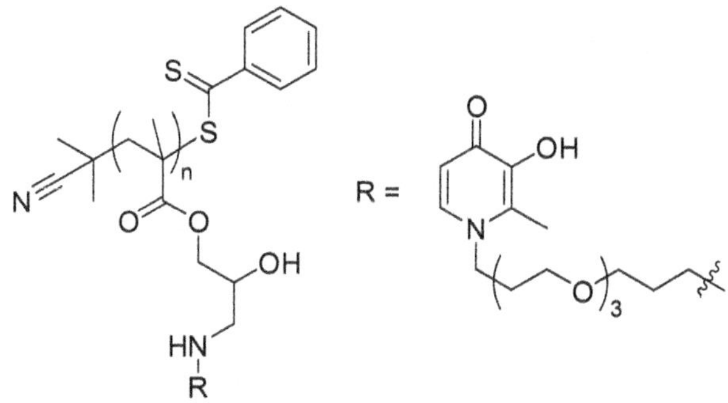

Fig. 8.8 Representative RAFT-PGMA water soluble polymer with pegylated 3-hydroxypyridin-4-one conjugative group R

against MRSA among the polymers tested with a 12 μM concentration achieving a bactericidal rate of 100%. The lower M_n counterpart (M_n = 13 400) of the representative water soluble polymer showed reduced bactericidal activity and inhibition was observed at a 48 μM concentration. This suggested that the density of the iron chelating units on the macromolecular scaffold determines the antimicrobial potency.

The polymeric chelators described thus far have molecular weights that disallow them to be taken up through the gastrointestinal tract, potentially prolonging their drug half life and their limited antimicrobial utility was likely due to their lack of water solubility. An aqueous environment exists for a microbial cell and the gastrointestinal lumen. The previous polymeric chelators are multi-component and sensitive to the choice in scaffold, linker, and binding moiety that manifest their water solubility (Fig. 8.9). The development of highly water soluble chelating polymers would potentially lead to a new horizon of therapeutic applications, in addition to topological applications. Conducting the polymerization in aqueous media would also increase the safety profile of the polymer and render it more economically viable. RAFT polymerization is an attractive method as it can occur in a wide range of solvents (including water), with high functional group tolerance and in the absence of metals. In addition, RAFT synthesis affords control of the polymer molecular weight with low polydispersity.

RAFT synthesized 3-hydroxypyridin-4-one polyvinylpyrrolidone co-polymers that have been developed are essentially two-component and are highly water-soluble and exhibit strong antimicrobial activity for a wider range of pathogens (Ang et al. 2018). The lead compound, DIBI, has exhibited activity against various groups of microorganisms and cancer cells (Holbein and Mira de Orduña 2010; Islam et al. 2016; Thorburn et al. 2017; Parquet et al. 2018; Holbein et al. 2011) and exhibits a lack of toxicity in murine models (Arora et al. 2018; Savage et al. 2018). The 3-hydroxypyridin-4-one chelator (MAHMP, Fig. 8.10) was designed for direct co-polymerization with water soluble monomers, such as *N*-vinylpyrrolidone (NVP) used for the main backbone of DIBI and this provides the inherent water solubility.

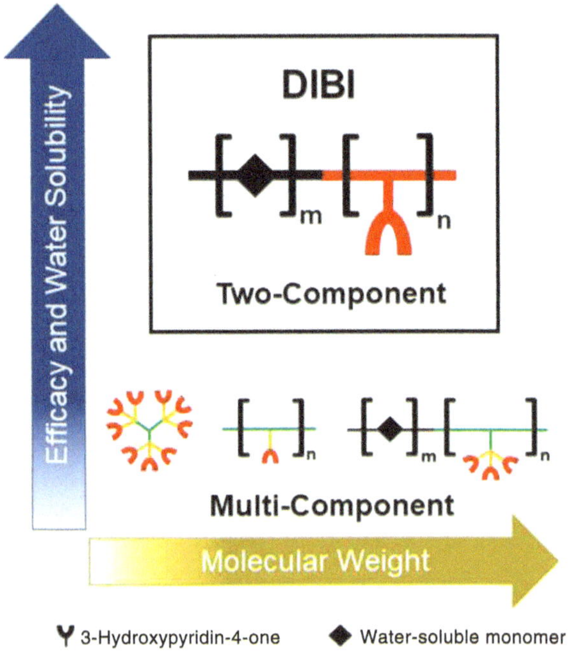

Fig. 8.9 Illustration comparing previously reported polymeric chelators and DIBI. Different colours highlight structural components for each polymeric chelator

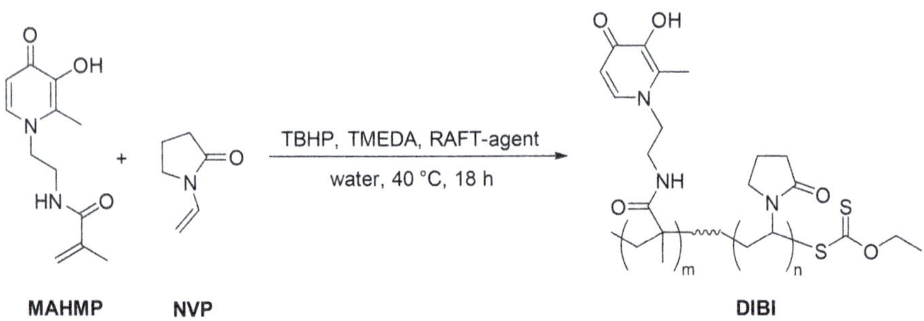

Fig. 8.10 Synthesis of DIBI (Mn: 7.5 kDa, Mw: 9 kDa, PDI: 1.2); TBHP = tert-butyl hydroperoxide, TMEDA = *N,N,N′,N′*-tetramethylethylenediamine, and RAFT agent = 2-[(ethoxymethanethioyl)sulfanyl]-2-methylpropanoic acid. (Adapted from Ang et al. 2018)

Polyvinylpyrrolidone (PVP) is ubiquitous in the medical field and being the main backbone of DIBI, it can attribute for the high water solubility and low toxicity profile of the metal chelating polymer. The earliest use of PVP was as a plasma volume expander for trauma victims post the 1950s and later in a wide variety of medical applications (Bühler 2005), such as a binder for pharmaceutical tablets, excipient for contact lens solutions and for the synthesis of dialysis membranes. The

RAFT polymerizations of MAHMP-co-PVP polymers were carried out using commercially available *N*-vinylpyrrolidone in mild aqueous conditions that gave moderate to high recover of the co-polymers (55–88% yield). The lowest polymer recovery was related to the highest incorporation of MAHMP into the co-polymer. DIBI has an average content of MAHMP of 13 mol% or 24 mass%, with a good polymer recovery of 85%. DIBI also exhibits high water solubility and the highest mass fraction in water tested was 70% w/w without the use of organic solvents (Ang et al. 2018), unlike the RAFT synthesized PGMA polymers that required DMSO for the dissolution of their polymers (Li et al. 2016).

DIBI inhibited all three classes of microbes exhibiting very low Minimum Inhibitory Concentrations (MICs). The molecular weight of DIBI as measured by Gel Permeation Chromatography (GPC) was 9 kDa with a polydispersity index of 1.2 and it has a total iron capacity of 338 μmol of iron per gram of co-polymer. With the other MAHMP-PVP co-polymers, MICs were lowered upon increasing the incorporation of MAHMP. The MIC of DIBI was lower by 2–3 orders of magnitude in comparison to its MAHMP monomer and to deferiprone against ATCC reference strains of *S. aureus*, *A. baumannii*, and *C. albicans*. PVP (10 kDa) was used as a control as it does not contain iron chelating moieties and did not exhibit any antimicrobial effect.

The antimicrobial efficacy of this 3-hydroxypyridin-4-one containing polymeric chelator is not fully explained by its iron binding capacity, size, and water solubility alone. DIBI had a lower iron binding capacity and molecular weight than previously reported water soluble RAFT PGMA polymers. As an example, the most potent water soluble RAFT PGMA polymer had a molecular weight of 50 kDa and an iron binding capacity of 843 μmol of iron per gram of polymer. The lower molecular weight and binding capacity of DIBI (10 kDa and 338 μmol) did not compromise its efficacy against MRSA having a MIC of 4 μM in comparison to 12 μM of the most potent water soluble RAFT PGMA polymer. With the 3-hydroxypyridin-4-one dendrimers (Zhou et al. 2014) the iron chelating capacity was higher than that of deferiprone, however alone they did not outperform deferiprone in antimicrobial activity. In combination with norfloxacin (at 0.5 μg/mL), the concentration of dendrimer used was high (500 μg/mL) in comparison to that needed for the RAFT synthesized polymers, to completely inhibit the growth of *S. aureus* (Zhou et al. 2014). The polymers described above were all water soluble; however, they varied in polymeric structure.

The choice of scaffold and metal binding group influence the water solubility of polymeric chelators. The hydrogen bonding groups of the polymers containing hexadentate 3-hydroxypyridin-4-one chelators and respective scaffolds render the polymers water soluble. The same is the case for DIBI that has amide groups that are a part of the MAHMP linkage and the PVP backbone that enable a highly water soluble polymer. Within the suite of RAFT PGMA polymers (Li et al. 2016) the only two water soluble polymers produced incorporated 3-hydroxypyridin-4-one conjugated group that had a pegylated amine group.

In addition to the characteristics above, the structure of a polymeric chelator following the binding of iron is likely congruent to their antimicrobial activity. The

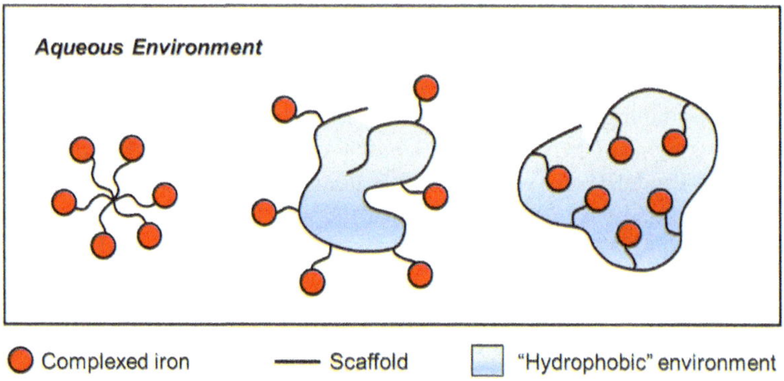

Fig. 8.11 Hypothetical folding scenarios of 3-hydroxypyridin-4-one polymeric chelators following iron binding

antimicrobial polymeric materials reported so far have their metal chelating moieties anchored in different ways. The dendrimers have the metal chelating moieties stemming from a central scaffold (Zhou et al. 2014) whereas in the linear polymers, they are appended along a backbone (Zhou et al. 2015a; Li et al. 2016; Ang et al. 2018). The hexadentate 3-hydroxypyridin-4-one chelators contain hydrogen bonding groups that would facilitate the complexed iron to point towards the surrounding aqueous environment. With the dendrimers, this would be more apparent as the chelators are fixed in position. The iron binding moieties of the RAFT PGMA polymers with pegylated side chains would be susceptible to point into the surrounding aqueous environment, in addition to the backbone having limited water solubility. With DIBI, the reverse is exhibited, its backbone is more highly water soluble than the chelating groups and upon iron binding, the complex could be masked by the PVP backbone and thus the iron is physically hidden from microbes. From this, different folding architectures can be speculated that discern the interplay of the complexed iron relating to the polymeric structure and surrounding aqueous environment (Fig. 8.11). It can be hypothesized that in addition to the polymeric chelators being unrecognizable by microbes, the inaccessibility of the complexed iron can be instrumental to the antimicrobial efficacy. This feature of DIBI appears to account for its very high antimicrobial activity, i.e., >1000X higher than deferiprone or its component MAHMP monomer.

8.5.3 Low Host Toxicity

New higher molecular weight (>1500 Da) chelators should have less host toxicity issues than those known low molecular weight (<1500 Da) hematological chelators (deferoxamine, deferiprone, deferasirox) on the basis that these larger molecules do not readily enter into host cells to directly affect host intracellular iron pools but rather primarily affect extracellular iron pools being accessed by microbial invaders. To date, relatively few of the new microbial specific iron chelator candidates reviewed above, have been tested for their host toxicity, except in the case of polymeric DIBI (Parquet et al. 2019). Testing using the Organization for Economic Co-operation and Development (OECD)-prescribed oral and systemic toxicity testing protocols in male and female rats has exhibited no observable adverse effects (NOAEL) from DIBI with 14 day repeated oral or systemic dosing at the highest doses tested (1000 mg/kg/day oral and 200 mg/kg/day intravenous) (Parquet et al. 2019).

It is also important to note that unlike the use of hematological chelators used to treat iron overload disorders that require long term use, iron sequestration anti-infective therapeutics would likely be used only on a relatively short term basis, i.e., to treat active infection. This therapy approach for iron sequestrants therefore would be somewhat analogous to the therapeutic regimens now used for conventional antibiotics. This treatment approach would lessen the prospect for disruption of normal host iron homeostasis that might occur with prolonged use of an iron sequestrant.

8.6 Antibiotic Resistance and Microbial Iron Needs

8.6.1 Resistance Mechanisms

Antibiotic resistance results from several discrete mechanisms that can arise within a microbe or be acquired from other microbes by transfer of genetic material (for a recent review (Schroeder et al. 2017)). The main antibiotic resistance mechanisms are summarized in Table 8.3. From these various possibilities, it can be appreciated that antibiotic resistance can be due to antibiotic degradation by the microbe, systems to thwart antibiotic uptake into microbes or mutational changes leading to altered target structures to which antibiotics are no longer effective. Of importance is that these various mechanisms all require some degree of microbial growth and/or microbial metabolic or synthetic activities for their expression. Therefore, these mechanisms would each have varying degrees of dependence on the activity of iron dependent enzymes. Thus, iron withdrawal that would restrict adequate production and supply of these iron dependent microbial enzymes could also affect expression of these resistance mechanisms. Examples of key iron dependent enzymes are ribonucleotide reductase needed for DNA repair/synthesis; cytochrome oxidase needed for ATP energy production or citrate aconitase needed in the TCA cycle. Deficiencies in these critical enzymes could be expected to generally suppress the expression of the various antibiotic resistance mechanisms.

Table 8.3 Main mechanisms of antibiotic resistance and known and possible effects of iron withdrawal

Resistance mechanism	Nature of resistance	(Reference)	Likely affected by iron withdrawal?
Antibiotic neutralization	Enzymes produced by microbes modify/degrade antibiotic rendering it inactive	β-lactam degradation and aminoglycoside modifications (Wright 2005); metallo-β-lactamase, and aminoglycoside acetyltransferase in *A. baumannii*	Presumably yes as enzyme induction requires RNA and protein synthesis utilizing iron dependent enzymes
Antibiotic target modification	Mutations providing altered non-sensitive microbial target	Mupirocin resistance in *S. aureus* from altered insensitive isoleucine-tRNA synthetase target (Liu et al. 2017)	Presumably yes as low iron can suppress Fe-dependent ribonucleotide reductase levels as needed for DNA synthesis and repair
Antibiotic efflux pumps	Reduced intracellular antibiotic concentration, exclusion from cell	Ciprofloxacin and other fluoroquinolone efflux in *P. aeruginosa* (Lubelski et al. 2007; Amaral et al. 2013)	Yes, iron withdrawal can affect energy production by iron-dependent enzymes and iron insufficiency causes membrane instability (Prasad et al. 2006)
Physical resistance to antibiotic delivery into microbes	Biofilm growth physically protecting microbes within biofilm	*P. aeruginosa* biofilm displays resistance (Gupta et al. 2016)	Yes, iron withdrawal can suppress biofilm formation and also disrupt established biofilm growth (Post et al. 2019)
Metabolic mutation; persister cells	Slower growth and reduced electron transport reduces antibiotic sensitivity	*S. aureus* small colony variants – hemin/menadione and thymidine auxotrophs display multiple resistance (Proctor et al. 1998, 2014)	Yes, deferiprone-Gallium active against *S. aureus* SCVs, particularly hemin auxotrophs (Richter et al. 2017)

8.6.2 Antibiotic Resistance Is Separate to Microbial Iron Needs

Important for potential iron withdrawal therapies for antibiotic resistant infections are that the various mechanisms leading to antibiotic resistance do not also lead to changes (in particular reduction) in microbial iron requirements, i.e. over those of their antibiotic sensitive counterparts, i.e., antibiotic resistance does not alter iron needs or sensitivity to iron withdrawal by a chelator. This appears to be the case and the results summarized in Table 8.4 demonstrate this point broadly. Here, iron needs as reflected by sensitivity to iron withdrawal using hydroxypyridinone chelators are

Table 8.4 Antibiotic resistant and sensitive microbial pathogens share similar susceptibilities to iron withdrawal by different hydroxypyridinone (HPO) chelators

Microbial pathogen	Clinical isolate	Antibiotic sensitivity or resistance	Antibiotic type: MIC μM	HPO chelator type: MIC μM
Acinetobacter baumannii	LAC-4	Multiple Resistance	CIP: 193[a] GEN: 134[a]	DIBI: 0.2[a]
	ATCC19606	Sensitive	CIP: 3[a] GEN: 16.7[a]	DIBI: 0.2[a] DFP: 575[b] DFP: 920[c]
	LAC-15	Multiple Resistance	GEN: 4.2[a] CIP: >772[a] CST: >443 [a]	DIBI: 0.2[a]
	ATCC17978	Sensitive	CIP: 3[a] GEN: 2.1[a] CST: 1.7 [a]	DFP: 460[c] DIBI: 0.2[a]
Staphylococcus aureus	ATCC43300	MRSA Multiple Resistance	AMP: 92[d]	DFP: 287[e] DIBI: 0.2[e]
	ATCC25923	Sensitive	AMP: 2.0 [f] MUP: 0.5[g]	DFP: 287[e] DIBI: 0.2[e]
	CDC0563	MUP Resistant	MUP: 1023[h]	DIBI 0.2[h]
	CDC0563-MupA	MUP Sensitive plasmid-less clone	MUP: 6[h]	DIBI 0.2[h]
Candida albicans	LP1158-07	FLU Resistant	FLU: >209[i]	DIBI 0.2[i]
	96113	FLU Sensitive	FLU: 1.6[i]	DIBI 0.2[i]
	SC5314	FLU Sensitive	FLU: 1.6[i]	DFP: 1149[i] DIBI: 0.2[i]

MIC (minimum inhibitory concentration), *CIP* (ciprofloxacin), *GEN* (gentamicin), *CST* (colistin), *AMP* (ampicillin), *MUP* (mupirocin), *FLU* (fluconazole), *DFP* (deferiprone), *DIBI* (HPO copolymer)

[a]Parquet et al. (2019)
[b]Ang et al. (2018)
[c]Thompson et al. (2012)
[d]Chhibber et al. (2014)
[e]Parquet et al. (2018)
[f]Kang et al. (2011)
[g]Sutherland et al. (1985)
[h]Allan et al. (2020)
[i]Savage et al. (2018)

shown for various microbial pathogens (both bacteria and fungi). These results show the sensitivity to an iron chelator of a clinical microbial isolate with a known (reported) antibiotic resistance (i.e., a high Minimum Inhibitory Concentration (MIC) for the particular antibiotic) in comparison to the chelator sensitivity of a related isolate with a known sensitivity to the same antibiotic (i.e., low MIC for the particular antibiotic). These results underscore several important aspects of using iron withdrawal as a therapy for antibiotic resistant microbial pathogens. In the case of isogenic *S. aureus* isolates, either a gain or a loss of mupirocin resistance resulted in no change in DIBI sensitivity and thus the iron requirement of the isolates.

Importantly, the presence or absence of resistance to broadly different antibiotics (i.e., different chemical classes of antibiotics) for broadly different microbes (both Gram positive and Gram negative) did not reflect changes in iron needs based on sensitivity to the hydroxypyridinone chelators tested.

The requirement of iron for growth has been tested and shown to be similar for both antibiotic sensitive and antibiotic resistant microbes including for example, isolates of *C. albicans* (Savage et al. 2018), *S. aureus* (Parquet et al. 2018) and *A. baumannii* (Parquet et al. 2019). These studies have shown microbial growth rates and response to iron are similar for antibiotic resistant isolates as compared to their antibiotic sensitive sister isolates.

Based on these various results, iron dependence of pathogenic microbes including antibiotic resistant isolates represent an Achilles' heel for microbes. Exploiting this susceptibility with new iron withdrawal agents that can complement innate host iron withdrawal defenses has substantial potential to address our antibiotic resistance infection problem.

8.6.3 Antibiotic Resistance, Persisters, Bacterial Stress Response and Implications for Iron Withdrawal

Bacterial responses to antibiotic exposure have important implications for antibiotic resistance development. Exposure of bacteria to antibiotics is known to trigger emergence of antibiotic resistant persister cells which may represent a minor subpopulation of an originally present, resistant phenotype that becomes positively enriched in the presence of the antibiotic (Michiels et al. 2016). Alternatively, antibiotic resistant persister Small Colony Variants (SCVs) can arise from accelerated mutations triggered by DNA damage resulting from exposure to an antibiotic. This response has been regarded as part of the generalized SOS stress response as observed from stress caused by various agents (Torres-Barcelo et al. 2015; Maslowska et al. 2019). Interestingly, intracellular free iron plays a role in the generation of Reactive Oxygen Species (ROS) but bacterial defense against ROS also requires catalase and superoxide dismutase both of which are iron dependent enzymes. Additionally, repair of DNA damage involves ribonucleotide reductase which is another enzyme that is iron dependent for activity.

SCV isolates obtained from clinical specimens following treatment of infected human patients with β-lactams and aminoglycosides often have menadione or hemin auxotrophy, whereas thymidine auxotrophy is typically seen in SCVs from patients treated with anti-folates (Proctor et al. 2014). Importantly, regardless of the initial drug treatment which induced the SCV phenotype, these variants often have cross resistance to other unrelated antibiotics due to their altered metabolism and electron gradient deficiency (Proctor et al. 1998; Garcia et al. 2013; Richter et al. 2017).

Bactericidal antibiotics such as ciprofloxacin induce oxidative stress that can damage iron sulfur clusters (Kohanski et al. 2007; Jensen et al. 2014). Substantial evidence that ciprofloxacin induces mutations leading to resistance via ROS- and iron dependent mechanisms has been obtained in *E. coli*, where *Δfur* and *ΔsodAB* knockout mutants, with loss of iron homeostasis control leading to accumulation of intracellular iron, or loss of superoxide dismutase activity, respectively, both had significantly higher rates of ciprofloxacin resistant mutations following ciprofloxacin exposure compared to wild type (Méhi et al. 2014). Ciprofloxacin and related fluoroquinoline antibiotic structures are known to bind iron (Kara et al. 1991; Heeb et al. 2010) and could hypothetically bring ROS-reactive iron into the bacterial cytoplasm following uptake.

Ciprofloxacin has been shown to be mutagenic in *S. aureus*, increasing both mutation rates and DNA recombination, via activation of RecA, which functions directly in DNA repair, as well as auto cleavage of repressor molecule LexA, allowing the induction of the SOS response, including the error prone UmuC type polymerase (Cirz et al. 2007; Schroder et al. 2013). Topoisomerase IV (GrlA) is the primary target of ciprofloxacin in Gram positive bacteria, and this enzyme functions in assisting DNA replication (along with DNA gyrase, the secondary CIP target). Thus, interference with GrlA leads to DNA damage that requires repair (Heeb et al. 2010). RecA repairs DNA by binding damaged DNA, and forming a stabilized nucleoprotein filament, which then acts as a template for repair, a process which is made possible in Gram positive bacteria by AddAB (RecBCD in Gram negatives), a nuclease which acts via an essential iron-sulfur cluster to bind DNA fragments and yields the RecA substrate (Yeeles et al. 2009).

Implicitly the above mechanisms leading to antibiotic resistance would require growth as well as metabolic and macromolecular synthesis activity and thus, would require adequate supply of key iron dependent enzymes. Therefore, iron sequestration sufficient to limit the adequate supply of some or all of these key enzymes might be expected to suppress these resistance mechanisms. However, there have been conflicting reports in the literature as to the influence of iron supply and the effects of iron chelators on both antibiotic activity and the formation of antibiotic resistant persister cells (reviewed by Ezraty and Barras 2016). These authors have pointed out the likely issues for these conflicting results stem from the different testing methods utilized.

Previous studies have often used chelator addition testing where small molecule iron chelators are added to ostensibly sequester iron *in situ* to then test for the effects on persister cell formation or +/− effects on antibiotic activity. We believe that this approach of addition of small molecule chelators to cultures to sequester iron *in situ* is problematic for a number of reasons. Small molecules including 2,2-dipyridyl, bathophenanthroline-sulfonate, deferoxamine and deferiprone do chelate iron but these are either relatively poor at inhibiting microbial growth, i.e., requiring rather high concentrations or, are totally ineffective at sequestering bio-available iron as measured by their effects on microbial growth restriction (see above Sect. 8.4.5). This problem has been demonstrated for *Candida albicans* (Holbein and Mira de Orduña 2010; Savage et al. 2018) and for various bacteria (Ang et al. 2018;

Thompson et al. 2012). Our view is that *in situ* chelation of iron with small molecule chelators that can readily enter microbial cells, i.e., those mentioned above, may not appropriately restrict iron availability to microbes and the results from their use should be interpreted with caution.

An alternate approach has been referred to as the medium approach (Ezraty and Barras 2016) and this has provided quite different results from the chelator addition approach. However, this too has recognized issues because Chelex-100 resin as has often been used to extract and physically remove iron from culture medium is not iron specific and is known to also affect various other trace essential metals.

We have overcome the above issues using two alternative approaches both of which employ novel chemically related iron selective 3-hydroxypyridin-4-one-functionalized chelating polymers. 3-Hydroxypyridin-4-one chelators are more specific for iron than imidodiacetate chelators such as EDTA and its chemical cousin resins, e.g., Chelex-100. For our first approach, a medium extraction based approach, FEC-1, a hydrophilic but water insoluble macroreticular resin, is used to selectively remove iron from the culture medium. The utility of this *ex situ* approach has been demonstrated by growth restoration upon re-addition of only iron to FEC-1 extracted media that would not otherwise support growth for *C. albicans* (Holbein and Mira de Orduña 2010), *S. aureus* (Parquet et al. 2018) and *A. baumannii* (Parquet et al. 2019). Our second approach employs use of FEC-1's close chemical cousin, DIBI which in contrast, is water soluble but being 9 kDa M_w cannot readily enter microbial cells. Thus, DIBI addition provides *in situ* iron sequestration as a soluble extracellular iron sink. DIBI has been shown to be >1000X more growth inhibitory than deferiprone, for example, only 0.2 μM DIBI was growth inhibitory for *A. baumannii* in contrast to deferiprone which required 575 μM for growth inhibition (Ang et al. 2018). DIBI at low concentrations has been shown not to interfere with antibiotic activity but rather it synergistically enhances activity of various antibiotics. Also, of significance is DIBI suppresses regrowth of antibiotic exposed bacteria.

8.7 Iron Withdrawal Is Effective for Antibiotic Resistant Microbes

8.7.1 Iron Chelators Inhibit Both Antibiotic Sensitive and Resistant Microbial Pathogens

A key requirement for the use of iron chelators against antibiotic resistant microbial pathogens is the need for adequate activity against these pathogens. Various iron chelators have been tested for their anti-microbial activities as reviewed in Sect. 8.4. However, in many of the studies reported the antibiotic resistance profiles of the test microorganisms were not reported and importantly, useful comparative results for a comparable antibiotic sensitive isolate were often not available. Synthetic hydroxypyridinone chelators have shown the most promise as new antimicrobials as was discussed in Sect. 8.5.1. Table 8.4 summarizes the reported sensitivities of various microbes to this class of chelators along with known (tested) antibiotic resistance attributes of the isolate tested. Both Minimum Inhibitory Concentration (MIC) data for key antibiotics and for the chelators are summarized. Multiple Drug Resistant (MDR) *A. baumannii* isolates had *in vitro* sensitivities to low M_w deferiprone (DFP) or to polymeric DIBI that were quite similar to those found for comparable antibiotic sensitive strains, tested under similar conditions. Important in this regard, is that resistance or sensitivity to members of widely different chemical classes of antibiotics, including fluoroquinolines (ciprofloxacin, CIP), aminoglycosides (gentamicin, GEN), polymyxins (colistin, CST), β-lactams (ampicillin, AMP), carboxylic acids (mupirocin, MUP) and azoles (fluconazole, FLU) for important Gram negative, Gram positive and fungal pathogens did not reflect significant differences in sensitivity to iron withdrawal by these hydroxypyridinone chelators. Thus, it appears that resistance to particular or to multiple antibiotics does not indicate altered microbial iron requirements or loss of sensitivity to iron withdrawal, i.e., through possible cross resistance to the chelators. Studies with other hydroxypyridinone class chelators including small molecule hexadentate monomers and their corresponding polymers indicate this aspect will likely hold true for additional bacterial pathogens including the *Enterobacteriaceae* (Zhou et al. 2015a, b). Unfortunately, the possible resistance characteristics of the additional bacterial species as tested by these authors were not reported and the needed comparison data to their antibiotic sensitive cohorts were not reported.

Based on the available evidence it appears reasonable to conclude that antibiotic resistant microbes have similar iron needs and thus, they will have similar sensitivity to iron withdrawal agents as their antibiotic sensitive counterparts.

8.7.2 *Iron Chelators Suppress Infection from Antibiotic Resistant Microbes*

Another key requirement for iron withdrawal agents regarding their potential use as anti-infective alternatives to antibiotics is their ability to suppress infection as caused by antibiotic resistant microbes, i.e. in addition to any demonstrated *in vitro* activity. This key aspect has seen only limited study to date, but a number of recent studies have demonstrated that novel chelators do possess useful *in vivo* anti-infective activities against antibiotic resistant pathogens. Fig. 8.12 summarizes findings from several such studies. The hydroxypyridinone DIBI has been shown to suppress both wound and nares topical infection with antibiotic resistant *S. aureus* in mice with 2 days of topical treatment (i.e., DIBI application to the wound or intranasally respectively) at approximately 10 μmol/kg per day. The wound infection model utilized for this study was first established to validate fusidic acid efficacy (Kugelberg et al. 2005) and the results with DIBI showed comparable bacterial burden reductions to that reported by these authors for fusidic acid. The nares

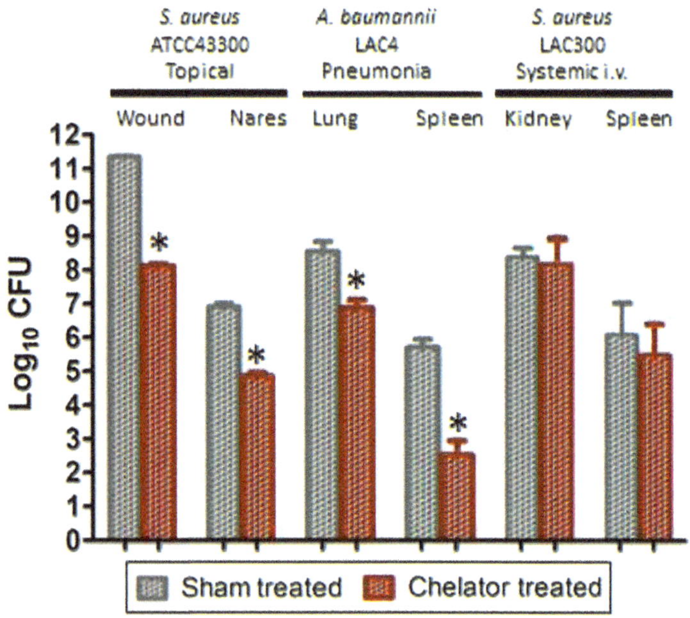

Fig. 8.12 Iron chelators suppress infection from both Gram positive and Gram negative antibiotic resistant bacteria
Mice infected topically with antibiotic resistant MRSA *S. aureus* ATCC 43300 on either skin wounds or on their anterior nares were treated with the chelator DIBI as described previously (Parquet et al. 2018) and bacterial burdens after 5 days were compared to sham treated (vehicle treated only) groups. The stars show significant reductions in bacterial burdens compared to the sham treatment. Mice infected intranasally with *A. baumannii* antibiotic resistant isolate LAC4 to initiate pneumonia followed by septicemia as reported by Parquet et al. (2019) were treated intranasally once with DIBI or sham treated with only vehicle and bacterial burdens after 24 h infection were determined for both lungs and spleens. The stars show significant reductions in bacterial burdens compared to the sham treatment. In other testing reported by Luo et al. (2014) mice were injected intravenously with *S. aureus* MRSA antibiotic resistant isolate LAC300 to initiate a systemic infection and bacterial burdens in kidneys and spleens were compared in groups treated with either Deferasirox (DEF) or placebo (sham treated). In those studies, DEF tended to reduce bacterial burdens but the results were not found to be statistically significant (the results as graphed are based only on estimates of bacterial burdens taken from the Luo publication). All these various infection studies show that iron chelators on their own can suppress infection for various antibiotic resistant bacterial infections

carriage model utilized was described by Chhibber et al. (2014) and DIBI was found to reduce nares burdens comparably or better than that reported for mupirocin, noting mupirocin is currently clinically used in man for decolonization of MRSA (Humphreys et al. 2016). Reductions of MRSA bacterial burdens with these discrete infections, i.e., in different body compartments of BALB/C mice, were significant as compared to sham treated controls. Separately, deferasirox (DEF) has been shown to suppress experimental systemic infection in mice caused by antibiotic resistant *S. aureus* MRSA including a vancomycin (VAN) resistant clinical isolate

(Luo et al. 2014). A 2-day intravenous treatment course with approximately 10 μmol/kg/day deferasirox resulted in a reduced (although not statistically significant) bacterial burden in both kidneys and spleens of infected mice (Fig. 8.12). Consistent with these various studies, *S. aureus* has been shown to upregulate its iron acquisition mechanisms during growth in the nares (Chaves-Moreno et al. 2016) and during systemic infection (Bacconi et al. 2017).

In a separate study of experimental pneumonia/septicemia in BALB/C mice caused by intranasal introduction of a hypervirulent antibiotic resistant isolate of *A. baumannii* DIBI reductions of *A. baumannii* bacterial burdens in both the lung and spleen (see Fig. 8.12) were comparable to those obtained with tigecycline (TGC) an antibiotic to which this isolate is highly susceptible (Parquet et al. 2019). Importantly, *A. baumannii* has also been shown to upregulate its iron acquisition systems during infection (Gaddy et al. 2012) indicating iron supply is important to this infection.

These various infection studies with antibiotic resistant bacteria demonstrate that growth of these bacteria during infection is at least partially iron restricted by host iron withdrawal defenses causing these pathogens to upregulate their iron acquisition mechanisms and in turn ensuring their sensitivity to iron sequestering chelator addition. Given the findings that iron chelators such as deferasirox or hydroxypyridinones suppress infection, it seems reasonable that these chelators might play a role in bolstering natural innate iron withdrawal defense mechanisms to various other infections.

8.7.3 Antimicrobial Iron Chelators Do Not Impede But Can Enhance Antibiotic Activities

Yet another important aspect in considering the use of iron withdrawal chelators as alternatives to antibiotics is that these, if co-administered with conventional antibiotics, should not interfere with the activities of antibiotics. A clear additional benefit would be that chelators through withdrawing microbial iron supplies would improve the activities of conventional antibiotics including towards antibiotic resistant isolates. These desired attributes have now been demonstrated in various studies.

Some of the first convincing evidence that iron withdrawal agents would not interfere but rather could positively affect antibiotic action for antibiotic resistant isolates was in relation to lactoferrin, the host iron binding defense protein for *S. aureus* isolates from bovine mastitis. Diarra et al. (2002) demonstrated that lactoferrin as naturally found in mammary and other body mucosal secretions, synergistically improved the activity of penicillin including against penicillin resistant isolates. This suggested a potential therapeutic use of lactoferrin along with antibiotics to treat bovine mastitis and this showed clinical promise (Lacasse et al. 2008). However, clinical use of lactoferrin (or other transferrin class proteins) has yet to prove practical, possibly due to issues related to larger scale collection and purification for use in man or other animals.

Synthetic chelators do offer better potential for large scale and more cost-effective production as well as for more robust safety and quality assurance. In this regard, studies by Moreau–Marquis et al. (2009) demonstrated that either of the clinically approved iron chelators deferoxamine (DFO) or deferasirox (DEF) in combination with tobramycin resulted in a 90% reduction in biofilm growth of antibiotic resistant *P. aeruginosa* while none of these agents were fully effective on their own. In addition, using checkerboard plate cross titration assays, Zarember et al. (2009) showed deferiprone (DFP) synergized in growth inhibition activity with ketoconazole against *Aspergillus fumigatus*. Novel hydroxypyridinone iron chelators such as MRH7 have also been shown to enhance antibacterial activity of ethambutol for *Mycobacterium avium* growing in macrophages, suggesting a potential for iron chelators to also address intracellular bacterial infections (Moniz et al. 2015).

To conclude as to a useful synergy between an iron chelator (or any other adjunct) with an antibiotic(s) the gold standard test is the time/kill kinetic assay as typically applied to test bactericidal antibiotics. In these tests, a somewhat reduced concentration of antibiotic or test chelator are typically used separately, i.e., so that each agent on its own does not provide complete killing when added to a relatively high number of rapidly growing log phase bacterial cells. This testing approach then allows a better assessment of the combined agent affects. It is important to note that while many antibiotics are bactericidal in action, chelators are fundamentally different in action. Chelators are not primarily bactericidal but deny access to growth essential iron and therefore killing by these agents would be delayed compared to bactericidal antibiotics and later, due to iron insufficiency, bacterial death would likely result from physiological apoptosis.

Both clinically approved DEF and hydroxypyridinone DIBI have been shown not to interfere with but to synergistically enhance antibiotic killing activity against various antibiotic resistant bacteria as discussed below. To allow a better appreciation of these kinetic kill studies, an example using gentamicin (GEN) with *A. baumannii* is shown in Fig. 8.13 (results as adapted from Parquet et al. 2019). Note for this testing, GEN was added at 1XMIC (i.e., at GEN minimum inhibitory concentration) and on its own this provided only partial initial killing followed by strong recovery growth to near control bacterial colony forming units (CFU)/mL by 24 h.

Importantly, this recovery growth phenomenon following antibiotic exposure has clinical relevance in relation to the development of antibiotic resistance. Antibiotics are usually administered at a relatively high dose, i.e., multiple of MIC but later during a treatment course, due to antibiotic clearance etc., concentrations can wane. Thus, if bacterial survivors are present under these conditions, they can more likely regrow. Additionally, this condition of suboptimal antibiotic concentration would favour selection and outgrowth of antibiotic resistant survivors.

Thus, while synergistic activity providing additional initial killing is important, the possible prevention of survivor regrowth following antibiotic exposure is also very important. In the example shown in Fig. 8.13 the chelator DIBI was also tested at a low concentration that was insufficient on its own to fully arrest growth of the rapidly dividing log phase cells, noting that the initial high number of bacterial cells would have been iron-replete and therefore iron withdrawal would be expected to ensue only after some continued growth/replication. However, the addition of both GEN and

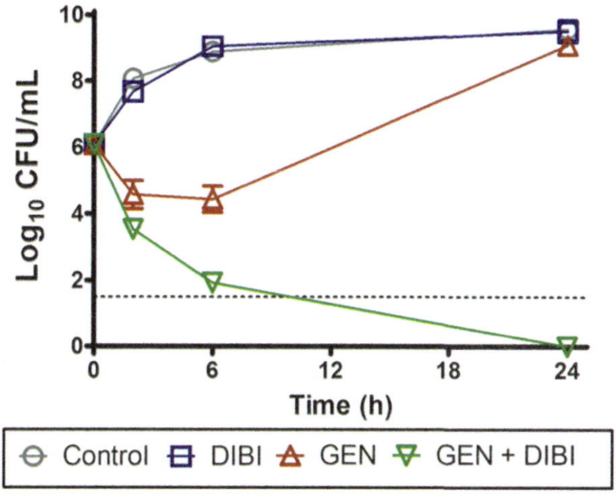

Fig. 8.13 Example of a time kill kinetic assay showing chelator enhancement of antibiotic killing and prevention of survivor re-growth
A. baumannii ATCC17978 which is sensitive to the aminoglycoside Gentamicin (GEN) (Minimum Inhibitory Concentration (MIC) = 1 μg/mL) was exposed to 0.5 μg/mL GEN (i.e., ½ MIC) and this caused only partial killing of the population followed by rapid recovery growth that reached near untreated control Colony Forming Units (CFU) levels by 24 h of exposure. The DIBI concentration used in this experiment was 20 μg/mL and this on its own did not affect total CFU by 24 h. It should be noted that a large rapidly growing iron replete bacterial population had been introduced at 0 h and gross effects of DIBI on bacterial numbers would not be expected under these test conditions. However, this DIBI treatment exhibited effects of iron withdrawal as evident when DIBI was applied in combination with GEN. The GEN/DIBI combination resulted in extensive and continued bacterial killing with no detectable CFU remaining at 24 h exposure. (Results adapted from Parquet et al. 2019)

DIBI showed a strong synergistic activity of the two agents with the combination providing continued killing which was complete by 24 h (no detectable CFU at 24 h).

The 24 h measurement point in a time/kill assay also has significance as it is generally accepted (i.e., defined by the American Society for Microbiology) that synergy of two anti-infectives is confirmed if there is ≥ 2 log CFU reduction provided by the combination by 24 h incubation, i.e., as compared to untreated control or to individual agent related CFU reductions at 24 h. In the example in Fig. 8.13, the combination of GEN+DIBI resulted in a >8 log reduction in bacterial CFU by 24 h. Note, had the combination proved to be antagonistic, then survivor/growth for the combination would have been higher than those for either GEN or DIBI alone.

Similar patterns of time/kill responses have been reported for MRSA using VAN and DEF (Luo et al. 2014), for *Vibrio vulnificus* using ciprofloxacin (CIP) and DEF (Neupane and Kim 2010), for *A. baumannii* using DIBI with various other antibiotics (Parquet et al. 2019) and for *S. aureus* using DIBI with various antibiotics (Parquet et al. 2018). The ability of different iron chelators to synergize with various antibiotics, i.e., as representative of various chemically distinct classes and for different genera of bacteria is of broad significance. We have summarized various findings demonstrating this in Table 8.5. Importantly, in all the cases tested, DEF or DIBI

Table 8.5 Synergy of iron withdrawal chelators with antibiotics as determined with time/kill kinetic assays

Bacterium tested	Antibiotic character	Antibiotic tested	Chelator tested	Log_{10} CFU at 24 h				Log_{10} change	Synergy[b]	Ref
				Control	Antibiotic	Chelator	Combination	combination[a]		
A. baumannii 17978	Sensitive	CIP	DIBI	9.79	7.99	9.39	5.41	−2.58	yes	c
A. baumannii 17978	Sensitive	GEN	DIBI	9.58	9.10	9.52	0	−9.10	yes	c
A. baumannii 17978	Sensitive	TGC	DIBI	10.03	8.88	9,80	4.10	−4.78	yes	c
A. baumannii 17978	Sensitive	CST	DIBI	9.79	9.30	9.39	1.78	−7.52	yes	c
A. baumannii LAC-4	MDR CIPresistant	CIP	DIBI	9.36	8.96	9.52	6.88	−2.16	yes	c
S. aureus LAC300	MRSA	VAN	DEF	11.5	11.3	8.7	5.5	−3.20	yes	d
S. aureus Mu50	VISA resistant	VAN	DEF	11.2	10.5	9.2	5.5	−3.70	yes	d
S. aureus 6538	sensitive	VAN	DIBI	8.06	6.57	6.83	4.87	−1.70	mild	e
S. aureus 43300	MRSA	MUP	DIBI	9.10	7.65	8.39	6.2	−1.45	mild	f
V. vulnificus 27562	Sensitive	CIP	DEF	10.0	8.70	6.60	3.80	−2.80	yes	g
V. vulnificus 33815	Sensitive	CIP	DEF	11.0	8.90	9.80	3.70	−6.10	yes	g
V. vulnificus CUH 42-14	Sensitive	CIP	DEF	11.0	10.0	6.10	3.80	−2.30	yes	g

CFU Colony Forming Units, *CIP* (ciprofloxacin), *GEN* (gentamicin); CST (colistin), *TGC* (tigecycline), *MUP* (mupirocin), *VAN* (vancomycin), *DEF* (deferasirox), *DIBI* (HPO copolymer), *MDR* multiple drug resistant, *MRSA* Methicillin resistant *S. aureus*, *VISA* Vancomycin resistant *S. aureus*

[a]+/- Log_{10} CFU change of combination over the higher of either antibiotic or chelator alone

[b]Synergy if change of combination ≥2 $-log_{10}$ CFU; weak synergy at <−2 but >−1 $-log_{10}$CFU

[c]Parquet et al. (2019)

[d]Luo et al. 2014 (values shown are estimated from authors Fig. 8.1b, d)

[e]Parquet et al. (2018)

[f]Allan et al. (2020)

[g]Neupane and Kim 2010 (values shown are only estimates from their Fig. 8.1)

did not impede antibiotic killing but typically improved or extended the antibiotic killing phase. When either DEF or DIBI was present with these various antibiotics, recovery growth was also greatly suppressed, noting that recovery growth was typically observed with only antibiotic exposure. Among the results above, killing with the chelator/antibiotic combinations was not always complete by 24 h but the combination treatment typically strongly restricted recovery. For some isolates (including antibiotic sensitive ones), the antibiotic/chelator pairs exhibited a less pronounced synergy (log_{10}CFU reduction >1 but <2) but antagonism was not found for any. The reader is encouraged to review the various time/kill results provided in these various studies given the importance of the synergistic interactions of iron chelators with conventionally used antibiotics.

On the basis of the various results summarized in Table 8.5 and results from other investigations mentioned above, new therapeutics that function to withdraw microbial iron have high potential to work in conjunction with conventional antibiotics for improving antibiotic responses, including against antibiotic resistant bacteria. There is also an important potential benefit for these chelator/antibiotic combinations as to reducing the very conditions that promote the opportunity for developing antibiotic resistance during infection. This important latter aspect is further discussed in future prospects below.

8.8 Prospects and Future Directions

New generation iron chelators especially those with 3-hydroxypyridin-4-one functionality have excellent potential to become stand-alone anti-infectives. Many of those proposed to date have yet to be adequately tested *in vitro* let alone for their *in vivo* antimicrobial efficacy or for their host toxicity and hopefully, such studies will now be forthcoming. Among the various candidates, the novel hydroxypyridinone copolymer, DIBI, has seen substantial development and has demonstrated a low toxicity profile for animals. It like other synthetic chelators such as deferasirox also appears to complement and boost the host's natural iron withdrawal defense mechanisms during various microbial infections. The prospect for microbes developing resistance to iron sequestering agents seems highly unlikely. Iron is not substitutable in an array of discrete iron dependent enzymes, these being irreplaceably needed by microbes. Genes for microbial siderophore production are generally chromosomal and not plasmid carried and there are many discrete genes needed to elaborate the complex siderophore chemical structures shown in this chapter. Interestingly, in this regard testing with DIBI has shown no evidence for resistance development to DIBI after multiple growth passages in the presence of a partially inhibitory concentration of DIBI that restricted but yet still permitted slowed growth of *S. aureus* (Allan et al. 2020). The various attributes of these novel chelators open the prospects for using new agents such as DIBI in several different therapeutic contexts and for various infections.

8.8.1 Prophylactics for Human Infection

Prophylactic decolonization of MRSA with mupirocin (MUP) for hospitalized patients is already employed and it has demonstrated a reduced incidence of post-operative infection (Humphreys et al. 2016). However, wider use of MUP has led to increased incidence of MUP resistance (Antonov et al. 2015) and therefore, it would be desirable to obtain clearance of staphylococci with alternative agents avoiding MUP. Recent studies (Allan et al. 2020) have shown that DIBI performs as well as mupirocin for experimental nares clearance of *S. aureus* in mice, providing proof of concept of it as an alternate to mupirocin for prophylactic decolonization of the nares.

8.8.2 Adjuncts with Antibiotics

Iron chelators have been shown to enhance antibiotic activity, with both deferasirox (DEF) and DIBI showing ability to synergistically enhance antibiotic activity *in vitro* and *in vivo*. Thus, DEF, DIBI and possibly other new antimicrobial chelators now in development have potential to serve as adjuncts to various conventional antibiotics. Such new adjunct formulations of existing antibiotics might serve to extend the usage life of conventional antibiotics and help address treatment needs for antibiotic resistant infections.

8.8.3 Suppression of Antibiotic Resistance Formation and Transfer

As was discussed above in Sect. 8.6.3, antibiotic resistant survivors and persister cells pose a significant problem with antibiotic therapy. For example, staphylococcal Small Colony Variants (SCVs) have been identified in various recurrent nosocomial infections (Onyango and Alreshidi 2018). SCVs can occur naturally as a slow growing bacterial subpopulation that displays antibiotic resistance and these can persist and grow in the presence of antibiotic therapy. SCVs also arise in response to oxidative stress or from antibiotics that induce DNA damage such as ciprofloxacin (Painter et al. 2015; Acker and Coenye 2017). Because iron chelators suppress microbial recovery growth following antibiotic exposure, they can be expected to impact outgrowth of antibiotic resistant clones including antibiotic resistant persister cells and SCV survivors.

Given the suppression of recovery growth observed when iron chelators such as DIBI are present with antibiotics; we have carried out preliminary studies (unpublished results) as to the effects of DIBI on antibiotic resistant SCV formation.

S. aureus ATCC25923 treated with ciprofloxacin (CIP) at 2XMIC (Minimum Inhibitory Concentration) to provide a substantial initial killing was then incubated for up to 96 h for periodic sampling of survivor growth. The survivor population became progressively enriched in SCVs as identified by their pin-point colony morphology on blood agar. These SCV clones were phenotypically stable following re-growth on blood agar containing no antibiotic, taking 48 h to produce visible isolated colonies (24 h longer than normal), suggesting that a genetic mutation had occurred. When DIBI was present alone or with CIP, few if any SCVs were recovered. Six clones from each test condition were then tested for their MICs to CIP, DIBI, and to other antibiotics, The CIP induced SCVs were found to have CIP MICs in the range of 1–2 μg/mL, i.e., representing a 4- to 16-fold increase in the MIC of the untreated control clones and therefore possessing CIP resistance. Interesting, the survivor population from the DIBI/CIP treatment was not enriched in SCVs and these survivor clones had normal CIP sensitivity. In addition, DIBI on its own did not result in any SCVs with survivors at 96 h showing normal colony morphology and normal CIP sensitivity. Interestingly, all the clones tested at 96 h regardless of the treatment applied, showed unaltered DIBI sensitivity, demonstrating no apparent formation of DIBI resistance when tested on its own or when with CIP. These encouraging studies are being pursued given their potential importance.

Interestingly, there appears to be a possible iron related basis for these findings. The polyphenolic flavonoid baicalein has been shown to significantly lower ciprofloxacin induced mutations, and to reduce RecA/LexA/UmuC expression, ROS generation, and ATP production (Peng et al. 2011). Baicalein acts a direct scavenger of radicals, and has antimicrobial effect attributed to inhibition of ATP synthase (Peng et al. 2011) but has also been characterized as an iron chelator that can form stable, inert complexes (Perez et al. 2009). Thus, a more effective iron chelator such as DIBI may have similar or stronger suppressing effects on ciprofloxacin induced mutations. Significantly, interference or inhibition of RecA has been proposed as an important strategic target for drug discovery to prevent repair of DNA damage induced by antibiotic treatment (Kohanski et al. 2007), so this potential mechanism of iron chelators warrants further confirmation and molecular characterization. It would be interesting to see if other iron withdrawing chelators also supress SCV formation given the potential benefit of preventing SCV or persister antibiotic resistance formation.

Horizontal transfer of antibiotic resistance genetic material by extrachromosomal DNA elements is a major mechanism for bacterial antibiotic resistance acquisition and spread in bacteria. For example, *S. aureus* antibiotic resistance genes are typically located on mobile genetic elements, particularly plasmids (Juhas 2015). Remarkably, plasmids examined from many strains isolated decades apart and on different continents appear to fall into three main families with high (98%) core homology, suggesting selective pressure has optimized plasmid content (Shearer et al. 2011). However, carrying plasmids is also known to present a fitness cost to a pathogen, i.e., in the absence of antibiotic exposure there is a tendency to shed plasmids to regain a fitness competitive growth edge (Peacock and Paterson 2014).

We hypothesized that appropriate iron withdrawal by novel chelators might increase (exacerbate) fitness costs for plasmid carrying antibiotic resistant bacteria and thus, might encourage plasmid loss. We have carried out simple preliminary testing to assess if DIBI exposure during bacterial growth might promote plasmid loss. Our testing with high level mupirocin resistant (MUP-A plasmid borne) MRSA isolates has shown that growth in a sub-inhibitory concentration of DIBI provides a slowed iron restricted growth and it does induce loss of the MUP-A plasmid at an elevated rate (unpublished results). These promising results warrant further investigation with other novel chelators, additional plasmid carrying antibiotic resistant isolates and with other bacteria, for example, *A. baumannii* carrying carbapenem resistance genes on plasmids. Should an iron chelator encourage plasmid antibiotic resistance loss or interfere with plasmid transfer it would open an important additional avenue to tackle antibiotic resistance in microbial pathogens.

8.8.4 Sepsis Therapy

Clinical treatment of sepsis is challenging for two reasons. First, antibiotic resistance of bacteria is increasing and along with this, incidence of sepsis is mounting as well. More concerning is until now there is no approved therapy available to treat the dysregulated immune response in sepsis. The only ever approved drug for sepsis therapy (drotrecogin alpha (activated) – Xigris®) was withdrawn from the market in 2011 (Martí-Carvajal et al. 2011). Therefore, there is a large unmet need to improve the outcome of this deadly disease. Preclinical data suggest promise for including iron sequestration agents in the therapy of sepsis in order to reduce bacterial growth, overcome antibiotic resistance, and dampen hyper-inflammatory Reactive Oxygen Species (ROS) production and tissue damage (Thorburn et al. 2017). However, the concept of reducing iron levels by iron sequestration agents often raises concerns by physicians and their patients, since physiologic iron levels are generally considered to be requires and optimal for health. However, we believe this may not apply for life-threatening conditions such as sepsis. Based on the available preclinical data, the combination of antibiotics and iron chelators has synergistic effects to fight infection and improve the immune response in sepsis (Islam et al. 2016). In addition, there is no doubt that under iron overload conditions, iron chelation is beneficial to reduce the risk of infections in humans (Schaible and Kaufmann 2004). Furthermore, because of the increased infection risk in the surgical patient, we encourage further investigation and development of iron sequestration agents in the perioperative prophylaxis regimen for infections.

8.9 Conclusions

The iron requirements and iron acquisition mechanisms of microbial pathogens are relatively distinct from antibiotic activity and antibiotic resistance mechanisms. These features provide the foundations for using iron withdrawal by iron sequestering chelators as a therapeutic means to suppress pathogen growth and address antibiotic resistant infection. Conventional clinically used iron chelators that were developed to treat hematological disorders in humans are not well suited for use as anti-infectives due to their limited antimicrobial activity and potential host toxicity issues. However, novel purpose designed antimicrobial higher molecular weight chelators based on 3-hydroxypyridin-4-one functionality can overcome these issues by primarily addressing iron pools that are accessed by microbes during infection and also by bolstering the innate host iron withdrawal mechanisms as already triggered to fight infection and without undue upset to overall host iron homeostasis. Furthermore, iron withdrawal antimicrobial chelators can enhance activities of conventional antibiotics extending their utility including for treatment of antibiotic resistant infections.

8.10 Dedication

This chapter is dedicated to the memory of Eugene D. Weinberg, Ph.D. (1922–2019). Gene was the father of iron and infection studies. His foundational review "Iron in Infection" (Weinberg 1978) spurred interest for research into pathogenesis and iron in many laboratories around the world and he was a mentor and friend to many.

References

Aali M., Dickson K, Zhou J, Holbein BE, Lehmann C (2019) Comparing the efficacy of the novel iron chelator, DIBI, with different classical iron chelators in murine poly-bacterial sepsis. Poster presented at: the 2019 annual meeting of the international anesthesia research society, Montréal, Canada

Acker HV, Coenye T (2017) The role of reactive oxygen species in antibiotic-mediated killing of bacteria. Trends Microbiol 25:456–466. https://doi.org/10.1016/j.tim.2016.12.008

Afeltra A, Caccavo D, Ferri GM, Addessi MA, De Rosa FG, Amoroso A, Bonomo L (1997) Expression of lactoferrin on human granulocytes: analysis with polyclonal and monoclonal antibodies. Clin Exp Immunol 109:279–285. https://doi.org/10.1046/j.1365-2249.1997.4351333.x

Allan DS, Del Carmen Parquet M, Savage KA, Holbein BE (2020) Iron sequestrant DIBI, a potential alternative for nares decolonization of methicillin-resistant Staphylococcus aureus, is anti-infective and inhibitory for mupirocin-resistant isolates. Antimicrob Agents Chemother 64. https://doi.org/10.1128/AAC.02353-19

Amaral L, Martins A, Spengler G, Molnar J (2013) Efflux pumps of Gram-negative bacteria: what they do, how they do it, with what and how to deal with them. Front Pharmacol 4:168. https://doi.org/10.3389/fphar.2013.00168

Ang MTC, Gumbau-Brisa R, Allan DS, McDonald R, Ferguson MJ, b Holbein BE, Bierenstiel M (2018) DIBI, a 3-hydroxypyridin-4-one chelator iron-binding polymer with enhanced antimicrobial activity. Med Chem Commun 9:1206–1212. https://doi.org/10.1039/C8MD00192H

Antonov NK, Garzon MC, Morel KD, Whittier S, Planet PJ, Lauren CT (2015) High prevalence of mupirocin resistance in Staphylococcus aureus isolates from a pediatric population. Antimicrob Agents Chemother 59:3350–3356. https://doi.org/10.1128/AAC.00079-15

Anzaldi LL, Skaar EP (2010) Overcoming the heme paradox: heme toxicity and tolerance in bacterial pathogens. Infect Immun 78:4977–4989. https://doi.org/10.1128/IAI.00613-10

Arora N, Caldwell A, Wafa K, Szczesniak A, Caldwell M, Al-Banna N, Sharawy N, Islam S, Zhou J, Holbein BE, Kelly MEM, Lehmann C (2018) DIBI, a polymeric hydroxypyridinone iron chelator, reduces ocular inflammation in local and systemic endotoxin-induced uveitis. Clin Hemorheol Microcirc 69:153–164. https://doi.org/10.3233/CH-189109

Bacconi M, Haag AF, Chiarot E, Donato P, Bagnoli F, Delany I, Bensi G (2017) In vivo analysis of Staphylococcus aureus-infected mice reveals differential temporal and spatial expression patterns of fhuD2. Infect Immun 85:e00270–e00217. https://doi.org/10.1128/IAI.00270-17

Bairwa G, Hee Jung W, Kronstad JW (2017) Iron acquisition in fungal pathogens of humans. Metallomics 9:215–227. https://doi.org/10.1039/c6mt00301j

Baman Balfour JA, Foster RH (1999) Deferiprone – a review of its clinical potential in iron overload in beta-thalassaemia major and other transfusion dependent diseases. Drugs 58:553–578. https://doi.org/10.2165/00003495-199958030-00021

Banin E, Vasil ML, Greenberg EP (2005) Iron and Pseudomonas aeruginosa biofilm formation. Proc Natl Acad Sci U S A 102:11076–11081. https://doi.org/10.1073/pnas.0504266102

Banin E, Lozinski A, Brady KM, Berenshtein E, Butterfield PW, Moshe M, Chevion M, Greenberg EP, Banin E (2008) The potential of desferrioxamine-gallium as an anti-Pseudomonas therapeutic agent. Proc Natl Acad Sci U S A 105:16761–16766. https://doi.org/10.1073/pnas.0808608105

Barrasa-Villar JI, Aibar-Remón C, Prieto-Andrés P, Mareca-Doñate R, Moliner-Lahoz J (2017) Impact on morbidity, mortality, and length of stay of hospital-acquired infections by resistant microorganisms. Clin Infect Dis 65:644–652. https://doi.org/10.1093/cid/cix411

Barton JC, Acton RT (2019) Hepcidin, iron, and bacterial infection. Vitam Horm 110:223–242

Bengtsson-Palme J, Kristiansson EDG, Larsson J (2018) Environmental factors influencing the development and spread of antibiotic resistance. FEMS Microbiol Rev 42:68–80. https://doi.org/10.1093/femsre/fux053

Bilitewski U, Blodgett JAV, Duhme-Klair AK, Dallavalle S, Laschat S, Routledge A, Schobert R (2017) Chemical and biological aspects of nutritional immunity-perspectives for new anti-infectives that target iron uptake systems. Angew Chem Int Ed Eng 56:14360–14382. https://doi.org/10.1002/anie.201701586

Britigan BE, Hayek MB, Doebbeling BN, Fick RBJ (1993) Transferrin and lactoferrin undergo proteolytic cleavage in the Pseudomonas aeruginosa-infected lungs of patients with cystic fibrosis. Infect Immun 61:5049–5055

Budzikiewicz H (2001) Siderophore-antibiotic conjugates used as trojan horses against Pseudomonas aeruginosa. Curr Top Med Chem 1:73–82. https://doi.org/10.2174/1568026013395524

Bühler V (2005) Polyvinylpyrrolidone excipients for pharmaceuticals – povidone. Springer-Verlag Berlin Heidelberg, New York

Cartwright GE, Lauritsen MA, Jones PJ, Merrill IM, Wintrobe MM (1946) The anemia of. J Clin Investig 25:65–80

Caza M, Kronstad JW (2013) Shared and distinct mechanisms of iron acquisition by bacterial and fungal pathogens of humans. Front Cell Infect Microbiol 3:80. https://doi.org/10.3389/fcimb.2013.00080

Ceci A, Baiardi P, Felisi M, Cappellini MD, Carnelli V, De Sanctis V, Galanello R, Maggio A, Masera G, Piga A, Schettini F, Stefano I, Tricta F (2002) The safety and effectiveness of deferiprone in a large-scale, 3-year study in Italian patients. Br J Haematol 118:330–336. https://doi.org/10.1046/j.1365-2141.2002.03554.x

Chan GC-F, Chan S, Ho P-L, Ha S-Y (2009) Effects of chelators (Deferoxamine, Deferiprone and Deferasirox) on the growth of Klebsiella pneumoniae and Aeromonas hydrophila isolated from transfusion-dependent thalassemia patients. Hemoglobin 33:352–360. https://doi.org/10.3109/03630260903211888

Chaves-Moreno D, Wos-Oxley ML, Jáuregui R, Medina E, Oxley APA, Pieper DH (2016) Exploring the transcriptome of Staphylococcus aureus in its natural niche. Nat Sci Rep 6:33174. https://doi.org/10.1038/srep33174

Chhibber S, Gupta P, Kaur S (2014) Bacteriophage as effective decolonising agent for elimination of MRSA from anterior nares of BALB/c mice. BMC Microbiol 14:212. https://doi.org/10.1186/s12866-014-0212-8

Chi-Fung Chan G, Chan S, Ho P-L, Ha S-Y (2009) Effects of chelators (deferoxamine, deferiprone and deferasirox) on the growth of Klebsiella pneumoniae and Aeromonas hydrophila isolated from transfusion-dependent thalassemia patients. Hemoglobin 33:352–360. https://doi.org/10.3109/03630260903211888

Chitambar CR (2016) Gallium and its competing roles with iron in biological systems. Biochim Biophys Acta 1863:2044–2053. https://doi.org/10.1016/j.bbamcr.2016.04.027

Chitambar CR (2017) The therapeutic potential of iron-targeting gallium compounds in human disease: from basic research to clinical application. Pharmacol Res 115:56–64. https://doi.org/10.1016/j.phrs.2016.11.009

Chitamber CR (2010) Medical applications and toxicities of gallium compounds. Int J Environ Res Public Health 7:2337–2367. https://doi.org/10.3390/ijerph7052337

Cirz R, Jones M, Gingles N, Minogue T, Jarrahi B, Peterson S, Romesberg F (2007) Complete and SOS-mediated response of Staphylococcus aureus to the antibiotic ciprofloxacin. J Bacteriol 189:531–539. https://doi.org/10.1128/JB.01464-06

Culyba MJ, Mo CY, Kohli RM (2015) Targets for combating the evolution of acquired antibiotic resistance. Biochemistry 54:3573–3582. https://doi.org/10.1021/acs.biochem.5b00109

Czaplewski L, R B, Clokie M, Dawson M, Fairhead H, Fischetti VA, Foster S, Gilmore BF, Hancock REW, Harper D, Henderson IR, Hilpert K, Jones BV, Kadioglu A, Knowles D, Ólafsdóttir S, Payne D, Projan S, Shaunak S, Silverman J, Thomas CM, Trust TJ, Warn P, Rex JH (2016) Alternatives to antibiotics—a pipeline portfolio review. Lancet Infect Dis 16:239–251. https://doi.org/10.1016/S1473-3099(15)00466-1

de Leseleuc L, Harris G, KuoLee R, Xu HH, Chen W (2014) Serum resistance, gallium nitrate tolerance and extrapulmonary dissemination are linked to heme consumption in a bacteremic strain of Acinetobacter baumannii. Int J Med Microbiol 304:360–369. https://doi.org/10.1016/j.ijmm.2013.12.002

de Locht M, Boelaert JR, Schneider Y-J (1994) Iron uptake from ferrioxamine and from ferrirhizoferrin by germinating spores of rhizopus microsporus. Biochem Pharmacol 47:1843–1850. https://doi.org/10.1016/0006-2952(94)90314-x

Diarra MS, Petitclerc D, Lacasse P (2002) Effect of lactoferrin in combination with penicillin on the morphology and the physiology of Staphylococcus aureus isolated from bovine mastitis. J Dairy Sci 85:1141–1149. https://doi.org/10.3168/jds.S0022-0302(02)74176-3

Dobbin PS, Hider RC, Hall AD, Taylor PD, Sarpong P, Porter JB (1993) Synthesis, physicochemical properties, and biological evaluation of N-substituted 2-Alkyl-3-hydroxy-4(1″)-pyridinones: orally active iron chelators with clinical potential. J Med Chem 36:2448–2458. https://doi.org/10.1021/jm00069a002

El-Gendy N, Qian J, Eshelman K, Rivera M, Berkland C (2015) Antibiotic activity of Iron-sequestering polymers. Biomacromolecules 16:1480–1488. https://doi.org/10.1021/bm5016392

Ellermann M, Arthur JC (2017) Siderophore-mediated iron acquisition and modulation of host-bacterial interactions. Free Radic Biol Med 105:68–78. https://doi.org/10.1016/j.freeradbiomed.2016.10.489

Ezraty B, Barras F (2016) The 'liaisons dangereuses' between iron and antibiotics. FEMS Microbiol Rev 40:418–435. https://doi.org/10.1093/femsre/fuw004

Foley TL, Simeonov A (2012) Targeting iron assimilation to develop new antibacterials. Expert Opin Drug Discovery 7:831–847. https://doi.org/10.1517/17460441.2012.708335

Friedman ND, Temkin E, Carmeli Y (2016) The negative impact of antibiotic resistance. Clin Microbiol Infect 22:416–422. https://doi.org/10.1016/j.cmi.2015.12.002

Frieria M, Kumarb K, Boutin A (2017) Antibiotic resistance. J Infect Public Health 10:369–378. https://doi.org/10.1016/j.jiph.2016.08.007

Gaddy JA, Arivett BA, McConnell MJ, López-Rojas R, Pachón J, Actis LA (2012) Role of acinetobactin-mediated iron acquisition functions in the interaction of Acinetobacter baumannii strain ATCC 19606T with human lung epithelial cells, Galleria mellonella caterpillars and mice. Infect Immun 80:1015–1024. https://doi.org/10.1128/IAI.06279-11

Ganz T (2018) Iron and infection. Int J Hematol 107:7–15. https://doi.org/10.1007/s12185-017-2385-z

Ganz T, Nemeth E (2015) Iron homeostasis in host defence and inflammation. Nat Rev Immunol 15:500–510. https://doi.org/10.1038/nri3863

Garcia L, Lemaire S, Kahl B, Becker K, Proctor R, Denis O, Tulkens P, Van Bambeke F (2013) Antibiotic activity against small colony variants of Staphylococcus aureus: review of in vitro, animal, and clinical data. J Antimicrob Chemother 68:1455–1465. https://doi.org/10.1093/jac/dkt072

Ghosh M, Miller PA, Mollmann U, Claypool WD, Schroeder VA, Wolter WR, Suckow M, Yu H, Li S, Huang W, Zajicek J, Miller MJ (2017) Targeted antibiotic delivery: selective siderophore conjugation with Daptomycin confers potent activity against multidrug resistant Acinetobacter baumannii both in vitro and in vivo. J Med Chem 60:4577–4583. https://doi.org/10.1021/acs.jmedchem.7b00102

Ghosh M, Lin YM, Miller PA, Mollmann U, Boggess WC, Miller MJ (2018) Siderophore conjugates of Daptomycin are potent inhibitors of Carbapenem resistant strains of Acinetobacter baumannii. ACS Infect Dis 4:1529–1535. https://doi.org/10.1021/acsinfecdis.8b00150

Giardina PJ, Grady RW (2001) Chelation therapy in beta-thalassemia: an optimistic update. Semin Hematol 38:360–366. https://doi.org/10.1016/s0037-1963(01)90030-7

Goss CH, Kaneko Y, Khuu L, Anderson GD, Ravishankar S, Aitken ML, Lechtzin N, Zhou G, Czyz DM, McLean K, Olakanmi O, Shuman HA, Teresi M, Wilhelm E, Caldwell E, Salipante SJ, Hornick DB, Siehnel RJ, Becker L, Britigan BE, Singh PK (2018) Gallium disrupts bacterial iron metabolism and has therapeutic effects in mice and humans with lung infections. Sci Transl Med 10:eaat7520. https://doi.org/10.1126/scitranslmed.aat7520

Gupta P, Sarkar S, Das B, Bhattacharjee S, Tribed P (2016) Biofilm, pathogenesis and prevention—a journey to break the wall: a review. Arch Microbiol 198:1–15. https://doi.org/10.1007/s00203-015-1148-6

Habgood MD, Liu ZD, Dehkordi LS, Khodr HH, Abbott J, Hider RC (1999) Investigation into the correlation between the structure of hydroxypyridinones and blood–brain barrier permeability. Biochem Pharmacol 57:1305–1310. https://doi.org/10.1016/s0006-2952(99)00031-3

Hancock REW, Nikaido H (1978) Outer membranes of gram negative bacteria. 19. Isolation from Pseudomonas-aeruginosa pao1 and use in reconstitution and definition of permeability barrier. J Bacteriol 136:381–390

Heeb S, Fletcher M, Chhabra S, Diggle S, Williams P, Camara M (2010) Quinolones: from antibiotics to autoinducers. FEMS Microbiol Rev 35:247–274. https://doi.org/10.1111/j.1574-6976.2010.00247.x

Heinz U, Hegetschweiler K, Acklin P, Faller B, Lattmann R, Schnebli HP (1999) 4-[3,5-Bis(2-hydroxyphenyl)-1,2,4-triazol-1-yl]- benzoic acid: a novel efficient and selective Iron(III)

complexing agent. Angew Chem Int Ed 38:2568–2570. https://doi.org/10.1002/(SICI)1521-3773(19990903)38:17<2568::AID-ANIE2568>3.0.CO;2-C

Heli H, Mirtorabi S, Karimian K (2011) Advances in iron chelation: an update. Expert Opin Ther Pat 21:819–856. https://doi.org/10.1517/13543776.2011.569493

Hershko C (2010) Pathogenesis and management of iron toxicity in thalassemia. Ann N Y Acad Sci 1202:1–9. https://doi.org/10.1111/j.1749-6632.2010.05544.x

Hider RC, Konga X (2010) Chemistry and biology of siderophores. Nat Prod Rep 27:637–657. https://doi.org/10.1039/b906679a

Holbein BE, Mira de Orduña R (2010) Effect of trace iron levels and iron withdrawal by chelation on the growth of Candida albicans and Candida vini. FEMS Microbiol Lett 307:19–24. https://doi.org/10.1111/j.1574-6968.2010.01956.x

Holbein BE, Feng M, Huber AL, Kidby DK (2011) Polymeric metal chelating compositions and methods of preparing same for controlling growth and activities of living cells and organisms. WIPO Pat., 2012167368A1, 2012

Holden VI, Bachman MA (2015) Diverging roles of bacterial siderophores during infection. Metallomics 7:986–995. https://doi.org/10.1039/c4mt00333k

Humphreys H, Becker K, Dohmen PM, Petrosillo N, Spencer M, van Rijen M, Wechsler-Fordos A, Pujol M, Dubouix A, Garau J (2016) Staphylococcus aureus and surgical site infections: benefits of screening and decolonization before surgery. J Hosp Infect 94:295e304. https://doi.org/10.1016/j.jhin.2016.06.011

Islam, S., S. Jarosch, J. Zhou, M. d. C. Parquet, J. T. Toguri, P. Colp, B. E. Holbein & C. Lehmann (2016) Anti-inflammatory and anti-bacterial effects of iron chelation in experimental sepsis. J Surg Res, 200, 266–273. DOI: https://doi.org/10.1016/j.jss.2015.07.001

Jensen P, Briales A, Brochmann R, Wang H, Kragh K, Kolpen M, Hempel C, Bjarnsholt T, Høiby N, Ciofu O (2014) Formation of hydroxyl radicals contributes to the bactericidal activity of ciprofloxacin against Pseudomonas aeruginosa biofilms. Pathog Dis 70:440–443. https://doi.org/10.1111/2049-632X.12120

Ji C, Miller PA, Miller MJ (2012) Iron transport-mediated drug delivery: practical syntheses and in vitro antibacterial studies of tris-catecholate siderophore-aminopenicillin conjugates reveals selectively potent antipseudomonal activity. J Am Chem Soc 134:9898–9901. https://doi.org/10.1021/ja303446w

Johnson EE, Wessling-Resnick M (2012) Iron metabolism and the innate immune response. Microbes Infect 14:207–216. https://doi.org/10.1016/j.micinf.2011.10.001

Johnstone TC, Nolan EM (2015) Beyond iron: non-classical biological functions of bacterial siderophores. Dalton Trans 44:6320–6339. https://doi.org/10.1039/c4dt03559c

Juhas M (2015) Horizontal gene transfer in human pathogens. Crit Rev Microbiol 41:101–108. https://doi.org/10.3109/1040841X.2013.804031

Kang H-K, Kim H-Y, Cha J-D (2011) Synergistic effects between silibinin and antibiotics on methicillin-resistant Staphylococcus aureus isolated from clinical specimens. Biotechnol J 6(11):1397–1408. https://doi.org/10.1002/biot.201000422

Kara M, Hasinoff B, McKay D, Campbell N (1991) Clinical and chemical interactions between iron preparations and ciprofloxacin. Br J Pharmacol 31:257–261. https://doi.org/10.1111/j.1365-2125.1991.tb05526.x

Katz L, Baltz RH (2016) Natural product discovery: past, present, and future. J Ind Microbiol Biotechnol 43:155–176. https://doi.org/10.1007/s10295-015-1723-5

Kelson AB, Carnevali M, Truong-Le V (2013) Gallium-based anti-infectives: targeting microbial iron-uptake mechanisms. Curr Opin Pharmacol 13:707–716. https://doi.org/10.1016/j.coph.2013.07.001

Khan A, Singh P, Srivastava A (2018) Synthesis, nature and utility of universal iron chelator – siderophore: a review. Microbiol Res 212-213:103–111. https://doi.org/10.1016/j.micres.2017.10.012

Kohanski M, Dwyer D, Hayete B, Lawrence C, Collins J (2007) A common mechanism of cellular death induced by bactericidal antibiotics. Cell 130:797. https://doi.org/10.1016/j.cell.2007.06.049

Kontoghiorghes GJ, Kolnagou A, Skiada A, Petrikkos G (2010) The role of Iron and Chelators on infections in Iron overload and non-Iron loaded conditions: prospects for the design of new antimicrobial therapies. Hemoglobin 34:227–239. https://doi.org/10.3109/03630269.2010.483662

Kugelberg E, Norstro T, Petersen TK, Duvold T, Andersson DI, Hughes D (2005) Establishment of a superficial skin infection model in mice by using Staphylococcus aureus and Streptococcus pyogenes. Antimicrob Agents Chemother 49:3435–3441. https://doi.org/10.1128/AAC.49.8.3435-3441.2005

Lacasse P, Lauzon K, Diarra MS, Petitclerc D (2008) Utilization of lactoferrin to fight antibiotic-resistant mammary gland pathogens. J Anim Sci 86:66–71. https://doi.org/10.2527/jas.2007-0216

Larsen R, Gozzelino R, Jeney V, Tokaji L, Bozza FA, Japiassú AM, Bonaparte D, Cavalcante MM, Chora Â, Ferreira A, Marguti I, Cardoso S, Sepúlveda N, Smith A, Soares MP (2010) A central role for free Heme in the pathogenesis of severe sepsis. Sci Transl Med 2:51ra71. https://doi.org/10.1126/scitranslmed.3001118

Lehmann C, Sharawi N, Al-Banna N, Corbett N, Kuethe JW, Caldwell CC (2014) Novel approaches to the development of anti-sepsis drugs. Expert Opin Drug Discovery 9:523–531. https://doi.org/10.1517/17460441.2014.905538

Lesic B, Foulon J, Carniel E (2002) Comparison of the effects of Deferiprone versus Deferoxamine on growth and virulence of Yersinia entercolitica. Antimicrob Agents Chemother 46:1741–1745. https://doi.org/10.1128/AAC.46.6.1741-1745.2002

Lessa JA, Parrilha GL, Beraldo H (2012) Gallium complexes as new promising metallodrug candidates. Inorg Chim Acta 393:53–63. https://doi.org/10.1016/j.ica.2012.06.003

Li J, Olaleye ED, Kong X, Zhou T, Ma Y, Osamah JJ, Rugaie A, Hider RC, Zhang G, Alsam S, Abbate V (2016) Macromolecular iron-chelators via RAFT-polymerization for the inhibition of methicillin-resistant Staphylococcus aureus growth. Polymer 87:64–72. https://doi.org/10.1016/j.polymer.2016.01.073

Link G, Konijn AM, Breuer W, Cabantchik ZI, Hershko C (2001) Exploring the "iron shuttle" hypothesis in chelation therapy: effects of combined deferoxamine and deferiprone treatment in hypertransfused rats with labeled iron stores and in iron-loaded rat heart cells in culture. J Lab Clin Med 138:130–138. https://doi.org/10.1067/mlc.2001.116487

Liu ZD, Hider RC (2002) Design of clinically useful iron(III)-selective chelators. Med Res Rev 22:26–64. https://doi.org/10.1002/med.1027

Liu X, Deng S, Huang J, Huang Y, Zhang Y, Yan Q, Wang Y, Li Y, Sun C, Xu J (2017) Dissemination of macrolides, fusidic acid and mupirocin resistance among Staphylococcus aureus clinical isolates. Oncotarget 8:58086–58097. https://doi.org/10.18632/oncotarget.19491

Lubelski J, Konings WN, Driessen AJM (2007) Distribution and physiology of ABC-type transporters contributing to multidrug resistance in bacteria. Microbiol Mol Biol Rev 71:463–476. https://doi.org/10.1128/MMBR.00001-07

Luepke KH, Suda KJ, Boucher H, Russo RL, Bonney MW, Hunt TD, Mohr JF (2017) Past, present, and future of antibacterial economics: increasing bacterial resistance, limited antibiotic pipeline, and societal implications. Pharmacotherapy 37:71–84. https://doi.org/10.1002/phar.1868

Luo G, Spellberg B, Gebremariam T, Lee H, Xiong YQ, French SW, Bayer A, Ibrahim AS (2014) Combination therapy with iron chelation and vancomycin in treating murine staphylococcemia. Eur J Clin Microbiol Infect Dis 33:845–851. https://doi.org/10.1007/s10096-013-2023-5

Martí-Carvajal AJ, Solà I, Lathyris D, Cardona AF (2011) Human recombinant activated protein C for severe sepsis. Cochrane Database Syst Rev 4:CD004388. https://doi.org/10.1002/14651858.CD004388.pub4

Maslowska KH, Makiela-Dzbenska K, Fijalkowska IJ (2019) The SOS system: a complex and tightly regulated response to DNA damage. Environ Mol Mutagen 60:368–384. https://doi.org/10.1002/em.22267

Maxton DG, I B, Reynolds AP, Catt SD, Peters TJ, Menzies IS (1986) Lactulose 51Cr-labelled ethylenediaminetetra-acetate, L-rhamnose and polyethyleneglycol 500 as probe markers for assessment in vivo of human intestinal permeability. Clin Sci 71:71–80. https://doi.org/10.1042/cs0710071

Méhi O, Bogos B, Csörgő B, Pál F, Nyerges A, Papp B, Pál C (2014) Perturbation of iron homeostasis promotes the evolution of antibiotic resistance. Mol Biol Evol 31:2793–2804. https://doi.org/10.1093/molbev/msu223

Michiels JE, Van dem Bergh B, Verstraten N, Michiels J (2016) Molecular mechanisms and clinical implications of bacterial persistence. Drug Resist Updat 29:76–89. https://doi.org/10.1016/j.drup.2016.10.002

Minandri F, Bonchi C, Frangipani E, Imperi F, Visca P (2014) Promises and failures of gallium as an antibacterial agent. Future Microbiol 9:379–397. https://doi.org/10.2217/fmb.14.3

Mobarra N, Shanaki M, Ehteram H, Nasiri H, Sahmani M, Mohsen S, Goudarzi M, Pourkarim H, Azad M (2016) A review on iron chelators in treatment of iron overload syndromes. Int J Hematol Oncol Stem Cell Res 10:239–247

Mohammadi Z, Xie S-X, Golub AL, Gehrke SH, Berkland C (2011) Siderophore-mimetic hydrogel for iron chelation therapy. J Appl Polym Sci 121:1384–1392. https://doi.org/10.1002/app.33562

Mollmann U, Heinisch L, Bauernfeind A, Kohler T, Ankel-Fuchs D (2009) Siderophores as drug delivery agents: application of the "Trojan Horse" strategy. Biometals 22:615–624. https://doi.org/10.1007/s10534-009-9219-2

Moniz T, Nunes A, Silva AMG, Queirós C, Ivanova G, Gomes MS, Rangel M (2013) Rhodamine labeling of 3-hydroxy-4-pyridinone iron chelators is an important contribution to target Mycobacterium avium infection. J Inorg Biochem 121:156–166. https://doi.org/10.1016/j.jinorgbio.2013.01.002

Moniz T, Silva D, Silva T, Gomes MS, Rangel M (2015) Antimycobacterial activity of rhodamine 3,4-HPO iron chelators against Mycobacterium avium: analysis of the contribution of functional groups and of chelator's combination with ethambutol. Med Chem Commun 6:2194–2203. https://doi.org/10.1039/C5MD00456J

Moreau-Marquis S, O'Toole GA, Stanton BA (2009) Tobramycin and FDA-approved iron chelators eliminate Pseudomonas aeruginosa biofilms on cystic fibrosis cells. Am J Respir Cell Mol Biol 41:305–31. https://doi.org/10.1165/rcmb.2008-0299OC

Movassaghi M, van der Donk WA (2018) Synthesis of antibiotics and related molecules. J Organomet Chem 83:6826–6828. https://doi.org/10.1021/acs.joc.8b01330

Mullard A (2014) Momentum builds around new antibiotic business models. Nat Rev 13:711–713. https://doi.org/10.1038/nrd4455

Nairz M, Dicht S, Schroll A, Haschka D, Tymoszuk P, Theurl I, Weiss G (2018) Iron and innate anti-microbialimmunity—depriving the pathogen, defending the host. J Trace Elem Med Biol 48:118–133. https://doi.org/10.1016/j.jtemb.2018.03.007

Naylor NR, Atun R, Zhu N, Kulasabanathan K, Silva S, Chatterjee A, Knight GM, Robotham JV (2018) Estimating the burden of anti-microbialresistance: a systematic literature review. Antimicrob Resist Infect Control 7:58. https://doi.org/10.1186/s13756-018-0336-y

Neumann W, Nolan EM (2018) Evaluation of a reducible disulfide linker for siderophore-mediated delivery of antibiotics. J Biol Inorg Chem 23:1025–1036. https://doi.org/10.1007/s00775-018-1588-y

Neumann W, Sassone-Corsi M, Raffatellu M, Nolan EM (2018) Esterase-catalyzed siderophore hydrolysis activates an enterobactin-ciprofloxacin conjugate and confers targeted antibacterial activity. J Am Chem Soc 140:5193–5201. https://doi.org/10.1021/jacs.8b01042

Neupane GP, Kim DM (2010) In vitro time-kill activities of ciprofloxacin alone and in combination with the iron chelator deferasirox against Vibrio vulnificus. Eur J Clin Microbiol Infect Dis 29:407–410. https://doi.org/10.1007/s10096-010-0875-5

Noinaj N, Buchanan SK, Cornelissen CN (2012a) The transferrin-iron import system from pathogenic Neisseria species. Mol Microbiol 86:246–257. https://doi.org/10.1111/mmi.12002

Noinaj N, Easley NC, Oke M, Mizuno N, Gumbart J, Boura E, Steere AN, Zak O, Aisen P, Tajkhorshid E, Evans RW, Gorringe AR, Mason AB, Steven AC, Buchanan SK (2012b) Structural basis for iron piracy by pathogenic Neisseria. Nature 483:53–58. https://doi.org/10.1038/nature10823

Nunes A, Podinovskaia M, Leite A, Gameiro P, Zhou T, Ma Y, Kong X, Schaible UE, Hider RC, Rangel M (2010) Fluorescent 3-hydroxy-4-pyridinone hexadentate iron chelators: intracellular distribution and the relevance to antimycobacterial properties. J Biol Inorg Chem 15:861–877. https://doi.org/10.1007/s00775-010-0650-1

Nurchi VM, Crisponi G, Pivetta T, Donatoni M, Remelli M (2008) Potentiometric, spectrophotometric and calorimetric study on iron(III) and copper(II) complexes with 1,2-dimethyl-3-hydroxy-4-pyridinone. J Inorg Biochem 102:684–692. https://doi.org/10.1016/j.jinorgbio.2007.10.012

Olivieri NF, Sabouhanian A, Gallie BL (2019) Single-center retrospective study of the effectiveness and toxicity of the oral iron chelating drugs deferiprone and deferasirox. PLoS One 14:e0211942. https://doi.org/10.1371/journal.pone.0211942

Onyango LA, Alreshidi MM (2018) Adaptive metabolism in staphylococci: survival and persistence in environmental and clinical settings. J Pathog 2018:1092632. https://doi.org/10.1155/2018/1092632

Painter KL, Strange E, Parkhill J, Bamford KB, Armstrong-James D, Edwards AM (2015) Staphylococcus aureus adapts to oxidative stress by producing H_2O_2-resistant small-colony variants via the SOS response. Infect Immun 83:1830–1844. https://doi.org/10.1128/IAI.03016-14

Palmer LD, Skaar EP (2016) Transition metals and virulence in bacteria. Annu Rev Genet 50:67–91. https://doi.org/10.1146/annurev-genet-120215-035146

Paoli CJ, Reynolds MA, Sinha M, Gitlin M, Crouser E (2018) Epidemiology and costs of sepsis in the United States-an analysis based on timing of diagnosis and severity level. Crit Care Med 46:1889–1897. https://doi.org/10.1097/CCM.0000000000003342

Parquet M d C, Savage KA, Allan DS, Davidson RJ, Holbein BE (2018) Novel iron-chelator DIBI inhibits Staphylococcus aureus growth, suppresses experimental MRSA infection in mice and enhances the activities of diverse antibiotics in vitro. Front Microbiol 9:1811. https://doi.org/10.3389/fmicb.2018.01811

Parquet M d C, Savage KA, Allan DS, Ang MTC, Chen W, Logan SM, Holbein BE (2019) Antibiotic resistant Acinetobacter baumannii is susceptible to the novel iron-sequestering anti-infective DIBI in vitro and in experimental pneumonia in mice. Antimicrob Agents Chemother 63:e00855–e00819. https://doi.org/10.1128/AAC.00855-19

Peacock SJ, Paterson GK (2014) Mechanisms of methicillin resistance in Staphylococcus aureus. Annu Rev Biochem 84:577–601. https://doi.org/10.1146/annurev-biochem-060614-034516

Pélissier MA, Marteau P, Pochart P (2007) Antioxidant effects of metronidazole in colonic tissue. Dig Dis Sci 52:40–44. https://doi.org/10.1007/s10620-006-9231-0

Peng Q, Zhou S, Yao F, Hou B, Huang Y, Hua D, Zheng Y, Qian Y (2011) Baicalein suppresses the SOS response system of Staphylococcus aureus induced by ciprofloxacin. Cell Physiol Biochem 28:1045–1050. https://doi.org/10.1159/000335791

Perez C, Wei Y, Guo M (2009) Iron-binding and anti-Fenton properties of baicalein and baicalin. J Inorg Biochem 103:326–332. https://doi.org/10.1016/j.jinorgbio.2008.11.003

Post SJ, Shapiro JA, Wuest WM (2019) Connecting iron acquisition and biofilm formation in the ESKAPE pathogens as a strategy for combatting antibiotic resistance. Med Chem Commun 10:505–512. https://doi.org/10.1039/C9MD00032A

Prasad T, Chandra A, Mukhopadhyay CK, Prasad R (2006) Unexpected link between iron and drug resistance of Candida spp.: iron depletion enhances membrane fluidity and drug diffusion, leading to drug-susceptible cells. Antimicrob Agents Chemother 50:3597–3606. https://doi.org/10.1128/AAC.00653-06

Proctor R, Kahl B, von Eiff C, Vaudaux P, Daniel P, Lew D, Peters G (1998) Staphylococcal small colony variants have novel mechanisms for antibiotic resistance. Clin Infect Dis 27:S68–S74. https://doi.org/10.1086/514906

Proctor R, Kriegeskorte A, Kahl B, Becker K, Löffler B, Peters G (2014) Staphylococcus aureus small colony variants (SCVs): a roadmap for the metabolic pathways involved in persistent infections. Front Cell Infect Microbiol 4:1–8. https://doi.org/10.3389/fcimb.2014.00099
Qiu D-H, Huang Z-L, Zhou T, Shen C, Hider RC (2011) In vitro inhibition of bacterial growth by iron chelators. FEMS Microbiol Lett 314:107–111. https://doi.org/10.1111/j.1574-6968.2010.02153.x
Rangel-Vega A, Bernstein LR, Mandujano-Tinoco EA, Garcia-Contreras SJ, Garcia-Contreras R (2015) Drug repurposing as an alternative for the treatment of recalcitrant bacterial infections. Front Microbiol 6:282. https://doi.org/10.3389/fmicb.2015.00282
Raymond KN, Muller G, Matzanke BF (1984) Complexation of iron by siderophores: a review of their solution and structural chemistry and biological function. Top Curr Chem 58:49–102
Richter K, Thomas N, Zhang G, Prestidge C, Coenye T, Wormald P, Vreugde S (2017) Deferiprone and gallium-protoporphyrin have the capacity to potentiate the activity of antibiotics in Staphylococcus aureus small colony variants. Front Cell Infect Microbiol 7:280. https://doi.org/10.3389/fcimb.2017.00280
Robins-Browne RM, Prpic JK (1983) Desferrioxamine and systemic yersiniosis. Lancet 2:1372. https://doi.org/10.1016/s0140-6736(83)91136-4
Robins-Browne RM, Prpic JM (1985) Effects of iron and desferrioxamine on infections with Yersinia enterocolitica. Infect Immun 47:774–779
Roosenberg JM 2nd, Miller MJ (2000) Total synthesis of the siderophore danoxamine. J Organomet Chem 65:4833–4838. https://doi.org/10.1021/jo000050m
Roosenberg JM 2nd, Lin YM, Lu Y, Miller MJ (2000) Studies and syntheses of siderophores, microbial iron chelators, and analogs as potential drug delivery agents. Curr Med Chem 7:159–197. https://doi.org/10.2174/0929867003375353
Savage KA, Parquet MC, Allan DS, Davidson RJ, Holbein BE, Lilly EA, Fidel PLJ (2018) Iron restriction to clinical isolates of Candida albicans by the novel chelator DIBI inhibits growth and increases sensitivity to azoles in vitro and in vivo in a murine model of experimental vaginitis. Antimicrob Agents Chemother 62:e02576–e02517. https://doi.org/10.1128/AAC.02576-17
Schaible UE, Kaufmann SH (2004) Iron and microbial infection. Nat Rev Microbiol 2:946–953. https://doi.org/10.1038/nrmicro1046
Schaible UE, Collins HL, Priem F, Kaufmann SH (2002) Correction of the iron overload defect in beta-2-microglobulin knockout mice by lactoferrin abolishes their increased susceptibility to tuberculosis. J Exp Med 196:1507–1513. https://doi.org/10.1084/jem.20020897
Schroder W, Goerke S, Wolz C (2013) Opposing effects of aminocoumarins and fluoroquinolones on the SOS response and adaptability in Staphylococcus aureus. J Antimicrob Chemother 68:529–538. https://doi.org/10.1093/jac/dks456
Schroeder M, Brooks BD, Brooks AE (2017) The complex relationship between virulence and antibiotic resistance. Gen Dent 8:39. https://doi.org/10.3390/genes8010039
Shearer JES, Wireman J, Hostetler J, Forberger H, Borman J, Gill J, Sanchez S, Mankin A, LaMarre J, Lindsay JA, Bayles K, Nicholson A, O'Brien F, Jensen SO, Firth N, Skurray RA, Summers AO (2011) Major families of multiresistant plasmids from geographically and epidemiologically diverse staphylococci. Genes Genomes Genetics 1:581–590. https://doi.org/10.1534/g3.111.000760
Sheldon JR, Heinrichs DE (2015) Recent developments in understanding the iron acquisition strategies of gram positive pathogens. FEMS Microbiol Rev 39:592–630. https://doi.org/10.1093/femsre/fuv009
Sheldon JR, Laakso HA, Heinrichs DE (2016) Iron acquisition strategies of bacterial pathogens. Microbiol Spectr 4. https://doi.org/10.1128/microbiolspec
Singer M, Deutschman CS, Seymour CW, Shankar-Hari M, Annane D, Bauer M, Bellomo R, Bernard GR, Chiche JD, Hotchkiss RS, Coopersmith CM, Levy MM, Marshall JC, Martin GS, Opal SM, Rubenfeld GD, van der Poll T, Vincent JL, Angus DC (2016) The third international consensus definitions for sepsis and septic shock (Sepsis-3). JAMA 315:801–810. https://doi.org/10.1001/jama.2016.0287

Singh S, Epemolu RO, Dobbin PS, Tilbrook GS, Ellis BL, Damani LA, Hider RC (1992) Urinary metabolic profiles in human and rat of 1,2-dimethyl- and 1,2-diethyl-substituted 3-hydroxypyridin-4-ones. Drug Metab Dispos 20:256–261

Sohnle PG, Hahn BL, Karmarkar R (2001) Effect of metals on Candida albicans growth in the presence of chemical chelators and human abscess fluid. J Lab Clin Med 137:284–289. https://doi.org/10.1067/mlc.2001.113577

Stintzi A, Barnes C, Xu J, Raymond KN (2000) Microbial iron transport via a siderophore shuttle: a membrane transport system. Proc Natl Acad Sci 97:10691–10696. https://doi.org/10.1073/pnas.200318797

Stojiljkovic I, Kumar V, Srinivasan N (1999) Non-iron metalloporphyrins: potent antibacterial compounds that exploit haem/Hb uptake systems of pathogenic bacteria. Mol Microbiol 31:429–442. https://doi.org/10.1046/j.1365-2958.1999.01175.x

Streater M, Taylor PD, Hider RC, Porter J (1990) Novel 3-hydroxy-2(1H)-pyridinones. Synthesis, iron(III)-chelating properties and biological activity. J Med Chem 33:1749–1755

Sutherland R, Boon RJ, Griffin KE, Masters PJ, Slocombe B, White AR (1985) Antibacterial activity of Mupirocin (Pseudomonic acid), a new antibiotic for topical use. Antimicrob Agents Chemother 27:495–498. https://doi.org/10.1128/aac.27.4.495

Tacke F, Nuraldeen R, Koch A, Strathmann K, Hutschenreuter G, Trautwein C, Strnad P (2016) Iron parameters determine the prognosis of critically Ill patients. Crit Care Med 44:1049–1058. https://doi.org/10.1097/CCM.0000000000001607

Thompson MG, Corey BW, Si Y, Craft DW, Zurawski D (2012) Antibacterial activities of iron chelators against common nosocomial pathogens. Antimicrob Agents Chemother 56:5419–5421. https://doi.org/10.1128/AAC.01197-12

Thompson MG, Truong-Le V, Alamneh YA, Black CC, Anderl J, Honnold CL, Pavlicek RL, Abu-Taleb R, Wise MC, Hall ER, Wagar EJ, Patzer E, Zurawski DV (2015) Evaluation of gallium citrate formulations against a multidrug-resistant strain of Klebsiella pneumoniae in a murine wound model of infection. Antimicrob Agents Chemother 59:6484–6493. https://doi.org/10.1128/AAC.00882-15

Thorburn T, Aali M, Kostek L, LeTourneau-Paci C, Colp P, Zhou J, Holbein BE, Hoskin D, Lehmann C (2017) Anti-inflammatory effects of a novel iron chelator, DIBI, in experimental sepsis. Clin Hemorheol Microcirc 67:241–250. https://doi.org/10.3233/CH-179205

Tomaras AP, Crandon JL, McPherson CJ, Banevicius MA, Finegan SM, Irvine RL, Brown MF, O'Donnell JP, Nicolau DP (2013) Adaptation-based resistance to siderophore-conjugated antibacterial agents by Pseudomonas aeruginosa. Antimicrob Agents Chemother 57:4197–4207. https://doi.org/10.1128/AAC.00629-13

Tomaras AP, Crandon JL, McPherson CJ, Nicolau DP (2015) Potentiation of antibacterial activity of the MB-1 siderophore-monobactam conjugate using an efflux pump inhibitor. Antimicrob Agents Chemother 59:2439–2442. https://doi.org/10.1128/AAC.04172-14

Torres-Barcelo C, Kojadinovic M, Moxon R, MacLean RC (2015) The SOS response increases bacterial fitness, but not evolvability, under a sublethal dose of antibiotic. Proc R Soc B 282:20150885. https://doi.org/10.1098/rspb.2015.0885

Ventola CL (2015) The antibiotic resistance crisis part 1: causes and threats. Pharma Ther 40:277–283

Wandersman C, Delepelaire P (2004) Bacterial iron sources: from siderophores to hemophores. Annu Rev Microbiol 58:611–647. https://doi.org/10.1146/annurev.micro.58.030603.123811

Ward PP, Uribe-Luna S, Conneely OM (2002) Lactoferrin and host defense. Biochem Cell Biol 80:95–102. https://doi.org/10.1139/o01-214

Weinberg ED (1978) Iron and infection. Microbiol Rev 42:45–66

Weinberg ED (2009) Iron availability and infection. Biochim Biophys Acta 1790:600–605. https://doi.org/10.1016/j.bbagen.2008.07.002

Wilson BR, Bogdan AR, Miyazawa M, Hashimoto K, Tsuji Y (2016) Siderophores in iron metabolism: from mechanism to therapy potential. Trends Mol Med 22:1077–1090. https://doi.org/10.1016/j.molmed.2016.10.005

Workman DG, Hunter M, Dover LG, Tétard D (2016) Synthesis of novel Iron(III) chelators based on triaza macrocycle backbone and 1-hydroxy-2(H)-pyridin-2-one coordinating groups and their evaluation as anti-microbialagents. J Inorg Biochem 160:49–58. https://doi.org/10.1016/j.jinorgbio.2016.04.018

Wright GD (2005) Bacterial resistance to antibiotics: enzymatic degradation and modification. Adv Drug Deliv Rev 57:1451–1470. https://doi.org/10.1016/j.addr.2005.04.002

Xie Y-Y, Liu M-S, Hu P-P, Kong X-L, Qiu D-H, Xu J-L, Hider RC, Zhou T (2013) Synthesis, physico-chemical properties, and anti-microbialevaluation of a new series of iron(III) hexadentate chelators. Med Chem Res 22:2351–2359. https://doi.org/10.1007/s00044-012-0229-1

Xu B, Kong X-L, Zhou T, Qiu D-H, Chen Y-L, Liu M-S, Yang R-H (2011) Synthesis, iron(III)-binding affinity and in vitro evaluation of 3-hydroxypyridin-4-one hexadentate ligands as potential anti-microbialagents. Bioorg Med Chem Lett 21:6376–6380. https://doi.org/10.1016/j.bmcl.2011.08.097

Yeeles J, Cammack R, Dillingham M (2009) An iron-sulfur cluster is essential for the binding of broken DNA by AddAB-type helicase-nucleases. J Biol Chem 284:7746–7755. https://doi.org/10.1074/jbc.M808526200

Yokel RA, Fredenburg AM, Meurer KA, Skinner TL (1995) Influence of lipophilicity on the bioavailability and disposition of orally active 3-hydroxypyridin-4-one metal chelators. Drug Metab Dispos 23:1178–1180

Zarember KA, Cruz AR, Huang C-Y, Gallin JI (2009) Antifungal activities of natural and synthetic iron chelators alone and in combination with azole and polyene antibiotics against Aspergillus fumigatus. Anti-microb Agents Chemother 53:2654–2656. https://doi.org/10.1128/AAC.01547-08

Zheng T, Nolan EM (2014) Enterobactin-mediated delivery of beta-lactam antibiotics enhances antibacterial activity against pathogenic Escherichia coli. J Am Chem Soc 136:9677–9691. https://doi.org/10.1021/ja503911p

Zhou T, Neubert H, Liu DY, Liu ZD, Ma YM, Kong XL, Luo W, Mark S, Hider RC (2006) Iron binding dendrimers: a novel approach for the treatment of haemochromatosis. J Med Chem 49:4171–4182. https://doi.org/10.1021/jm0600949

Zhou T, Ma Y, Kong X, Hider RC (2012) Design of iron chelators with therapeutic application. Dalton Trans 41:6371–6389. https://doi.org/10.1039/C2DT12159J

Zhou Y-J, Zhang M-X, Hider RC, Zhou T (2014) In vitro anti-microbialactivity of hydroxypyridinone hexadentate-based dendrimeric chelators alone and in combination with norfloxacin. FEMS Microbiol Lett 355:124–130. https://doi.org/10.1111/1574-6968.12465

Zhou Y-J, Kong X-L, Li J-P, Ma Y-M, Hider R-C, Zhou T (2015a) Novel 3-hydroxypyridin-4-one hexadentate ligand-based polymeric iron chelator: synthesis, characterization and anti-microbialevaluation. Med Chem Commun 6:1620–1625. https://doi.org/10.1039/C5MD00264H

Zhou Y-J, Liu M-S, Osamah AR, Kong X-L, Alsam S, Battah S, Xie Y-Y, Hider RC, Zhou T (2015b) Hexadentate 3-hydroxypyridin-4-ones with high iron(III) affinity: design, synthesis and inhibition on methicillin resistant Staphylococcus aureus and Pseudomonas strains. Eur J Med Chem 94:8–21. https://doi.org/10.1016/j.ejmech.2015.02.050

Zhou T, Chena K, Kong L-M, Liu M-S, Mac Y-M, Xie Y-Y (2018) Synthesis, iron binding and anti-microbialproperties of hexadentate 3-hydroxypyridinones-terminated dendrimers. Bioorg Med Chem Lett 28:2504–2512. https://doi.org/10.1016/j.bmcl.2018.05.058

Chapter 9
Phage Biotechnology to Mitigate Antimicrobial Resistance in Agriculture

Aruni Premaratne, Hui Zhang, Ran Wang, Nalini Chinivasagam, and Craig Billington

Abstract The prevalence of key antibiotic resistant bacteria was reported by the World Health Organization in 2014 and they found very high rates of resistance in all regions of the globe. The United States Centres for Disease Control has also estimated that 20% of the two million antibiotic resistant infections in the US are linked to agricultural use. Antibiotics provide a vital function in reducing mortality in humans and animals, so their efficacy must be protected by coordinated action across multiple sectors, including agriculture. Alongside better antibiotic stewardship, a key to achieving this goal must be the development of new antimicrobial agents. For agriculture, a renewed focus on intensification, food security and reduced food loss also provide additional pressures on controlling bacterial infections and spoilage. Here, we discuss the potential of a new class of antimicrobial agents, phages, as a replacement or supplement, to some of the conventional antibiotics currently used in agriculture. We show that phages have many of the desirable properties needed to control bacterial diseases in agriculture including efficacy, low levels of resistance, lack of cross-resistance to antibiotics, biodegradability and narrow target range.

In poultry, studies of *Campylobacter* and *Salmonella* biocontrol have demonstrated that optimal timing for phage application is likely 24–48 h prior to slaughter, up to 5 log reductions in caecal counts may be achieved, and that phage resistance is low and transient. Use of phages in market swine has shown that they are able to reduce *Salmonella* carriage in tonsils and caeca by up to 3 logs and reduce overall carriage by 50%. Reductions in the shedding of *Clostridium* and *E. coli* in piglets

A. Premaratne · C. Billington (✉)
Institute of Environmental Science and Research, Christchurch, New Zealand
e-mail: Craig.Billington@esr.cri.nz

H. Zhang · R. Wang
Jiangsu Academy of Agricultural Sciences, Nanjing, China

N. Chinivasagam
Queensland Department of Agriculture and Fisheries, Brisbane, Australia

H. Panwar et al. (eds.), *Sustainable Agriculture Reviews 49*, Sustainable Agriculture Reviews 49, https://doi.org/10.1007/978-3-030-58259-3_9

have also been observed following phage application. Phages have shown efficacy in reducing *Staphylococcus aureus* infections in mouse models of mastitis and have reduced disease progression by up to 81% in cows' udders. Calves were protected from diarrhoea onset and death due to *E. coli* and *Salmonella* infection where phages were administered. Complete suppression of wilting was observed when phages were applied to tomato and a 50% reduction when applied in rice wilt. For soft rot disease associated with potatoes, a 94% reduction in rotten tissue was seen in plants treated with phages. Up to 90% reductions in *Erwinia* were achieved with phage treatment of flowers for fireblight. Additionally, the use of phages may provide new opportunities to agricultural industries to control pathogens not currently effectively controlled by antibiotics or other treatments. However, it is evident that application of phages to each system needs to be tailored and optimised, and that some systems are more challenging for phage use than others (e.g. poultry appear more suited than beef cattle). Whilst there are few phage products available currently, it is likely we will see a rapid rise in their use in the coming years.

Keywords Phage · Biocontrol · Agriculture · Biotechnology · Antimicrobial resistance · Poultry · Pigs · Cattle · Plant disease · One health

9.1 Introduction

The World Health Organization (WHO) reported the prevalence of key antibiotic resistant bacteria of international concern in 2014 and found very high rates of resistance (up to 84% of isolates for methicillin, 49% for fluoroquinolones, 81% for third generation cephalosporins, and 60% for penicillin) in all regions of the globe (World Health Organisation 2014). The US Centres for Disease Control (CDC) has also estimated that 20% of the two million antibiotic resistant infections in the US are linked to agricultural use (ASM 2019). The global impact of antibiotic resistance has been estimated to cause up to ten million deaths and cost US$100 trillion by 2050, if left unchecked (MacLean and San Millan 2019).

In late 2016, in response to this extraordinary crisis, the United Nations General Assembly called upon the WHO, the Food and Agriculture Organization of the United Nations (FAO), and the World Organisation for Animal Health to develop a global stewardship and development framework (World Health Organisation 2017). This call recognized the need to co-ordinate action against antimicrobial resistance in agriculture, animals, humans and the environment in a "One Health" approach (Mwangi et al. 2016).

However, the use of antimicrobials such as antibiotics cannot simply be stopped as they provide a vital function in reducing mortality in humans and animals. One of the crucial recommendations in the WHO draft framework, therefore, was to develop new antimicrobial agents for use in agriculture and other sectors. Here, we discuss the potential of a new class of antimicrobial agents, bacteriophages (phages), as a replacement or supplement, to some of the conventional antibiotics currently used in agriculture. Moreover, the use of phages may provide new opportunities to agricultural industries to control pathogens not currently effectively controlled by antibiotics or other treatments.

Phages are viruses that specifically infect and multiply in bacteria and are probably the most numerous organisms on the planet. Most of them belong to the order *Caudovirales* and possess an icosahedral head, a tail and double stranded DNA. Depending on their lifestyle, phages can be classified as either virulent and temperate. Virulent phages obligately follow a lytic cycle that involves multiplication within the bacterial cell and then lysis of the cell wall to release progeny phage. Temperate phages can insert their DNA into the bacterial host genome, or plasmids, and replicate until induction of the lytic cycle, which is usually caused by cellular stress (García et al. 2010; Rivas et al. 2010; Love et al. 2018).

Infection of the bacterial cell is mediated by phage tail anti receptors that recognize specific bacterial cell wall receptors. After adsorption to the cell, phages eject their DNA into the cell where is transcribed and translated by host cell enzymes. Phage enzymes then harness cell resources to produce daughter phages. Near the end of the replicative cycle phage enzymes (endolysins) are produced which lyse the cell wall from within to release the newly formed particles. It is this cell lysis which gives phages an ability to kill bacteria and act as antimicrobials. Unlike conventional antimicrobials, one phage can produce up to several hundred daughter phages per cell so there is an amplification of the antimicrobial activity (García et al. 2010; Rivas et al. 2010; Love et al. 2018). An illustration of the phage lytic cycle is shown in Fig. 9.1.

Since their discovery at the turn of the twentieth century, phages were used to treat bacterial infections. Firstly, this was human patients suffering dysentery and later to treat wounds both in the battlefield and in civilian life. The political complications following the Second World War left Eastern countries with limited supplies of antibiotics, which further spurred phage research, particularly in what is now The Republic of Georgia. The success of antibiotics during the post-war years meant phage research was limited in Western countries (Brüssow 2005). More recently, phages have been used to treat agricultural animal diseases (Smith and Huggins 1983) and this growing interest in the use of phages has now been spurred on again by the emergence of antibiotic resistance.

The scope of potential uses of phages as alternatives to antibiotics for the control of bacteria in agriculture and food production is vast. So, to limit the size of this article we have chosen to not discuss the use of phages in aquaculture and postharvest food safety and to exclude discussion of phage endolysins. If the reader is interested in these topics, then other recent reviews are available (García et al. 2010; Defoirdt et al. 2011; Love et al. 2018).

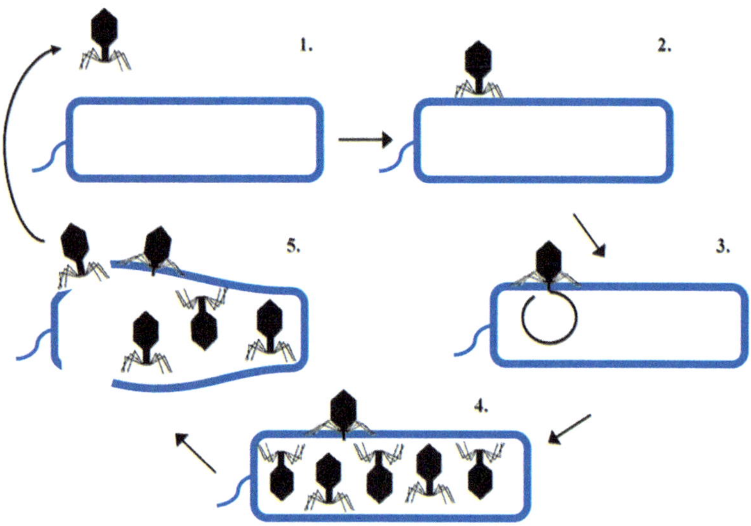

Fig. 9.1 The virulent phage lytic lifecycle. Lytic life cycle of a virulent tailed phage (not to scale). (1) phage nears the bacterial cell; (2) phage contacts and binds to cell receptors; (3) phage binds irreversibly and ejects nucleic acid into the cell, where it is transcribed and translated; (4) numerous progeny phages are assembled; (5) endolysins degrade the bacterial cell wall releasing progeny phages

9.2 Application of phages in Agriculture

9.2.1 Poultry

Campylobacter jejuni and selected *Salmonella* serovars play a major role in human disease but colonise chickens with no deleterious effects on the bird (Shaughnessy et al. 2009). *Campylobacter* is a commensal in poultry though the organism's colonisation pattern in commercial broilers is not well understood (Conlan et al. 2007), thus controlling the organism in broiler flocks is a challenge. The organism's prevalence in slaughter aged broiler flocks can reach 100% on selected farms (Sahin et al. 2015). Studies have estimated that a 3 log reduction in *Campylobacter* numbers in the intestines of infected birds at slaughter, can contribute to a 90% reduction in public health risks (Crotta et al. 2017). Thus, there is a need to address on-farm *Campylobacter* control in an acceptable manner.

The leading *Salmonella* serovars of concern in the US are *S.* Enteritidis (45.7%) and *S.* Typhimurium (15.8%) (European Food Safety Authority 2016). Some of these serovars such as *S.* Enteritidis, *S.* Heidelberg (Foley et al. 2013) and *S.* Typhimurium (Crabb et al. 2018) can be present in poultry. Routes for on-farm transmission can be the hatchery (Stern 2008) or sources such as feed (Veldman et al. 1995). A meta-analysis of European surveys for pathogen prevalence in poultry meat across 21 countries attributes 33% to *Campylobacter* and 7% to *Salmonella*

(Goncalves-Tenorio et al. 2018). More specifically, the European Union States have reported the highest number of *Salmonella* non-compliant samples to be of poultry meat origin (5.1–6.8%) in comparison to table eggs (0.6%) (European Food Safety Authority 2016).

Campylobacter is responsible for around 1.3 million infections in the USA, with resistance to the common drug of choice for treatment – ciprofloxacin increasing from 13% in 1997 to 25% in 2011 (Centers for Disease Control 2013). Non-typhoidal *Salmonella* is responsible for 1.2 million illnesses in the USA, with resistance to the antibiotics of choice ceftriaxone (3%), ciprofloxacin (3%) or multiple classes of other drugs of relevance (5%) (Centers for Disease Control 2013).

Antibiotics are used on chicken farms (Mehdi et al. 2018). In the 1970s and 1980s, concerns about an increase in the antibiotic resistant *Salmonella* and *Campylobacter* and multi drug resistant (MDR) forms of *Salmonella* and *E. coli* led some countries to withdraw the use of antibiotics as growth promotants (Blackall 2019). Amongst other strategies, such as addressing public health, infection management and antibiotic stewardship, protecting the food supply at the farm or plant level is a vital step (Centers for Disease Control 2013). Reducing pathogen entry to the human food chain from intensively farmed poultry can play a contributory role in addressing human disease risks from MDR pathogens.

The use of phages as a biocontrol agent on farmed poultry is an option to meet this challenge. Phages are host specific, can replicate in the host and are a safe option for controlling *Campylobacter* and *Salmonella* (Hudson et al. 2005). An understanding of host concentrations and inactivation patterns for *Salmonella* and *Campylobacter* in foods has been addressed (Bigwood et al. 2009b). Phages have been shown to be commonly present in chicken and other foods indicating on-going consumer exposure (Tsuei et al. 2007) and thus would likely be a safe and acceptable option to be used with poultry. Connerton et al. (2011) in a review have highlighted the potential of using *Campylobacter* phages for broilers either on-farm or on food, via bio-sanitisation, to reduce *Campylobacter* numbers. Overseas models have suggested that phages have the greatest potential to reduce *Campylobacter* levels in the live chicken (Havelaar et al. 2007). But, to date, there are no commercial phage preparations against *Campylobacter*.

Research is on-going to achieve reductions in pathogen levels on farms for *Salmonella* (Sukumaran et al. 2016; Grant et al. 2017) and *Campylobacter* (Atterbury et al. 2003; Carrillo et al. 2005; El-Shibiny et al. 2009; Firlieyanti et al. 2016). Addressing pathogen levels on poultry farms can target the reduction of pathogen numbers entering the food chain. Figure 9.2 illustrates potential pathways for pathogen movement and points at which phage based interventions have been adopted to enable the reduction of pathogen loads along the human food chain. These include the use of phages at the hatchery (*Salmonella*), on-farm to reduce colonisation (*Campylobacter*, *Salmonella*) also as a feed additive (*Salmonella*) or at the plant as a carcass rise (*Salmonella*, *Campylobacter*) and finally in composted dairy waste (*Salmonella*). These approaches collectively contribute to reducing pathogen levels in a safe and sustainable manner.

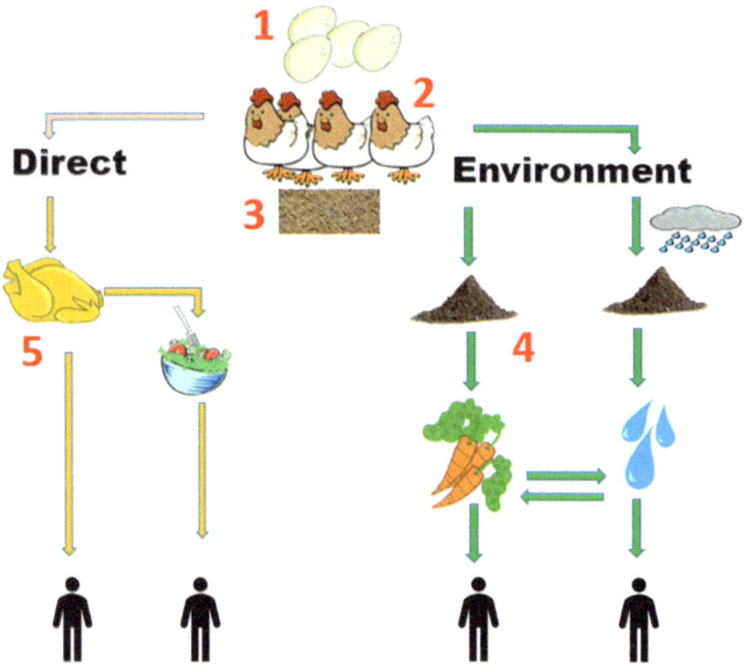

Fig. 9.2 Phage biocontrol at points of *Campylobacter* and *Salmonella* transmission in poultry farm to humans. Reduce horizontal transfer of *Salmonella* from the incubator to hatchers (1) using phage spray to fertile eggs (Henriques et al. 2013). Reduce bird colonisation (2) by phage oral administration (Colom et al. 2015; Carvalho et al. 2010). Use phage as an alternative feed additive (3) in their diet to improve growth (Kim et al. 2013). Reduce carcass contamination (4) using phage spray/wash (Goode et al. 2003; Duc et al. 2018). Use phage to manage waste/compost (5) to prevent reinfection (Heringa et al. 2010).

Campylobacter phages belong to the Myoviridae family with lytic phages from two groupings, from a total of four, having proven application in poultry (Connerton et al. 2011). The phages against *Salmonella* are lytic phages belonging to the Myoviridae, Siphoviridae and Podoviridae families (Zhang et al. 2010; Hakdong et al. 2012). The phage bacteria relationship is a natural association in the chicken gut. Lower levels of *Campylobacter* have been shown to be naturally present in the caeca of chickens (5.1 log CFU/g) in the presence of autochthonous *Campylobacter* phages compared to those chickens lacking phages in the caeca (6.9 log CFU/g) (Atterbury et al. 2005). Commercial broiler flock environments (Connerton et al. 2004) and free range poultry environments (Carrillo et al. 2007) are a source of phages against either *C. jejuni* and/or *C. coli*. Environmentally exposed mature organic birds (73 days) can also be a source of diverse phages (El-Shibiny et al. 2005). A diverse range of *Campylobacter* phages has been isolated from broilers and their farming environments adopting conventional, free range and litter re-use practices (Estella et al. 2015). Thus, *Campylobacter* phages are already a part of commercial farming and can likely form the basis for phage biocontrol in a safe and acceptable manner.

In contrast to *Campylobacter*, where there are only two species of concern, *Salmonella* has over 2600 serovars, a factor that needs consideration when considering phages suitable for biocontrol of the multiple *Salmonella* serovars which can be present in poultry at one time (Rivera et al. 2018). To address this diversity, Rivera et al. (2018) screened backyard poultry systems that had a history of *Salmonella* infections and isolated phages with a wide host range. Lytic phages were isolated from several sites, with *S.* Enteritidis proving to be a good host for phage isolation. Free range poultry environments can be a source of *Salmonella* phages (Fiorentin et al. 2004). Broad spectrum *Salmonella* phages have been isolated from sources such as sewage which has a wider source input (Akhtar et al. 2014) and dairy farms (Moreno Switt et al. 2013). Thus, as with *Campylobacter*, *Salmonella* phages can be sourced from the farming environment to adopt more "natural" biocontrol options.

Two tables follow which summarise other relevant recent literature on phage biocontrol on *Campylobacter* (Table 9.1) and *Salmonella* in poultry (Table 9.2), each highlighting outcomes and potential areas or further work. Generally, this work represents studies undertaken under controlled laboratory experimental conditions. Some experiments under commercial farming conditions, which are the minority, are also described.

The studies reviewed for poultry have provided an insight into the use of phages as a biocontrol option to reduce the levels of both *Salmonella* and *Campylobacter*. Unlike antibiotics, phage biocontrol has very specific targets and can achieve significant reductions in pathogens, though repeatability and deployment can be challenging and so there is a need for ongoing research to exploit its full potential. For poultry, future work should include a better understanding of phage resistance in the bird gut and aspects of virulence genes (Kittler et al. 2013). Selection of phage combinations that target a broad host range is another area that may require further work (Fischer et al. 2013). The potential for phages to eradicate antibiotic resistant strains is another area of interest (Janez et al. 2014). Scale-up of phage production to commercial scale and the use of suitable strains capable of producing high phage titres in a safe manner is another area that would require further work (Janež and Loc-Carrillo 2013). Whilst studies suggest the administration of phages 2 days before slaughter being the most effective, which also allows time for phage replication and minimises host resistance (El-Shibiny et al. 2009), there is a need for specific details of these options. The selection, timing and method of delivery are also key factors for attaining successful phage therapy in chickens (Atterbury et al. 2007) that need to be addressed for large commercial applications. Finally, before widespread commercial use, there is a need for more trials in commercial farming environments with naturally colonised birds (Janez et al. 2014).

Table 9.1 Experimental and farm studies on *Campylobacter* biocontrol in chickens

Experimental studies – *Campylobacter*				
Model	Bacteria	Phage	Outcome	References
20 day old broilers	*C. jejuni* (8 log CFU)	5, 7 and 9 log PFU of 2 phage cocktail (day 25)	Highest reductions 24 h and 48 h after treatment. 0.5–5 log CFU/g reduction over 5 days. Low phage resistance (<4%) and resistant mutants are unfit	Loc Carrillo et al. (2005)
10 day old chickens	*C. jejuni* (5 log CFU)	9–10 log PFU of single phage type (days 7–10)	Delayed colonisation	Wagenaar et al. (2005)
32 day old chickens	*C. jejuni* (5 log CFU)	10–11 log PFU of 2 phage cocktail (for 6 days)	Initial 3 log reduction. After 5 days, 1 log less than control	Wagenaar et al. (2005)
21 day old broilers	*C. jejuni* (8 log CFU)	Single phage type, PFU not stated (day 25)	Phage resistance via genomic rearrangements is transient and a fitness cost to the organism	Scott et al. (2007)
20 day old broilers	*C. jejuni* or *C. coli* (8 log CFU)	9 or 7log PFU of single phage type	2 log reduction in *C. jejuni* in 48 h with 7 log PFU phage dose. Higher dose (9 log PFU) needed for similar reduction of *C. coli*. Isolates acquired low resistance (2%). Group 2 phages have broad-spectrum infective potential	El-Shibiny et al. (2009)
Six day old chicks	*C. jejuni* (4 log CFU/ml)	7 log PFU/ml of 4 phage cocktail. Second group received a single phage only	Phage cocktail and single phage significantly reduced *C. jejuni* in weeks 1–4. Maximum reduction2.8 log CFU/g. observed resistance (43% single phage; 24% cocktail) did not impact on *C. jejuni* reductions. Phage persisted in birds up to 42 days	Fischer et al. (2013)
24 day old chickens	*C. jejuni* (7 log CFU)	7 log PFU of 2-phage cocktail	2.4 log CFU/g reduction in *C. jejuni*. Most effective 2 days post-treatment. Selectively targeted *Campylobacter* and no impact on other microbiota	Richards et al. (2019)
Commercial on-farm study – *Campylobacter*				
36-, 32- & 31 day broilers	Naturally colonised by *C. jejuni*	5.8–7.5 logPFU/bird of 4 phage cocktail.	Either reduction or no-effect on *C. jejuni* counts across 3 trials (days 1–4). Significant reductions (>3.2 log in the caeca) in trial 1 at slaughter. Significant reductions in trial 3, but group contaminated by naturally occurring phages. Recommended phage application at 1–4 days prior to slaughter	Kittler et al. (2013)

Table 9.2 Experimental and farm studies of *Salmonella* biocontrol in chickens

Experimental studies – *Salmonella*				
Host	Bacteria	Phage	Outcome	References
Day old chicks	*S.* Enteritidis via contact birds (9–10 log CFU/g caeca by day 7)	11 log PFU/bird of 3 phage cocktail (day 7)	3.5 fold reduction in *S.* Enteritidis compared to control (day 5). Reductions continued at 10, 15, 20 and 25 days	Fiorentin et al. (2005)
Day old chicks	*S.* Enteritidis (3.95log CFU/ chick)	8 log PFU/chick of single phage type or 2 phage cocktail (1 h post-challenge)	Reductions in *Salmonella* at 24 h, but not 48 h. Persistent reductions not observed	Andreatti et al. (2007)
Mature birds (36 days)	*S.* Enteritidis, *S.* Hadar, or *S.* Typhimurium (8 log CFU)	9 or 11 log PFU/bird of single phage type/bird.	*S.* Enteritidis reduced by >4.2 log CFU by 24 h *S.* Typhimurium reduced by 2.19 log CFU by 24 h. No effect of phage treatment against *S.* Hadar. Observed resistance dependent on phage titre i.e. higher dose higher resistance	Atterbury et al. (2007)
1 day old layer chicks	*S.* Enteritidis (7 log CFU/g) administered or via contact birds	5,7 or 9 log PFU/g feed of single phage type (21 days)	All treatments reduced *S.* Enteritidis in the intestines. 9 log PFU/g treatment resulted in 70% of contact birds with no detectable intestinal *Salmonella* 3 weeks after treatment. Both 7 log and 9 log PFU/g treatments reduced environmental contamination by 33–50%. Phages may protect against horizontal spread of *Salmonella* in the production environment	Lim et al. (2012)
Pathogen free chicks	*S.* Enteritidis or *S.* Typhimurium (5 log CFU/ chick on day 2)	12 log PFU/chick for *S.* Enteritidis and ~ 11 log PFU/chick for *S.* Typhimurium (days 1, 2, 3, 6, 8, 10, 13 & 15) Undefined phage cocktail used	Between days 7 and 15 all chicks were cleared of both *Salmonella* serovars	Nabil et al. (2018)
Commercial on-farm study – *Salmonella*				
Two control and two test broiler houses (~34,000 chickens)	*Salmonella* infection detected in house	~8 log PFU/ mLSalmoFREE®6-phage cocktail (days 18, 26/27, 34/35)	*Salmonella* levels reduced at pre-harvest stage. Reductions of *Salmonella* in second trial difficult to assess due to cross contamination of phages. Phage resistance not common	Clavijo et al. (2019)

9.2.2 Pigs

Antibiotics are commonly added to pig feed for growth and/or disease prevention in many countries. In 2011, more than 80% of pig farms in China were reported to add antibiotics in feed, drinking water or premixed feeds (Jing and Hu 2011). However, globally the use of oxytetracycline, sulfadiazine and other antibiotics in pig rearing has increased pathogen drug resistance and so now these drugs fail to effectively prevent diseases in swine. Furthermore, excessive intake of antibiotics can lead to direct damage in liver, kidney and blood in farmed animals. For these reasons, antibiotic use is now strictly regulated for disease prevention and therapy in animal husbandry in most countries.

It has been estimated that a ban on the use of antibiotics in the pig industry would lead to an increased farming cost of US$6 or more per pig (Jing and Hu 2011). So, finding alternatives to antibiotics is of great concern to the animal husbandry industry. Application of antibiotics leads to increases in animal growth and feed utilization rate by reducing subclinical infections, inhibition of competing bacteria for nutrition, enhancing host immunity and increasing beneficial microbial flora. Therefore, the search for antibiotic substitutes has concentrated on these aspects. At present, the most promising research fields include the application of phages, probiotic bacteria and bacteriocins. In this section, we review the application of phages as substitutes for antibiotics in pig breeding and pork processing.

Multi drug resistant (MDR) bacteria can enter the food chain when antibiotics are used in farm animals, therefore in the European Union (EU), the use of antibiotics as growth promoters is banned and is limited to therapeutic applications only (Vigre et al. 2008). In China, antibiotic feed additives for animals will be withdrawn in 2020 (China Ministry of Agriculture and Rural Areas 2019). However, even in the absence of antibiotic selective pressure, swine reared in antibiotic free production systems are continually exposed to persistent MDR bacteria such as MDR isolates of *Salmonella* Typhimurium (Boyen et al. 2008).

Phages have the potential to be sustainable alternatives to antibiotics used against such pathogens since they are compatible with food use, with the flexibility that they can be applied therapeutically or for sanitization purposes (Skurnik and Strauch 2006; Hanlon 2007). Generally recognized as safe (GRAS) status has been granted in the US for the use of a number of phage products as sanitization agents on ready-to-eat foods (Monk et al. 2010). Phages are being evaluated for use as 'processing aids' under EU legislation (Directive 89/107/EEC) and would be applied during manufacturing as long as any residues did not have an ongoing technological effect on the finished product. The responsibility for safety, in this case, would lie with the manufacturer, as Regulation (EC) No. 178/2002 states it is the manufacturers' responsibility to ensure the final product is safe for human consumption (von Jagow and Teufer 2007).

Phage intervention strategies have been used to control various *Salmonella* serovars including Enteritidis and Typhimurium, with experiments highlighting their potential use for biosanitization (Goode et al. 2003; Carey-Smith et al. 2006;

Bigwood et al. 2009a; Sillankorva et al. 2009) and for phage therapy of infected animals (Fiorentin et al. 2005; Atterbury et al. 2007; Wall et al. 2010). Early work by Lee and Harris (2001, 2002) demonstrated the potential for application of FelixO1 phage to reduce concentrations of *S.* Typhimurium in tonsils and caeca of young (4 week old) pigs. Reductions in *S.* Typhimurium of ~2–3 log CFU were also achieved in market weight swine following application of a phage cocktail (Wall et al. 2010).

More recently, Albino et al. (2014) isolated phages from a pig farm active against *Salmonella* Typhimurium serotypes Abony, Enteritidis, Typhi, and Typhimurium. A pool of six phages was given to 30 pigs (weight 90-100 kg) at various concentrations (10^3–10^9 PFU/ml) which had been orally inoculated (10^5 CFU/ml) with *S.* Typhimurium 2 days prior. *Salmonella* was detected in 28/30 of the faecal samples from the control pigs and 17/30 pigs given phages. These results indicate that the phages were responsible for reducing the colonization of *Salmonella* in pigs from 93% to 56%.

Experiments by Callaway et al. (2011) also demonstrated reduced carriage of *S.* Typhimurium in smaller weaned (~10 kg) pigs following phage application. A cocktail of two phages was given by oral dose (3×10^9 PFU) to half (24/48) of a group of pigs inoculated (2×10^{10} CFU) with *S.* Typhimurium 24 h prior. Following enrichment for *Salmonella*, 23/24 control pigs were positive, but only 13/24 phage treated were positive. Significant reductions in *Salmonella* concentrations were noted in the caecum and rectum of phage treated pigs. The concentration of bacteria shed was also reduced in the phage treated group, but this was not significantly different.

Application of a phage cocktail was able to reduce *S.* Typhimurium levels on artificially contaminated pig skin (Hooton et al. 2011). The phage cocktail (PC1) comprised four distinct anti *Salmonella* phages; SH17, SH18, SH19 and Felix 01. *S.* Typhimurium U288 counts were reduced to undetectable levels (>99% reduction) following the application of PC1 to pigskin. The trial provides proof of concept that the application of phage cocktails to pig skin can reduce levels of the most prevalent *S.* Typhimurium serovar in pigs and suggests phage cocktails could be used post slaughter to reduce *Salmonella* contamination of pig carcasses.

Stability of phages is a factor that needs to be ensured so that the phages can be stored, transported and delivered via the oral route to pigs. To address this challenge, a microencapsulated phage cocktail was administered to pig feed (Saez et al. 2011). Pigs were fed a microencapsulated phage cocktail daily for 5 days and compared to pigs receiving phages by oral gavage or no treatment (total = 21 pigs). Pigs in the phage treated group were less likely to shed *S.* Typhimurium at 2 h and 4 h post challenge than pigs given gavage and or no treatment ($p < 0.05$). Concentrations of *S.* Typhimurium in the ileum and cecum were also lower than control pigs. It was concluded that the feeding of microencapsulated phages is a practical and effective means of reducing *Salmonella* colonization and shedding in pigs.

Escherichia coli has developed resistance against many antibiotics that are used in human and veterinary medicine, including pigs (Stedt et al. 2014). The early experiments of Smith and Huggins (1983) first demonstrated the potential of phages to treat *E. coli* diarrhoea in piglets (< 1-day-old). Whereby either a mixture of two phages, or a single phage, were tested for control of an experimentally induced *E. coli* O20 infection. Phage treated piglets had much reduced concentrations of *E. coli* at 3 h post treatment (7 log CFU/g faeces vs 9 log CFU/g) and 7 h post treatment (5 log CFU/g vs 9 log CFU/g) compared to controls. All phage treated piglets survived, whereas the majority of control piglets did not.

More recently, weaned pigs with an experimentally induced enterotoxigenic *E. coli* O149:H10 diarrhoea were treated with phages, both individually and as a seven phage cocktail (Jamalludeen et al. 2009). Administration of phages was either shortly after challenge (10^{10} CFU) or 24 h later, following the onset of diarrhoea. Six phages (10^{10} PFU), each individually administered shortly after challenge, produced a significant difference in weight change, duration and severity of diarrhoea, and extent of shedding over 6 days. A cocktail of three phages was tested shortly after *E. coli* challenge, with co-treatment of florfenicol to reduce competing flora and oral administration of sodium bicarbonate to neutralise stomach pH, and was found to significantly reduce the severity of diarrhoea and the diarrhoea score. Phage therapy of pigs after disease onset was trialled using a mixture of two phages and again improvements in weight change, duration and severity of diarrhoea, and the extent of shedding were observed compared to controls. This work suggests that phage treatment for *E. coli* diarrhoea in pigs may be a promising approach.

Another cause of diarrhoeal disease in piglets and young pigs are *Clostridium* spp. Lee et al. (2016) have examined the potential for phages to control *Clostridium* and other coliforms in suckling pigs and crossbred sows. The authors used a commercial phage preparation (CTCBIO Inc., Seoul, Republic of Korea; 10^9 PFU/g) containing three *E. coli* specific phages and two *C. perfringens* specific phages. Addition of the phages in suckling piglet's diets led to an increase in the number of weaned piglets, increased body weight at weaning and increased average daily weight gain. Supplementation of sow's diets with phages decreased faecal *Clostridium* shedding at day 14 and coliform shedding was significantly lower at the end of the experiment (day 21). For suckling piglets, *Clostridium* and coliform shedding was reduced at both day 14 and day 21. This work highlights the potential for phages to replace antibiotics as growth promotants in pigs.

Salem et al. (2015) have also demonstrated an association between the prevalence of phages and *Yersinia enterocolitica* and *Y. pseudotuberculosis* in pigs in Finland. While these species are not considered to cause disease in pigs, they are significant to the pork industry as consumption of undercooked pig meat can cause human foodborne illness. Further work has been undertaken to characterise the phages from the earlier study (Salem and Skurnik 2018), which could be used in future for biocontrol experiments to reduce the concentrations of these foodborne pathogens on pigs prior to slaughter.

Phages are promising alternatives for the replacement of antibiotics in pig production. Applications include biocontrol pig diseases, promotion of weight gain, and reduction, or elimination, of transmission of foodborne pathogens to humans via pig meat. In particular, it has proven to be very challenging to replace antibiotic use during weaning of piglets and so phages could be a very valuable addition to animal husbandry and veterinary practice in this common agricultural practice.

9.2.3 Dairy Cows and Beef Cattle

Common bacterial diseases in dairy cows are clinical and subclinical mastitis, metritis, retained placenta, diarrhoea, lameness and respiratory diseases (Gutierrez et al. 2019). Mastitis is a common disease in dairy cows and is caused predominantly by *Staphylococcus* spp. Enterotoxigenic *E. coli* (ETEC) causes calf diarrhoea, which has a severe economic impact on beef and dairy farmers due to its high mortality and morbidity rates (Gutierrez et al. 2019). It is challenging to treat these pathogens in bovines as there is global pressure to reduce antibiotic use on farms and many strains have developed antibiotic resistance.

9.2.3.1 Mastitis

Bovine mastitis is an inflammation of the mammary gland and udder tissues of cows. It affects the quality and quantity of milk production and causes severe economic loss to dairy farmers worldwide. Mastitis is caused by contagious pathogens such as *Staphylococcus* spp., *Streptococcus* spp. or by environmental pathogens such as *E. coli*. In addition to pathogens, it can also be caused or promoted by injury, allergies and neoplasia's (Barrera-Rivas et al. 2017). *Staphylococcus aureus* is responsible for about one third of cases of clinical and subclinical mastitis (Saglam et al. 2017). Mastitis can be treated with antibiotics but the ability to acquire resistance to multiple antibiotics makes *S. aureus* challenging to treat (Barrera-Rivas et al. 2017). A survey in Mexico of 36 *S. aureus* strains from cow milk with subclinical mastitis identified that more than 90% of isolates were resistant to six or more antibiotics, 77% to cefuroxime, 81% to tetracycline, and 100% were resistant to penicillin, dicloxacillin, cefotaxime, ampicillin and cephalothin. However, 100% of these isolates were susceptible to phages demonstrating the potential of phages to combat antibiotic resistant mastitis causing pathogens (Varela-Ortiz et al. 2018). Similarly, Son et al. (2010) found that multiple drug resistant *S. aureus* isolates from milk in Korea were sensitive to phages.

Both *in vitro* and *in vivo* studies have indicated that either individual phage or phage cocktails could be effective in treating *S. aureus* and methicillin resistant *S. aureus* (MRSA) (Ganaie et al. 2018; Iwano et al. 2018, and Table 9.3). Due to the difficulties working with large animals, much *in vivo* work on mastitis phage biocontrol has been undertaken using mice as a model organism for cows. The efficacy of two phages (vBSM-A1 and vBSP-A2) was tested by Geng et al. (2019) in a mouse lactation model. Lactating mice (10–14 days post-partum) were inoculated with *S. aureus* and 4 h later treated with the phages individually or as a cocktail. A reduction in *S. aureus* numbers was observed in phage treated mice, along with

Table 9.3 Phage biocontrol of bovine mastitis

Model	Bacteria	Treatment	Observation	References
Lactating mouse	*S. aureus*	2 phage cocktail	Reduced bacterial count (>4log CFU). Reduced scores for gland pathology and histology	Breyne et al. (2017)
Lactating mouse	*S. aureus*	2 phages individually and as a cocktail	Improved mammary pathology and reduced bacterial counts	Geng et al. (2019)
Lactating mouse	*S. aureus*	1 phage (ϕSA012)	Significant reductions in CFU and reduced mammary gland inflammation	Iwano et al. (2018)
Bovine mammary epithelial cells (MAC-T)	*S. aureus*	1 phage (vB_SauM_JS25)	Significant reductions in intracellular counts	Zhang et al. (2017)
Cow udder	*S. aureus*	1 phage (phage K)	Non-significant (16.7%) elimination of infection in udder quarters	Gill et al. (2006a)
Cow udder	*S. aureus*	3 phage cocktail	Reduction in disease progression (70–81%)	https://milksa.co.za/research/dairy-rd-in-sa/biological-control-mastitis-cows-using-bacteriophages
Cow udder	*S. aureus, P. aeruginosa* and others	3 phage cocktail	Qualitative reduction in infected udders (66%)	Shende et al. (2017)
Bovine mammary epithelial cells (MAC-T)	*E. coli*	4 phage cocktail	Reduction in mammary cell adhesion (98.0–99.7%) and invasion (74.3–98.1%)	Porter et al. (2016)

significant improvements in mammary pathology. The effectiveness of the phage cocktail was greater than either phage alone, and the effect was comparable to a positive control treated with the antibiotic ceftiofur (Geng et al. 2019).

Another two phage cocktail was tested in a murine lactation model by Breyne et al. (2017). Mice (10–14 days post-partum) were injected in the fourth abdominal mammary gland pair with 3.4×10^2 CFU/gland *S. aureus.* Phage treated groups received an intramammary dose of 3×10^7 PFU4h later. Testing of glands 24 h later revealed a significant 4.3 log reduction in *S. aureus* count in phage treated glands compared to the control, with the antibiotic cefalonium achieving a 6.7 log reduction. Gross pathology and histology gradings of glands were also significantly reduced compared to the untreated control for both phage and antibiotic treated groups.

Iwano et al. (2018) tested the efficacy of a single phage (ϕSA012) against *S. aureus* in another lactating mouse model. The left and right fourth mammary glands of mice, 7–10 days after parturition, were injected with 25 μl *S. aureus* (10^3-10^5 CFU) and subsequently injected with 25 μl ϕSA012 (10^5–10^7 PFU) into the mammary gland or 100 μl ϕSA012 (4×10^7PFU) intraperitoneally or intravenously. Groups of lactating mice were euthanized on days 2 and 4, and the glands tested to determine the number of CFU. There were reductions in CFU but no significant effect of phage treatment when 10^5CFU were challenged in the mice, likely due to a large inflammatory response to the bacterium damaging the glands. At the lower inoculum (10^3CFU), there was less inflammation and treatment with phages did lead to significant reductions in *S. aureus* by all three administration routes. Controls demonstrated that phages did not induce inflammation in the glands.

Whilst *S. aureus* is typically an extracellular pathogen it does have the potential for invasion of mammalian cells, and this lifestyle may be a factor in the survival and persistence of the bacteria in bovine and human infections such as mastitis. Zhang et al. (2017) tested the ability of phages to treat intracellular infections. They found that phages could be internalised, by phagocytosis, into cells from a bovine mammary cell line (MAC-T) at low rates (12%) and were able to infect and kill *S. aureus* when internalised.

However, phage treatments for *S. aureus* in cow udders have given mixed results. Holstein cows with naturally occurring subclinical *S. aureus* mastitis were treated with intramammary infusion of phage K (1.25×10^{11}PFU/day, 5 days) during lactation (Gill et al. 2006a). Three of 18 quarters (16.7%) were cured in the phage treated group and none of the 20 control group quarters was cured (no significant difference). In further experiments, infusion of phages into quarters resulted in an increased somatic cell count in the milk and PFU counts indicated there was significant degradation or inactivation of the phage occurring. Further work by the same group suggested that adsorption of milk whey proteins to the *S. aureus* cell surface appeared to inhibit phage attachment and hinder cell lysis (Gill et al. 2006b).

Milk South Africa published a study of phage treatment of *S. aureus* mastitis in dairy cows udders (https://milksa.co.za/research/dairy-rd-in-sa/biological-control-mastitis-cows-using-bacteriophages; Accessed 16/09/2019). A three phage cocktail (3.9×10^9PFU) was tested in a series of trials (28 cows in three trials) to cure natural cases of *S. aureus* mastitis. Treated cows were sampled daily for 1 week during treatment and 2 weeks after treatment. Results showed that mastitis was reduced by 73% in trial 1, 70% in trial 2 and 81% in trial 3 compared to the control (40% glycerol solution), as measured by area under disease progression curve (AUDPC) measurement. There was also a variable increase (up to 2 log) in the amount of phage detected in milk, suggesting some phage replication was occurring *in vivo*. However, there is no further information on the status of the project.

Another group in India have also reported applying phages to control mixed species (*S. aureus* and *P. aeruginosa*) mastitis in cows not responding to antibiotic therapy (Shende et al. 2017). A three phage cocktail was applied by intramammary infusion (6 ml 3 × 10^{12} PFU/ml) to six cows similarly to the protocol of Gill et al. (2006a) described above. Four of the six cases were cured of infection by day 10 (66%) as measured by qualitative assessment (Shende et al. 2017).

Initial work to investigate the potential of phage for biocontrol of *E. coli* associated mastitis has been undertaken by Porter et al. (2016). A bovine mammary epithelial cell (MAC-T) assay was used to test if phages (4 phage cocktail; 10^8 PFU/well) could stop cell attachment and invasion by three mastitic *E. coli* strains (10^6CFU/well). Pre-treatment of the cell line with the phage cocktail significantly reduced mammary cell adhesion by the three *E. coli* strains (by 98.0, 99.6, and 99.7%) and intracellular survival in mammary cells (by 88.3, 98.1, and 74.3%).

Phages active against other mastitis causing pathogens such as *Streptococcus* spp. and *Klebsiella* spp. have been isolated (Russell et al. 1969; Hill and Brady 1989; Amiri Fahliyani et al. 2018), but to date, there is no evidence that these have been tested in animal models or bovines.

9.2.3.2 Other Human and Bovine Pathogens

Most strains of *E. coli* are harmless to bovines and humans, but some strains produce Shiga toxins which can cause foodborne disease in humans. Shiga toxin producing strains of *E. coli* (STEC) can cause bloody diarrhoea including haemorrhagic colitis and HUS (haemolytic uremic syndrome). The most prevalent STEC are serotypes O157:H7, O26, O103, O121, O111 and O45, and these are considered adulterants in food (US Food Safety and Inspection Service 2012). Ruminants, especially cattle, are the main reservoir for STEC. Beef carcasses can be contaminated with faecal matter containing STEC via hides during slaughter and consumption of raw or undercooked beef can lead to food poisoning (Sabouri et al. 2017; Abdelsattar et al. 2019).

Antibiotics can be used to reduce shedding of STEC but are not highly effective as many strains are resistant to antibiotics. So post harvest beef carcass safety measures, including hide wash cabinets for hide-on carcasses, steam vacuuming of hide-off carcasses, organic acids and hot water-sprays are used to reduce the contamination of carcasses (Tolen et al. 2018). However, post slaughter decontamination of STEC on carcasses is resource intensive and not always completely effective. Phages have been examined as an alternative intervention in beef cattle for this purpose. The phages can be applied to hides just before slaughter to minimise carcass cross contamination or be delivered orally and rectally to reduce shedding of STEC in faeces. Most cattle are infected at an early stage of the production cycle at less than 12 weeks old, so it has been recommended that treatment should be targeted at calves (Gutierrez et al. 2019).

Experiments where a 4-phage phage cocktail was delivered orally, rectally, and both orally and rectally (3.3 × 10^{11} PFU, 1.5 × 10^{11} PFU, 4.8 × 10^{11} PFU respectively) to cattle did not achieve a significant reduction of *E. coli* O157:H7 numbers in faeces compared to the untreated control (Rozema et al. 2009). Rivas et al. (2010) demonstrated reductions in *E. coli* O157:H7 within a rumen model when dosed with two O157-specific phages, but again, when the phages were applied to live animals there was no significant reduction in faecal shedding of *E. coli* O157:H7 compared to control animals. A plausible explanation for these results may be that orally administered phages are inactivated by stomach acids. To overcome this, an encapsulated 4 phage cocktail (Ephage; 10^{10} PFU/day in bolus or 10^{11} PFU/day in feed) was administered orally to steers inoculated with *E. coli* O157:H7 (10^{11} CFU). Although shedding of *E. coli* O157:H7 was significantly reduced by 14 days in bolus-fed steers, overall there was no decrease in the concentration of *E. coli* O157:H7 shed by either Ephage treatment (Stanford et al. 2010).

Some studies have also been undertaken on the feasibility of using phages to treat STEC on cattle hides prior to slaughter. Arthur et al. (2016) tested the commercial phage product Finalyse (Elanco, US) applied (10^{10}PFU/head) in one gallon of water/head with a dwell time of at least 1 h to ~300 cattle, with an equal number of untreated controls. Analysis of hide and carcass samples for *E. coli* O157:H7 revealed a prevalence of 51.8% in phage treated animals compared to 57.6% in the controls. In carcass samples, the *E. coli* O157 prevalence was 17.1% from phage treated animals compared to 17.6% in samples from untreated animals. So, neither sample type showed significant reductions in concentrations of *E. coli* O157:H7 associated with phage use. Another commercial phage preparation (Passport Food Safety Solutions, US) for control of STEC O157 and non-O157 was tested by Tolen et al. (2018) on detached hides. Phage treatment (~10^8 PFU/ml) resulted in small 0.4–0.7 log CFU/cm^2 reductions (inoculum 10^8CFU/ml) in *E. coli* O157, O121, and O103. But serotypes O111 and O45 did not show any significant reduction.

So, whilst there have been some positive signs, the overall efficacy of phage against STEC either by oral/rectal or hide treatment has been mostly negative. Reasons for this are not fully clear but factors may include the presence of substantial amounts of competing microflora, an association of STEC with mucosa making the bacterium inaccessible, and presence of faeces and other biomaterials sequestering phage.

Some strains of enterotoxigenic *E. coli* are also a threat to new-born calves where they can induce life threatening diarrhoea. Smith and Huggins (1983) applied a two phage cocktail (2×10^{11} PFU) to 8-16 h old calves infected with (3×10^9 CFU) *E. coli* O9:K30,99. They found calves treated with the cocktail 1-8 h after infection were protected from diarrhoea onset and death, whilst delay of phage treatment until diarrhoea began almost always resulted in death. In addition, naïve calves fed faeces from phage excreting calves were protected from establishment of *E. coli* infection and remained healthy. More recently, work has been undertaken looking at phage control of *Salmonella* infections in calves (Shirley 2016). Three pairs of 5–7 week old calves were inoculated with *S.* Enteritidis (~10^{10} CFU) and at the onset of fever, one of the pairs of calves was administered a 7 phage cocktail (7×10^{10} PFU) each day for 5 days. One of the phage treated calves showed reduced shedding and recovered, whilst the other treated calf did not recover and was euthanised. Other control animals had equal or intermediate symptoms to the latter calf. The phage treated calf showed the least shedding of *Salmonella* amongst all calves and phage were detected in faeces and peripheral lymph nodes, which indicate that this may be a promising approach for therapy.

There is clearly still much work to be undertaken for phage therapy of bacterial pathogens in dairy cows and beef cattle. The most promising applications under development are those for cow mastitis and, possibly, treatment of calves. Whereas, applications for phages to control STEC in beef cattle are going to require much more intensive research to come to fruition.

9.2.4 Horticulture

A narrow range of antibiotics are used for horticulture and the total volumes used are lower compared to other agricultural sectors, however, their use does likely result in contamination of soils and waterways due to overspray (Thanner et al. 2016). Streptomycin is the main antibiotic in use for plant disease control globally and is used for pathogens such as *Erwinia amylovora* (fire blight of apple and pear), *Pseudomonas syringae* (flower and fruit infections of apple and pear) and *Xanthomonas campestris* (bacterial spot of tomato and pepper) (Sundin and Wang 2018). Despite a ban on antibiotic use for control of plant diseases by the European Union, streptomycin is used for fire blight management in Austria, Germany, and Switzerland under controls (Thanner et al. 2016; Sundin and Wang 2018). Some other antibiotics used in horticulture include oxytetracycline (bacterial spot of peach and nectarine), gentamicin (fire blight and vegetable diseases), oxolinic acid (fire blight) and kasugamycin (rice plant diseases, fire blight, kiwifruit canker) (Woodcock 2016; Sundin and Wang 2018).

In 2017 the FAO convened a meeting of technical experts to discuss antimicrobial resistance (AMR) and foods of plant origin (FAO 2018). Key findings from this meeting were that AMR genes, including those coding for resistance to drugs used to treat human and animal infections, are found in bacteria isolated from plant based foods. Furthermore, experiments where the lettuce was inoculated with antibiotic resistant bacteria and fed to mice, also shows that produce is a potential vector for transmission of antibiotic resistance to humans (ASM 2019). Whilst the extent to which antimicrobial use in horticulture selects for the emergence and maintenance of AMR bacteria in plant based systems is unknown, it is evident that pathogenic bacteria (both AMR and non-AMR) need to be controlled by better management strategies, including the application of new technologies such as phages.

There have been a variety of bacterial diseases of horticultural plants that have been assessed for phage biocontrol (Table 9.4). Fire blight, as may be expected being one of the key diseases currently controlled by antibiotics, has been the subject of several studies. Gasic et al. (2014) isolated seven phages specific to the fire blight causative organism *Erwinia amylovora* in Serbia. Phage Ea2 was selected for biocontrol experiments in pear and apple flowers. The phage (10^8 PFUml^{-1}) was

Table 9.4 Summary of phage biocontrol experiments on plant diseases

Crop	Bacterial Disease	Causative Bacteria	Treatment	Outcome	References
Apple/Pear/ Quince	Fire blight	*Erwinia amylovora*	3 phage cocktail	Significant reduction of concentration on flowers (65–84%)	Schwarczinger et al. (2017)
Apple/Pear	Fire blight	*Erwinia amylovora*	One phage	Significant reduction of symptoms on flowers and reduction of symptoms on pear slices	Gasic et al. (2014)
Apple/Pear	Fire blight	*Erwinia amylovora*	4 phages separately	Reduction of concentration on apple flowers (40–90%) and symptoms on pear slices	Müller et al. (2011)
Grape	Pierce's	*Xylella fastidiosa*	4 phage cocktail	Reduction in symptoms on leaves and CFU at inoculum sites (3 log)	Das et al. (2015)
Grapefruit	Citrus canker	*Xanthomonas axonopodis* pv. *citri*	4 phage cocktail	Reduction in disease symptoms (27–87%)	Balogh et al. (2008)
Kiwifruit	Canker	*Pseudomonas syringae* pv. *actinidiae*	One phage	Reduction in leaf necrosis (80%)	Oh (2018)
Leek	Blight	*Pseudomonas syringae* pv. *Porri*	6 phage cocktail	Some reductions but results not significant	Rombouts et al. (2016)
Lettuce	Soft rot	*Pectobacterium carotovorum* subsp. *carotovorum*	One phage	Reduced incidence of soft rot (~75%)	Lim et al. (2013)
Mushroom	Brown blotch	*Pseudomonas tolaasii*	3 phage cocktail	Formation of blotches completely inhibited	Kim et al. (2011)
Onion	Leaf blight	*Xanthomonas axponpodis* pv. *Allii*	5 phage cocktail	Reduction in disease severity (11–35%)	Lang et al. (2007)
Orange	Citrus spot	*Xanthomonas axponpodis* pv. *citrumelo*	3 phage cocktail	Reduction in disease symptoms (35–48%)	Balogh et al. (2008)
Pepper (Paprika)	Black spot	*Xanthomonas euvesicatoria*	One phage	Reduction in lesions (15.2–67.9%)	Gasic et al. (2018)

(continued)

Table 9.4 (continued)

Crop	Bacterial Disease	Causative Bacteria	Treatment	Outcome	References
Potato	Soft rot	*Dickeya solani, Pectobacterium carotovorum, Pectobacterium wasabiae*	2 phages separately or as a cocktail	Reduction of maceration in slices (80%) and whole tuber (95%)	Czajkowski et al. (2015)
Potato	Soft rot	*Dickeya solani*	9 phages separately	Reduction of tuber maceration (up to 50%)	Czajkowski et al. (2014)
Potato	Soft rot	*Dickeya solani*	One phage	Reduction of plants infected (up to 93%)	Czajkowski et al. (2017)
Potato	Soft rot	*Dickeya solani*	6 phage cocktail	Reduction in diseased tissue (75.3%) and disease incidence (47.6%)	Carstens et al. (2018)
Potato	Soft rot/ black leg	*Pectobacterium atrosepticum*	3 phage cocktail	Reduction in rotten tissue (94.2%)	Buttimer et al. (2018)
Potato	Wilt	*Ralstonium solanacearum*	6 phage cocktail	Reduction in wilting (20%)	Wei et al. (2017)
Potato	Common scab	*Streptomyces scabies*	One phage	Reduced tuber surface lesions (94.8%)	McKenna et al. (2001)
Geranium (potato model)	Soft rot	*Dickeya dadantii*	2 phages separately	Complete suppression of symptoms	Soleimani-Delfan et al. (2015)
Radish	Common scab	*Streptomyces scabies*	2 phages separately	Reduction of symptoms in seedlings	Goyer (2005)
Rice	Wilt	*Xanthomonas oryzae* pv. *oryzae*	6 phage cocktail	Reduced incidence of disease (50.1–53.7%)	Chae et al. (2014)
Tomato	Wilt	*Ralstonium solanacearum*	One phage	Suppression or delay in wilting	Bae (2012)
Tomato	Wilt	*Ralstonium solanacearum*	One phage	Complete suppression of wilting	Fujiwara et al. (2011)
Tomato	Wilt	*Ralstonium solanacearum*	One phage	Complete suppression of wilting	Elhalag et al. (2018)
Tomato	Spot	*Xanthomonas campestris* pv. *vesicatoria*	6 phage cocktail	Reduction in disease progression (16.5–41.5%)	Obradovic et al. (2004)
Tomato	Speck	*Pseudomonas syringae* pv. *tomato*	47 phages separately	7/47 phages suppressed disease incidence >50%	Cement et al. (2018)
Tomato	Spot	*Xanthomonas perforans*	8 phages separately	Reduction in disease severity (21–56%)	Balogh et al. (2018)

applied to flowers at the same time as *E. amylovora* inoculation, 2 h before, or 2 h after. Application of the phage 2 h before *E. amylovora* inoculation and at the same time as *E. amylovora* inoculation significantly reduced fire blight symptom development, however, there was no significant effect when phages were applied 2 h after *E. amylovora* inoculation.

Twelve phages active against *E. amylovora* were isolated in Hungary from blighted apple, pear and quince trees (Schwarczinger et al. 2017). A three phage cocktail (ϕH2A, ϕH5K, ϕH7B; 10^{10} PFU ml^{-1}) was tested for a reduction in *E. amylovora* numbers (10^5 CFU ml^{-1}) in apple flowers (total volume applied 20 μl). The flowers (15 flowers/treatment) were incubated at a relative humidity of 80% at 24/21 °C (day/night) for 4 days. The phage cocktail reduced *E. amylovora* significantly (65–84%) compared to untreated controls for all the apple and quince cultivars tested. The same phage cocktail was then tested on unripe pear fruit slices. Where 10 ml phage cocktail (10^{10} PFU ml^{-1}) was used to soak the pear slices for 5 min each and dried slices were inoculated with 10 μl (10^5 CFU ml^{-1}) of *E. amylovora*. Slices were incubated at 28 °C in the dark for 4 days. Pear slices were then ranked for symptoms according to a bonitation scale. Symptom severity was reduced on both cultivars tested compared to positive controls.

Bacterial canker of kiwifruit trees, which is caused by *Pseudomonas syringae* pv. *Actinidiae* (*Psa*), is an issue worldwide with control options limited apart from antibiotics and copper (Woodcock 2016; Oh 2018; Wojtus et al. 2019; Yin et al. 2019). So alternative methods need to be developed. Oh (2018) have isolated 77 phages active against *Psa* strains from soils in South Korean kiwifruit orchards. Phage cocktails (3–5 phages; 10^7–10^8 PFU ml^{-1}) were sprayed onto 1 month old grafted kiwifruit trees in a greenhouse 3 h before inoculation with *Psa* (10^8 CFU ml^{-1}). Treatment with phages protected kiwifruit trees from *Psa* at a similar level to streptomycin treatment, with an 80% reduction in leaf necrosis measured compared to untreated controls at 27 days post inoculum.

Xylella fastidiosa subsp. *fastidiosa* causes Pierce's Disease and is a significant issue for the US wine industry (Das et al. 2015). Transmission is via sap-feeding insects and it colonizes the xylem of host plants forming clogging biofilms. Disease control methods are often only partially successful, with the most widely used practice being the application of systemic insecticides such as neonicotinoids. However, these chemicals have been associated with bee colony collapse disorder, so new methods are required. Phage biocontrol has been explored for this purpose (Das et al. 2015). A cocktail of four phages (Sano, Salvo, Prado, Paz; 40 μl 10^{10} $PFUml^{-1}$) was applied to 21 grapevines and tested for therapeutic and prophylactic biocontrol efficacy against *X. Fastidiosa* (40 μl 10^9 CFU ml^{-1} injected at two locations/plant). At weeks 8 and 12 (5 and 9 weeks post-treatment) the level of *X. fastidiosa* was significantly lower (10–1000×) in treated grapevines compared to non-treated grapevines. Non-treated grapevines began to show symptoms from week 4, with all grapevines exhibiting typical *X. fastidiosa* symptoms by week 7–8. Phage treated grapevines had no symptoms after week 4 (1-week post treatment) and were asymptomatic for the remainder of the experiment. In studies where grapevines were treated with the phage cocktail prophylactically, pathogen levels reached up to

10^3 CFU/site at weeks 8and 12 post treatment, compared to up to 10^6 CFU/site in non-prophylactically treated grapevines. Phage treated grapevines showed no *X. fastidiosa* symptoms at week 8 or 12.

Asiatic citrus canker is caused by *Xanthomonas axonopodis* pv. *Citri* is a significant disease of citrus impacting fruit yield and quality (Balogh et al. 2008). Integrated pest management is used for its control including the use of mixtures of fungicides and copper solutions, but these chemicals impact the soil and increase long term resistance so alternatives such as phage biocontrol are warranted. Balogh et al. (2008) have tested the use of phages against *X. axonopodis* in both Duncan grapefruit and Valencia orange plants. Duncan grapefruit plants grown in glasshouses were treated with a four phage cocktail (CP2, ϕXac2005–1, ccϕ7, ccϕ13; 10^8–10^9 PFU/ml) in the evening and the next morning inoculated with *X. axonopodis* (10^6–10^8 CFU/ml). Then disease severity was measured in the plants 3–4 weeks later. In 4 of 5 experiments, there was a significant reduction in disease severity recorded compared to the control. Combination of phages with either skim milk, to prolong *in planta* phage stability, or copper-mancozeb treatment were not as effective as phages alone in reducing disease symptoms. Further trials on the use of phages for both grapefruit and orange citrus canker were conducted in commercial nurseries using naturally infected plants (Balogh et al. 2008). Phage treatment significantly reduced disease progression on Valencia oranges in two trials (48 & 35%). However, there was no significant effect on grapefruit plants. Phage treatment also demonstrated significant control of citrus spot caused by a phage sensitive strain but was not more effective than copper-mancozeb.

Tomato is another fruit crop vulnerable to many bacterial diseases and has been the subject of a number of phage biocontrol experiments (Table 9.4). Tomato wilt caused by *Ralstonium solanacearum* is a devasting disease with limited treatment options due to a ban on methyl bromide use and ineffectiveness of other chemicals (Bae 2012). The effects of the Podovirus PE204 on biocontrol of *R. solanacearum* on tomato plants were measured either with co-inoculation, prophylactic treatment or post-challenge (Bae 2012). Co-inoculation of PE204 (10^8PFU/ml) with *R. solanacearum* completely inhibited bacterial wilt occurrence. Addition of a wetting agent (0.1% Silwet L-77) to the phage solution did not inhibit biocontrol potential. Conversely, prophylactic phage treatment 1 day prior to bacterial challenge was unable to control bacterial wilt. Treatment 1 day post challenge was able to delay wilt development for approximately 3 days. A different approach was taken by Fujiwara et al. (2011), where tomato seedlings were grown in peat pellets soaked in 10^{10} PFU phage ϕRSL1 for 1 month, followed by another 10^{10} PFU phage inoculum. Two days later, root tips were cut and dipped in 10^8 CFU *R. solanacearum.* Symptoms were then graded in treated and control plants for up to 18 days. No phage treated plants wilted at 18 days post challenge, but all control plants were wilted at this time.

In the US, antibiotics and copper based chemicals have been used to control bacterial spot in tomato (Balogh et al. 2018). The antibiotic streptomycin was used extensively, but within a few years strains developed resistance. Subsequent use of copper solutions also led to resistance to that bactericide. So alternate interventions, such as phages, are needed to prevent crop losses (Balogh et al. 2018). Eight phages (PFU) were separately tested for biocontrol ability against spot causing bacterium *Xanthomonas perforans* in tomato plants. A variable reduction in disease severity (21–56%) was noted for each of the phage treatments. Another cause of tomato spot is the bacterium *Xanthomonas campestris* pv. *vesicatoria* and phage biocontrol using a commercial product (Agriphage; Omnilytics, Salt Lake City, US) has been tested against this species (Obradovic et al. 2004). Agriphage contained six different phages and was formulated with additives to prolong phage activity. The phage preparation (~10^{10} PFU/ml) was applied twice per week at dusk to plants experimentally infected with 10^8 CFU/ml *X. campestris.* Phage treatment significantly reduced disease severity and appeared to increase yield (not statistically significant) compared to copper-mancozeb treatment. In two following experiments, where phages were suspended in skimmed milk and sucrose, further improvements in spot disease control were recorded, but yields were not improved.

Tomato speck is a bacterial disease caused by *Pseudomonas syringae* pv. *tomato* (Pst) and causes decreased yield, defoliation, flower abortion and fruit damage. Pst is a commercial threat to tomato growing in Turkey and researchers there have investigated the use of 47 phages as alternatives to antibiotics (streptomycin) and fungicides/bactericides (mancozeb/copper) (Cement et al. 2018). Tomato seeds were dipped into a Pst suspension (10^8CFU/ml) for 30 min and dried for 24 h. For each trial, 150 pathogen treated tomato seeds were immersed into a phage solution (10^8 PFU/ml), mixed for 30 min, dried overnight and sown in pots with sterile soil. Ten days after germination each cotyledon was examined for speck symptoms. In trial 1, with seeds treated with 10 individual phages, the incidence and severity of Pst were reduced 6.2–39.1% and 8.6–51.4%, respectively. In trial 2, using 15 individual phages the incidence and severity of Pst were more variable and reduced 5.3–100% and 18.5–100%, respectively. Four of 15 phages had no significant effect. In trial 3, using14 individual phages, half the phages (7) had no significant effect and the remaining phages reduced the disease incidence and severity up to 35.8% and 44.3%, respectively. In the final trial of eight phages, only two phages produced a significant effect, producing 45.6–50.9% and 50.5–59.1% reductions in incidence and severity, respectively.

Soft rot is one of the most destructive bacterial diseases in agriculture that is estimated to affect 15–30% of crop production. Potato tuber soft rot and blackleg caused by soft rot Enterobacteriaceae, *Pectobacterium* spp. and *Dickeya* spp. result in losses in crop production worldwide (Carstens et al. 2018). Attempts to control blackleg, soft rot and other diseases in potato tubers have often been ineffective since the ban on antibiotics (streptomycin, tetracycline and vancomycin) and mercury based pesticides, due to the absence of effective alternatives (Czajkowski et al. 2014; Soleimani-Delfan et al. 2015).

Historically, *Pectobacterium* sp. have been the most problematic rot diseases of potato in temperate regions. *Pectobacterium atrosepticum* causes potato blackleg and soft rot, and biocontrol of induced soft rot (100 μl 10^7 CFU/ml *P. atrosepticum*) was assessed in whole tubers using a three phage cocktail (100 μl 10^7 PFU/ml). The weight of rotten tissue was 5.4(±3.1) g in controls and 0.3(±0.5) g in phage cocktail treated tubers, indicating this may be an effective treatment (Buttimer et al. 2018). However, the emergence and rapid spread of a new genetic clade of *Dickeya*, now named *Dickeya solani,* over the last 15 years is causing significant crop losses and so urgent action is required for its control.

A cocktail of six phages was tested for biocontrol of *D. solani* in a potato maceration assay; tubers were damaged by penetration with a steel rod, treated with phages (5×10^8 PFU/ml per phage) or water, inoculated with *D. solani* (10^9 CFU/ml), wrapped and incubated in the dark for 5 days (Carstens et al. 2018). Phage treatment significantly reduced disease incidence by >0.5 g macerated tissue (75.3% reduction) and disease severity (93.3 to 48.9%). However, biocontrol did not completely eliminate the infection from all tubers. Czajkowski et al. (2014) also treated sliced potato tubers experimentally infected by *D. solani* with nine separate phages. Seven of these phages were able to reduce potato tuber maceration to at least 50% of the untreated controls. Another series of experiments by this group also demonstrated phage biocontrol of multispecies rot (*P. carotovorum* subsp. *carotovorum, D. solani, P. wasabiae*) in potato slice and whole tuber assays (Czajkowski et al. 2015).

Biocontrol of rot in potato plants infected by *D. solani* using a single phage type (ϕD5) was undertaken by Czajkowski et al. (2017). In the first series of experiments, *in vitro* potato plants were inoculated with 10 μl of ϕD5 (10^{10}PFU/ml) and incubated at 20–22°C for 24 h. Plants were then inoculated with 10 μl *D. solani* (10^6CFU/ml) and monitored for 10 days. There was a significant difference in both numbers of infected plants (~92% decrease) and concentration of the pathogen (~2.5 log CFU decrease) in the phage treated groups. In the second series of experiments, potato plants were grown in potting mix for 2 weeks and treated with a suspension of ϕD5 (10^8PFU/ml). One week later, the potting mix was inoculated with 10^6CFU/ml *D. solani*. There was a significant difference in both numbers of infected plants (~93% decrease) and concentration of the pathogen (~1.5 log CFU decrease) in the phage treated groups. Together these data suggest ϕD5 may help protect potato from developing *D. solani* soft rot.

The withdrawal of most antibiotics and reductions in the availability of several other bactericidal agricultural compounds traditionally used for horticulture has led to great challenges for the industry in controlling bacterial pathogens. The use of phages for biocontrol of horticultural disease is a promising alternative to these compounds, but it is clear that much work still remains to be undertaken to reach similar levels of efficacy, including focussing on application methods, and persistence and effectiveness in the field.

9.3 Conclusions

Antibiotics provide a vital function in reducing mortality in humans and animals, so their efficacy must be protected in an era of rising, and potentially catastrophic, antimicrobial resistance in bacteria. Therefore, new antimicrobial agents for use in agriculture, medicine and other sectors must be developed urgently. For agriculture, a renewed focus on intensification, food security and reduced food loss provide additional pressures. Here, we have discussed the potential of a new class of antimicrobial agents, phages, as a replacement or supplement, to some of the conventional antibiotics currently used in agriculture. We have shown that phages have many of the desirable properties needed to control bacterial diseases in agriculture including efficacy, low levels of resistance, lack of cross resistance to antibiotics, biodegradability and narrow target range. Moreover, the use of phages may provide new opportunities to agricultural industries to control pathogens not currently effectively controlled by antibiotics or other treatments. However, it is evident that application of phages to each system needs to be tailored and optimised, and that some systems are more challenging for phage use than others (e.g. poultry appear more suited than beef cattle). Whilst there are few phage products available currently, it is likely we will see a rapid rise in their use in the coming years.

References

Abdelsattar AS, Abdelrahman F, Dawoud A, Connerton IF, El-Shibiny A (2019) Encapsulation of *E. coli* phage ZCEC5 in chitosan–alginate beads as a delivery system in phage therapy. AMB Express 9(1):87. https://doi.org/10.1186/s13568-019-0810-9

Akhtar M, Viazis S, Diez-Gonzalez F (2014) Isolation, identification and characterization of lytic, wide host range bacteriophages from waste effluents against *Salmonella enterica* serovars. Food Control 38:67–74. https://doi.org/10.1016/j.foodcont.2013.09.064

Albino LAA, Rostagno MH, Húngaro HM, Mendonça RCS (2014) Isolation, characterization, and application of bacteriophages for *Salmonella* spp. biocontrol in pigs. Foodborne Pathog Dis. https://doi.org/10.1089/fpd.2013.1600

Amiri Fahliyani S, Beheshti-Maal K, Ghandehari F (2018) Novel lytic bacteriophages of *Klebsiella oxytoca* ABG-IAUF-1 as the potential agents for mastitis phage therapy. FEMS Microbiol Lett 365(20). https://doi.org/10.1093/femsle/fny223

Andreatti RL, Higgins JP, Higgins SE, Gaona G, Wolfenden AD, Tellez G, Hargis BM (2007) Ability of bacteriophages isolated from different sources to reduce *Salmonella enterica* serovar Enteritidis *in vitro* and *in vivo*. Poult Sci 86(9):1904–1909. https://doi.org/10.1093/ps/86.9.1904

Arthur TM, Kalchayanand N, Agga GE, Wheeler TL, Koohmaraie M (2016) Evaluation of bacteriophage application to cattle in lairage at beef processing plants to reduce *Escherichia coli* O157:H7 prevalence on hides and carcasses. Foodborne Pathog Dis 14(1):17–22. https://doi.org/10.1089/fpd.2016.2189

ASM (2019) Plants – not just antibiotic-fed poultry and livestock – may be transmitting superbugs to people. https://www.asm.org/Press-Releases/2019/June/Plants-Not-Just-Antibiotic-Fed-Poultry-and-Lives

Atterbury RJ, Connerton PL, Dodd CER, Rees CED, Connerton IF (2003) Isolation and characterization of *Campylobacter* bacteriophages from retail poultry. Appl Environ Microbiol 69(8):4511–4518. https://doi.org/10.1128/aem.69.8.4511-4518.2003

Atterbury RJ, Dillon E, Swift C, Connerton PL, Frost JA, Dodd CER, Rees CED, Connerton IF (2005) Correlation of *Campylobacter* bacteriophage with reduced presence of hosts in broiler chicken ceca. Appl Environ Microbiol 71(8):4885–4887. https://doi.org/10.1128/AEM.71.8.4885-4887.2005

Atterbury RJ, Van Bergen MAP, Ortiz F, Lovell MA, Harris JA, De Boer A, Wagenaar JA, Allen VM, Barrow PA (2007) Bacteriophage therapy to reduce *Salmonella* colonization of broiler chickens. Appl Environ Microbiol 73(14):4543–4549. https://doi.org/10.1128/aem.00049-07

Bae JY (2012) Biocontrol potential of a lytic bacteriophage PE204 against bacterial wilt of tomato. J Microbiol Biotechnol 22(12):1613–1620. https://doi.org/10.4014/jmb.1208.08072
Balogh B, Canteros BI, Stall RE, Jones JB (2008) Control of citrus canker and citrus bacterial spot with bacteriophages. Plant Dis 92:1048–1052. https://doi.org/10.1094/PDIS-92-7-1048
Balogh B, Nga NTT, Jones JB (2018) Relative level of bacteriophage multiplication *in vitro* or in phyllosphere may not predict *in planta* efficacy for controlling bacterial leaf spot on tomato caused by *Xanthomonas perforans*. Front Microbiol 9. https://doi.org/10.3389/fmicb.2018.02176
Barrera-Rivas CI, Valle-Hurtado NA, González-Lugo GM, Baizabal-Aguirre VM, Bravo-Patiño A, Cajero-Juárez M, Valdez-Alarcón JJ (2017) Bacteriophage therapy: an alternative for the treatment of *Staphylococcus aureus* infections in animals and animal models. In: Enany S, Alexander LEC (eds) Frontiers in *Staphylococcus aureus*. IntechOpen. https://doi.org/10.5772/65761
Bigwood T, Hudson JA, Billington C (2009a) Influence of host and bacteriophage concentrations on the inactivation of food-borne pathogenic bacteria by two phages. FEMS Microbiol Lett 291:59–64. https://doi.org/10.1111/j.1574-6968.2008.01435.x
Bigwood T, Hudson JA, Billington C (2009b) Influence of host and bacteriophage concentrations on the inactivation of food-borne pathogenic bacteria by two phages. FEMS Microbiol Lett 291(1):59–64. https://doi.org/10.1111/j.1574-6968.2008.01435.x
Blackall P (2019) Why is antibiotic use in poultry being challenged. Poultry Health Conference, Bangkok Bangkok, Thailand, 7–8 May
Boyen F, Haesebrouck F, Maes D, Van Immerseel F, Ducatelle R, Pasmans F (2008) Non-typhoidal *Salmonella* infections in pigs : a closer look at epidemiology, pathogenesis and control. Vet Microbiol 130(1):1–19. https://doi.org/10.1016/j.vetmic.2007.12.017
Breyne K, Honaker RW, Hobbs Z, Richter M, Zaczek M, Spangler T, Steenbrugge J, Lu R, Kinkhabwala A, Marchon B, Meyer E, Mokres L (2017) Efficacy and safety of a bovine-associated *Staphylococcus aureus* phage cocktail in a murine model of mastitis. Front Microbiol 8:2348. https://doi.org/10.3389/fmicb.2017.02348
Brüssow H (2005) Phage therapy: the *Escherichia coli* experience. Microbiology 151(7):2133–2140. https://doi.org/10.1099/mic.0.27849-0
Buttimer C, Hendrix H, Lucid A, Neve H, Noben JP, Franz C, O'Mahony J, Lavigne R, Coffey A (2018) Novel N4-like bacteriophages of *Pectobacterium atrosepticum*. Pharmaceuticals 11(2). https://doi.org/10.3390/ph11020045
Callaway TR, Edrington TS, Brabban AD, Kutter EM, Karriker L, Stahl C, Wagstrom E, Anderson RC, Poole TL, Genovese KJ, Kreuger N, Harvey R, Nisbet DJ (2011) Evaluation of phage treatment as a strategy to reduce *Salmonella* populations in growing swine. Foodborne Pathog Dis 8(2):261–266. https://doi.org/10.1089/fpd.2010.0671
Carey-Smith G, Billington C, Hudson JA, Heinemann JA (2006) Isolation and characterisation of bacteriophages infecting *Salmonella* with respect to potential use in biocontrol and their co-existence with the host. FEMS Microbiol Lett 258(2):182–186. https://doi.org/10.1111/j.1574-6968.2006.00217.x
Carrillo CL, Atterbury RJ, El-Shibiny A, Connerton PL, Dillon E, Scott A, Connerton IF (2005) Bacteriophage therapy to reduce *Campylobacter jejuni* colonization of broiler chickens. Appl Environ Microbiol 71(11):6554–6563. https://doi.org/10.1128/aem.71.11.6554-6563.2005
Carrillo CML, Connerton PL, Pearson T, Connerton IF (2007) Free-range layer chickens as a source of *Campylobacter* bacteriophage. Anton Leeuw Int J Gen Mol Microbiol 92(3):275–284. https://doi.org/10.1007/s10482-007-9156-4
Carstens AB, Djurhuus AM, Kot W, Jacobs-Sera D, Hatfull GF, Hansen LH (2018) Unlocking the potential of 46 new bacteriophages for biocontrol of *Dickeya Solani*. Viruses-Basel 10(11). https://doi.org/10.3390/v10110621
Carvalho CM, Gannon BW, Halfhide DE, Santos SB, Hayes CM, Roe JM, Azeredo J (2010) The *in vivo* efficacy of two administration routes of a phage cocktail to reduce numbers of *Campylobacter coli* and *Campylobacter jejuni* in chickens. BMC Microbiol 10:232. https://doi.org/10.1186/1471-2180-10-232

Cement A, Saygili H, Horuz S, Aysan Y (2018) Potential of bacteriophages to control bacterial speck of tomato (*Pseudomonas syringae* pv. *tomato*). Fresenius Environ Bull 27(12A):9366–9373

Centers for Disease Control (2013) Antibiotic resistance threats in the United States, 2013. http://www.cdc.gov/drugresistance/pdf/arthreats-2013-508.pdf. Accessed 30 Aug 2019

Chae JC, Hung NB, Yu SM, Lee HK, Lee YH (2014) Diversity of bacteriophages infecting *Xanthomonas oryzae* pv. *oryzae* in paddy fields and its potential to control bacterial leaf blight of rice. J Microbiol Biotechnol 24(6):740–747. https://doi.org/10.4014/jmb.1402.02013

China Ministry of Agriculture and Rural Areas (2019) Chinese national policies. http://www.moa.gov.cn/. Accessed 13 Sept 2019

Clavijo V, Baquero D, Hernandez S, Farfan JC, Arias J, Arevalo A, Donado-Godoy P, Vives-Flores M (2019) Phage cocktail SalmoFREE reduces *Salmonella* on a commercial broiler farm. Poult Sci. https://doi.org/10.3382/ps/pez251

Colom J, Cano-Sarabia M, Otero J, Cortes P, Maspoch D, Llagostera M (2015) Liposome-encapsulated bacteriophages for enhanced oral phage therapy against *Salmonella* spp. Appl Environ Microbiol 81(14):4841–4849. https://doi.org/10.1128/aem.00812-15

Conlan AJ, Coward C, Grant AJ, Maskell DJ, Gog JR (2007) *Campylobacter jejuni* colonization and transmission in broiler chickens: a modelling perspective. J R Soc Interface 4(16):819–829. https://doi.org/10.1098/rsif.2007.1015

Connerton PL, Loc Carrillo CM, Swift C, Dillon E, Scott A, Rees CE, Dodd CE, Frost J, Connerton IF (2004) Longitudinal study of *Campylobacter jejuni* bacteriophages and their hosts from broiler chickens. Appl Environ Microbiol 70(7):3877–3883. https://doi.org/10.1128/AEM.70.7.3877-3883.2004

Connerton PL, Timms AR, Connerton IF (2011) *Campylobacter* bacteriophages and bacteriophage therapy. J Appl Microbiol 111(2):255–265. https://doi.org/10.1007/s10482-007-9156-4

Crabb HK, Allen JL, Devlin JM, Firestone SM, Wilks CR, Gilkerson JR (2018) *Salmonella* spp. transmission in a vertically integrated poultry operation: clustering and diversity analysis using phenotyping (serotyping, phage typing) and genotyping (MLVA). PLoS One 13(7):e0201031. https://doi.org/10.1371/journal.pone.0201031

Crotta M, Georgiev M, Guitian J (2017) Quantitative risk assessment of *Campylobacter* in broiler chickens – assessing interventions to reduce the level of contamination at the end of the rearing period. Food Control 75:29–39. https://doi.org/10.1016/j.foodcont.2016.12.024

Czajkowski R, Ozymko Z, Lojkowska E (2014) Isolation and characterization of novel soilborne lytic bacteriophages infecting *Dickeya* spp. biovar 3 ('*D. solani*'). Plant Pathol 63(4):758–772. https://doi.org/10.1111/ppa.12157

Czajkowski R, Ozymko Z, de Jager V, Siwinska J, Smolarska A, Ossowicki A, Narajczyk M, Lojkowska E (2015) Genomic, proteomic and morphological characterization of two novel broad host lytic bacteriophages φpd10.3 and φpd23.1 infecting pectinolytic *Pectobacterium* spp. and *Dickeya* spp. PLoS One 10(3):e0119812. https://doi.org/10.1371/journal.pone.0119812

Czajkowski R, Smolarska A, Ozymko Z (2017) The viability of lytic bacteriophage phi D5 in potato-associated environments and its effect on *Dickeya solani* in potato (*Solanum tuberosum* L.) plants. PLoS One 12(8). https://doi.org/10.1371/journal.pone.0183200

Das M, Bhowmick TS, Ahern SJ, Young R, Gonzalez CF (2015) Control of Pierce's disease by phage. PLoS One 10(6). https://doi.org/10.1371/journal.pone.0128902

Defoirdt T, Sorgeloos P, Bossier P (2011) Alternatives to antibiotics for the control of bacterial disease in aquaculture. Curr Opin Microbiol 14(3):251–258. https://doi.org/10.1016/j.mib.2011.03.004

Duc HM, Son HM, Honjoh K, Miyamoto T (2018) Isolation and application of bacteriophages to reduce *Salmonella* contamination in raw chicken meat. LWT-Food Sci Technol 91:353–360. https://doi.org/10.1016/j.lwt.2018.01.072

Elhalag K, Nasr-Eldin M, Hussien A, Ahmad A (2018) Potential use of soilborne lytic *Podoviridae* phage as a biocontrol agent against *Ralstonia solanacearum*. J Basic Microbiol 58(8):658–669. https://doi.org/10.1002/jobm.201800039

El-Shibiny A, Connerton PL, Connerton IF (2005) Enumeration and diversity of campylobacters and bacteriophages isolated during the rearing cycles of free-range and organic chickens. Appl Environ Microbiol 71(3):1259–1266. https://doi.org/10.1128/AEM.71.3.1259-1266.2005

El-Shibiny A, Scott A, Timms A, Metawea Y, Connerton P, Connerton I (2009) Application of a group II *Campylobacter* bacteriophage to reduce strains of *Campylobacter jejuni* and *Campylobacter coli* colonizing broiler chickens. J Food Prot 72(4):733–740. https://doi.org/10.4315/0362-028x-72.4.733

Estella H, Rodrigues H, Weyand C Diallo I, Chinivasagam HN (2015) Isolation and distribution of Campylobacter bacteriophages in chickens and the farming environment across varying litter management practices in Australia. Campylobacter, Helicobacter and related organisms (CHRO), Rotorua New Zealand, CHRO Conference 2015

European Food Safety Authority (2016) The European Union summary report on trends and sources of zoonoses, zoonotic agents and food-borne outbreaks in 2015. European Centre for Disease Prevention Control. EFSA J 14(12):e04634. https://doi.org/10.2903/j.efsa.2016.4634

FAO (2018) Antimicrobial resistance and foods of plant origin. Summary report of an FAO meeting of experts FAO antimicrobial resistance working group. http://www.fao.org/3/BU657en/bu657en.pdf

Fiorentin L, Vieira ND, Barioni Júnior W, Barros S (2004) *In vitro* characterization and *in vivo* properties of Salmonellae lytic bacteriophages isolated from free-range layers. Revista Brasileira de Ciência Avícola 6(2):121–128. https://doi.org/10.1590/s1516-635x2004000200009

Fiorentin L, Vieira ND, Barioni W Jr (2005) Oral treatment with bacteriophages reduces the concentration of *Salmonella* Enteritidis PT4 in caecal contents of broilers. Avian Pathol 34(3):258–263. https://doi.org/10.1080/01445340500112157

Firlieyanti AS, Connerton PL, Connerton IF (2016) Campylobacters and their bacteriophages from chicken liver: the prospect for phage biocontrol. Int J Food Microbiol 237:121–127. https://doi.org/10.1016/j.ijfoodmicro.2016.08.026

Fischer S, Kittler S, Klein G, Gluender G (2013) Impact of a single phage and a phage cocktail application in broilers on reduction of *Campylobacter jejuni* and development of resistance. PLoS One 8(10). https://doi.org/10.1371/journal.pone.0078543

Foley SL, Johnson TJ, Ricke SC, Nayak R, Danzeisen J (2013) *Salmonella* pathogenicity and host adaptation in chicken-associated serovars. Microbiol Mol Biol Rev 77(4):582–607. https://doi.org/10.1128/mmbr.00015-13

Fujiwara A, Fujisawa M, Hamasaki R, Kawasaki T, Fujie M, Yamada T (2011) Biocontrol of *Ralstonia solanacearum* by treatment with lytic bacteriophages. Appl Environ Microbiol 77(12):4155–4162. https://doi.org/10.1128/aem.02847-10

Ganaie MY, Qureshi S, Kashoo Z, Wani SA, Hussain MI, Kumar R, Maqbool R, Sikander P, Banday MS, Malla WA, Mondal P, Khan RIN (2018) Isolation and characterization of two lytic bacteriophages against *Staphylococcus aureus* from India: newer therapeutic agents against Bovine mastitis. Vet Res Commun 42(4):289–295. https://doi.org/10.1007/s11259-018-9736-y

García P, Rodríguez L, Rodríguez A, Martínez B (2010) Food biopreservation: promising strategies using bacteriocins, bacteriophages and endolysins. Trends Food Sci Technol 21(8):373–382. https://doi.org/10.1016/j.tifs.2010.04.010

Gasic K, Ivanovic M, Kuzmanovic N, Prokic A, Obradovic A, Sevic M (2014) Bacteriophage of *Erwinia amylovora* – host range and fire blight control potential. XIII International Workshop on Fire Blight. F. Rezzonico, T. H. M. Smits and E. Holliger 1056:123–126

Gasic K, Kuzmanovic N, Ivanovic M, Prokic A, Sevic M, Obradovic A (2018) Complete genome of the *Xanthomonas euvesicatoria* specific bacteriophage Kϕ1, its survival and potential in control of pepper bacterial spot. Front Microbiol 9. https://doi.org/10.3389/fmicb.2018.02021

Geng H, Zou W, Zhang M, Xu L, Liu F, Li X, Wang L, Xu Y (2019) Evaluation of phage therapy in the treatment of *Staphylococcus aureus*-induced mastitis in mice. Folia Microbiol (Praha). https://doi.org/10.1007/s12223-019-00729-9

Gill JJ, Pacan JC, Carson ME, Leslie KE, Griffiths MW, Sabour PM (2006a) Efficacy and pharmacokinetics of bacteriophage therapy in treatment of subclinical *Staphylococcus aureus* mastitis in lactating dairy cattle. Antimicrob Agents Chemother 50(9):2912–2918. https://doi.org/10.1128/AAC.01630-05

Gill JJ, Sabour PM, Leslie KE, Griffiths MW (2006b) Bovine whey proteins inhibit the interaction of *Staphylococcus aureus* and bacteriophage K. J Appl Microbiol 101(2):377–386. https://doi.org/10.1111/j.1365-2672.2006.02918.x

Goncalves-Tenorio A, Silva BN, Rodrigues V, Cadavez V, Gonzales-Barron U (2018) Prevalence of pathogens in poultry meat: A meta-analysis of european published surveys. Foods (Basel, Switzerland) 7(5). https://doi.org/10.3390/foods7050069

Goode D, Allen VM, Barrow PA (2003) Reduction of experimental Salmonella and campylobacter contamination of chicken skin by application of lytic bacteriophages. Appl Environ Microbiol 69(8):5032–5036. https://doi.org/10.1128/aem.69.8.5032-5036.2003

Goyer C (2005) Isolation and characterization of phages Stsc1 and Stsc3 infecting *Streptomyces scabiei* and their potential as biocontrol agents. Can J Plant Pathol 27(2):210–216. https://doi.org/10.1080/07060660509507218

Grant A, Parveen S, Schwarz J, Hashem F, Vimini B (2017) Reduction of *Salmonella* in ground chicken using a bacteriophage. Poult Sci 96(8):2845–2852. https://doi.org/10.3382/ps/pex062

Gutierrez D, Fernandez L, Rodriguez A, Garcia P (2019) Role of bacteriophages in the implementation of a sustainable dairy chain. Front Microbiol 10:12. https://doi.org/10.3389/fmicb.2019.00012

Hakdong S, Ju-Hoon L, Hyeryen K, Younho C, Sunggi H, Sangryeol R (2012) Receptor diversity and host interaction of bacteriophages infecting *Salmonella enterica* serovar Typhimurium. PLoS One 7(8):e43392. https://doi.org/10.1371/journal.pone.0043392

Hanlon GW (2007) Bacteriophages: an appraisal of their role in the treatment of bacterial infections. Int J Antimicrob Agents 30(2):118–128. https://doi.org/10.1016/j.ijantimicag.2007.04.006

Havelaar AH, Mangen M-JJ, de Koeijer AA, Bogaardt M-J, Evers EG, Jacobs-Reitsma WE, van Pelt W, Wagenaar JA, de Wit GA, van der Zee H, Nauta MJ (2007) Effectiveness and efficiency of controlling *Campylobacter* on broiler chicken meat. Risk Anal 27(4):831–844. https://doi.org/10.1111/j.1539-6924.2007.00926.x

Henriques A, Sereno R, Almeida A (2013) Reducing *Salmonella* horizontal transmission during egg incubation by phage therapy. Foodborne Pathog Dis 10(8):718–722. https://doi.org/10.1089/fpd.2012.1363

Heringa SD, Kim J, Jiang X, Doyle MP, Erickson MC (2010) Use of a mixture of bacteriophages for biological control of *Salmonella enterica* strains in compost. Appl Environ Microbiol 76(15):5327–5332. https://doi.org/10.1128/aem.00075-10

Hill AW, Brady CA (1989) A note on the isolation and propagation of lytic phages from *Streptococcus uberis* and their potential for strain typing. J Appl Microbiol 67(4):425–431. https://doi.org/10.1111/j.1365-2672.1989.tb02513.x

Hooton SPT, Atterbury RJ, Connerton IF (2011) Application of a bacteriophage cocktail to reduce *Salmonella* Typhimurium U288 contamination on pig skin. Int J Food Microbiol 151(2):157–163. https://doi.org/10.1016/j.ijfoodmicro.2011.08.015

Hudson JA, Billington C, Carey-Smith G, Greening G (2005) Bacteriophages as biocontrol agents in food. J Food Prot 68(2):426–437. https://doi.org/10.4315/0362-028x-68.2.426

Iwano H, Inoue Y, Takasago T, Kobayashi H, Furusawa T, Taniguchi K, Fujiki J, Yokota H, Usui M, Tanji Y, Hagiwara K, Higuchi H, Tamura Y (2018) Bacteriophage ϕsa012 has a broad host range against *Staphylococcus aureus* and effective lytic capacity in a mouse mastitis model. Biology (Basel) 7(1). https://doi.org/10.3390/biology7010008

Jamalludeen N, Johnson RP, Shewen PE, Gyles CL (2009) Evaluation of bacteriophages for prevention and treatment of diarrhea due to experimental enterotoxigenic *Escherichia coli* O149 infection of pigs. Vet Microbiol 136:135–141. https://doi.org/10.1016/j.vetmic.2008.10.021

Janež N, Loc-Carrillo C (2013) Use of phages to control *Campylobacter* spp. J Microbiol Methods 95:68–75. https://doi.org/10.1016/j.mimet.2013.06.024

Janez N, Kokosin A, Zaletel E, Vranac T, Kovac J, Vuckovic D, Mozina SS, Serbec VC, Zhang Q, Accetto T, Podgornik A, Peterka M (2014) Identification and characterisation of new

Campylobacter group III phages of animal origin. FEMS Microbiol Lett 359(1):64–71. https://doi.org/10.1111/1574-6968.12556
Jing S, Hu Z (2011) Application of antibiotic substitutes in pig feeding. Northern Animal Husbandry Oct 5th 2011
Kim M-H, Park S-W, Kim Y-K (2011) Bacteriophages of *Pseudomonas tolaasii* for the biological control of brown blotch disease. J Korean Soc Appl Biol Chem 54(1):99–104. https://doi.org/10.3839/jksabc.2011.014
Kim KH, Lee GY, Jang JC, Kim JE, Kim YY (2013) Evaluation of anti-SE bacteriophage as feed additives to prevent *Salmonella enteritidis* (SE) in Broiler. Asian Australas J Anim Sci 26(3):386–393. https://doi.org/10.5713/ajas.2012.12138
Kittler S, Fischer S, Abdulmawjood A, Gluender G, Klein G (2013) Effect of bacteriophage application on *Campylobacter jejuni* loads in commercial broiler flocks. Appl Environ Microbiol 79(23):7525–7533. https://doi.org/10.1128/aem.02703-13
Lang JM, Gent DH, Schwartz HF (2007) Management of *Xanthomonas* leaf blight of onion with bacteriophages and a plant activator. Plant Dis 91(7):871–878. https://doi.org/10.1094/pdis-91-7-0871
Lee N, Harris DL (2001) The effect of bacteriophage treatment to reduce the rapid dissemination of *Salmonella typhimurium* in pigs. Swine Res Rep 2000(50):196–197. http://lib.dr.iastate.edu/swinereports_2000/50
Lee N, Harris DL (2002) Potential of bacteriophage application as an intervention strategy against *Salmonella* in pigs, Iowa State University Extension Program Report. Iowa State University. ASL-R692, Ames
Lee SH, Hosseindoust AR, Kim JS, Choi YH, Lee JH, Kwon IK, Chae BJ (2016) Bacteriophages as a promising anti-pathogenic option in creep-feed for suckling piglets: targeted to control *Clostridium* spp. and coliforms faecal shedding. Livest Sci 191:161–164. https://doi.org/10.1016/j.livsci.2016.08.003
Lim T-H, Kim M-S, Lee D-H, Lee Y-N, Park J-K, Youn H-N, Lee H-J, Yang S-Y, Cho Y-W, Lee J-B, Park S-Y, Choi I-S, Song C-S (2012) Use of bacteriophage for biological control of *Salmonella* Enteritidis infection in chicken. Res Vet Sci 93(3):1173–1178. https://doi.org/10.1016/j.rvsc.2012.06.004
Lim JA, Jee S, Lee DH, Roh E, Jung K, Oh C, Heu S (2013) Biocontrol of *Pectobacterium carotovorum* subsp *carotovorum* using bacteriophage PP1. J Microbiol Biotechnol 23(8):1147–1153. https://doi.org/10.4014/jmb.1304.04001
Loc Carrillo C, Atterbury RJ, El-Shibiny A, Connerton PL, Dillon E, Scott A, Connerton IF (2005) Bacteriophage therapy to reduce Campylobacter jejuni colonization of broiler chickens. Appl Environ Microbiol 71(11):6554–6563
Love M, Bhandari D, Dobson R, Billington C (2018) Potential for bacteriophage endolysins to supplement or replace antibiotics in food production and clinical care. Antibiotics 7(1):17. https://doi.org/10.3390/antibiotics7010017
MacLean RC, San Millan A (2019) The evolution of antibiotic resistance. Science 365(6458):1082–1083. https://doi.org/10.1126/science.aax3879
McKenna F, El-Tarabily KA, Hardy GESJ, Dell B (2001) Novel *in vivo* use of a polyvalent *Streptomyces* phage to disinfest *Streptomyces scabies*-infected seed potatoes. Plant Pathol 50(6):666–675. https://doi.org/10.1046/j.1365-3059.2001.00648.x
Mehdi Y, Létourneau-Montminy M-P, Gaucher M-L, Chorfi Y, Suresh G, Rouissi T, Brar SK, Côté C, Ramirez AA, Godbout S (2018) Use of antibiotics in broiler production: global impacts and alternatives. Anim Nutr 4(2):170–178. https://doi.org/10.1016/j.aninu.2018.03.002
Monk AB, Rees CD, Barrow P, Hagens S, Harper DR (2010) Bacteriophage applications: where are we now? Lett Appl Microbiol 51:363–369. https://doi.org/10.1111/j.1472-765X.2010.02916.x
Moreno Switt AI, Orsi RH, den Bakker HC, Vongkamjan K, Altier C, Wiedmann M (2013) Genomic characterization provides new insight into *Salmonella* phage diversity. BMC Genomics 14(1). https://doi.org/10.1186/1471-2164-14-481

Müller I, Lurz R, Kube M, Quedenau C, Jelkmann W, Geider K (2011) Molecular and physiological properties of bacteriophages from North America and Germany affecting the fire blight pathogen *Erwinia amylovora*. Microb Biotechnol 4(6):735–745. https://doi.org/10.1111/j.1751-7915.2011.00272.x

Mwangi W, de Figueiredo P, Criscitiello MF (2016) One health : addressing global challenges at the nexus of human, animal, and environmental health. PLoS Pathog 12(9):e1005731. https://doi.org/10.1371/journal.ppat.1005731

Nabil NM, Tawakol MM, Hassan HM (2018) Assessing the impact of bacteriophages in the treatment of *Salmonella* in broiler chickens. Infect Ecol Epidemiol 8(1):1539056. https://doi.org/10.1080/20008686.2018.1539056

Obradovic A, Jones JB, Momol MT, Balogh B, Olson SM (2004) Management of tomato bacterial spot in the field by foliar applications of bacteriophages and SAR inducers. Plant Dis 88(7):736–740. https://doi.org/10.1094/pdis.2004.88.7.736

Oh CS (2018) Phage therapy to manage bacterial canker in kiwifruit caused by *Pseudomonas syringae* pv. *actinidiae*. Phytopathology 108(10):S1.254

Porter J, Anderson J, Carter L, Donjacour E, Paros M (2016) *In vitro* evaluation of a novel bacteriophage cocktail as a preventative for bovine coliform mastitis. J Dairy Sci 99(3):2053–2062. https://doi.org/10.3168/jds.2015-9748

Richards PJ, Connerton PL, Connerton IF (2019) Phage biocontrol of *Campylobacter jejuni* in chickens does not produce collateral effects on the gut microbiota. Front Microbiol 10(476). https://doi.org/10.3389/fmicb.2019.00476

Rivas L, Coffey B, McAuliffe O, McDonnell MJ, Burgess CM, Coffey A, Ross RP, Duffy G (2010) *In vivo* and *ex vivo* evaluations of bacteriophages e11/2 and e4/1c for use in the control of *Escherichia coli* O157:H7. Appl Environ Microbiol 76(21):7210–7216. https://doi.org/10.1128/aem.01530-10

Rivera D, Toledo V, Di Pillo F, Duenas F, Tardone R, Hamilton-West C, Vongkamjan K, Wiedmann M, Switt AIM (2018) Backyard farms represent a source of wide host range *Salmonella* phages that lysed the most common *Salmonella* serovars. J Food Prot 81(2):272–278. https://doi.org/10.4315/0362-028X.JFP-17-075

Rombouts S, Volckaert A, Venneman S, Devlercq B, Vandenheuvel D, Allonsius CN, Van Malderghem C, Jang HB, Briers Y, Noben JP, Klumpp J, Van Vaerenbergh J, Maes M, Lavigne R (2016) Characterization of novel bacteriophages for biocontrol of bacterial blight in leek caused by *Pseudomonas syringae* pv. *porri*. Front Microbiol 7. https://doi.org/10.3389/fmicb.2016.00279

Rozema EA, Stephens TP, Bach SJ, Okine EK, Johnson RP, Stanford K, McAllister TA (2009) Oral and rectal administration of bacteriophages for control of *Escherichia coli* O157:H7 in feedlot cattle. J Food Prot 72(2):241–250. https://doi.org/10.4315/0362-028x-72.2.241

Russell H, Norcross NL, Kahn DE (1969) Isolation and characterization of *Streptococcus agalactiae* bacteriophage. J Gen Virol 5(2):315–317. https://doi.org/10.1099/0022-1317-5-2-315

Sabouri S, Sepehrizadeh Z, Amirpour-Rostami S, Skurnik M (2017) A minireview on the *in vitro* and *in vivo* experiments with anti-*Escherichia coli* O157:H7 phages as potential biocontrol and phage therapy agents. Int J Food Microbiol 243:52–57. https://doi.org/10.1016/j.ijfoodmicro.2016.12.004

Saez AC, Zhang J, Rostagno MH, Ebner PD (2011) Direct feeding of microencapsulated bacteriophages to reduce *Salmonella* colonization in pigs. Foodborne Pathog Dis 8(12):1269–1274. https://doi.org/10.1089/fpd.2011.0905

Saglam AG, Sahin M, Celik E, Celebi O, Akca D, Otlu S (2017) The role of staphylococci in subclinical mastitis of cows and lytic phage isolation against *Staphylococcus aureus*. Vet World 10(12):1481–1485. https://doi.org/10.14202/vetworld.2017.1481-1485

Sahin O, Kassem II, Shen ZQ, Lin J, Rajashekara G, Zhang QJ (2015) *Campylobacter* in poultry: ecology and potential interventions. Avian Dis 59(2):185–200. https://doi.org/10.1637/11072-032315-Review

Salem M, Skurnik M (2018) Genomic characterization of sixteen *Yersinia enterocolitica*-infecting Podoviruses of pig origin. Viruses 10(4). https://doi.org/10.3390/v10040174

Salem M, Virtanen S, Korkeala H, Skurnik M (2015) Isolation and characterization of *Yersinia*-specific bacteriophages from pig stools in Finland. J Appl Microbiol 118(3):599–608. https://doi.org/10.1111/jam.12722

Schwarczinger I, Nagy JK, Kunstler A, Szabo L, Geider K, Kiraly L, Pogany M (2017) Characterization of *Myoviridae* and *Podoviridae* family bacteriophages of *Erwinia amylovora* from Hungary – potential of application in biological control of fire blight. Eur J Plant Pathol 149(3):639–652. https://doi.org/10.1007/s10658-017-1214-9

Scott A, Timms A, Connerton P, Carrillo C, Radzum K, Connerton I (2007) Genome dynamics of *Campylobacter jejuni* in response to bacteriophage predation. PLoS Pathog 3(8):1142–1151. https://doi.org/10.1371/journal.ppat.0030119

Shaughnessy RG, Meade KG, Cahalane S, Allan B, Reiman C, Callanan JJ, O'Farrelly C (2009) Innate immune gene expression differentiates the early avian intestinal response between *Salmonella* and *Campylobacter*. Vet Immunol Immunopathol 132(2–4):191–198. https://doi.org/10.1016/j.vetimm.2009.06.007

Shende R, Hirpurkar S, Sannat C (2017) Therapeutic utility of bacteriophage in bovine mastitis. Int J Livest Res 7(10):141–147. https://doi.org/10.5455/ijlr.20170707051745

Shirley JF (2016) Development toward a bovine *Salmonella* model and a bacteriophage treatment cocktail to reduce *Salmonella* peripheral lymph node carriage in calves. Auburn University. Master of Science

Sillankorva S, Pleteneva E, Shaburova O, Santos S, Carvalho C, Azeredo J, Krylov V (2009) *Salmonella* Enteritidis bacteriophage candidates for phage therapy of poultry. J Appl Microbiol 108(4):1175–1186. https://doi.org/10.1111/j.1365-2672.2009.04549.x

Skurnik M, Strauch E (2006) Phage therapy: facts and fiction. Int J Med Microbiol 296(1):5–14. https://doi.org/10.1016/j.ijmm.2005.09.002

Smith HW, Huggins MB (1983) Effectiveness of phages in treating experimental *Escherichia coli* diarrhoea in calves, piglets and lambs. J Gen Microbiol 129:2659–2675. https://doi.org/10.1099/00221287-129-8-2659

Soleimani-Delfan A, Etemadifar Z, Emtiazi G, Bouzari M (2015) Isolation of *Dickeya dadantii* strains from potato disease and biocontrol by their bacteriophages. Braz J Microbiol 46(3):791–797. https://doi.org/10.1590/s1517-838246320140498

Son JS, Kim EB, Lee SJ, Jun SY, Yoon SJ, Kang SH, Choi YJ (2010) Characterization of *Staphylococcus aureus* derived from bovine mastitis and isolation of two lytic bacteriophages. J Gen Appl Microbiol 56(4):347–353

Stanford K, McAllister TA, Niu YD, Stephens TP, Mazzocco A, Waddell TE, Johnson RP (2010) Oral delivery systems for encapsulated bacteriophages targeted at *Escherichia coli* O157:H7 in feedlot cattle. J Food Prot 73(7):1304–1312. https://doi.org/10.4315/0362-028x-73.7.1304

Stedt J, Bonnedahl J, Hernandez J, McMahon BJ, Hasan B, Olsen B, Drobni M, Waldenström J (2014) Antibiotic resistance patterns in *Escherichia coli* from gulls in nine European countries. Infect Ecol Epidemiol 4:1–10. https://doi.org/10.3402/iee.v4.21565

Stern NJ (2008) *Salmonella* species and *Campylobacter jejuni* cecal colonization model in broilers. Poult Sci 87(11):2399–2403. https://doi.org/10.3382/ps.2008-00140

Sukumaran AT, Nannapaneni R, Kiess A, Sharma CS (2016) Reduction of *Salmonella* on chicken breast fillets stored under aerobic or modified atmosphere packaging by the application of lytic bacteriophage preparation SalmoFresh™. Poult Sci 95(3):668–675. https://doi.org/10.3382/ps/pev332

Sundin GW, Wang N (2018) Antibiotic resistance in plant-pathogenic bacteria. Annu Rev Phytopathol 56(1):161–180. https://doi.org/10.1146/annurev-phyto-080417-045946

Thanner S, Drissner D, Walsh F (2016) Antimicrobial resistance in agriculture. MBio 7(2):e02227–e02215. https://doi.org/10.1128/mBio.02227-15

Tolen TN, Xie Y, Hairgrove TB, Gill JJ, Taylor TM (2018) Evaluation of commercial prototype bacteriophage intervention designed for reducing O157 and non-O157 shiga-toxigenic

Escherichia coli (STEC) on beef cattle hide. Foods (Basel, Switzerland) 7(7):114. https://doi.org/10.3390/foods7070114

Tsuei A-C, Carey-Smith GV, Hudson JA, Billington C, Heinemann JA (2007) Prevalence and numbers of coliphages and *Campylobacter jejuni* bacteriophages in New Zealand foods. Int J Food Microbiol 116(1):121–125. https://doi.org/10.1016/j.ijfoodmicro.2006.12.028

US Food Safety and Inspection Service (2012) Shiga toxin-producing *Escherichia coli* in certain raw beef products [Docket No. FSIS-2010-0023]. Federal Register, 77

Varela-Ortiz DF, Barboza-Corona JE, Gonzalez-Marrero J, Leon-Galvan MF, Valencia-Posadas M, Lechuga-Arana AA, Sanchez-Felipe CG, Ledezma-Garcia F, Gutierrez-Chavez AJ (2018) Antibiotic susceptibility of *Staphylococcus aureus* isolated from subclinical bovine mastitis cases and *in vitro* efficacy of bacteriophage. Vet Res Commun 42(3):243–250. https://doi.org/10.1007/s11259-018-9730-4

Veldman A, Vahl HA, Borggreve GJ, Fuller DC (1995) A survey of the incidence of *Salmonella* species and Enterobacteriaceae in poultry feeds and feed components. Vet Rec 136(7):169–172. https://doi.org/10.1136/vr.136.7.169

Vigre H, Larsen PB, Andreasen M, Christensen J, Jorsal SE (2008) The effect of discontinued use of antimicrobial growth promoters on the risk of therapeutic antibiotic treatment in Danish farrow-to-finish pig farms. Epidemiol Infect 136(1):92–107. https://doi.org/10.1017/S095026880700814X

von Jagow C, Teufer T (2007) Which path to go? Eur Food Feed Law Rev 2(3):136–145

Wagenaar JA, Van Bergen MAP, Mueller MA, Wassenaar TM, Carlton RA (2005) Phage therapy reduces *Campylobacter jejuni* colonization in broilers. Vet Microbiol 109(3–4):275–283. https://doi.org/10.1016/j.vetmic.2005.06.002

Wall SK, Zhang J, Rostagno MH, Ebner PD (2010) Phage therapy to reduce preprocessing *Salmonella* infections in market-weight swine. Appl Environ Microbiol 76(1):48–53. https://doi.org/10.1128/aem.00785-09

Wei CH, Liu JL, Maina AN, Mwaura FB, Yu JP, Yan CH, Zhang RF, Wei HP (2017) Developing a bacteriophage cocktail for biocontrol of potato bacterial wilt. Virol Sin 32(6):476–484. https://doi.org/10.1007/s12250-017-3987-6

Wojtus JK, Frampton RA, Warring S, Hendrickson H, Fineran PC (2019) Genome sequence of a jumbo bacteriophage that infects the kiwifruit phytopathogen *Pseudomonas syringae* pv. *actinidiae*. Microbiol Resour Announc 8(22):e00224-19. https://doi.org/10.1128/mra.00224-19

Woodcock SD (2016) A review of research and development undertaken on Psa. KVH (Kiwifruit Vine Health). www.kvh.org.nz

World Health Organisation (2014) Antimicrobial resistance: global report on surveillance. World Health Organisation, Geneva. Isbn 978 92 4 156474 8

World Health Organisation (2017) Global framework for development and stewardship to combat antimicrobial resistance – draft roadmap, WHO/EMP/IAU/2017.08. World Health Organization, Geneva

Yin YJ, Ni PE, Deng BH, Wang SP, Xu WP, Wang DP (2019) Isolation and characterisation of phages against *Pseudomonas syringae* pv. *actinidiae*. Acta Agric Scand Sect B Soil Plant Sci 69(3):199–208. https://doi.org/10.1080/09064710.2018.1526965

Zhang JY, Kraft BL, Pan YY, Wall SK, Saez AC, Ebner PD (2010) Development of an anti-*Salmonella* phage cocktail with increased host range. Foodborne Pathog Dis 7(11):1415–1419. https://doi.org/10.1089/fpd.2010.0621

Zhang L, Sun L, Wei R, Gao Q, He T, Xu C, Liu X, Wang R (2017) Intracellular *Staphylococcus aureus* control by virulent bacteriophages within MAC-T bovine mammary epithelial cells. Antimicrob Agents Chemother 61(2). https://doi.org/10.1128/AAC.01990-16

Chapter 10
The Role of Vaccines in Combating Antimicrobial Resistance

Kathrin U. Jansen, William C. Gruber, Raphael Simon, James Wassil, and Annaliesa S. Anderson

Abstract The introduction of new classes of antibiotics, and the high use of antimicrobials in healthcare, agriculture, and the food industry, have all contributed to accelerate the development of antimicrobial resistance (AMR) in bacterial species and dissemination of antibiotic resistant bacterial strains worldwide. At present, the dramatic rise in AMR among important human bacterial pathogens is reaching a state of global crisis threatening a return to the pre-antibiotic era. AMR, already a significant burden on public health and economies, is anticipated to grow even more severe in the coming decades.

The utility of vaccines to fight AMR has been broadly recognized. Several licensed vaccines, targeting both bacterial (*Haemophilus influenzae*, *Streptococcus pneumoniae*, *Salmonella enterica* serotype Typhi) and viral (influenza virus, rotavirus) pathogens, have already proven their anti-AMR benefits by reducing unwarranted antibiotic consumption and antibiotic resistant bacterial strains and by promoting herd immunity, thereby protecting indirectly even segments in a population that have not been or cannot be vaccinated. It is further encouraging that a number of new investigational vaccines, with a potential to reduce the spread of multi drug resistant bacterial pathogens, are in various stages of clinical development. Nevertheless, vaccines as a tool to combat AMR remain underappreciated and unfortunately underutilized. Global mobilization of public health and industry resources is key to maximizing the use of licensed vaccines, and the development of new prophylactic vaccines could have a profound impact on reducing AMR.

Keywords Pathogen · Serotype · Bacterial infection · Viral infection · Vaccination · Immune response · Herd immunity · Antibiotic resistance · Multi drug resistance ·

K. U. Jansen · W. C. Gruber · R. Simon · A. S. Anderson (✉)
Pfizer Vaccine Research and Development, Pearl River, NY, USA
e-mail: annaliesa.anderson@pfizer.com

J. Wassil
Pfizer Patient and Health Impact, Collegeville, PA, USA

Present Address: Vaxcyte, Foster City, CA, USA
e-mail: jimwassil@yahoo.com

H. Panwar et al. (eds.), *Sustainable Agriculture Reviews 49*, Sustainable Agriculture Reviews 49, https://doi.org/10.1007/978-3-030-58259-3_10

Extensive drug resistance · *Haemophilus influenzae* · *Clostridioides difficile* · *Streptococcus pneumoniae* · Group B streptococcus · *Enterobacteriaceae* · *Staphylococcus aureus* · *Salmonella* · Respiratory syncytial virus · Live attenuated vaccine · Whole cell vaccine · Subunit vaccine · Conjugate vaccine · Carbohydrate vaccine

Abbreviations

AMR	Antimicrobial resistance
BCG	Bacillus Calmette Guérin
CARB-X	Combating Antibiotic Resistant Bacteria Biopharmaceutical Accelerator
CDC	Centers for Disease Control and Prevention
CRM_{197}	Cross-reactive material 197
EU	European Union
GAVI	Global Alliance for Vaccines and Immunization
GBS	Group B streptococcus
Hib	*Haemophilus influenzae* type b
HIV	Human immunodeficiency virus
IgA	Immunoglobulin A
IgG	Immunoglobulin G
NDM-1	New Delhi metallo-β-lactamase 1
PCV	Polysaccharide conjugate vaccine
RSV	Respiratory syncytial virus
UK	United Kingdom
U.S.	United States
WHO	World Health Organization

10.1 Introduction

Our struggle against infectious diseases over millennia has been captured in the earliest historical records (Shokeir and Hussein 1999). Global epidemics and pandemics such as the black plague, smallpox, and the 1918 Spanish flu, and outbreaks of cholera and typhoid have had profound impact resulting in significant morbidity and mortality throughout history (Cunha and Cunha 2006). Before the age of modern medicine and vaccines, the perils of illness in early life due to maladies such as *Haemophilus influenzae* type b (Hib) meningitis, diphtheria, measles, and whooping cough made it such that many children did not survive to adolescence (Centers for Disease Control and Prevention 1999). In addition, a myriad of events that at present are generally medically manageable with appropriate care, such as surgery, or preventable, such as contracting tetanus from a wound, were very often fatal. Improvements in effective sanitation and hygiene practices and nutrition led to concomitant increases in life expectancy. However, these gains eventually plateaued; the development of effective vaccines and the discovery of antibiotics pushed life expectancy to the unprecedented levels seen today (Centers for Disease Control and Prevention 2017). The rise in antimicrobial resistance (AMR) among important human bacterial pathogens thus represents an alarming global crisis with threats to return to the pre-antibiotic era and to have a significant adverse effect on public health in the coming decades.

Active and passive vaccination strategies to prevent infectious disease were already in use prior to the discovery of the first antibiotic, penicillin, in 1928 (Graham and Ambrosino 2015; Plotkin 2014). Whole cell inactivated typhoid vaccine was administered to British troops during the Boer War in South Africa to prevent the frequent outbreaks of *Salmonella enterica* serotype Typhi that ravaged deployed military personnel (Steele et al. 2016). Similarly, immunotherapy with horse immunoglobulin preparations was routinely used to prevent and treat diphtheria and tetanus prior to the introduction of antibiotics (Fig. 10.1) (Graham and Ambrosino 2015). Vaccines are effective in preventing infections by induction of a typically broad polyclonal antibody and/or cellular immune responses specifically targeted to the pathogen of concern. Hence, unlike current antibiotics, vaccines

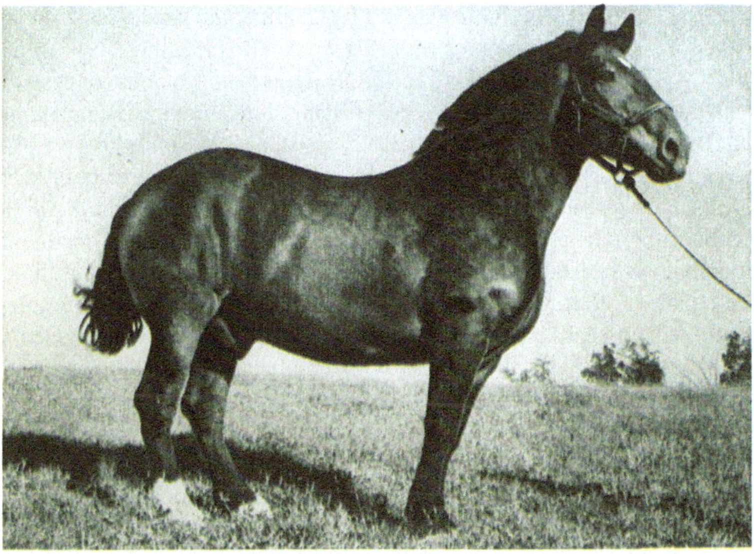

Fig. 10.1 Immunoglobulins for passive vaccination prior to antibiotic discovery. "Jumbo" lived at the Lederle laboratory site (later Wyeth, then Pfizer) and was recognized as a prolific producer of serum for use in pneumonia and tetanus antitoxin prophylaxis and therapy. Copyright [Kathrin U. Jansen, William C. Gruber, Raphael Simon, James Wassil, and Annaliesa S. Anderson] 2020

cannot cause "bystander" microbial resistance or induce resistance in the pathogens targeted. The following chapter explores the evidence, rationale, and opportunity for vaccines to reduce and prevent AMR and combat the rise of multi drug resistant bacterial pathogens.

10.2 Antimicrobial Resistance Is an Urgent Public Health Threat

Antimicrobial resistance predates the age of humans, as bacteria and the eukaryotic fungi and molds from which many antibiotics have been derived have been engaged in a chemical arms race for millennia as they compete for ecological niches. Ancient AMR genes have been found in bacteria recovered from ice cores dating back thousands of years, for which the collection of genes harbored by environmental isolates has been termed in aggregate the antibiotic "resistome" (Perry et al. 2016). The introduction of antibiotics in the 1940s and 1950s placed evolutionary pressure on microorganisms to adapt developing AMR. Indeed, introduction of each new antibiotic class since has been reliably met with the expansion of resistance. Moreover, this trend has accelerated over time, with recognition of the shortening of the intervals from introduction of a new antibiotic to first documented cases of resistance. While it took approximately 5 years to see resistance to penicillin after its introduction in 1943, with the introduction of novel antibiotics in the 1980s, including amoxicillin, ciprofloxacin, linezolid, and tigecycline, the time to first documented resistance was only a few months (Pray 2008). AMR spread has been further exacerbated by the global engines of economic growth in an interconnected world. Globalization has served as a vehicle for transmission, allowing emerging antibiotic resistant microbial strains and associated resistance plasmids to spread rapidly across continents. This phenomenon is illustrated well by the spread of fluoroquinolone resistant *Clostridioides* (previously known as *Clostridium) difficile* 027 epidemic lineages (He et al. 2013; Peng et al. 2017), as well as methicillin and fluoroquinolone resistant *Staphylococcus aureus* strains detected in clinical trial isolates (Holden et al. 2013) (Fig. 10.2). The excessive and irresponsible use of antimicrobials in healthcare, agriculture, and the food industry has fueled the dramatic rise of AMR globally (https://www.combatamr.org/amr-review-antimicrobial-resistance). In human medicine alone, global consumption of antibiotics rose by nearly 40% between the years 2000 and 2010 (Van Boeckel et al. 2014).

Recognition of this looming threat has spurred a call to action across the globe. In 2013, the United States (U.S.) Centers for Disease Control and Prevention (CDC) published a list cataloging antibiotic resistant pathogens in the U.S. (Centers for Disease Control and Prevention 2013a), which stratified 18 pathogens into urgent, serious, and concerning threat tiers based on the threat they pose to human health and urgency of the need for new and effective modalities for their treatment and prevention. This list was updated in 2019 (Centers for Disease Control and

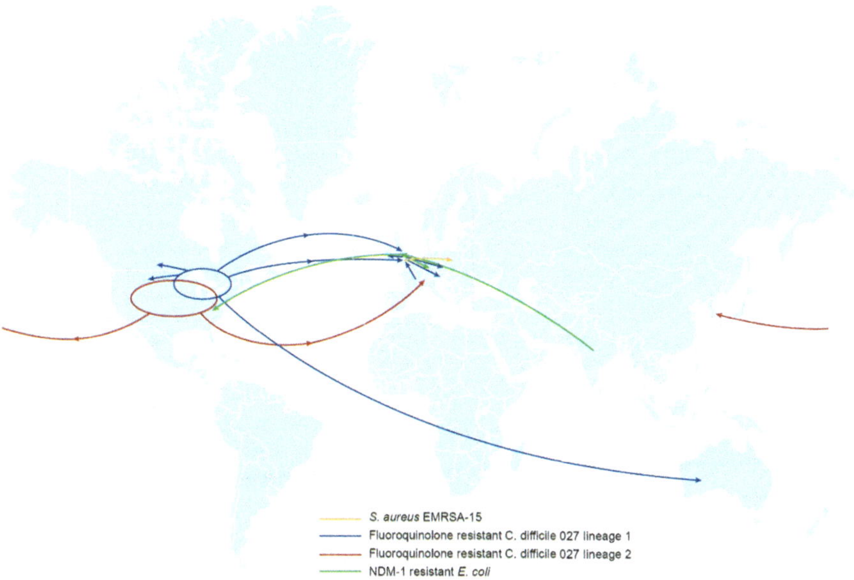

Fig. 10.2 Examples of the worldwide spread of multi drug resistant microbes. Acquisition of antibiotic resistance genes and global connectivity led to the rapid spread of epidemic antibiotic resistant strains such as EMRSA-15 *S. aureus* (Aanensen et al. 2016), fluoroquinolone resistant *C. difficile* 027 (He et al. 2013), and NDM-1 producing *E. coli* (Nordmann et al. 2011) across the globe. EMRSA-15, epidemic methicillin resistant *S. aureus* 15 strain; NDM-1, New Delhi metallo-β-lactamase 1. (Reproduced from Jansen and Anderson 2018)

Prevention 2019) to include two additional "urgent threats" (*Candida auris* and carbapenem resistant *Acinetobacter*), remove one pathogen (vancomycin resistant *S. aureus*), and add a new tier ("watch list") that included azole resistant *Aspergillus fumigatus* and drug resistant microbes *Mycoplasma genitalium* and *Bordetella pertussis* (Table 10.1). The 2019 CDC report also detailed higher estimates of antibiotic resistance among reported pathogens in the U.S. relative to the 2013 report, based on a more robust data set and methodology (Centers for Disease Control and Prevention 2019). A global priority list of antibiotic resistant pathogens was also established by the World Health Organization (WHO) in 2017. Using data from multiple sources and systems, and applying a multi criteria decision analysis method, the WHO stratified 12 genera of bacteria into three priority tiers: critical, high, and medium (Table 10.1) (World Health Organization 2017a). Global antibiotic resistance levels associated with major bacterial pathogens are shown in Fig. 10.3 (Jansen et al. 2018).

Pathogens of the highest priority on both lists include *Acinetobacter baumannii*, *Pseudomonas aeruginosa*, and members of the *Enterobacteriaceae* family (primarily *Klebsiella* spp. and *Escherichia coli*) (Table 10.1). These ominous public health threats are important causes of hospital based, or nosocomial infections and have demonstrated resistance to a large number of antibiotics, including carbapenems

Table 10.1 Stratification of antibiotic resistant microbial pathogens according to the CDC and WHO guidelines

CDC		WHO	
Urgent threats	Carbapenem resistant *Acinetobacter*	Critical priority	*Acinetobacter baumannii*, carbapenem resistant
	Candida auris		*Pseudomonas aeruginosa*, carbapenem resistant
	Clostridioides difficile		
	Carbapenem resistant *Enterobacteriaceae*		*Enterobacteriaceae**, carbapenem resistant, 3rd-generation cephalosporin resistant
	Drug resistant *Neisseria gonorrhoeae*		
Serious threats	Drug resistant *Campylobacter*	High priority	*Enterococcus faecium*, vancomycin resistant
	Drug resistant *Candida*		*Staphylococcus aureus*, methicillin resistant, vancomycin intermediate and resistant
	Extended spectrum β-lactamase producing *Enterobacteriaceae*		*Helicobacter pylori*, clarithromycin resistant
	Vancomycin resistant *Enterococcus*		*Campylobacter*, fluoroquinolone resistant
	Multi drug resistant *Pseudomonas aeruginosa*		*Salmonella* spp., fluoroquinolone resistant
	Drug resistant non-typhoidal *Salmonella*		*Neisseria gonorrhoeae*, 3rd-generation cephalosporin resistant, fluoroquinolone resistant
	Drug resistant *Salmonella* serotype Typhi		
	Drug resistant *Shigella*		
	Methicillin resistant *Staphylococcus aureus*		
	Drug resistant *Streptococcus pneumoniae*		
	Drug resistant *Mycobacterium tuberculosis*		
Concerning threats	Erythromycin resistant Group A streptococcus	Medium priority	*Streptococcus pneumoniae*, penicillin nonsusceptible
	Clindamycin resistant Group B streptococcus		*Haemophilus influenzae*, ampicillin resistant
			Shigella spp., fluoroquinolone resistant

(continued)

Table 10.1 (continued)

CDC		WHO	
Watch list	Azole resistant *Aspergillus fumigatus*		
	Drug resistant *Mycoplasma genitalium*		
	Drug resistant *Bordetella pertussis*		

Adapted from Centers for Disease Control and Prevention (2019) and World Health Organization (2017a)
**Enterobacteriaceae* include: *Klebsiella pneumoniae*, *Escherichia coli*, *Enterobacter* spp., *Serratia* spp., *Proteus* spp., *Providencia* spp., and *Morganella* spp.
CDC Centers for Disease Control and Prevention, *WHO* World Health Organization

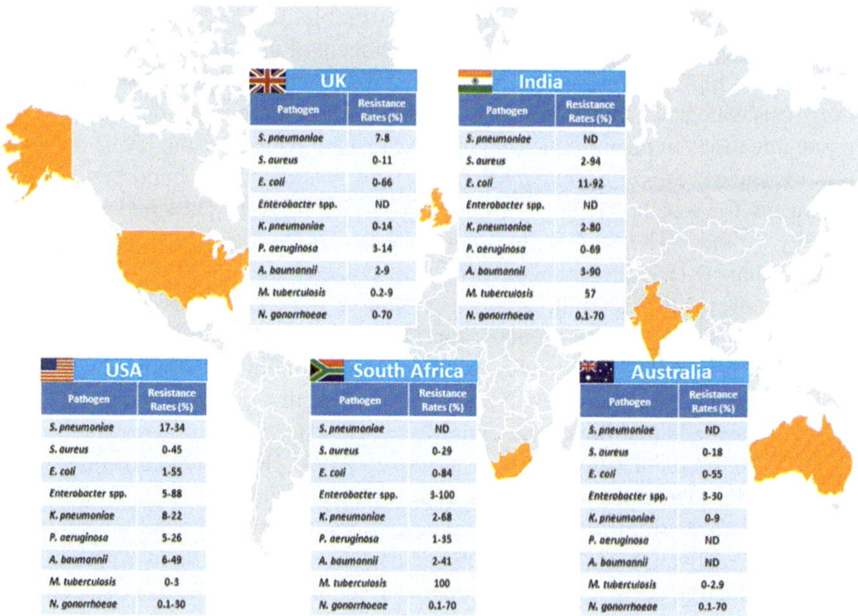

Fig. 10.3 Antibiotic resistance levels associated with major bacterial pathogens across the globe. Data shown are from 2000–2014 and represent the percentage of isolates (the range) tested that are resistant to each antibiotic class used for each pathogen (pathogen specific), not taking into account the proportion of strains that are resistant to more than one antibiotic class. For all pathogens except *M. tuberculosis* and *N. gonorrhoeae*, data were obtained from the Center for Disease Dynamics, Economics & Policy (https://resistancemap.cddep.org). For *M. tuberculosis*, data were obtained from WHO Drug Resistant TB Surveillance & Response – Supplement: Global Tuberculosis Report 2014 (World Health Organization 2014a). For *N. gonorrhoeae*, data were obtained from the World Health Organization Global Gonococcal Antimicrobial Surveillance Program which covers strains analyzed between 2011 and 2014 (http://www.who.int/reproductive-health/topics/rtis/gonococcal_resistance/en/). *ND* no data provided. Copyright [Kathrin U. Jansen, William C. Gruber, Raphael Simon, James Wassil, and Annaliesa S. Anderson] 2020

and third generation cephalosporins (World Health Organization 2017a; https://www.who.int/en/news-room/detail/27-02-2017-who-publishes-list-of-bacteria-for-which-new-antibiotics-are-urgently-needed). These highlighted pathogens cause a wide range of diseases, including pneumonia, urinary tract infection, bacteremia, and wound infections (Gaynes et al. 2005). *E. coli*, a clinically ubiquitous Gram negative bacterium, is the most common cause of urinary tract infections, with over 6 million cases occurring in the U.S. each year (Russo and Johnson 2003). Carbapenem resistant *Enterobacteriaceae*, with *Klebsiella* spp. being the major contributor, are a scourge in hospitals, where they are difficult to control through routine infectious disease protocols, and generally require treatment with toxic antibiotics such as colistins. Other pathogens of concern identified by the CDC and WHO include those responsible for diarrheal and enteric illness (*C. difficile*, *Helicobacter pylori*, *Campylobacter*, *Salmonella* spp., *Shigella* spp.) or sexually transmitted disease (*Neisseria gonorrhoeae*) (Table 10.1). Vancomycin resistant *Enterococcus faecium*, an important causative agent of urinary tract infections, was classified as high priority, as was *S. aureus*, a pathogen that frequently shows multi drug resistance and can cause a wide range of ailments ranging from skin and soft tissue infections to pneumonias and invasive disease. Due to rising levels of antibiotic resistance, *Streptococcus pneumoniae* and *H. influenzae*, important invasive pathogens for which effective vaccines are available, were classified as medium priority by the WHO, and *S. pneumoniae* was classified as serious threat by the CDC (Table 10.1). Both pathogens will be discussed later in this chapter.

A notable AMR bacterial pathogen present on the CDC list is *Mycobacterium tuberculosis* (Table 10.1) (Centers for Disease Control and Prevention 2019). Indeed, *M. tuberculosis* has the highest global burden of infected individuals of any single pathogen (approximately 2 billion people), with a devastatingly high prevalence in lower and middle income countries where extensively drug resistant strains are a major problem (Raviglione et al. 2012; World Health Organization 2018). Additionally, tuberculosis is exacerbated in patients with acquired immune deficiency syndrome (https://www.who.int/news-room/fact-sheets/detail/tuberculosis), for which reactivation of the latent tuberculosis disease and/or rapid progression of primary infection occurs due to an impaired T-cell immunity (Walker et al. 2013).

Molecular mechanisms of resistance to different classes of antibiotics associated with major bacterial pathogens and survival strategies have been reviewed (Walsh 2000) and are schematically shown in Fig. 10.4a. Importantly, AMR can transfer across bacterial species and geographies rapidly. For example, the plasmid residing antibiotic resistance gene NDM-1 (New Delhi metallo-β-lactamase 1) arose in India and was brought to Europe by patients who had become colonized with NDM-1 *Enterobacteriaceae* after travel to India for surgical procedures (Walsh et al. 2011; Yong et al. 2009). NDM-1 was subsequently transferred to other Gram negative species across Europe, conferring resistance to all antibiotic agents except colistin and tigecycline (Fig. 10.2) (Nordmann et al. 2011; Walsh et al. 2011; Yong et al. 2009). Worldwide, AMR is a significant and growing cause of mortality. It is estimated that at least 700,000 people die of infections with AMR pathogens every year, with up to 50,000 deaths occurring in the U.S. and Europe alone (O'Neill

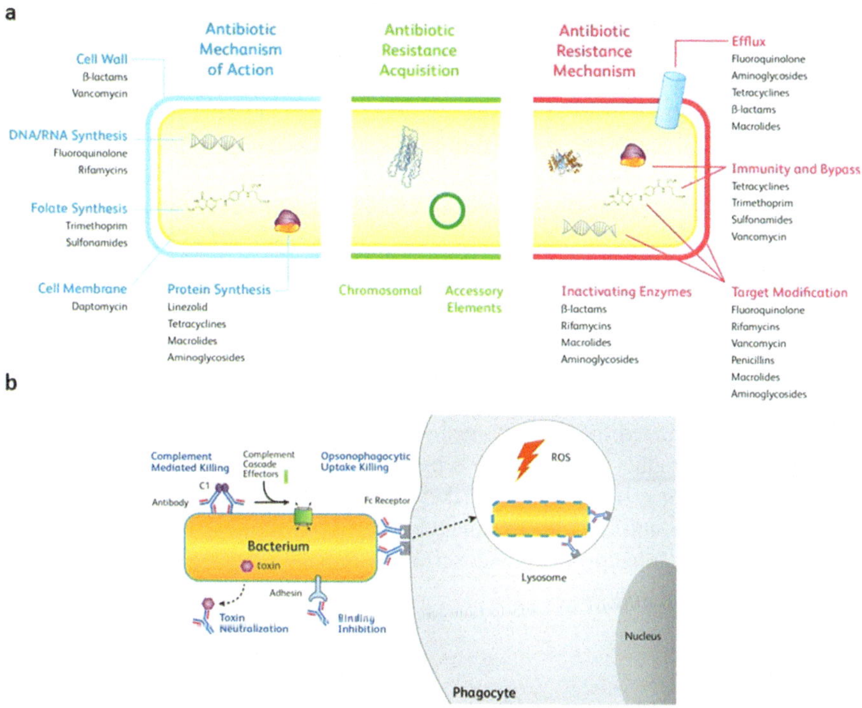

Fig. 10.4 Molecular mechanisms of action for antibiotics compared to vaccines. (**a**) Antibiotics either kill bacteria (bactericidal) or stop them from growing (bacteriostatic) by four main mechanisms: preventing DNA/RNA synthesis; preventing folate synthesis, which prevents nucleic acid synthesis; destroying the cell wall/membrane; and targeting ribosomes to prevent protein synthesis. Antibiotic resistance mechanisms neutralize the mechanism of action for the antibiotic. Resistance mechanisms can be acquired through horizontal transfer from plasmids and other genetic elements donated by bacteria that are co-localized with the pathogen. Alternatively, resistance can occur through vertical transmission via chromosomal mutations. These resistance mechanisms include the expression of enzymes such as the β-lactamases which inactivate the antibiotics (β-lactams); the expression or overexpression of efflux pumps which remove the antibiotic from the bacteria; the modification of the target so that it is no longer susceptible to the antibiotic; and using bypass mechanisms to circumvent antibiotic toxicity, including modification of the cell surface to prevent antibiotic entry or direct modification of antibiotics to prevent target engagement (Kohanski et al. 2010; Levy and Marshall 2004). (**b**) In contrast to antibiotics, vaccines exert their action via immune pathways, eliciting antigen specific polyclonal antibodies that can either neutralize bacterial virulence factors such as toxins or adhesins, or engage effector arms to kill the bacteria through mechanisms including the complement cascade or opsonophagocytic uptake into phagocytes (Forthal 2014). *ROS* reactive oxygen species. Copyright [Kathrin U. Jansen, William C. Gruber, Raphael Simon, James Wassil, and Annaliesa S. Anderson] 2020

2014). The mortality rates due to AMR are greater than those due to tetanus, cholera, and measles combined, and not much lower than those caused by common afflictions such as diarrheal disease or diabetes (O'Neill 2016a). With rates of resistance continuing at their current pace, it is estimated that annually, 10 million people worldwide will succumb to an AMR infection by 2050, exceeding the number of deaths from cancer (O'Neill 2016a).

AMR also represents a major economic burden on healthcare systems. In the European Union (EU), the costs associated with management of antibiotic resistant infections and productivity losses were estimated to be about €1.5 billion per year based on 2007 data (European Medicines Agency; European Centre for Disease Prevention and Control 2009; World Health Organization 2015) and are expected to be about €1.1 billion per year between 2015 and 2050 (The Organisation for Economic Co-operation and Development (OECD) 2019). In the U.S. alone, at least two million infections a year are caused by bacteria that are resistant to at least first line antibiotics. Costs to treat these infections were estimated to exceed 20 billion U.S. dollars each year (Centers for Disease Control and Prevention 2013a). Financial and analytical organizations such as Klynveld Peat Marwick Goerdeler and RAND Europe have estimated that a continued increase in resistance could reduce world gross domestic product by 2% to 3.5% by 2050 (KPMG LLP 2014; O'Neill 2014; Taylor et al. 2014a). If no action is taken against AMR, the cost in terms of lost global production until 2050 is estimated to be 100 trillion U.S. dollars. AMR is thus an immense global problem with serious implications for public health, healthcare systems, and economies.

10.3 Vaccines Are an Important Underutilized Tool to Help Address the Antimicrobial Resistance Problem

To address the AMR crisis, a number of international organizations, including the WHO, the United Nations General Assembly, the World Bank, the G7, the G20, and the EU, as well as the U.S. and United Kingdom (UK) governments have been urgently developing strategic action plans to address the rising AMR issues (G7 Summit 2015; Tagliabue and Rappuoli 2018). In 2015, the WHO published a Global Action Plan on AMR that outlines five key objectives: (1) improve awareness and understanding of AMR through effective communication, education, and training; (2) strengthen the knowledge and evidence base through surveillance and research; (3) reduce the incidence of infection through effective sanitation, hygiene, and prevention measures; (4) optimize the use of antimicrobial medicines in human and animal health; and (5) develop the economic case for sustainable investment that takes account of the need of all countries to increase investment in new medicines, diagnostic tools, vaccines, and other interventions (World Health Organization 2015). Similar goals were set by the CDC in the 5-year US National Action Plan for Combating Antibiotic Resistant Bacteria (Centers for Disease Control and Prevention 2015) and by the U.S. National Vaccine Advisory Committee (National Vaccine Advisory Committee 2016). Other recommendations to employ vaccines as a tool to address AMR were made by the Review on Antimicrobial Resistance, commissioned by the UK government and the Wellcome Trust, which indicated the need for intensifying research and development into new and improved effective antimicrobial therapies along with vaccines (O'Neill 2016a). In addition, experts participating in the Chatham House Workshop, convened by the UK Centre on Global Health Security (London, UK) in 2017, reviewed current knowledge and activities on the role of vaccines in combating AMR and discussed how to influence national and international policies to properly recognize the anti-AMR vaccine contribution (Chatham House 2017; Clift and Salisbury 2017). More importantly, they produced a seminal priority list of vaccines needed to effectively combat AMR.

Each of these proposals emphasizes the importance of effective antimicrobials, but it is also important to recognize the difficulty of such an endeavor, as no new classes of antibiotics have been introduced over the past 15 years and there are few candidates in the pipeline (O'Neill 2016a). Additionally, new antimicrobials are placed on the WHO reserve list, limiting their use. These factors make the development of new antimicrobials commercially unattractive for pharmaceutical companies. On the other hand, the research and development pipelines for prophylactic infectious disease vaccines are on the rise (Shen and Cooke 2019; World Health Organization 2019a), providing valuable opportunities to prevent disease caused by AMR pathogens.

In considering the role of vaccines in AMR prevention, it is important to note that the mechanisms of action of vaccines and antibiotics are fundamentally different (Fig. 10.4). First, antibiotics classically treat established infections and disease, whereas vaccines classically prevent infections from happening in the first place. The mode of action for antibiotics centers on interference with a pathogen's physiology, addressing usually a single biological target (Kohanski et al. 2010). Antimicrobial prophylaxis has established value in prevention of some infections including surgical infections, perinatal newborn Group B streptococcus and recurrent urinary tract infections, among others (Ahmed et al. 2017; Bratzler et al. 2013; Di Renzo et al. 2015), but at a cost – the potential for enabling AMR of the targeted pathogen or bystander organisms with pathogenic potential. By comparison, vaccines induce protective immune responses that are pathogen specific and target one or multiple bacterial virulence factors such as toxins or adhesins, either neutralizing them or engaging the effector arms of the immune system to kill the bacterial pathogen through complement and/or opsonophagocytosis (Forthal 2014). Prophylactic antibiotics are administered in anticipation of a pathogen or pathogens that might cause disease. The current antibiotic treatment paradigm dictates administration of an antibiotic once infection is suspected, with a change of the antimicrobial following empiric observation if the patient's condition does not improve, or a specific pathogen is identified. The broad spectrum action of antibiotics is beneficial when the etiology of the infection is not or cannot be identified; however, antibiotics also kill bystander bacteria and microbial flora, making the patient vulnerable to dysbiosis and outgrowth of resistant disease causing pathogens, as well as promote selection for bacteria to develop AMR.

In contrast to antibiotics, prophylactic vaccines are species specific and prevent the infection or disease, thus reducing both antibiotic use and spread of resistant bacterial strains. Unlike antimicrobials, vaccines are not inducing antibiotic resistance. Bacteria can evolve compensatory mutations, including, for example,

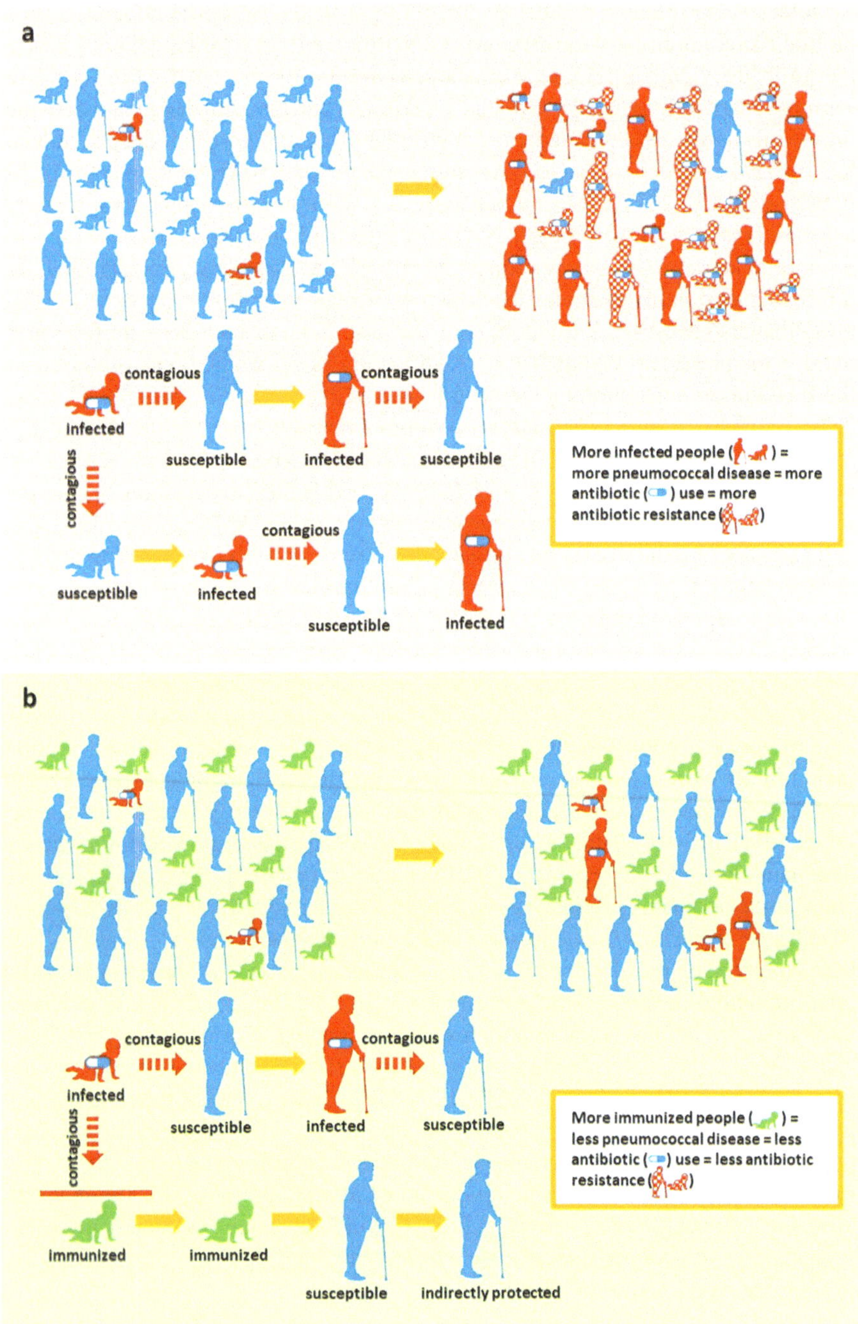

Fig. 10.5 High vaccination rates promote herd immunity for *S. pneumoniae*, thus decreasing antibiotic use and consequent spread of antimicrobial resistance. (**a**) When a population is not immunized against *S. pneumoniae*, most members are susceptible to the pathogen. A susceptible individual

expression of enzymes such as β-lactamases which inactivate β-lactams, upregulation of efflux pumps that cause removal of the antibiotic, or direct modification of the antibiotic target site through mutation. Vaccines, by comparison, act through immune pathways, and the polyclonal nature of vaccine induced immune responses limits escape mutants. Although vaccine immunity may fade over time due to waning of the specific host immune response (Kennedy and Read 2017), functional immunity can be restored following re-immunization with a booster dose, and that can be done repeatedly over one's lifetime. Resistance against vaccine mediated immunity develops rarely. However, in some instances such as *S. pneumoniae*, replacement of vaccine preventable serotypes with non-vaccine preventable serotypes that also cause disease has been observed (Weinberger et al. 2011). An example of loss of vaccine antigen expression possibly due to immune pressure is seen for *B. pertussis*, where strains that did not produce pertactin (Hegerle and Guiso 2014) emerged after the whole cell based *B. pertussis* vaccine was replaced with an acellular vaccine containing fewer pertussis antigens but including pertactin. These strains, believed to have competitive evolutionary advantage in vaccinated individuals compared to pertactin positive strains (Safarchi et al. 2015), may have emerged due to a more limited range of immunity elicited by the acellular vaccine (Octavia et al. 2012). Otherwise, with the notable exception of influenza that undergoes antigenic drift and shift in viral surface glycoproteins (Kim et al. 2018), there are very few examples whereby human pathogens have overcome vaccine-mediated immunity due to antigenic evolution.

Vaccination can affect AMR both directly and indirectly. Bacterial vaccines directly reduce antibiotic use through prevention of bacterial infections, and thus selection for AMR strains. Viral vaccines also diminish antibiotic use through avoidance of unwarranted antibiotic prescriptions as well as through prevention of secondary bacterial infections. Additionally, bacterial vaccines decrease circulation of resistant strains in vaccinated populations in regions with adequate vaccine coverage. In such settings, vaccines are known to induce herd immunity, an indirect vaccine phenomenon that leads to protection of even unvaccinated individuals in a vaccinated population. The relation between vaccination and herd immunity and the effect of immunization on the spread of AMR are schematically shown in Fig. 10.5,

Fig. 10.5 (continued) who becomes infected can therefore spread the pathogen to other susceptible individuals, so that over time a large proportion of the population is infected, requiring antibiotic treatment to clear the infection. Widespread antibiotic use, however, drives an increase in antibiotic resistant bacteria, which can rapidly spread. Proportions of individuals with antimicrobial resistance shown are consistent with pre-pneumococcal conjugate vaccine values for antibiotic nonsusceptible invasive pneumococcal disease rates in children younger than 5 years and adults 65 years of age and older in the U.S. (Kyaw et al. 2006; Pilishvili et al. 2010). (**b**) Widespread immunity at the population level against *S. pneumoniae* interrupts transmission of the pathogen, so that spread of pneumococcal disease is prevented. This results in much lower overall antibiotic use in the population, thus stemming further development of antibiotic resistance. Furthermore, susceptible members of the population, including those who have not or cannot be immunized (e.g., immunocompromised), are now protected (herd immunity). Copyright [Kathrin U. Jansen, William C. Gruber, Raphael Simon, James Wassil, and Annaliesa S.Anderson] 2020

using pneumococcal disease as an example. In the following sections of this chapter, we will discuss examples of proven anti-AMR benefits of licensed vaccines, review the status of new vaccine candidates with potential against AMR, and outline challenges and prospects related to the use of vaccines as a tool to reduce prevent AMR.

10.4 Vaccines Have Reduced Incidence and Evolution of Antimicrobial Resistant Bacterial Pathogens

There are several well-documented and epidemiologically supported examples whereby both bacterial and viral vaccines have impacted AMR. Additionally, vaccine strategies have been purposefully used to combat the rise of an AMR pathogen.

10.4.1 Vaccines Reduce Circulating Antibiotic Resistant Strains and Antibiotic Use

10.4.1.1 *Haemophilus influenzae* Type b Vaccine

H. influenzae is an invasive bacterial pathogen that can cause severe infection characterized by pneumonia, septicemia, and meningitis, where mortality occurs in up to 5% of infected individuals (https://www.cdc.gov/hi-disease/about/index.html). Hib microbes account for 95% of all strains that cause invasive disease following infection with *H. influenzae* (Immunization Action Coalition 2019). The polyribosyl phosphate capsule of Hib is an important virulence factor and protective antigen, and conjugate vaccines based on the polyribosyl phosphate capsule are highly efficacious. Prior to the introduction of Hib conjugate vaccines into the routine infant immunization schedule in 1987, first in the U.S. and then globally, Hib was a devastating pathogen in infants and young children. At that time, incidence rates of Hib disease (including bacterial meningitis and other invasive diseases) in children younger than 5 years ranged from 49 to 601 per 100,000 in some populations (Peltola et al. 1990; Ward et al. 1986). In the U.S. between 1978 and 1981, the incidence of invasive Hib disease was estimated to be approximately 500 cases per 100,000 (1 in 200) in children younger than 5 years (Cochi et al. 1985). In addition, a steady increase in β-lactam resistance among invasive Hib isolates had been observed starting in the early 1970s (Tristram et al. 2007), mediated by bacterial expression of β-lactamases and/or, to a lesser extent, modified penicillin binding proteins (Tristram et al. 2007). For example, a study by the CDC has demonstrated that among a collection of 40 *H. influenzae* clinical isolates, more than a quarter were resistant to ampicillin (Thornsberry and Kirven 1974). In the UK, resistance for *H. influenzae* isolates to ampicillin (and β-lactamase expression) did rapidly increase between 1977 and 1981, from 1.6% to 6.2% (almost 4-fold) (Morrissey et al. 2008). In the late 1990s, global surveillance studies, such as PROTECT and Alexander, found that approximately 16% of all Hib strains worldwide were β-lactamase positive, however with large variation between countries, from 1.8% in Italy to 65% in South Korea (Hoban and Felmingham 2002; Jacobs 2003; Jacobs et al. 2003).

The development and deployment of Hib capsular polysaccharide conjugate vaccines as part of routine childhood immunizations rapidly reduced the incidence of Hib disease (Adam et al. 2010; Centers for Disease Control and Prevention (CDC) 2002; Peltola et al. 1999). According to the CDC reported Active Bacterial Core Surveillance data from 2014, the invasive Hib disease incidence was 0.19 per 100,000 for children younger than 5 years, the value below the Healthy People 2020 objective of 0.27 per 100,000 (Centers for Disease Control and Prevention 2016), indicating a dramatic reduction in the disease rates due to Hib vaccination. Similarly, vaccine introduction in the UK in 1992 resulted in a near elimination of Hib disease in children younger than 5 years within just a few years. Comparable successes were observed globally (Hargreaves et al. 1996). Moreover, global use of the Hib vaccine turned the tide against growing Hib antibiotic resistance. Shortly after introduction of Hib conjugate vaccines worldwide, significant decreases in β-lactamase positive clinical isolates were observed (Heilmann et al. 2005), although in some countries (such as Japan) (Hasegawa et al. 2003), the prevalence of these resistant strains may have been decreasing before vaccine implementation. The impact of Hib conjugate vaccines on AMR strains was also confirmed in studies that have shown a correlation between Hib vaccine use and a reduction in resistance to one or more antibiotics. For example, in a 10-year Italian study, after universal introduction of Hib vaccine in 1999, a 50% decrease in resistance to ampicillin and related antibiotics among clinical isolates across all ages was observed (Giufre et al. 2011).

10.4.1.2 Pneumococcal Conjugate Vaccines

S. pneumoniae continues to be a leading global cause of serious illness among unvaccinated children and adults. In 2005, the WHO estimated that 1.6 million deaths were caused by this pathogen annually (http://www.who.int/ith/diseases/pneumococcal/en/). In the 1990s, before the introduction of the 7-valent pneumococcal capsular polysaccharide conjugate vaccine (PCV7, Prevnar®) into the childhood immunization program, ~63,000 cases of invasive pneumococcal disease occurred each year in the U.S. (Feldman and Anderson 2016). Importantly, at this time resistance to penicillin and other classes of antibiotics also emerged among *S. pneumoniae* isolates in the U.S. The CDC's pneumococcal surveillance study demonstrated a more than 60-fold increase in penicillin resistance during the period between 1979–1987 and 1992 in the U.S. (Breiman et al. 1994). Further increase in resistance among pneumococcal strains was seen by 1993–1994, of which 14.1% were penicillin nonsusceptible, 3.2% were penicillin resistant, and 25.5% were nonsusceptible to more than one antimicrobial agent (Butler et al. 1996).

Introduction of polysaccharide conjugate vaccines (PCVs), initially covering 7 (PCV7; Wyeth 2000) and subsequently 13 (PCV13, Prevnar 13®; Pfizer 2010) pneumococcal serotypes, had a tremendous success in the U.S. with more than 90% efficacy against invasive pneumococcal disease observed in the primary target population of children younger than 5 years (Cohen et al. 2017). Importantly, PCVs protected against both antibiotic susceptible and resistant isolates. Several studies in the U.S. have analyzed the laboratory confirmed data from the population based Active Bacterial Core Surveillance system to evaluate changes in invasive pneumococcal disease rates following introduction of PCVs. One of those analyses, performed on the data from 1996 to 2004, found that after introduction of PCV7 in the U.S., rates of penicillin nonsusceptible infections with serotypes included in the vaccine fell by 87% (5.0–0.7 cases per 100,000) for any ages, 98% (61.5–1.2 cases per 100,000) for children younger than 2 years, and 79% (12.3–2.6 cases per 100,000) for adults 65 years of age and older. Additionally, the rate of infection with strains of *S. pneumoniae* showing reduced susceptibility to multiple antibiotics dropped by 59% for people of all ages (Kyaw et al. 2006). Another study reported that only seven years after introduction of PCV7, ~211,000 cases of invasive pneumococcal disease caused by the seven serotypes covered by PCV7 (including antibiotic resistant strains) were prevented not only in children but also in individuals of all ages. The incidence of invasive pneumococcal disease caused by PCV7-type strains decreased by 94% (15.5–1.0 cases per 100,000) for all age groups, 100% (81.9–0.4 cases per 100,000) for children younger than 5 years, and 92% (33.7–2.7 cases per 100,000) for adults 65 years of age and older (Pilishvili et al. 2010). Between 1998 and 2008, rates of penicillin nonsusceptible invasive pneumococcal disease caused by all pneumococcal serotypes decreased by 64% for children younger than 5 years (12.1–4.4 cases per 100,000) and 45% for adults 65 years of age and older (4.8–2.6 cases per 100,000), with a similar reduction for invasive pneumococcal disease nonsusceptible to multiple antibiotics (Hampton et al. 2012).

A subsequent study on the impact of PCV13 on antibiotic nonsusceptible invasive pneumococcal disease in the U.S. also demonstrated decreased rates of antibiotic nonsusceptible invasive pneumococcal disease caused by serotypes included in PCV13 but not in PCV7 between 2009 (immediately before PCV13 was introduced) and 2013: from 6.7 to 2.2 per 100,000 for all ages, from 6.5 to 0.5 per 100,000 in children younger than 5 years, and from 4.4 to 1.4 per 100,000 in adults 65 years of age and older (Tomczyk et al. 2016) (Fig. 10.6). Marked decreases were also observed for rates of multi drug nonsusceptible invasive pneumococcal disease. Furthermore, following the introduction of PCV13, the annual incidence of antibiotic nonsusceptible invasive pneumococcal disease in children younger than 5 years in the U.S. was reduced from 2010 through 2013 by a range of 63%–83% for strains resistant to macrolides, cephalosporins, tetracyclines, and penicillins, indicating direct impact on circulating AMR strains (Tomczyk et al. 2016).

Surveillance studies in other countries have also shown a considerable impact of PCVs on invasive pneumococcal disease rates. For example, in South Africa, between 2009 and 2012, penicillin nonsusceptible invasive pneumococcal disease rates had declined by 47% after three years of PCV7 use in children younger than

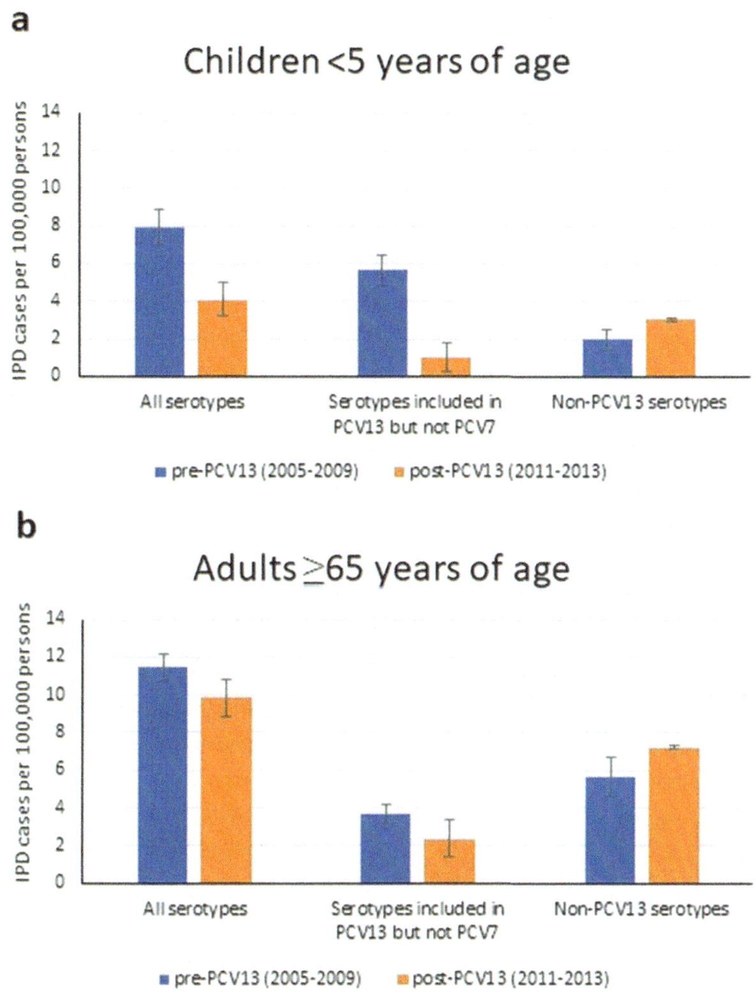

Fig. 10.6 Reduction of antimicrobial resistance after broad rollout of PCV13. Data presented show average annual rates of antibiotic nonsusceptible invasive pneumococcal disease (IPD) of the vaccine- and non-vaccine type, with standard deviations in (**a**) vaccinated (children younger than 5 years) and (**b**) non-vaccinated (adults 65 years of age and older) populations, prior to (2005–2009) and following (2011–2013) introduction of PCV13 vaccine. (Adapted from Tomczyk et al. 2016). Copyright [Kathrin U. Jansen, William C. Gruber, Raphael Simon, James Wassil, and Annaliesa S. Anderson] 2020

2 years (von Gottberg et al. 2014). Subsequent analyses revealed that between 2008 and 2015, rates of invasive pneumococcal disease caused by penicillin susceptible and nonsusceptible pneumococcal isolates decreased by 61% and 91%, respectively, for children younger than 2 years, and by 42% and 72%, respectively, for all ages (von Gottberg et al. 2016).

Numerous studies demonstrate that antibiotic use was also reduced following PCV introduction. For example, with introduction of PCV7 in 2000 in the U.S., antibiotic prescription for acute otitis media in children younger than 2 years fell by 42% from 1997–1999 to 2004 (Zhou et al. 2008). Another study, conducted in Northern California, indicated that up to 35 antibiotic prescriptions per 100 children were prevented with PCV7 vaccination from the first vaccine dose to the age of 3.5 years, from which the authors suggested that approximately 1.4 million antibiotic prescriptions are preventable by PCV in the U.S. annually (Fireman et al. 2003). In Germany, there were 539,000 fewer antibiotic prescriptions due to pneumonia in children 0–10 years of age between 2007 and 2014 (Chatham House 2017). Similarly, after the introduction of PCV10 in the Netherlands in 2011, prescription of antibiotics for respiratory infection in children 2–7 years of age was reduced by up to 24% from 2002 to 2013 (Gefenaite et al. 2014). An international group of experts estimated that overall, universal coverage with PCV could avert up to 11.4 million days of antibiotic therapy for pneumonia caused by *S. pneumoniae* annually in children younger than 5 years, a 47% reduction in the 75 countries included in the analysis (Laxminarayan et al. 2016).

In addition, pneumococcal conjugate vaccination has been found to reduce pneumonia cases misattributed to respiratory viral infection in the setting of co-incident secondary pneumococcal lower respiratory tract infection. In a large randomized, placebo-controlled study in South Africa, a 9-valent PCV prevented 31% (95% confidence interval, 15–43%) of pneumonias attributed to influenza A and parainfluenza viruses and respiratory syncytial virus (RSV) in fully immunized infants, with the effect presumed due to otherwise undiagnosed contemporaneous pneumococcal infection (Madhi et al. 2004).

10.4.1.3 Typhoid Conjugate Vaccine

Typhoid vaccines also provide a contemporary example of how a vaccine can be used to prevent dissemination of an AMR pathogen. *S.* Typhi is the causative agent of typhoid enteric fever, a potentially life-threatening disease. In 2000, *S.* Typhi caused approximately 21.7 million illnesses and 216,000 deaths worldwide (Crump et al. 2004). Typhoid fever remains a common infectious disease in low- and middle-income countries, causing approximately 11.9 million cases and 129,000 deaths in 2010 according to the International Vaccine Institute (Mogasale et al. 2014), although the true disease burden is likely underestimated. In the U.S., endemic disease has been essentially eradicated due to improvements in water sanitation, and most cases of typhoid are travel-associated. The CDC has categorized *S.* Typhi as being of serious concern as an antibiotic resistance threat, as 74% of *S.* Typhi infections had partial or full resistance to ciprofloxacin in 2017, and resistance to other antibiotics was also observed (Centers for Disease Control and Prevention 2019). The discovery in 2016, in the Sindh province of Pakistan, of an extensively drug resistant haplotype 58 clone of *S.* Typhi, resistant to first- and second-line antibiotics as well as third-generation cephalosporins, thus evoked particular alarm

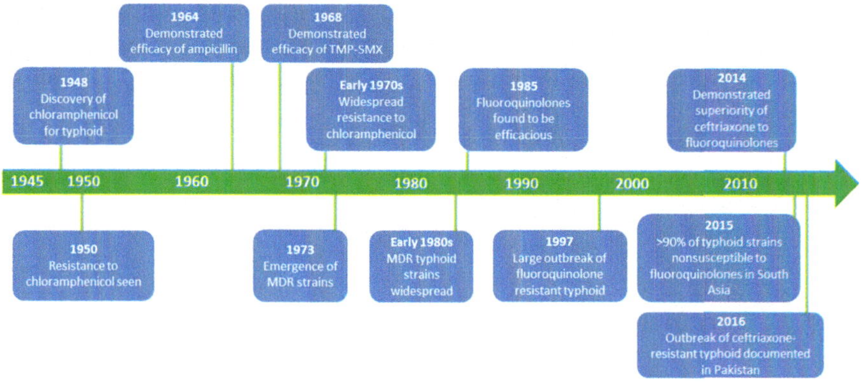

Fig. 10.7 **Timeline of acquisition of antibiotic resistance by *S.* Typhi.** *MDR* multi drug resistant, *TMP-SMX* trimethoprim-sulfamethoxazole. (Adapted from Andrews et al. 2018)

(Fig. 10.7) (Andrews et al. 2018). Since recognition of its emergence, the ongoing major typhoid outbreak with this clone has affected more than 5200 people witihin the Sindh region (https://www.who.int/csr/don/27-december-2018-typhoid-pakistan/en/; Qamar et al. 2018). Analysis of the extensively drug resistant isolate indicated that the clone emerged by a single step transformation of multi drug resistant *S.* Typhi through acquisition of a promiscuous plasmid encoding resistance to fluoroquinolones and third generation cephalosporins previously identified in other enteric bacteria (Klemm et al. 2018). Since H58 is the dominant global clonotype, if left unchecked, extensively drug resistant H58 *S.* Typhi has the capacity to cause a global public health crisis (Klemm et al. 2018; Levine and Simon 2018). Fortunately, there are several licensed typhoid vaccines, including the recently WHO prequalified Vi capsular conjugate vaccine Typbar-TCV™ manufactured by Bharat Biotech (India), that is the first and only typhoid vaccine approved for use in children and infants younger than 2 years (Sahastrabuddhe and Saluja 2019). In response to the outbreak, and due to the limited treatment options and risk for rapid spread of this extensively drug resistant typhoid clone, Pakistani authorities launched an emergency typhoid vaccination campaign in the most affected areas, using Typbar-TCV vaccine (Bhatti 2019; https://www.who.int/csr/don/27-december-2018-typhoid-pakistan/en/).

Vi-conjugate vaccines have also been used in response to a typhoid outbreak in Zimbabwe, Africa with *S.* Typhi isolates manifesting high levels of multi drug resistance and reduced fluoroquinolone susceptibility (N'Cho et al. 2019), whereby a vaccination campaign with the conjugate vaccine was carried out in February-March 2019, targeting children 6 months to 15 years of age. Three months after initiation of the vaccination effort, surveillance for febrile cases with suspected typhoid in the worst affected communities revealed a complete absence of typhoid cases among 24 children who provided blood cultures, compared with 23 of 109

(21%) positive blood cultures seen in a study directly preceding the start of the campaign. This vaccine intervention effort was the first attempt to control a typhoid outbreak in Africa through vaccination and the first use of the typhoid Vi-conjugate vaccine in the continent (Olaru et al. 2019).

These examples of the purposeful use of a vaccine to control an outbreak with an AMR pathogen thus represents a new paradigm in public health, that may be extended to other pathogens in the future.

10.4.2 Vaccines Mediate Herd Immunity

Herd immunity is the protection conferred through broad vaccine coverage at the population level, to members of the community who are not vaccinated, cannot be vaccinated, or do not mount effective immune responses following vaccination. As a critical threshold of vaccinated individuals is reached, indirect protection can be conferred to unvaccinated individuals within the community through prevention of transmission and reduced pathogen spread. High vaccination rates at the population level are needed to achieve herd immunity and can both reduce transmission of AMR pathogens and limit antibiotic use by non-vaccinated individuals (Fig. 10.5b). Significant herd immunity has been achieved by both Hib and pneumococcal conjugate vaccines, driven in part by the reduction of nasopharyngeal colonization with pathogens expressing vaccine serotypes. Infant immunization with Hib vaccines led to a rapid fall in the rates of invasive Hib infections worldwide, in both vaccinated and unvaccinated children, an effect attributed to decreased carriage and transmission among young children (Steinhoff and Goldblatt 2003).

The introduction of PCV7 and PCV13 in pediatric vaccination programs has had significant impact on reduction of vaccine type invasive pneumococcal disease in both unvaccinated pediatric and adult populations, particularly elderly (65 years of age and older), due to the herd effect. This has been attributed to both the reduction in bacterial carriage and a substantial decrease in the incidence of invasive pneumococcal disease (Cohen et al. 2017). As described in Sect. 10.4.1, analyses of invasive pneumococcal disease cases identified through the U.S. Active Bacterial Core Surveillance system demonstrated significant reductions in the rates of penicillin nonsusceptible infections for the all-ages population as well as adults 65 years of age and older, which were associated with serotypes included in PCV7 (between late 1990s and middle-to-late 2000s) (Hampton et al. 2012; Kyaw et al. 2006; Pilishvili et al. 2010) and PCV13 (between middle 2000s and early 2010s) (Fig. 10.6b) (Tomczyk et al. 2016).

In other countries, the invasive pneumococcal disease rates also reduced after PCV7 introduction: by 8.8% for adults 65 years of age and older (Denmark 2010) (Ingels et al. 2012) and 70% for the entire adult population (Taiwan 2012) (Lai et al. 2014). Similar effects were observed for pneumonia disease (Tsaban and Ben-Shimol 2017). In South Africa, rates of invasive pneumococcal disease caused by PCV7 serotypes fell by 57% for young adults (25–44 years of age, 2009–2012) (von

Gottberg et al. 2014). Rates of invasive pneumococcal disease caused by penicillin-susceptible and -nonsusceptible pneumococcal isolates also significantly decreased for the all-ages population between 2008 and 2015, as previously described in Sect. 10.4.1 (von Gottberg et al. 2016). Substantial reductions in invasive pneumococcal disease and pneumonia disease rates through herd immunity were also associated with PCV10 and PCV13 immunization in countries using these vaccines (Tsaban and Ben-Shimol 2017), as seen, for example, by the 61% reduction in invasive pneumococcal disease in adults 65 years of age and older in Ontario, Canada (Rudnick et al. 2013).

10.4.3 Preventing Antimicrobial Resistance Using Viral Vaccines

Although they do not directly generate antibacterial immunity, viral vaccines are an important tool for containment of AMR. First, they help prevent viral disease and thus avoid the inappropriate use of antibiotics. Additionally, bacterial infections are common secondary complications following some viral diseases and may even cause concurrent viral-bacterial superinfections that can be reduced by vaccination against a bacterial pathogen (Madhi et al. 2004). Vaccination against viral pathogens thus prevents secondary bacterial infections that may be antibiotic resistant. Influenza virus and rotavirus vaccines represent prominent examples of approved vaccines with these anti AMR benefits.

10.4.3.1 Influenza Virus Vaccine

An estimated 3–5 million cases of influenza occur each year worldwide, causing 290,000 to 650,000 respiratory deaths (Iuliano et al. 2018; https://www.who.int/en/news-room/fact-sheets/detail/influenza-(seasonal)). Due to the constant evolution of influenza viruses, the WHO Global Influenza Surveillance and Response System closely monitors circulating influenza virus types. Live-attenuated, inactivated, and recombinant influenza vaccines, targeting influenza A and B, are produced annually to match changes in the hemagglutinin proteins contained in the strains expected to circulate in the following influenza season (https://www.who.int/en/news-room/fact-sheets/detail/influenza-(seasonal)). The elderly population, people with chronic pulmonary or cardiovascular conditions, and immunocompromised individuals are at greatest risk for severe influenza disease and disease complications (Mertz et al. 2013). Recovery from influenza infection is accompanied by an overt risk for secondary bacterial respiratory infections (Prasso and Deng 2017), thus further amplifying the morbidity and mortality due to influenza (Kash and Taubenberger 2015). Among influenza patients who developed pneumonia, up to 75% were confirmed to have a secondary bacterial infection (Zambon 2001). *S. pneumoniae*, *H. influenzae*, and *S. aureus* are reported as the most common causes of secondary bacterial infections associated with influenza (Joseph et al. 2013; Morris et al. 2017). Vaccination against influenza thus indirectly protects against these bacterial pneumonias that may be antibiotic resistant.

Acute otitis media is another common secondary bacterial infection associated with influenza (Kash and Taubenberger 2015), and there is evidence that the incidence of this infection and associated antibiotic use can also be reduced through influenza vaccination. In a prospective, blinded study in children 6–60 months old in Turkey (N = 119), the frequency of acute otitis media in the influenza vaccinated group was significantly reduced compared with the unvaccinated control group (2.3% versus 5.2%, approximately 50% reduction) during the influenza season (Ozgur et al. 2006). In a prospective, randomized study conducted in Italy in children 1–5 years of age and prone to acute otitis media (N = 180), immunization with a trivalent virosomal-adjuvanted inactivated influenza vaccine significantly reduced the mean number of antibiotic courses (13.2% effectiveness, $p < 0.001$) as well as the mean number of acute otitis media episodes (54.8% effectiveness, $p = 0.03$), with the latter likely contributing to the reduction in antibiotic use (Marchisio et al. 2009). In a Phase 3 randomized multinational study in children 6–36 months old in Europe (N = 12,018), immunization with an inactivated quadrivalent influenza vaccine reduced the risk for antibiotic use by 71% in Europe, 36% in Asia Pacific, and 59% in Central America compared with the control group, during 5 consecutive influenza seasons (Dbaibo et al. 2020). Analyses of pooled data from 24,046 children 6–83 months old, collected in 8 randomized clinical trials in the U.S., Europe, and Asia, have demonstrated high efficacy of live attenuated influenza vaccine against influenza associated acute otitis media compared with placebo (85%; 95% confidence interval, 78.3–89.8%) or trivalent inactivated influenza vaccine (54%; 95% confidence interval, 27.0–71.7%). In children who became infected despite being vaccinated, the relative reduction in the development of acute otitis media in the vaccinated population was 38.2% (95% confidence interval, 11.0–58.2%) compared with placebo (Block et al. 2011). Children vaccinated with live attenuated influenza vaccine also had a decreased incidence of all-cause acute otitis media compared with placebo: 12.4% (95% confidence interval, 2.0–21.6%) reduction in year 1 and 6.2% (95% confidence interval, -12.4–21.7%) reduction in year 2, with the estimated 12 month effectiveness of the vaccine compared with placebo of 7.5% (95% confidence interval, -2.4–16.2%) (Heikkinen et al. 2013).

Globally, the influenza season represents the period of greatest antibiotic use, in part due to the frequent inappropriate prescription of antibiotics for respiratory tract infections caused by viral pathogens. For example, in the U.S., nearly half of all antibiotic prescriptions are written for respiratory illnesses associated with pathogens such as influenza that are not susceptible to antibiotics (Fleming-Dutra et al. 2016). Reduction in infection through vaccination thus reduces antibiotic use. Indeed, the study conducted in Canada using national health and prescription survey systems demonstrated convincingly that introduction of universal influenza vaccination to everyone over 6 months of age in Ontario resulted in reduced influenza associated antibiotic prescriptions from 17.9 to 6.4 per 1000 people (a reduction of

~64%) compared to other Canadian provinces where the use of influenza vaccines was limited to at-risk populations (Kwong et al. 2009). A self control study in the UK that analyzed data on children 2–4 years old from The Health Improvement Network database (N = 33,137) found that children vaccinated with a live attenuated influenza vaccine had 14.5% fewer amoxicillin prescriptions during the period of influenza vaccine immunity compared with other winter seasons (Hardelid et al. 2018). By protecting against flu, even moderately effective seasonal influenza vaccines can prevent inappropriate antibiotic prescriptions for respiratory infections of viral origin. In the season of 2017–2018, the influenza vaccination coverage in the U.S. was 37.1% among adults and 57.9% among children 6 months through 17 years of age, leaving ample room for improvement (https://www.cdc.gov/flu/fluvaxview/coverage-1718estimates.htm). Implementation of national universal influenza vaccination programs, improvement of existing vaccines towards increased breadth of efficacy to an extended repertoire of viral strains, higher efficacy in older adults and young children, and development of universal influenza vaccines would provide further impact in the fight against AMR.

10.4.3.2 Rotavirus Vaccine

Diarrheal disease is a second leading cause of mortality and morbidity among children younger than 5 years, and children in low income countries are particularly affected (https://www.who.int/en/news-room/fact-sheets/detail/diarrhoeal-disease). Diarrheal illness can be caused by bacterial, viral, or parasitic organisms. Among diarrheal pathogens, rotavirus is a leading cause of severe diarrheal disease in infants and young children (https://www.who.int/immunization/diseases/rotavirus/en/). Two oral rotavirus vaccines are currently licensed for infants in the U.S.: RotaTeq® and Rotarix® (https://www.cdc.gov/rotavirus/vaccination.html), and two more are approved internationally and are WHO prequalified (https://www.who.int/immunization/diseases/rotavirus/en/). Rotavirus vaccines have had a significant public health impact on the incidence and severity of childhood diarrheal disease. Efficacy of RotaTeq and Rotarix ranges from 80 to 100% in industrialized countries, including Latin America (Giaquinto et al. 2011; Linhares et al. 2008; Vesikari et al. 2007), and 39–77% in developing countries, such as Africa and Asia (Madhi et al. 2010; Zaman et al. 2010). There is also evidence of herd protection from rotavirus vaccine to unvaccinated children (Patel et al. 2011; Pollard et al. 2015). As infection with rotavirus can lead to inappropriate antibiotic use if a misdiagnosis of bacterial infection is given (e.g., enterotoxigenic *E. coli* or *Vibrio cholerae*) or if treatment is sought based on symptoms (in many countries, patients can receive antibiotics from pharmacists without being given a prescription), implementation of national rotavirus vaccination programs worldwide would benefit containment of AMR by reducing inappropriate antibiotic prescriptions in countries endemic for these bacterial pathogens.

10.5 Vaccines Under Development with Potential to Reduce Antimicrobial Resistance

Given the proven success of licensed vaccines in combating AMR, sustained efforts are being directed towards the development of new and improved vaccines targeting pathogens that exhibit increased antibiotic resistance, are associated with high antibiotic use, and are considered priority organisms by the WHO and the CDC (Centers for Disease Control and Prevention 2019; World Health Organization 2017a). In the following sections, we will discuss select examples of vaccines under development that target pathogens with demonstrated propensity to acquire antibiotic resistance, and thus hold promise in further reducing AMR (Table 10.2).

10.5.1 Bacterial Vaccines in Late-Stage Clinical Development

10.5.1.1 *Clostridioides difficile* Vaccines

C. difficile, a Gram positive anaerobic, spore forming bacillus, is the main cause of nosocomial infectious diarrhea in industrialized countries (Guerrant et al. 1990; Kelly et al. 1994; Kyne and Kelly 1998; Magill et al. 2014; McFarland 1995). *C. difficile* infection frequently occurs consequent to antibiotic use, whereby ablation of the normal flora and the accompanying dysbiosis following antibiotic treatment make available an intestinal niche that *C. difficile* colonizes. Pathogenesis is mediated primarily by two large clostridial glucosylating toxins, toxin A (TcdA) and toxin B (TcdB) (Kuehne et al. 2010), which modify intracellular signaling pathways in intestinal epithelial cells, causing cytotoxicity, inflammation, and diarrhea (Voth and Ballard 2005).

C. difficile infection accounts for 20–30% of cases of diarrhea that develops after antibiotic use, and is the most commonly recognized cause of infectious diarrhea in healthcare settings (Cohen et al. 2010). *C. difficile* is carried in approximately 1–3% of healthy adults and approximately 16–35% of hospital inpatients on antibiotic treatment (Aslam et al. 2005). As many as 50% or more of hospitalized patients colonized by *C. difficile* are asymptomatic carriers (Cohen et al. 2010). According to the CDC's national estimate, there were 223,900 cases of *C. difficile* infection related to antibiotic use and antibiotic resistance in 2017 in the U.S., along with 12,800 associated deaths (Centers for Disease Control and Prevention 2019). Older adults (65 years of age and older) are at increased risk for *C. difficile* infection, particularly when exposed to healthcare settings (Bartlett and Gerding 2008; Bauer et al. 2011; Leffler and Lamont 2015; Pepin et al. 2005; Simor 2010). Although most patients experiencing a first episode of *C. difficile* infection respond well to standard antibiotic treatment (McDonald et al. 2018), approximately 15–35% of patients suffer from at least one recurrence (Gerding et al. 2008; Leffler and Lamont 2015; Louie et al. 2011), often leading to a vicious

Table 10.2 Examples of vaccine candidates in active clinical development with the potential to reduce antimicrobial resistance

Vaccine name	Organization	Vaccine type	Vaccine composition	Stage	NCT	Status	Study population	Reference
Clostridioides difficile								
PF-06425090	Pfizer	Toxoid	Genetically-/chemically-inactivated toxins A and B	Phase 3	NCT03090191	Ongoing	Adults at risk of developing *C. difficile* infection, ≥50 years	https://clinicaltrials.gov/
VLA84	Valneva	Toxoid	Recombinant fusion protein consisting of truncated toxins A and B	Phase 2	NCT02316470	Completed	Healthy adults, ≥50 years	https://clinicaltrials.gov/
GSK2904545A	GSK	Toxoid	Recombinant F2 antigen	Phase 1	NCT04026009	Ongoing	Healthy adults, 18-45 and 50-70 years	https://clinicaltrials.gov/
Streptococcus pneumoniae								
V114	Merck	Conjugate (15-valent)	Capsular polysaccharides of *S. pneumoniae* conjugated to CRM_{197}	Phase 3	NCT03480763	Completed	Healthy adults, ≥50 years	https://clinicaltrials.gov/
					NCT03480802	Completed	Healthy adults, ≥18 years	
					NCT03692871	Ongoing	Healthy infants	
20vPnC	Pfizer	Conjugate (20-valent)	Capsular polysaccharides of *S. pneumoniae* conjugated to CRM_{197}	Phase 3	NCT03760146	Completed	Pneumococcal vaccine-naïve adults, ≥18 years	https://clinicaltrials.gov/
					NCT04382326	Ongoing	Healthy infants	
					NCT04379713			
Pneumosil	Serum Institute of India	Conjugate (10-valent)	Capsular polysaccharides of *S. pneumoniae* conjugated to CRM_{197}	Phase 3	NCT03896477	Suspended	Healthy infants, 42-56 days	Moffitt and Malley (2016); https://clinicaltrials.gov/

(continued)

Table 10.2 (continued)

Vaccine name	Organization	Vaccine type	Vaccine composition	Stage	NCT	Status	Study population	Reference
GSK2830929A, GSK2830930A	GSK	Conjugate (11- and 12-valent)	Capsular polysaccharides of *S. pneumoniae* conjugated to non-typeable *H. influenzae* protein D (PHiD-CV)	Phase 2	NCT01616459	Completed	Healthy infants, 6-12 weeks	Carmona Martinez et al. (2019); https://clinicaltrials.gov/
GSK2189242A	GSK	Conjugate/ subunit (bivalent)	Recombinant PhtD and PlyD1 of *S. pneumoniae* plus PHiD-CV	Phase 2	NCT01204658	Completed	Healthy infants, 6-14 weeks	Prymula et al. (2017); https://clinicaltrials.gov/
ASP3772	Affinivax	Complex (MAPS)	Capsular polysaccharides and proteins of *S. pneumoniae*	Phase 1/2	NCT03803202	Ongoing	Healthy adults, 18-85 years	http://affinivax.com/vaccine-pipeline/; https://clinicaltrials.gov/
Unspecified	Sanofi	Subunit (trivalent)	Recombinant PhtD, PcpA, and PlyD1 of *S. pneumoniae*	Phase 1	NCT01444352	Completed	Healthy adults, 18-50 years	Kamtchoua et al. (2013); https://clinicaltrials.gov/
PATH-wSP	PATH/Boston Children's Hospital	Inactivated whole cell	Mutation inactivated whole cell *S. pneumoniae*	Phase 2	NCT02097472	Completed	Healthy toddlers and adults, 12 months to 45 years	Moffitt and Malley (2016); https://clinicaltrials.gov/
Group B streptococcus								
GBSIII-TT	NIAID	Conjugate (monovalent)	Capsular polysaccharide of GBS serotype III conjugated to TT	Phase 2	NCT00128219	Completed	Healthy non-pregnant women, 18-40 years	Hillier et al. (2019); https://clinicaltrials.gov/

GBSII-TT/III-TT	Baylor College of Medicine	Conjugate (bivalent)	Capsular polysaccharide of GBS serotypes II and III conjugated to TT	Phase 2	N/A	Completed	Healthy adults, 18-45 years	Baker et al. (2003)
GBS-NN	Minervax ApS	Subunit (bivalent)	Recombinant fusion of N-terminal domains of GBS Rib and Alpha C surface proteins	Phase 1	NCT02459262	Completed	Healthy non-pregnant women, 18-40 years	Rose et al. (2018); https://clinicaltrials.gov/
					NCT03807245	Completed		
GBS trivalent vaccine	GSK	Conjugate (trivalent)	Capsular epitopes of GBS serotypes Ia, Ib, and III conjugated to CRM_{197}	Phase 2	NCT02270944	Completed	Healthy non-pregnant women, 18-40 years	Leroux-Roels et al. (2019), Leroux-Roels et al. (2016); https://clinicaltrials.gov/
				Phase 2	NCT02690181		Healthy non-pregnant women, 22-46 years	
GBS6	Pfizer	Conjugate (hexavalent)	Capsular epitopes of GBS serotypes Ia, Ib, II, III, IV, and V conjugated to CRM_{197}	Phase 2	NCT03765073	Ongoing	Healthy non-pregnant and pregnant women, 18-40 years	https://clinicaltrials.gov/
Escherichia coli								
ExPEC4V/EcoXyn-4V or JNJ-63871860	LimmaTech (formerly GlycoVaxyn) and Janssen	Conjugate (tetravalent)	O-antigens of *E. coli* serotypes O1A, O2, O6A, and O25B individually bioconjugated to rEPA	Phase 1	NCT02289794	Completed	Healthy women with a history of recurrent UTIs, 18-70 years	Frenck Jr. et al. (2019), Huttner et al. (2017); https://clinicaltrials.gov/
				Phase 2	NCT02546960	Completed	Healthy adults, ≥18 years	

(continued)

Table 10.2 (continued)

Vaccine name	Organization	Vaccine type	Vaccine composition	Stage	NCT	Status	Study population	Reference
Mycobacterium tuberculosis								
Multiple vaccines	Multiple	Genetically modified BCG, whole cell inactivated, subunit, recombinant vector		Phase 1-3	Multiple	Various	Various	Andersen and Scriba (2019), Khoshnood et al. (2018) World Health Organization (2018); https://clinicaltrials.gov/
Shigella								
CVD 1208S	University of Maryland	Live attenuated	Live attenuated *S. flexneri* 2a strain	Phase 1	N/A	Completed	Healthy adults, 18-45 years	Kotloff et al. (2007)
WRSS1	WRAIR	Live attenuated	Live attenuated *S. sonnei*	Phase 2	N/A	Completed	Healthy men, 18-22 years	Orr et al. (2005)
SsWC	WRAIR	Inactivated	Whole-cell formalin-inactivated trivalent *S. sonnei*	Phase 1	N/A	Completed	Healthy adults, 18-50 years	McKenzie et al. (2006)
S. sonnei-rEPA	WRAIR	Conjugate	O-antigen of *S. sonnei* conjugated to rEPA	Phase 3	N/A	Completed	Healthy men, 18-22 years	Cohen et al. (1997)
SF2a-TT15	Institut Pasteur	Conjugate	Synthetic repeats of *S. flexneri* type 2a O-antigen conjugated to TT	Phase 1	NCT02797236	Completed	Healthy adults, 18-45 years	Barel and Mulard (2019); https://clinicaltrials.gov/
GVXNS D133	LimmaTech	Conjugate	Bioconjugate of *S. dysenteriae* type 1 O-antigen and rEPA	Phase 1	NCT01069471	Completed	Healthy adults, 18-50 years	Hatz et al. (2015)

Flexyn2a	LimmaTech	Conjugate	Bioconjugate of *S. flexneri* type 2a O-antigen and rEPA	Phase 1	NCT02388009	Completed	Healthy adults, 18-50 years	Riddle et al. (2016); https://clinicaltrials.gov/
				Phase 2b	NCT02646371			
1790GAHB	GSK	Subunit (GMMA)	OMV vaccine for *S. sonnei*	Phase 2a	NCT02676895	Completed	Healthy adults, 18-45 years	Obiero et al. (2017); https://clinicaltrials.gov/
					NCT03089879			
Invaplex 50	Naval Medical Research Center/ WRAIR	Subunit	Complex of IpaB/C/D with *S. flexneri* 2a LPS	Phase 1	NCT00082069	Completed	Healthy adults, 18-40 years	Riddle et al. (2011), Tribble et al. (2010); https://clinicaltrials.gov/
				Phase 1	N/A		Healthy adults, 18-45 years	
Non-typhoidal *Salmonella*								
CVD 1000	University of Maryland	Conjugate	Conjugates of O-antigen and flagellin from *S.* Typhimurium and *S.* Enteritidis, formulated with Typbar-TCV™	Phase 1	NCT03981952	Ongoing	Healthy adults, 18-45 years	Baliban et al. (2018); https://clinicaltrials.gov/
Paratyphoid *Salmonella*								
CVD 1902	University of Maryland	Live attenuated	Live attenuated *S.* Paratyphi A strain 9150	Phase 1	NCT01129453	Completed	Healthy adults, 18-45 years	Wahid et al. (2019); https://clinicaltrials.gov/

(continued)

Table 10.2 (continued)

Vaccine name	Organization	Vaccine type	Vaccine composition	Stage	NCT	Status	Study population	Reference
Staphylococcus aureus								
4C-Staph	GSK	Subunit	Csa1A (Sur2), FhuD2, EsxA/EsxB, HlAH35L	Phase 1	NCT01160172	Completed	Healthy adults, 18-40 years	Mancini et al. (2016); https://clinicaltrials.gov/
NDV-3	NovaDigm	Subunit	Recombinant N-terminal portion of Als3p of *Candida albicans*		NCT03455309	Completed	Men at increased risk for *S. aureus* colonization and disease, 17-35 years	Schmidt et al. (2012); https://clinicaltrials.gov/
Respiratory syncytial virus								
ResVax	Novavax	Nanoparticle	Recombinant RSV-F protein in nanoparticles	Phase 3	NCT02624947	Completed	Healthy third-trimester pregnant women, 18-40 years	https://clinicaltrials.gov/

RSV vaccine	Pfizer	Subunit	Engineered soluble pre-fusion site Ø–stabilized RSV F trimers	Phase 3	NCT04424316	Ongoing	Healthy third-trimester pregnant women, 18-49 years	Schmoele-Thoma et al. (2019); https://clinicaltrials.gov/
				Phase 2	NCT03529773	Ongoing	Healthy adults, 18-49 and 50-85 years	
					NCT03572062	Ongoing	Healthy older adults, 65-85 years	
					NCT04071158	Completed	Healthy non-pregnant women, 18-49 years	
					NCT04032093	Ongoing	Healthy third-trimester pregnant women, 18-49 years	
GSK3003891A	GSK	Subunit	Engineered soluble pre-fusion site Ø–stabilized RSV F trimers	Phase 2	NCT02360475 NCT02753413	Completed	Healthy non-pregnant women, 18-45 years	Beran et al. (2018); https://clinicaltrials.gov/
VRC-RSVRGP084-00VP (DS-Cav1)	NIAID	Subunit	Engineered soluble pre-fusion site Ø–stabilized RSV F trimers	Phase 1	NCT03049488	Completed	Healthy adults, 18-50 years	Crank et al. (2019); https://clinicaltrials.gov/
Multiple vaccines	Multiple	Subunit, recombinant vector, live-attenuated		Phase 1-2	Multiple	Various	Healthy children and adults	Jares Baglivo and Polack (2019); PATH (2019)

(continued)

Table 10.2 (continued)

Vaccine name	Organization	Vaccine type	Vaccine composition	Stage	NCT	Status	Study population	Reference
Human immunodeficiency virus								
Multiple vaccines	Multiple	Subunit, recombinant vectors		Phase 1-3	Multiple	Various	Various	Hsu and O'Connell (2017), Trovato et al. (2018)
Influenza virus								
M-001 (universal flu vaccine)	BiondVax	Subunit	Recombinant protein containing 9 B-cell and T-cell conserved epitopes from influenza A and B HA, NP, and M1	Phase 3	NCT03450915	Ongoing	Healthy adults, ≥50 years	https://clinicaltrials.gov/
VTP-100	Vaccitech	Recombinant vector	Recombinant influenza A NP and M1 in MVA vector	Phase 2b	NCT03880474	Ongoing	Healthy adults, ≥18 years	https://clinicaltrials.gov/
VAL-506440	Moderna	mRNA	mRNA of H10N8 HA in lipid nanoparticles	Phase 1	NCT03076385	Completed	Healthy adults, 18-64 years	Bahl et al. (2017), Feldman et al. (2019); https://clinicaltrials.gov/
VAL-339851	Moderna	mRNA	mRNA of H7N9 HA in lipid nanoparticles	Phase 1	NCT03345043	Ongoing	Healthy adults, 18-49 years	

20vPnC 20-valent pneumococcal conjugate vaccine, *Als3p* agglutinin like sequence 3 protein, *BCG* Bacillus Calmette Guérin, CRM_{197} cross reactive material 197, *GBS* Group B streptococcus, *GMMA* generalized modules for membrane antigens vaccine delivery system, *GSK* GlaxoSmithKline, *HA* hemagglutinin, *LPS* lipopolysaccharide, *M1* matrix protein, *MAPS* multiple antigen presenting system, *mRNA* messenger ribonucleic acid, *MVA* modified vaccinia virus Ankara, *N/A* not available, *NCT* ClinicalTrials.gov identifier, *NIAID* National Institute of Allergy and Infectious Diseases, *NP* nucleoprotein, *OMV* outer membrane vesicle, *PATH* Program for Appropriate Technology in Health, *PcpA* pneumococcal choline binding protein A, *PHiD-CV* pneumococcal polysaccharide protein D-conjugate vaccine, *PhtD* pneumococcal histidine triad protein D, *PlyD1* pneumolysoid, *rEPA* recombinant *Pseudomonas aeruginosa* exotoxin A, *RSV* respiratory syncytial virus, *TT* tetanus toxoid, *UTI* urinary tract infection, *WRAIR* Walter Reed Army Institute of Research

cycle requiring additional antibiotic use. Risk factors for recurrence include failure to mount a protective immune response and infection with a hypervirulent strain (Kyne et al. 2001). Over the past 20 years, the incidence, severity, and mortality of *C. difficile* infection, including hospital-associated outbreaks, have increased in both the U.S. and Europe (McDonald et al. 2018; Wiegand et al. 2012). Emergence of hypervirulent pathogenic strains such as BI/NAP1/027, an increased use of antibiotics that disrupt the intestinal microflora, improved detection methods, and an increased exposure to spores in healthcare facilities all contribute to the observed *C. difficile* infection escalation (Donskey 2017; Gerding 2004; Lessa et al. 2015; Polage et al. 2015).

C. difficile strains are resistant to many antibiotics commonly used to treat various infections, including tetracyclines, erythromycin, penicillins, cephalosporins, and fluoroquinolones (He et al. 2013; Johanesen et al. 2015; Spigaglia 2016; Tenover et al. 2012). The current treatment recommendation for *C. difficile* infection is oral vancomycin or fidaxomicin for non-severe or severe cases and oral or rectal vancomycin, stand-alone or concomitant with intravenous metronidazole for fulminant cases (McDonald et al. 2018). However, the antibiotic regimen that is required to clear *C. difficile* can cause development of AMR (Freeman et al. 2015; Spigaglia et al. 2011). Moreover, treatment options for *C. difficile* infection are becoming limited due to the emergence of AMR. Indeed, *C. difficile* strains originally treatable with metronidazole have shown increased minimum inhibitory concentration values in several studies (Adler et al. 2015; Freeman et al. 2015; Moura et al. 2013). A recent systematic literature review and meta-analysis found resistance of *C. difficile* to vancomycin is increasing as well (Saha et al. 2019). Given this burden of *C. difficile* infection and the rapid global spread of epidemic and antibiotic resistant strains, the CDC has classified *C. difficile* as an urgent antibiotic resistance threat (Centers for Disease Control and Prevention 2019). A vaccine against *C. difficile* would both protect against disease and, importantly, limit the need for antibiotic use to treat the infection, thus also limiting antibiotic resistance.

The toxins that mediate *C. difficile* infection, TcdA and TcdB, can be neutralized by antibodies (Giannasca et al. 1999; Kyne et al. 2001; Lowy et al. 2010; Wilcox et al. 2017), and bezlotoxumab, a recently approved anti-TcdB monoclonal antibody, has been found to prevent *C. difficile* infection recurrence (Merck 2016). Since *C. difficile* infection pathogenesis is toxin mediated, and toxoid based vaccines have protected against other toxin mediated diseases (such as tetanus, diphtheria, or anthrax), vaccines to protect against *C. difficile* infection have focused on the development of neutralizing antibody responses against TcdA and TcdB. Four investigational vaccines have progressed to clinical development. A chemically inactivated toxoid based vaccine (ACAM-CDIFF) developed by Sanofi Pasteur was assessed in a Phase 3 trial (NCT01887912, https://clinicaltrials.gov/), but the study was terminated due to the low probability that it would meet its primary objective, leading to discontinuation of the program (Sanofi 2017). Another vaccine candidate, VLA84, developed by Valneva, is a recombinant fusion protein comprising fragments of the receptor binding domains of

TcdA and TcdB separated by a 4-amino acid linker (Tian et al. 2012). This vaccine candidate completed Phase 2 evaluation in 2017 (NCT02316470, https://clinicaltrials.gov/); however, it has not yet progressed to Phase 3 studies (https://valneva.com/research-development/clostridium-difficile/). GlaxoSmithKline is also initiating clinical studies with a toxin fragment approach (NCT04026009). Currently, the most advanced vaccine candidate is PF-06425090, developed by Pfizer, which is in a Phase 3 trial (https://clinicaltrials.gov/ct2/show/NCT03090191; https://www.pfizer.com/science/find-a-trial/nct03090191). It is comprised of a bivalent toxoid formulation of *C. difficile* toxins A and B that are each genetically and chemically inactivated (Vidunas et al. 2016). If licensed and universally recommended, a *C. difficile* vaccine would provide an important tool for preventing AMR, as vaccinated individuals would be protected from *C. difficile* infection, thus reducing the associated antibiotic use and selection of multi drug resistant bacterial species.

10.5.1.2 *Streptococcus pneumoniae* Vaccines

Following introduction of PCV13, as a result of the significant effectiveness on both carriage and invasive disease, serotypes not included in the vaccine have become responsible for the majority of invasive pneumococcal disease cases in Europe and North America (Balsells et al. 2017; Kyaw et al. 2006). To help address this major unmet medical need, several pneumococcal conjugate vaccines with higher valencies are being developed, including 15-valent (Merck) and 20-valent polysaccharide conjugate formulations (Pfizer) that are currently undergoing Phase 3 evaluation in healthy adults and infants (NCT03480763, NCT03480802, NCT03692871, NCT03760146, NCT03760146, NCT04382326, NCT04379713) (https://clinicaltrials.gov/). If successful, these vaccines will have the potential to further reduce the burden of pneumococcal diseases globally. While the most prevalent pathogenic pneumococcal serotypes had been included in the approved PCV vaccine, with over 90 defined pneumococcal serotypes, there still remains a large unmet medical need to increase protection through vaccination with extended serotype coverage vaccines. An approach that has been undertaken to address this need is the use of conserved epitopes of pneumococcal surface proteins such as proteins A and C, adhesin A, pneumolysin, histidine triad proteins, and choline binding protein A (Alderson 2016; Moffitt and Malley 2016). Several investigational pneumococcal conjugate and subunit vaccines utilizing this approach are in clinical development (Table 10.2) (Alderson 2016; Moffitt and Malley 2016), including a bivalent vaccine containing pneumococcal histidine triad protein D and pneumolysoid 1 (GlaxoSmithKline) (Prymula et al. 2017) and a trivalent vaccine containing pneumococcal histidine triad protein D, pneumolysoid 1, and pneumococcal choline-binding protein A (Sanofi) (Kamtchoua et al. 2013). Alternatively, a pneumococcal vaccine candidate being developed by Affinivax comprises a macromolecular complex designed as the multiple antigen presenting system for increased immunogenicity, where subunit and conjugate approaches are merged and pneumococcal proteins are used as the carrier for pneumococcal capsular polysaccharides (Zhang et al. 2013; http://affinivax.com/vaccine-pipeline/). This vaccine is currently under Phase 1/2 evaluation in young as well as elderly adults (NCT03803202) (https://clinicaltrials.gov/).

10.5.1.3 Group B streptococcus Vaccines

Streptococcus agalactiae, also known as Group B streptococcus (GBS), is an encapsulated Gram positive bacterium common in the intestinal tract that also asymptomatically colonizes the vaginal mucosa (women) and rectum (women and men) of approximately 25% of the population. GBS can cause invasive infections, including pneumonia, meningitis, bacteremia, and sepsis across all age groups. According to the CDC's national estimate, in 2016 there were 31,000 cases of invasive GBS disease, causing 1700 deaths (Centers for Disease Control and Prevention 2019).

Pregnant women and their infants are particularly vulnerable to GBS infection. Asymptomatic maternal GBS carriage during pregnancy is a risk factor for endometritis, chorioamnionitis, sepsis, and preterm labor in the mother and for GBS related bloodstream infection, meningitis, pneumonia, and stillbirth in the baby. GBS disease presenting within the first 90 days of life is particularly devastating (https://www.cdc.gov/groupbstrep/about/fast-facts.html). In the U.S. and some other high income countries, GBS related disease incidence has been reduced by screening pregnant women for vaginal colonization and then treating carriers with antibiotics during labor, a process known as intrapartum antibiotic prophylaxis. Approximately 25% of pregnant women are reported to undergo intrapartum antibiotic prophylaxis in the U.S. and even higher rates are seen in other countries such as Canada (Simioni et al. 2016). While proven effective for prevention of GBS disease in newborns (Braye et al. 2018), intrapartum antibiotic prophylaxis has not impacted acquisition of late onset GBS disease occurring more than 7 days after birth and compromises the establishment of the normal flora that neonates would otherwise acquire during passage through the birth canal, that is important for development of a healthy microbiome. Intrapartum antibiotic prophylaxis also has the capacity to induce AMR among constituents of the vaginal microflora. Given the growing recognition of the importance of the microbiome for human health, these findings and perhaps yet-to-be-discovered intrapartum antibiotic prophylaxis induced changes of the maternal and newborn intestinal microbiota should prompt additional research to assess the potential risks to subsequent health of mother and baby (Braye et al. 2018).

Although GBS resistance to penicillin is low, approximately 10% of the maternal population report penicillin allergies, leading to the administration of macrolide antibiotics as an alternative. However, the prevalence of macrolide resistance in GBS has been rising in recent years, ranging from 7 to 25% in the U.S. and Canada to over 60% in Asia, leaving physicians with vancomycin among the few options for use in mothers with macrolide resistant GBS (Lu et al. 2014; Schrag et al. 2002). In the U.S., although the incidence of early onset disease in infants has been decreasing consequent to intrapartum antibiotic prophylaxis intervention, the proportion of GBS infections resistant to erythromycin and clindamycin has increased steadily since 2000. The CDC estimated that in 2016, 58% of GBS isolates tested were erythromycin resistant and 42% were clindamycin resistant. Furthermore, clindamycin resistant GBS was estimated to be associated with 13,000 illnesses and 720 deaths (Centers for Disease Control and Prevention 2019). The CDC recognizes GBS as a concerning AMR threat (Centers for Disease Control and Prevention 2019). An effective maternal GBS vaccine administered to the mother would thus not only protect against maternal and infant GBS infections, but also reduce AMR.

GBS expresses a capsular polysaccharide, and anti-capsular serotype-specific immunoglobulin G (IgG) antibodies have been shown to kill GBS by opsonophagocytosis. Among the 10 documented GBS capsular serotypes, only a subset are associated with the majority of disease (Baker et al. 2014; Mukesi et al. 2019). Investigational GBS vaccines based on the capsular polysaccharide are thus being pursued that may be used as maternal vaccines to be administered to pregnant women, inducing functional antibodies that would be transferred across the placenta during the third trimester of pregnancy and protect neonates from GBS disease. Several Phase 2 studies have been conducted with GBS capsular polysaccharide conjugate vaccines (NCT00128219, NCT02459262, NCT02270944, NCT02690181, NCT03170609). These include mono- and bivalent vaccines (Baker et al. 2003; Hillier et al. 2019; Rose et al. 2018), a trivalent vaccine (Leroux-Roels et al. 2019; Leroux-Roels et al. 2016), and a hexavalent vaccine (Buurman et al. 2019; https://clinicaltrials.gov/). The hexavalent GBS vaccine being developed by Pfizer is comprised of serotypes Ia, Ib, II, III, IV, and V, representing the dominant serotypes associated with GBS disease worldwide, conjugated to cross-reactive material 197 (CRM_{197}) used as a carrier protein (Buurman et al. 2019). The GBS6 capsule polysaccharide vaccine (Pfizer) is currently being evaluated in a Phase 2 trial (NCT03765073) in healthy non-pregnant and pregnant women (https://clinicaltrials.gov/). Additionally, an alternative vaccine candidate, a GBS-NN bivalent subunit vaccine (Minervax ApS), comprising a fusion of recombinant N-terminal domains of the GBS Rib and Alpha C surface proteins, has been evaluated in two Phase 1 trials in healthy non-pregnant women (NCT02459262, NCT03807245) (https://clinicaltrials.gov/).

10.5.2 Bacterial Vaccines in Early Stage Clinical or Pre-clinical Development

10.5.2.1 *Enterobacteriaceae* Vaccines

Enterobacteriaceae are a large family of Gram negative microbes that include both normal components of the gut flora and pathogens, with substantial AMR in some prominent family members. Carbapenem resistant *Enterobacteriaceae* are given critical priority by the WHO (World Health Organization 2017a) and are considered an urgent threat by the CDC (Centers for Disease Control and Prevention 2019). *E. coli* and *Klebsiella pneumoniae* pose the greatest concerns because they have high levels of resistance to third generation cephalosporins and extended spectrum β-lactam antibiotics. *E. coli* infections are also associated with high levels of fluoroquinolone resistance, and *K. pneumoniae* isolates highly resistant to carbapenems have caused frequent nosocomial outbreaks. Both species are part of the normal intestinal flora but can cause serious illness. *E. coli* is the most frequent cause of urinary tract infections, including cystitis and pyelonephritis, both community acquired and nosocomial, and bloodstream infections at all ages. *E. coli* may also be associated with intra abdominal infections such as peritonitis as well sepsis and meningitis in neonates. Notably, certain pathotypes of *E. coli* are also leading causative agents of foodborne infections worldwide. *K. pneumoniae* poses a similar problem; however, it tends to infect more vulnerable individuals including pre-term infants and patients with impaired immune systems, diabetes, or suffering from alcohol abuse, and those receiving advanced medical care. Multi drug resistant *Enterobacteriaceae* have recently achieved greater attention due to the rapid global spread of NDM-1 producing strains (Walsh et al. 2011; Yong et al. 2009), with associated spread of this gene to other Gram negative species (Nordmann et al. 2011). With the recent discovery of *E. coli* strains harboring the MCR-1 plasmid-1 conferring resistance to the last line antibacterial colistin (McGann et al. 2016), there is concern that strains containing both MCR-1 and NDM-1 may emerge, resulting in untreatable infections.

Capsular polysaccharides are an important virulence factor of extraintestinal *E. coli*; however, the predominant capsule types such as K1 and K5 are structurally homologous to human glycans and are hence not suitable as vaccine targets. Vaccine approaches for *E. coli* have thus focused on lipopolysaccharides (or O-antigens) (Huttner et al. 2017; Poolman and Wacker 2016). Although *E. coli* can express more than 180 different O-antigen serotypes, only a subset are associated with the majority of pathogenic strains (Poolman and Wacker 2016). Investigators at the Swiss Serum and Vaccine Institute and the Walter Reed Army Institute of Research assessed a 12-valent formulation of *E. coli* lipopolysaccharides derived O polysaccharide linked to recombinant *P. aeruginosa* exoprotein A as a carrier, targeting the dominant serotypes associated with disease. Phase 1 clinical studies conducted in the 1990s confirmed that measurable antibody levels and rises in functional activity were induced against all 12 O-antigen types included in the vaccine (Cross et al. 1994). A vaccine targeting extraintestinal pathogenic *E. coli*, containing 4 O-antigen bioconjugates (ExPEC4V/EcoXyn-4V or JNJ-63871860), is being developed by LimmaTech (formerly GlycoVaxyn) and Janssen (van den Dobbelsteen et al. 2016) and has been evaluated in Phase 1 and 2 trials (NCT02289794, NCT02546960), including healthy women between 18 and 70 years of age with a history of recurrent urinary tract infections (Frenck Jr. et al. 2019; Huttner et al. 2017). Sequoia Pharmaceuticals is developing a vaccine candidate based on the *E. coli* type I fimbrial adhesin protein (FimH) (Langermann et al. 2000) that has been assessed in a

Phase 1 trial (https://sequoiasciences.com/uti-vaccine-program). Investigators at the Swiss Serum and Vaccine Institute assessed purified *Klebsiella* capsule polysaccharides in Phase 1 clinical studies where they were found as safe and well tolerated, with measurable induction of anti-capsular IgG (Cryz Jr. et al. 1986; Edelman et al. 1994). While this vaccine was not pursued in efficacy studies with active immunization, it was used in combination with a *Pseudomonas* vaccine component (discussed in *Pseudomonas* vaccines later in this section) to generate a hyperimmune intravenous immunoglobulin formulation that was assessed among intensive care patients (Donta et al. 1996) where a possible trend towards efficacy against *Klebsiella* infection was noted, although this was not statistically significant. Vaccines containing inactivated strains of bacteria have also been explored. Clinical efficacy has been reported with commercially available Uromune® (a mixture of *E. coli*, *K. pneumoniae*, *Enterococcus faecalis*, and *Proteus vulgaris*) and SolcoUrovac® (6 *E. coli* strains mixed with *Proteus mirabilis*, *K. pneumoniae*, *Morganella morganii*, and *E. faecalis*) when tested against recurrent urinary tract infections (Nesta and Pizza 2018).

10.5.2.2 Other Gram Negative Bacterial Vaccines

Gram negative carbapenem resistant *A. baumannii* and carbapenem resistant *P. aeruginosa* are listed by the WHO as critical priority pathogens (World Health Organization 2017a). *A. baumannii* and *P. aeruginosa* infections are both associated with healthcare settings and though they do not cause high rates of infection, they are characterized by high levels of antibiotic resistance and associated morbidity. Both pathogens cause pneumonia and bloodstream infections in hospital settings, especially in critically ill patients (Centers for Disease Control and Prevention 2019; Jones 2010). Risk factors for *P. aeruginosa* infections include severe burns, cystic fibrosis, mechanical ventilation, catheterization, and immunocompromise (Gellatly and Hancock 2013). According to CDC estimates, there were 8500 infections and 700 deaths associated with carbapenem resistant *A. baumannii* and 32,600 infections and 2700 deaths associated with multi drug resistant *P. aeruginosa* in 2017 in the U.S. (Centers for Disease Control and Prevention 2019). Rates of carbapenem resistance among *P. aeruginosa* have been increasing, with recent estimates in the U.S. and Europe ranging from 17.8 to 19.2% (World Health Organization 2017b). Some strains of carbapenem resistant *A. baumannii* and multi drug resistant *P. aeruginosa* are resistant to nearly all antibiotics (Centers for Disease Control and Prevention 2019).

Vaccines targeting *Acinetobacter* are in early pre-clinical development (Gagneux-Brunon et al. 2018). However, questions remain regarding appropriate antigen selection for an *A. baumannii* vaccine (Chen 2015) and the adequacy of animal models to predict human protection (Alving 2002). In addition, clinical studies would be challenging: though this pathogen is a voracious pathogen, it occurs infrequently and affects populations for which vaccination would be a challenge.

Several investigational vaccines against *P. aeruginosa* have reached clinical development. Pathogenic *P. aeruginosa* can express either of two serotypes of flagellin, termed FlaA and FlaB. Vaccines based on FlaA and FlaB were immunogenic and well-tolerated when administered to healthy adult volunteers (Doring et al. 1995). When such a vaccine was assessed in patients with cystic fibrosis, partial protection was seen against infection (relative risk 0.66 in vaccinated compared to placebo) (Doring et al. 2007); however, this vaccine was not pursued further. *P. aeruginosa* expresses up to 21 different O-antigen serotypes, for which 8–10 are associated with the majority of infections. Researchers at the Swiss Serum and Vaccine Institute generated an octavalent conjugate formulation comprised of the 8 most common *P. aeruginosa* O-types linked individually to recombinant *P. aeruginosa* exoprotein A, a pathogen relevant carrier protein. Preliminary clinical studies with monovalent O polysaccharide recombinant *P. aeruginosa* exoprotein A conjugate formulations found that robust opsonic antibody and toxin neutralizing activity were induced following vaccination (Cryz Jr. et al. 1987). Phase 1 clinical studies conducted at the University of Maryland in volunteers immunized with the octavalent formulation in parallel with a 24-valent *Klebsiella* capsular polysaccharide formulation revealed induction of IgG titers specific to all the administered polysaccharide antigens (Edelman et al. 1994). Efficacy trials conducted in cystic fibrosis patients immunized with the octavalent conjugate vaccine revealed, however, that this vaccine did not offer significant protection against infection with *P. aeruginosa* in this population (Cryz Jr. et al. 1997).

Protection against infection was also assessed among intensive care patients who upon admission were passively administered the aforementioned intravenous immunoglobulin preparation derived from volunteers immunized with the octavalent *P. aeruginosa* conjugate along with the 24-valent *Klebsiella* capsule polysaccharide formulation (Donta et al. 1996). Although there was no evidence of protective efficacy against *Pseudomonas*, it was theorized that this may have been attributable in part to possible administration of sub-protective levels of antibody, thus it remains to be determined whether anti-O polysaccharide antibodies would protect otherwise healthy individuals against pseudomonal infection. An outer membrane protein based vaccine designated as VLA43 (formerly known as IC43) generated by fusion of the surface loops of outer membrane proteins OprI and OprF (Valneva) showed promising results in a Phase 2 study (NCT00876252). In preliminary studies, the vaccine had an acceptable safety profile, increased antibody levels upon vaccination, and reduced mortality, but did not reduce rates of infection in patients in an intensive care unit on mechanical ventilation (Rello et al. 2017). Unfortunately, results from the subsequent confirmatory Phase 2/3 study (NCT01563263) did not confirm significantly reduced mortality in vaccinated patients (Valneva 2016; https://clinicaltrials.gov/ct2/show/NCT01563263?term=NCT01563263&rank=1). Several additional whole cell and subunit vaccine candidates have recently been evaluated in early stage pre-clinical studies (Hegerle et al. 2018; Meynet et al. 2018; Zhang et al. 2018).

10.5.2.3 *Mycobacterium tuberculosis* Vaccines

M. tuberculosis is the etiologic cause of tuberculosis, a disease that is one of the top 10 causes of death worldwide and the leading cause of death by a single infectious agent. Exposure to *M. tuberculosis* usually results in asymptomatic infection, but 5–15% of infected individuals will develop tuberculosis in their lifetime, and immunocompromised individuals, including those with human immunodeficiency virus (HIV), malnutrition, or diabetes, and tobacco users are at a much higher risk. Over 90% of tuberculosis cases occur in low- and middle-income countries. The WHO estimates that 1.8 billion people – close to one quarter of the world's population – are infected with *M. tuberculosis* globally. In 2017, an estimated 10 million people became ill from tuberculosis (including 1 million children), of which 1.6 million died (World Health Organization 2018) (https://www.tballiance.org/why-new-tb-drugs/global-pandemic).

Active, drug-susceptible tuberculosis disease is successfully treated with antibiotics, and an estimated 54 million lives were saved through tuberculosis diagnosis and treatment between 2000 and 2017. However, tuberculosis therapy is an extended process lasting from six months to over two years and rates of compliance are an ongoing concern. While the disease burden caused by tuberculosis is gradually falling globally and mortality rates decreased by 42% between 2000 and 2017 (World Health Organization 2018), multi drug resistant tuberculosis remains a public health crisis and a health security threat (Koch et al. 2018). In 2017, there were an estimated 558,000 new cases of tuberculosis with resistance to rifampicin, the most effective first line drug, of which 82% had multi drug resistant tuberculosis (defined as tuberculosis that is resistant to both rifampicin and isoniazid). Extensively drug resistant tuberculosis, a more advanced manifestation of AMR, is defined as multi drug resistant tuberculosis plus resistance to at least one drug in both of the two most important classes of medicines in a multi drug resistant tuberculosis regimen: fluoroquinolones and second line injectable agents such as amikacin, capreomycin, or kanamycin (World Health Organization 2018). In 2017, approximately 8.5% of multi drug resistant tuberculosis cases had extensively drug resistant phenotypes, and extensively drug resistant tuberculosis has been identified in more than 127 countries. Only 55% of multi drug resistant tuberculosis patients are successfully treated worldwide. AMR leads to longer treatment regimens, prolonged periods of contagiousness, and higher mortality in populations infected with tuberculosis (World Health Organization 2018; https://www.who.int/news-room/fact-sheets/detail/tuberculosis; https://www.tballiance.org/why-new-tb-drugs/global-pandemic).

Bacillus Calmette Guérin (BCG) vaccine, the only available tuberculosis vaccine and in use for almost 100 years, is composed of an attenuated strain of *Mycobacterium bovis* and used to vaccinate >90% of newborns in endemic countries where vaccination results in a reduction of disseminated disease and mortality in young children. Re-administering BCG vaccine does not provide additional protection after a childhood dose, however, and BCG vaccine does not prevent the reactivation of latent tuberculosis to pulmonary disease in the nearly one third of the human population that is already infected and at risk. Given these shortcomings of BCG vaccine, several more modern vaccine approaches are being pursued (Khoshnood et al. 2018; Raviglione et al. 2012) that may have a profound impact on tuberculosis disease morbidity and mortality and assist in stemming AMR, through prevention of the initial infection as well as reduction of reactivation of latent infection. Examples of such approaches include improved priming with genetically modified BCG, use of alternative inactivated whole cell mycobacterial preparations, elaboration of subunit vaccines including novel adjuvant formulations, and use of vaccines based on recombinant viral vectors. Using these approaches, several new vaccines are being investigated and developed, often by consortia of pharmaceutical companies and academic institutions (Andersen and Scriba 2019; Khoshnood et al. 2018). The recombinant, double mutant BCG vaccine, VPM1002 (Max Planck Institute, Vakzine Projekt Management, Serum Institute of India, TB Vaccine Initiative), is undergoing Phase 2/3 evaluation (NCT03152903) in adults who have been successfully cured of category 1 pulmonary tuberculosis, to determine efficacy of a single dose of the vaccine against tuberculosis recurrence (https://clinicaltrials.gov/ct2/show/NCT03152903?term=NCT03152903&rank=1). Another live attenuated whole cell tuberculosis vaccine candidate, MTBVAC (Biofabri, Universidad de Zaragoza, TB Vaccine Initiative), is designed for prophylactic and post-exposure immunization (Aguilo et al. 2017). Safety and immunogenicity of MTBVAC are being evaluated in two Phase 2 trials: in adults with or without latent tuberculosis (NCT02933281) and in newborns (NCT03536117) (https://clinicaltrials.gov/).

There are also several investigational tuberculosis vaccines based on inactivated whole cell bacteria that have reached Phase 3 clinical development. These include heat killed *Mycobacterium vaccae*, a non-pathogenic species sharing many common antigens with *M. tuberculosis*. The inactivated *M. vaccae* candidate, developed by Anhui Zhifei Longcom (China), is registered in China as adjunct immunotherapy for patients with drug susceptible tuberculosis (World Health Organization 2018). In a Phase 3 study (NCT00052195), the *M. vaccae* vaccine administered in five intradermal doses was well tolerated and had low but significant (39%) efficacy against tuberculosis in individuals infected with HIV who had previously received BCG vaccine (Khoshnood et al. 2018; von Reyn et al. 2010). Another completed Phase 3 study (NCT01979900) evaluated the efficacy and safety of the *M. vaccae* vaccine to prevent tuberculosis in high risk groups; results from this study have not yet been disseminated, however (Andersen and Scriba 2019; https://clinicaltrials.gov/ct2/show/NCT01979900?term=NCT01979900&rank=1). The MIP vaccine (Cadila, Indian Council of Medical Research), whole cell heat inactivated *Mycobacterium indicus pranii*, has also been assessed in a Phase 3 trial as an adjunct immunotherapy to anti tubercular treatment for pulmonary tuberculosis. Significantly higher rates of sputum culture conversion (culture turning bacilli negative for an initially culture positive patient who had completed treatment; the proposed measure of disease cure) were seen in patients receiving MIP intradermally, suggesting a role for MIP in clearance of detectable bacilli and, potentially, disease cure (Sharma et al. 2017). DAR-901, the vaccine candidate comprised of a heat inactivated non-tuberculous mycobacterium related to *M. vaccae* (Dartmouth, Geisel

School of Medicine, Global Health Innovative Technology Fund), is currently being evaluated in a Phase 2 trial (NCT02712424) as a booster vaccine to prevent tuberculosis in adolescents (https://clinicaltrials.gov/ct2/show/NCT02712424?term=NCT02712424&rank=1). RUTI® (Archivel Farma) is a detoxified vaccine candidate based on fragmented *M. tuberculosis* cells, intended to be used as a therapeutic vaccine in combination with a short, intensive antibiotic treatment (World Health Organization 2018). Safety and immunogenicity of RUTI in patients with multi drug resistant tuberculosis favorably responding to the standard multi drug resistant tuberculosis treatment are being evaluated in a Phase 2 trial (NCT02711735, https://clinicaltrials.gov/).

Live vectored vaccines expressing immunodominant recombinant antigen 85A that is shared by *M. tuberculosis* and BCG have also been assessed in clinical studies. Ad5Ag85A, based on a recombinant adenovirus, is being developed by McMaster University (Hamilton, Ontario, Canada) and is in early stage clinical development, undergoing Phase 1 clinical evaluation (NCT02337270) in healthy individuals primed with BCG vaccine (https://clinicaltrials.gov/). Another vaccine candidate, MVA85A, comprises a modified vaccinia virus Ankara expressing recombinant antigen 85A and was developed by the University of Oxford (Oxford, UK). This vaccine was assessed in a pivotal Phase 2b study (NCT00953927) where it was given as a booster to South African infants previously vaccinated with BCG vaccine. Unfortunately, MVA85A failed to improve protection against tuberculosis infection compared to BCG vaccine alone in vaccinated infants (Tameris et al. 2013) and was subsequently abandoned.

Adjuvanted subunit vaccine candidates for tuberculosis are being clinically tested as booster vaccines to prevent active or recurrent tuberculosis disease (Andersen and Scriba 2019). Two vaccines, H4:IC31 and H56:IC31, comprised of multiple mycobacterial antigens including Ag85B and formulated with the adjuvant IC31, are in Phase 2 development (NCT02075203, NCT03512249). One of these, H4:IC31 (Sanofi-led consortium), has demonstrated partial efficacy (30.5%) against sustained *M. tuberculosis* infection (based on rates of conversion in interferon gamma release assays) in high risk adolescents primed with BCG vaccine (Nemes et al. 2018; http://www.aeras.org/candidates). Another multicomponent subunit vaccine candidate, ID93+GLA-SE (Infectious Disease Research Institute, Quratis), has been evaluated in a Phase 2 trial in adults with cured tuberculosis (NCT02465216), where it was found to elicit both humoral and cellular immune responses (Penn-Nicholson et al. 2018). An upcoming Phase 2b study will assess prevention of tuberculosis recurrence in the same population (https://clinicaltrials.gov/ct2/show/NCT02465216?term=ID93%2BGLA-SE&rank=4). The most promising of the subunit tuberculosis vaccine candidates is M72, developed by GlaxoSmithKline (Rixensart, Belgium) and containing two proteins shared by *M. tuberculosis* and BCG. M72, adjuvanted with AS01E, a liposomal based adjuvant system containing the immunostimulants monophosphoryl lipid A and the saponin QS-21 from *Quillaja saponaria* Molina (Garcon and Di Pasquale 2017), was evaluated in a Phase 2b study (NCT01755598) and demonstrated an overall 54% efficacy for prevention of pulmonary tuberculosis in HIV negative adults 18–50 years of age with latent *M. tuberculosis* infection (Van Der Meeren et al. 2018). Despite this encouraging result, and the large numbers of people who could be helped by this vaccine, it is clear that more work is needed to develop a vaccine that can have broader efficacy for a larger population demographic. It is also apparent that immune approaches to prevent re-activation of latent infection as opposed to preventing the initial infection may provide benefits to curb disease (https://www.who.int/immunization/research/development/tuberculosis/en/).

10.5.2.4 *Shigella* Vaccines

Shigella are important human enteric pathogens that cause gastroenteritis ranging from self-limiting intestinal cramping and fever to dysentery characterized by severe diarrhea with mucus containing bloody stool. In the U.S., shigellosis is a reportable infection, with the CDC estimating approximately 450,000 cases occurring annually, of which there are 77,000 antibiotic resistant infections and fewer than 5 deaths (Centers for Disease Control and Prevention 2019). In lower- and middle-income counties, *Shigella* is one of the top 5 causes of moderate to severe diarrhea in children less than 5 years old and contributes to excess mortality and growth impairment (Kotloff et al. 2013). *Shigella* spp. are also identified as priority pathogens by the CDC due to widespread resistance to ampicillin and trimethoprim-sulfamethoxazole and rising resistance to ciprofloxacin and azithromycin (Centers for Disease Control and Prevention 2019). *Shigella* are classified into species and serotypes based on structural differences in the O polysaccharides of lipopolysaccharide. There are four major species: *S. dysenteriae*, *S. boydii*, *S. flexneri*, and *S. sonnei*. Among these, several serotypes are disproportionately found as causative agents of disease, including the single *S. sonnei* and *S. flexneri* serotypes 2a, 3a, and 6 (Baker and The 2018).

Multiple pre-clinical vaccine candidates have been described for *Shigella*, including whole cell vaccines, purified outer membrane vesicle vaccines, protein subunit vaccines, and glycoconjugates, of which several have progressed to clinical studies (Barel and Mulard 2019; Mani et al. 2016). Following the hypothesis that antibodies against *Shigella* O polysaccharides are protective against *Shigella* disease, researchers at the U.S. National Institutes of Health developed a series of *Shigella* O polysaccharide based glycoconjugates (Chu et al. 1991; Kubler-Kielb et al. 2010; Pozsgay et al. 1993; Robbins et al. 1991; Robbins et al. 2009; Robbins and Schneerson 1990). This included a candidate *S. sonnei* conjugate with recombinant *P. aeruginosa* exoprotein A that was assessed in an efficacy trial among military recruits in Israel in the early 1990s, where it was found to provide ~74% protection against culture confirmed *S. sonnei* shigellosis (Cohen et al. 1997). Based on this landmark study, other *Shigella* O polysaccharide conjugate vaccines have been developed and advanced to clinical studies, including a construct comprised of synthetic O polysaccharide repeats conjugated to tetanus toxoid developed by the Pasteur Institute that was recently tested in a first-in-human trial (NCT02797236) (Barel and Mulard 2019). LimmaTech has developed a bioconjugate comprised of

S. dysenteriae O1 O-antigen linked to recombinant *P. aeruginosa* exoprotein A. This bioconjugate vaccine elicited a favorable safety profile and significant increases in anti-lipopolysaccharide IgG levels in a Phase 1 study in the U.S. (Hatz et al. 2015). In order to provide broad coverage, an O polysaccharide based *Shigella* vaccine would need to include, however, the four primary serotypes (*S. sonnei* and *S. flexneri* 2a, 3a, and 6). Hence, these prior monovalent constructs represent iterative advances towards an ultimate multivalent formulation that could be used to prevent shigellosis.

Several whole cell *Shigella* vaccines have been tested in clinical studies. A live attenuated *S. flexneri* 2a vaccine strain developed at the University of Maryland Center for Vaccine Development and Global Health, generated by mutations in the guanosine biosynthetic locus (*guaBA*) and *sen-set* virulence genes, was found to be well tolerated and immunogenic in a Phase 1 trial among North American volunteers, where it induced significant levels of serum anti-O polysaccharide IgG and fecal IgA (Kotloff et al. 2007). A separate live attenuated *S. sonnei* vaccine strain engineered by deletion of the *virG* plasmid virulence gene was tested in Israeli volunteers, where it induced measurable levels of lipopolysaccharide specific IgG and IgA antibody secreting cells, albeit with moderate diarrhea in some volunteers (Orr et al. 2005). A whole cell formalin inactivated preparation of *Shigella* developed by the U.S. military has also progressed through Phase 1 clinical testing where volunteers administered the vaccine by the oral route generated increased serum anti-lipopolysaccharide IgG and IgA titers, as well as intestinal IgA detectable in stool (McKenzie et al. 2006). The GlaxoSmithKline Vaccines Institute for Global Health has developed an outer membrane vesicle vaccine based on shed membrane vesicles, termed Generalized Membrane Module Antigens, that has progressed through Phase 2 clinical studies in Kenya, where it was found to be safe and significantly increased levels of anti-lipopolysaccharide IgG antibodies among volunteers in this *Shigella* endemic setting (Obiero et al. 2017). The type III secretion proteins of *Shigella*, IpaB and IpaD, are important virulence factors for which antibodies generated against these antigens could interfere with the ability of *Shigella* to inject virulence proteins into the host cytosol, a requisite step for infection. The U.S. Army has designed a subunit vaccine comprised of a complex of IpaB/D with *S. flexneri* 2a lipopolysaccharide (Invaplex), that was assessed for safety and immunogenicity after intranasal administration (Riddle et al. 2011; Tribble et al. 2010). Immunization with this formulation was generally well tolerated and induced both systemic and mucosal immune responses against the vaccine antigens.

10.5.2.5 Non-typhoidal and Paratyphoid *Salmonella* Vaccines

Non-typhoidal *Salmonella* is the second most common cause of bacterial gastroenteritis in the U.S., and the most frequent cause of hospitalizations and death due to bacterial enteric disease. Surveillance by the CDC estimated that between 2015 and 2017, 1.35 million cases of salmonellosis occurred annually, resulting in 26,500 hospitalizations and 420 deaths (Centers for Disease Control and Prevention 2019).

It is also a frequent cause of multi-state outbreaks due to contaminated food products. Despite intensive efforts to reduce transmission through the food supply, rates of non-typhoidal *Salmonella* have remained stable or risen year after year (Tack et al. 2019) (https://www.cdc.gov/foodnet/reports/prelim-data-intro-2018.html). Non-typhoidal *Salmonella* gastroenteritis is characterized by cramping, fever, and bloody diarrhea, for which progression to invasive disease represents a life-threatening complication. In sub-Saharan Africa, invasive non-typhoidal *Salmonella* disease with genomically divergent *Salmonella* isolates is widespread among infants and toddlers, with case fatality rates of up to 25% (Feasey et al. 2012, 2016; Kingsley et al. 2009). Non-typhoidal *Salmonella* gastroenteritis is generally self limiting and the standard of care does not call for antibiotic treatment; however, invasive disease requires urgent antimicrobial therapy.

In the U.S., rates of non-typhoidal *Salmonella* resistance to antibiotics such as ciprofloxacin have been increasing in recent years, prompting inclusion of non-typhoidal *Salmonella* in the CDC priority list as a serious threat (Centers for Disease Control and Prevention 2019). The CDC estimated that between 2015 and 2017, 212,500 antibiotic resistant non-typhoidal *Salmonella* infections occurred annually in the U.S., resulting in 70 deaths (Centers for Disease Control and Prevention 2019). In sub-Saharan Africa, widespread resistance to multiple standard of care antibiotics is prevalent among invasive isolates (Marks et al. 2017).

Despite decades of research into a protective vaccine for non-typhoidal *Salmonella*, yielding multiple candidates that have demonstrated efficacy in preclinical studies, only a single non-typhoidal *Salmonella* vaccine has progressed to clinical studies. WT05, a live attenuated *S. enterica* serotype Typhimurium generated by deletion of the *aroC* and *ssaV* genes, was orally administered to volunteers where it was shed for up to 23 days but poorly induced anti-O polysaccharide antibodies (Hindle et al. 2002). A trivalent glycoconjugate vaccine intended for use in sub-Saharan Africa, comprised of conjugates of O polysaccharides and flagellin from the two dominant circulating *S. enterica* serotypes, Typhimurium and Enteritidis, formulated with Typbar-TCV, inducing functional antibodies in preclinical studies (Baliban et al. 2018), is poised to enter first-in-human trials (NCT03981952). Since acquisition of antibodies against *S.* Typhimurium O polysaccharides in early life is accompanied by reduced incidence of disease, it is anticipated that vaccination with O polysaccharide conjugates during infancy will protect against invasive non-typhoidal *Salmonella* infection (Nyirenda et al. 2014). Other vaccine constructs for which clinical studies are planned include non-typhoidal *Salmonella* Generalized Membrane Module Antigens and O polysaccharide conjugates with CRM_{197} developed by the GlaxoSmithKline Vaccines Institute for Global Health.

Paratyphoid fever, caused by *S. enterica* serotypes Paratyphi A, B, or C, is clinically indistinguishable from typhoid enteric fever. Among the three paratyphoid serotypes, *S.* Paratyphi A is the most common and is endemic to South and Southeast Asia and parts of Africa and Latin America (GBD 2017 Typhoid and Paratyphoid Collaborators 2019). Along with *S.* Typhi, *S.* Paratyphi A has developed increasing resistance to fluoroquinolones and ciprofloxacin (Parry et al. 2019). While efficacious typhoid vaccines are licensed and available for use, there are no *S.* Paratyphi A vaccines.

The successful strategies that have led to the currently available typhoid vaccines have been similarly employed for the development of an *S.* Paratyphi A vaccine, including the use of live attenuated vaccine strains and glycoconjugates as platforms (World Health Organization 2014b). Researchers at the University of Maryland Center for Vaccine Development and Global Health genetically attenuated *S.* Paratyphi A strain 9150 through deletion of the *guaBA* and *clpPX* (regulatory protease) loci. This live attenuated vaccine strain was administered in a dose escalating Phase 1 trial to North American volunteers, where it was safe and well tolerated even at the highest doses of 10^{10} colony forming units, where induction of circulating anti-lipopolysaccharide antibody secreting cells was seen (Wahid et al. 2019). Unlike *S.* Typhi, *S.* Paratyphi A does not express a capsule and hence the surface polysaccharide is the lipopolysaccharide associated O-antigen. Pioneering efforts by investigators at the U.S. National Institutes of Health led to the development of glycoconjugates based on *S.* Paratyphi A lipopolysaccharide derived O polysaccharides conjugated to tetanus toxoid. Different variants of these conjugates were tested in age de-escalating Phase 1 and 2 trials in Vietnam among adults, adolescents, and young children, where they demonstrated a favorable safety profile and were found to induce robust anti-O polysaccharide IgG levels that were maximal after a single dose, and correlated with serum bactericidal activity. Based on these initial favorable findings, pre-clinical development of an *S.* Paratyphi A O polysaccharide conjugate with CRM_{197} has been undertaken by the GlaxoSmithKline Vaccines Institute for Global Health (Micoli et al. 2012). The International Vaccine Institute in South Korea has also reported pre-clinical development of conjugates of *S.* Paratyphi A O polysaccharide linked to diphtheria toxoid as the carrier (Ali et al. 2014). Clinical studies have not yet been announced for these conjugates; however, an ultimate formulation would need to include coverage for typhoid that is co-endemic in the same areas, bears similar risk factors and disease pathology, and is also an AMR priority.

10.5.2.6 *Staphylococcus aureus* Vaccines

The Gram positive bacterium *S. aureus* is a common commensal component of human microflora; however, upon breaching a mucosal or epithelial barrier, it becomes an opportunistic pathogen capable of causing various skin and soft tissue infections as well as invasive life threatening disease. *S. aureus* is common in both community and hospital settings, where it can cause a range of outcomes, including bacteremia, toxic shock syndrome, infectious endocarditis, osteomyelitis, and pneumonia (Dayan et al. 2016; Tong et al. 2015).

S. aureus treatment can be complicated by resistance to β-lactams and other classes of antibiotics. Infections caused by methicillin resistant *S. aureus* are harder to treat than infections with methicillin sensitive strains and are associated with prolonged hospital stays and increased morbidity and mortality. Notably, the CDC estimates that methicillin resistant *S. aureus* contributes to over 70,000 cases of invasive disease and 9000 deaths per year in the U.S. alone (https://www.cdc.gov/mrsa/healthcare/inpatient.html). Overall, there were 323,700 estimated cases of methicillin resistant *S. aureus* infections in hospitalized patients and 10,600 deaths in 2017 (Centers for Disease Control and Prevention 2019). Prophylactic use of antibiotics, including topical mupirocin that targets *S. aureus,* has been used to decolonize body surfaces such as the nasal mucosa prior to periods of heightened risk, including undergoing major surgery; however, this can contribute to resistance (Dayan et al. 2016). Both the CDC and the WHO have placed methicillin resistant *S. aureus* on their priority lists, highlighting the significance of AMR in this microbial species (Centers for Disease Control and Prevention 2019; World Health Organization 2017a). *S. aureus* has the propensity to develop resistance even to newer antibiotics that have been introduced, such as linezolid, a Gram positive bacterium protein synthesis inhibiting drug introduced in 2000 (Endimiani et al. 2011), and daptomycin, a Gram positive membrane disrupting drug introduced in 2003 (Marty et al. 2006). *S. aureus* glycopeptide resistance is currently a source of concern, as this class of antibiotics, including vancomycin, is one of the main resources for combating infections caused by methicillin resistant *S. aureus*. Reduced susceptibility to vancomycin, a drug commonly used to treat otherwise resistant strains, was first described in 1996 in Japan (Hiramatsu et al. 1997b). Thereafter, an *S. aureus* isolate with acquired heterogeneous resistance to vancomycin was characterized (Hiramatsu et al. 1997a). To date, strains of methicillin resistant *S. aureus* with acquired resistance to vancomycin are rare; however, widespread and often uncontrolled empirical vancomycin use, particularly during elective surgeries, could further drive resistance. This has already been documented in the emergence of vancomycin resistant enterococci and vancomycin intermediate *S. aureus* (Caroom et al. 2013; Gaviola et al. 2016; Neu 1992). Given the high disease burden and resistance among *S. aureus* isolates to many classes of antibiotics, a strong rationale exists to develop effective vaccines to protect individuals against this species and to reduce AMR, especially in the older adult population who are at higher risk of disease and more often undergo hospitalization.

As the mechanisms of protection for *S. aureus* are incompletely understood, this has challenged the development of vaccines, and despite extensive efforts there is currently no licensed vaccine to prevent *S. aureus* infection. *S. aureus* can express a capsule polysaccharide for which two types – CP5 and CP8 – predominate (Arbeit et al. 1984). Nabi Biopharmaceuticals assessed a bivalent vaccine formulation composed of capsule polysaccharides from serotypes 5 and 8, each individually conjugated to nontoxic recombinant *P. aeruginosa* exotoxin A. While a post-hoc analysis revealed potential short term efficacy against CP8-expressing strains in a study in hemodialysis patients, this finding was not confirmed in an expanded trial (Fattom et al. 2015). Investigators at Merck developed the *S. aureus* surface protein iron surface determinant B as a protein subunit vaccine and assessed this construct for efficacy in patients undergoing elective cardiothoracic surgery. There was no evidence of protection seen in this study, and a safety signal was seen, with higher rates of mortality in the vaccinated group compared to placebo, leading Merck to abandon further development of iron surface determinant B (McNeely et al. 2014). Pfizer developed a 4-component vaccine (SA4Ag) composed of *S. aureus* capsule polysaccharides serotypes 5 and 8 individually linked to non-toxic diphtheria protein CRM_{197} in formulation with two recombinant proteins, clumping factor A and manganese transporter C (also known as r305A), which are key to bacterial virulence and survival (Frenck Jr. et al. 2017). SA4Ag elicited robust functional immune responses and had an acceptable safety profile in an early Phase 1/2 study (NCT01364571) (Frenck Jr. et al. 2017; https://clinicaltrials.gov/). A large Phase 2b study (NCT02388165) was subsequently conducted to evaluate postoperative *S. aureus* infections in patients undergoing elective spinal surgery (https://clinicaltrials.gov/). Unfortunately, the results of a pre-planned interim analysis indicated low statistical probability to meet the pre-defined primary efficacy objective, leading to the company's decision to terminate the study and discontinue the program due to futility (Pfizer 2018).

Another 4-component vaccine targeting *S. aureus*, 4C-Staph (Novartis, now GlaxoSmithKline), comprised of five different staphylococcal proteins, including genetically detoxified alpha-toxin hemolysin, surface proteins FhuD2 and Csa1A, and EsxAB protein, a fusion of two secreted virulence factors EsxA and EsxB, administered with a Toll like receptor 7-stimulating adjuvant (Mancini et al. 2016), has been assessed in a Phase 1 study (NCT01160172). There is no further information on 4C-Staph clinical development (https://clinicaltrials.gov/ct2/results?cond=&term=NCT01160172&cntry=&state=&city=&dist). An investigational vaccine NDV-3, that is being developed by NovaDigm Therapeutics (http://www.novadigm.net/), contains the recombinant N-terminal portion of the *Candida albicans* agglutinin like sequence 3 protein, which has both sequence and structural homology with cell surface proteins of *S. aureus*, including a collagen binding protein (Sheppard et al. 2004). During Phase 1 evaluation in healthy individuals (NCT01273922), NDV-3 was safe and elicited robust humoral (IgG and IgA antibodies) as well as cellular (secretion of interferon gamma and interleukin-17A) immune responses (Schmidt et al. 2012). A randomized, placebo controlled Phase 2 trial (NCT03455309) has been conducted to evaluate the efficacy of NDV-3 in preventing *S. aureus* nasal colonization among a population of military recruits who are at increased risk for *S. aureus* colonization and disease (https://clinicaltrials.gov/). How the GlaxoSmithKline and NovaDigm approaches differ from previous approaches is not clear, however, and it appears that to develop a vaccine to prevent *S. aureus* infection, there needs to be a greater understanding of the pathophysiology of *S. aureus* disease and how a vaccine could neutralize the approaches that the bacteria uses to thwart the immune system.

10.5.3 Viral Vaccines Under Development

10.5.3.1 Respiratory Syncytial Virus Vaccines

RSV is the leading cause of bronchiolitis and viral pneumonia in infants and can lead to fatal respiratory distress, especially in neonates and young infants with underlying cardio-pulmonary disease. Globally, by 2 years of age nearly everyone has been infected with RSV (Glezen et al. 1986). Worldwide, RSV kills approximately 66,000–199,000 infants annually, with the vast majority of those deaths occurring in low- to middle-income countries (Nair et al. 2010). In the U.S., RSV is the leading cause of infant hospitalization, with approximately 50,000 admissions of children 12 months of age and younger occurring annually (American Academy of Pediatrics Committee on Infectious Diseases; American Academy of Pediatrics Bronchiolitis Guidelines Committee 2014). RSV also causes respiratory illness in older adults, with approximately 100,000 hospitalizations and 5000 deaths annually in the U.S. among adults 65 years of age and older (Falsey et al. 2005; Matias et al. 2014; Widmer et al. 2012; Zhou et al. 2012). In the U.S., RSV disease rates in older adults approach approximately half that of influenza (Falsey et al. 2005). Like influenza, RSV infection is associated with the development of bacterial superinfections (Hament et al. 1999; Rey-Jurado and Kalergis 2017), and animal models have elucidated potential mechanisms for lethal synergy between RSV and bacteria (Beadling and Slifka 2004). Secondary bacterial infections, including otitis media and pneumonia, require the use of antibiotics. Furthermore, as described for influenza earlier in this chapter, antibiotics are often prescribed inappropriately for treatment of symptoms of a viral disease before the etiological agent has been determined. This increases selective pressure for drug resistance, contributing to AMR.

There is no RSV vaccine currently licensed; however, if available, it would have the potential to reduce the inappropriate use of antibiotics in RSV infections and prevent bacterial superinfections. RSV vaccine development has been riddled with many failures, primarily due to an incomplete understanding of the structural and immunobiology of this important viral pathogen and technical difficulties in producing an effective vaccine. Currently, there are a variety of RSV vaccine candidates in clinical and pre-clinical development, including live attenuated, whole inactivated, particle based, subunit, nucleic acid, and recombinant vector based, incorporating different antigens (Jares Baglivo and Polack 2019; PATH 2019), with the most advanced summarized in Table 10.2. These vaccines are contemplated for use in maternal immunization to protect infants through maternally transferred antibodies, and young children and elderly through direct vaccination.

The trimeric RSV F surface glycoprotein which mediates the fusion of the viral membrane with that of the host cell is the primary target of protective neutralizing antibodies (Beeler and van Wyke Coelingh 1989; The IMpact-RSV Study Group 1998). Vaccine development has focused historically on the highly stable post-fusion form of RSV F, and this approach led to multiple failures in Phase 3 studies (Falsey et al. 2008; Simoes et al. 2001). Most recently, Novavax assessed the efficacy and safety of an RSV F based recombinant nanoparticle vaccine candidate (ResVax), administered with adjuvant in a global Phase 3 study (NCT02624947). The vaccine was delivered through maternal immunization and aimed to reduce the rate of medically significant RSV induced lower respiratory tract infection in infants through 90 days of life (https://clinicaltrials.gov/). The trial failed its pre-specified primary endpoint (Novavax 2019a, b).

The metastable pre-fusion RSV F protein (RSV pre-F) represents the form of the protein present on infectious virions and contains neutralizing epitopes eliciting more potent RSV neutralizing antibodies (McLellan et al. 2013; Mousa et al. 2017; Ngwuta et al. 2015). Recently, it is this form of the RSV F protein that has become the focus of RSV vaccine development. The RSV pre-F DS-Cav1 candidate developed by the National Institute of Allergy and Infectious Diseases comprises engineered soluble RSV F trimers with stabilized pre-F-unique site Ø (Sastry et al. 2017). The vaccine, with or without alum adjuvant, is under Phase 1 evaluation in healthy adults (NCT03049488) (https://clinicaltrials.gov/). The prospectively planned interim immunogenicity analysis found a more than 10-fold boost in serum neutralizing activity against both A and B subtypes of RSV following the first dose of the vaccine, which was associated with antibodies targeting pre-fusion epitopes of RSV F. These findings represent important clinical proof of concept for the structure-based RSV vaccine design approach (Crank et al. 2019).

Further engineering has been conducted by other groups to stabilize the RSV pre-F antigen, and several investigational subunit vaccines are undergoing clinical testing. Among these, GlaxoSmithKline has completed two separate Phase 2 studies (NCT02360475, NCT02753413) evaluating immunogenicity and safety of the RSV pre-F vaccine candidate in healthy, non-pregnant women 18–45 years of age (https://clinicaltrials.gov/). All tested formulations of the RSV pre-F vaccine were found to be safe and immunogenic, with boosting of pre-existing RSV immunity. At day 30 postimmunization, geometric mean titers of RSV-A neutralizing antibodies in the RSV pre-F vaccine recipients were 3.1–3.9-fold greater than the pre-immunization titers, compared with a 0.9-fold increase in the control vaccine group. Similarly, geometric mean titers of antibodies competing with palivizumab, an anti-RSV monoclonal antibody targeting the pre-F neutralizing site II (Johnson et al. 1997), in the RSV pre-F vaccine recipients were increased more than 14-fold compared with a non-significant 1.1-fold increase in the control vaccine group (Beran et al. 2018).

Another RSV pre-F subunit vaccine candidate is being developed by Pfizer to protect infants and older adults by maternal or direct immunization, respectively. This vaccine is currently evaluated in randomized, placebo controlled Phase 2 and Phase 3 studies in healthy young and older men and non-pregnant women (NCT03529773), older adults (NCT03572062), young non-pregnant women (NCT04071158), and pregnant women (NCT04032093, NCT04424316) (https://clinicaltrials.gov/). The initial results from the first-in-human Phase 1/2 study (NCT03529773) demonstrated that the vaccine was safe and immunogenic in adults 18–49 years of age, eliciting 10–20-fold increases in serum neutralizing antibody titers for both RSV A and RSV B observed one month post immunization

(Schmoele-Thoma et al. 2019). The excellent safety profile and strong immunogenicity of this vaccine candidate support its further development.

10.5.3.2 Next Generation Influenza Vaccines

Next generation influenza vaccines aim to provide broad protection against influenza, eliminating the need for yearly vaccine production campaigns of evolving serotypes. Approaches towards universal influenza vaccine development have been recently extensively reviewed (Elbahesh et al. 2019; Epstein 2018; Estrada and Schultz-Cherry 2019). Several universal (broadly protective) influenza vaccines are currently being evaluated in clinical studies. M-001 (BiondVax Pharmaceuticals), comprised of several proteins conserved across influenza strains, has recently advanced to a Phase 3 study in adults 50 years of age and older (NCT03450915). Another investigational vaccine, MVA-NP+M1, has elicited potent humoral and cell-mediated immune responses when co-administered with a seasonal influenza vaccine and, based on promising Phase 1 results (NCT00942071) (Antrobus et al. 2014), is currently being assessed in a Phase 2b study (NCT03880474). An alternative approach to influenza vaccine development lies in RNA based vaccines, which promise more rapid production and scalability (Scorza and Pardi 2018). One candidate of this type, using lipid nanoparticles as a delivery platform, has progressed to Phase 1 clinical evaluation (NCT03076385) following positive pre-clinical data, with interim results reporting robust immune responses and no obvious safety concerns (Bahl et al. 2017).

10.5.3.3 Human Immunodeficiency Virus Vaccines

HIV infection continues to be a major global public health issue. As reported by the WHO, more than 32 million people have died of HIV (https://www.who.int/en/news-room/fact-sheets/detail/hiv-aids) since the epidemic was first recognized in 1981 (Centers for Disease Control 1981). In 2018, there were approximately 37.9 million people living with HIV worldwide and 770,000 people died of HIV related causes. The African continent is most affected, with 25.7 million people living with HIV in 2018. The current treatment option for HIV infection is lifelong antiretroviral therapy. While antiretroviral therapy controls the virus and reduces transmission, it does not, however, eradicate the infection and is associated with substantial cost (https://www.who.int/en/news-room/fact-sheets/detail/hiv-aids). An effective universal prophylactic HIV vaccine would be a more sustainable approach to prevent HIV, but developing such a vaccine is challenging, due to the extreme virus diversity, incomplete understanding of mechanisms of immunity, and the challenges in designing immunogens to induce broadly neutralizing antibodies (Hsu and O'Connell 2017).

There are numerous investigational vaccines against HIV in pre-clinical and early clinical development, among which a few have progressed to clinical efficacy trials (Hsu and O'Connell 2017). So far, the only vaccine candidate to have demonstrated at least partial efficacy – 60% one year after vaccination and 31.2% during the 3.5 years after vaccination – for preventing HIV infection is RV144, a recombinant canarypox vector vaccine (ALVAC-HIV [vCP1521]), administered in a heterologous prime-boost regimen with four priming injections followed by two booster injections of a recombinant glycoprotein 120 subunit vaccine (AIDSVAX B/E) in a Phase 3 trial in Thailand (NCT00223080) (Rerks-Ngarm et al. 2009). The immune correlate analysis suggested that the RV144 vaccine efficacy is likely to be associated with the induction of functional antibodies to the V1V2 region of HIV envelope protein (Haynes et al. 2012). The RV144 vaccine, administered in two doses of ALVAC-HIV (vCP2438) at weeks 0 and 4 and then in three doses with bivalent subtype C gp120 protein adjuvanted with MF59 at weeks 12, 24, and 52, is currently undergoing pivotal Phase 2b/3 efficacy clinical evaluation (HVTN702, NCT02968849) in HIV-seronegative South African adults (National Institute of Allergy and Infectious Diseases (NIAID) 2016; https://clinicaltrials.gov/ct2/show/NCT02968849?term=HVTN+702&cond=HIV&rank=1).

HIV infection predisposes patients to opportunistic bacterial co-infections that require frequent use of antibiotics, stimulating development of multi drug resistance. People living with HIV are estimated to be 16–27 times more likely to develop tuberculosis than persons without the virus. Furthermore, tuberculosis is one of the leading causes of HIV-related deaths, with Sub-Saharan Africa accounting for approximately 86% of those in 2016. According to the WHO estimates, 862,000 HIV positive people worldwide fell ill with tuberculosis and 251,000 people died from HIV associated tuberculosis in 2018 (https://www.who.int/tb/areas-of-work/tb-hiv/en/). Other opportunistic co-infections in patients with HIV include respiratory diseases, sinusitis, bronchitis, otitis, and pneumonia. Bacterial pneumonia in HIV infected individuals occurs at higher incidence, is more severe, is associated with greater mortality, and may be the first manifestation of underlying HIV infection. Bacterial pneumonia can occur at any stage of HIV disease and at any CD4 T-cell count, but recurrent pneumonia (two or more episodes within a one-year period) is characteristic of acquired immune deficiency syndrome and is much more likely to be accompanied by bacteremia (up to ~55 times). *S. pneumoniae* and *Haemophilus* species are the most common causes of community acquired bacterial pneumonia in both HIV-positive and -negative populations; *P. aeruginosa* and *S. aureus* infections are also more frequent in HIV infected individuals (Burack et al. 1994; HIV.org 2020; Hirschtick et al. 1995; Polsky et al. 1986). Gram negative bacterial enteric infections also frequently occur in HIV infected individuals, with at least 10-fold greater incidence compared with the uninfected population and with the greatest rates in patients with acquired immune deficiency syndrome. In the U.S., enteric infections in HIV infected patients are most often caused by *Salmonella* (particularly *S.* Typhimurium and *S.* Enteritidis), *Shigella*, and *Campylobacter*, but diarrheagenic *E. coli*- and *C. difficile*-associated infections are also common (Angulo and Swerdlow 1995; Haines et al. 2013; Huang et al. 2006; Nelson et al. 1992; Sanchez et al. 2005).

The microbes causing opportunistic bacterial co-infections in HIV positive populations are priority pathogens and AMR threats. Multiple studies have reported the isolation of antibiotic resistant bacterial strains from HIV patients, including methicillin resistant *S. aureus* (Hidron et al. 2010), multi drug resistant *M. tuberculosis* (Campos et al. 2003), multi drug resistant *E. coli* (Vignesh et al. 2008), and expanded spectrum cephalosporin resistant non-typhoidal *Salmonella* (Miriagou et al. 2004). Vaccination against HIV would not only prevent this viral infection from occurring in the vaccinated individual, but could also potentially reduce the incidence of bacterial infections and, consequently, attendant antibiotic use and spread of antibiotic resistant strains.

10.6 Global Mobilization Utilizing Vaccines Against Antimicrobial Resistance

AMR is a global problem, and hence necessitates a global response. The utility of vaccines as a tool to combat AMR has been broadly recognized (Centers for Disease Control and Prevention 2015; O'Neill 2016a; World Health Organization 2015). Improving the use of vaccines as an anti AMR tool requires global mobilization of diverse resources from stakeholders across the public health spectrum, including governments, regulatory bodies, academia, the biopharmaceutical industry, healthcare professionals, policymakers, and funding bodies. At the 2016 World Economic Forum held in Davos, Switzerland, over 80 international pharmaceutical, biotech, diagnostic, and generic drug companies signed the Davos Declaration on Antibiotic Resistance, calling for collective action to create a sustainable market for antibiotics, vaccines, and diagnostics and encourage appropriate use of new and existing treatments (Review on Antimicrobial Resistance 2016).

To date, incremental but measurable progress has been attained towards the implementation of anti AMR goals. At the 70th World Health Assembly, the WHO, the Food and Agriculture Organization of the United Nations, and the World Organisation for Animal Health presented results of the first open survey of countries' national action plan preparedness on AMR based on the objectives of the WHO Global Action Plan on AMR adopted in 2015 (World Health Organization 2015). The results indicated that 77 countries had developed a multisectoral plan and 57 were in the process of developing one (The Lancet 2017).

In acknowledgement of the grave threat posed by antibiotic resistant bacteria, President Barack Obama in 2014 issued an Executive Order titled Combating Antibiotic Resistant Bacteria that identified antibiotic resistant bacteria as a national security priority and mobilized multiple branches of government to address AMR (The White House 2014). This culminated in the issuance of the National Strategy for Combating Antibiotic Resistant Bacteria, that is widely recognized as the Combating Antibiotic Resistant Bacteria report (The White House 2015). This document delineated 5 key strategic goals: (1) slow the development and spread of resistant bacteria; (2) strengthen one health surveillance efforts; (3) advance development and use of diagnostics to detect resistant bacteria; (4) accelerate research towards new antibiotics, other therapeutics, and vaccines; and (5) improve international collaboration and capacity for AMR research and development, prevention, surveillance, and control. This important unifying order at the highest level of government served to raise global awareness of the threat posed by antibiotic resistance and, importantly, initiated multiple programmatic and policy changes at the federal level related to AMR prevention and recognized the potential role vaccines could contribute to address AMR.

Furthermore, the recent UK Review on Antimicrobial Resistance made three key recommendations pertaining to vaccine innovation and uptake: (1) to use existing products more widely in humans and animals; (2) to sustain a viable market for vaccines; and (3) to renew the impetus for early research in vaccines useful for AMR (O'Neill 2016b). The UK Chatham House meeting (London, UK), which included vaccine experts, representatives of international and regional organizations with an interest in AMR, economists, and scientists from the vaccine industry, also indicated that vaccines could play a bigger role in reducing AMR. The group felt that increased use of current vaccines such as PCV, influenza vaccine, rotavirus vaccine, and Hib vaccine could have a significant impact on reducing the threat of AMR. They also drafted a seminal list of priority prophylactic vaccines that should be developed to help further address AMR (Chatham House 2017; Clift and Salisbury 2017).

Following the success of the Chatham House meeting, the UK Wellcome Trust solicited a report facilitated by the Boston Consulting Group to provide an independent assessment of the potential of vaccines to combat AMR, and encourage greater attention, focus, and funding for vaccine development that could tackle drug resistant pathogens included in the WHO Global Priority List of Antibiotic-Resistant Bacteria. Pathogens were assessed and ranked for priority for vaccine development based on their public health impact, feasibility of research and development, probability of successful development, and likelihood of uptake and recommendation for use in routine immunization programs (Boston Consulting Group 2019).

The Global Alliance for Vaccines and Immunization (GAVI), a public private global health partnership founded by the Bill & Melinda Gates Foundation in 2000, with contribution from many countries, high-net-worth individuals, and organizations, supports global childhood vaccination in lower- to middle-income countries (https://www.gavi.org/). As of 2019, GAVI had contributed to the immunization of more than 700 million children worldwide (https://www.gavi.org/). In addition to the millions of deaths prevented by vaccination, GAVI support has also benefited AMR prevention, as several of the vaccines with documented impact on AMR identified earlier in this chapter (e.g., pneumococcus, Hib [as part of a pentavalent vaccine], and rotavirus) are supported by GAVI for vaccination of children in low- to middle-income countries. Given the critical role vaccines play in addressing AMR, the impact of vaccination on AMR is now included in GAVI's evaluation criteria for their vaccine investment strategy (Mok 2018) and is an important component of their 5 year strategic plan where the alliance committed to continue to scale up vaccines for diseases prone to AMR while incentivizing research in other vaccines that can contribute to fight AMR (GAVI. The Vaccine Alliance 2017).

An increasing number of public private partnerships and consortia are being formed to coordinate efforts to address the threat of AMR using various strategies, including vaccines. For example, Combating Antibiotic Resistant Bacteria Biopharmaceutical Accelerator (CARB-X), a global non-profit partnership led by Boston University, is dedicated to accelerating global antibacterial innovation by investing in the development of new life saving products to combat the most dangerous drug resistant bacteria (https://carb-x.org/). CARB-X is funded by the U.S. Department of Health and Human Services Biomedical Advanced Research and Development Authority (part of the Office of the Assistant Secretary for Preparedness and Response), the Bill & Melinda Gates Foundation, the National Institute of Allergy and Infectious Diseases, the UK Wellcome Trust, the UK Government's Global Antimicrobial Resistance Innovation Fund, and Germany's Federal Ministry of Education and Research. By the end of 2018, the CARB-X portfolio included 33 research projects in seven countries globally (CARB-X 2017–2018). The 2019 CARB-X antibacterial treatment and prevention product portfolio includes projects dedicated to important bacterial pathogens, including multivalent *S. aureus* toxoid vaccine (Integrated BioTherapeutics), *Klebsiella* vaccine (Vaxxilon), and Group A streptococcus vaccine (SutroVax) (https://carb-x.org/).

10.7 Challenges and Future Prospects

10.7.1 Barriers to Maximizing Licensed Vaccine Use

Vaccines have been highly effective in reducing levels of infectious diseases and, by association, the accompanying use of antibiotics for many pathogens, yet there remain hurdles to global access and implementation. While vaccine use in high-income countries has reached high coverage rates for most vaccines, global implementation is dramatically lower with coverage rates of only 19–45% for many vaccines (Greenwood 2014). The barriers to maximizing licensed vaccine use in pediatric as well as adult populations are diverse, stemming from flaws in healthcare systems and regulatory policies to misperceptions causing noncompliance (Table 10.3) (Anonymous 2018; Esposito et al. 2014; Ventola 2016a, b). The healthcare and regulatory barriers may include variability in national immunization laws and regulations, insufficient vaccine supply, lack of knowledge for vaccine indications and contraindications, inadequate national prioritization and budget allocation for vaccination, and a lack of population based systems to collect and consolidate individual vaccination data.

Vaccine hesitancy – defined by reluctance to vaccinate despite the availability of vaccines and seen increasingly in the delay or refusal of parents to vaccinate their

Table 10.3 Selected public misconceptions and facts about vaccines

Misconceptions	Facts
Diseases had already begun to disappear before vaccines were introduced, because of better hygiene and sanitation.	Dramatic reduction in the incidence of infectious diseases (e.g., measles, polio, *Haemophilus influenzae* type b), following vaccine introduction, even in modern times when hygiene was not further improving, indicates the significant direct impact of vaccines.
	Decreased levels of primary and/or booster vaccination caused disease outbreaks or epidemics even in the countries where disease incidence was previously very low due to vaccines (e.g., measles in the U.S., pertussis in Great Britain, Sweden, and Japan, and diphtheria in the former USSR).
Vaccine preventable diseases have been virtually eliminated from my country, so there is no need for my child to be vaccinated.	Some vaccine preventable diseases are still prevalent in middle- and low-income countries across the globe and can be brought into any country by travelers.
	Without vaccination, a few imported cases may quickly become an epidemic.
	Vaccination directly protects vaccine recipients and indirectly protects a small population of people who cannot receive vaccination (due to allergies or immune-compromising conditions) through herd immunity.
The majority of people who get disease have been vaccinated.	No vaccine is 100% effective (most routine childhood vaccines are effective for 85%-95% of recipients).
	In a country such as the U.S., many more people are vaccinated than those who are not.
	Therefore, in the case of an outbreak, the number of people who had been vaccinated but did not respond (got a disease) will exceed those who had not been vaccinated and got a disease.
There are "hot lots" of vaccine that have been associated with more adverse events and deaths than others. Parents should find the numbers of these lots and not allow their children to receive vaccines from them.	In high-income countries such as the U.S. and the EU, vaccine safety systems are regulated by the FDA and the EMA, respectively, to ensure the highest possible quality and safety of vaccines (Centers for Disease Control and Prevention 2013b).
	Vaccines are made under Good Manufacturing Practices, that require strict quality guidelines and controls.
	Vaccines for use in middle- and low-income countries, purchased through GAVI and UNICEF, meet WHO safety and quality standards (World Health Organization 2019b).
	Adverse events reported following vaccination may be temporally associated with receipt of the vaccine but are not necessarily caused by the vaccine.

(continued)

Table 10.3 (continued)

Misconceptions	Facts
Vaccines cause many harmful side effects, illnesses, and even death – not to mention possible long-term effects we don't even know about.	Vaccines are very safe and tested through rigorous clinical studies, post-marketing commitments, and the Vaccine Adverse Event Reporting System and Vaccine Safety Datalink run by the CDC and the FDA (Centers for Disease Control and Prevention 2013b).
	In childhood, the risk of being seriously injured or killed due to a vaccine-preventable disease is far greater than risks associated with receipt of any vaccine.
	The vast majority of vaccine adverse events are minor and temporary (e.g., a sore arm or mild fever).
	The frequency of serious vaccine adverse events is low (on the order of one per thousands to one per millions of doses), and some are so rare that risk cannot be accurately assessed.
Giving a child multiple vaccinations for different diseases at the same time increases the risk of harmful side effects and can overload the immune system.	Children are naturally exposed to many foreign antigens every day, including bacteria and viruses introduced orally or from the air.
	Multiple studies have demonstrated conclusively that the recommended pediatric vaccines are as effective in combination as they are individually, and simultaneous vaccination with multiple vaccines has no adverse effect on the normal immune system.
	Combining more antigens in a single vaccine injection (e.g., measles-mumps-rubella and chickenpox) would require fewer shots and visits while providing the benefits of individual vaccines.
	The Institute of Medicine in the U.S. does not consider childhood combination vaccines immune suppressive (Institute of Medicine (US) Vaccine Safety Committee 1994).

Adapted from https://www.who.int/vaccine_safety/initiative/detection/immunization_misconceptions/en/; https://www.cdc.gov/vaccinesafety/

CDC Centers for Disease Control and Prevention, *EMA* European Medicines Agency, *EU* European Union, *FDA* Food and Drug Administration, *GAVI* Global Alliance for Vaccines and Immunization, *UNICEF* United Nations Children's Fund, *U.S.* United States, *USSR* Union of Soviet Socialist Republics, *WHO* World Health Organization

children – is recognized by the WHO as one of the top 10 threats to global health in 2019 (along with AMR) (https://www.who.int/emergencies/ten-threats-to-global-health-in-2019). Vaccine hesitancy has already caused a resurgence of several vaccine preventable infectious diseases, including the recent well documented outbreaks of measles in New York (https://www.cdc.gov/measles/cases-outbreaks.html) and polio in the Philippines (https://www.who.int/csr/don/24-september-2019-polio-outbreak-the-philippines/en/). In the Philippines, concerns with the dengue vaccine, Dengvaxia, have exerted an effect on polio vaccination rates, resulting in an outbreak after 19 years of the country being declared completely polio-free in 2000 (Thornton 2019). Reasons for vaccine hesitancy are complex and include concerns about vaccine safety as well as moral or religious beliefs. Disproven and erroneous associations of the measles-mumps-rubella and hepatitis B pediatric vaccines with the development of autism or chronic fatigue syndrome and multiple sclerosis, respectively (https://www.cdc.gov/vaccinesafety/concerns/autism.html; DeStefano et al. 2002; Glanz et al. 2018; Klein and Diehl 2004; Smith and Woods 2010; Taylor et al. 2014b), are well-known examples of dangerous misinformation that has negatively affected the perception of vaccines and put lives at risk. Another grave common vaccine misconception is that the seasonal influenza vaccine shot can cause influenza illness (https://www.cdc.gov/flu/prevent/misconceptions.htm). The unacceptably low influenza vaccination rate among young healthy people between 18 and 49 years of age (as low as 26% in 2017–2018) (https://www.cdc.gov/flu/fluvax-view/coverage-1718estimates.htm) impacts herd immunity and bears deadly consequences for the elderly who respond suboptimally to influenza vaccines and are at highest risk for flu related deaths that occur annually in the tens of thousands in this cohort (https://www.cdc.gov/flu/about/burden/2017-2018.htm). Additionally, negative public perception of vaccines can lead to consequent vaccine hesitancy, as in the case of Dengvaxia and polio vaccination in the Philippines (Thornton 2019).

Combating the rise in dangerous misinformation through social media and other channels has also opened up as another front on the war against infectious disease (Betsch et al. 2012; Tomeny et al. 2017). A retrospective analysis of online vaccine discourse activity during the 2016 U.S. presidential election revealed intentional malicious spread of anti vaccine messages on Twitter, amplifying anti vaccination messages through online public health misinformation (Broniatowski et al. 2018).

10.7.2 Efforts Towards Better Utilization of Vaccines to Optimize Their Impact on Antimicrobial Resistance and Future Prospects

At a time when the global community is fervently working to mobilize resources to counteract AMR, vaccine development and deployment has the potential to contribute to AMR prevention by decreasing overall antibiotic prescribing pressure.

Much remains to be done to increase global access to already licensed vaccines. Additionally, the importance of maintaining and creating new markets for vaccines cannot be understated. Global vaccine coverage could be improved by simultaneous licensure in developed and developing countries, faster rollout in countries with the largest birth cohorts, such as China and India, improving logistics for delivering vaccines to remote locations, increasing funding by ministries of health for vaccination programs, and lowering population reticence to vaccination. In addition to maximizing childhood vaccination coverage, adult vaccination programs should also be expanded by adopting adult vaccination as a healthcare priority at the national level and improving infrastructure.

Changes in regulatory laws and policies are also required, with formal consideration given to vaccination benefits in AMR reduction. Regulatory oversight of clinical studies, including post marketing commitment studies, provides robust vaccine benefit-risk assessments; however, these extensive data sets are at times not fully taken into consideration by vaccine recommending bodies in many countries. Thus, widespread access driven in part by reimbursement to healthcare providers of costs associated with the vaccine and its administration may be delayed. National advisory committees on immunization – multidisciplinary groups of national experts responsible for providing independent, evidence informed advice to policymakers and program managers on policy issues related to immunization and vaccines – would need to develop the Guidance for Industry that supports including AMR data in label updates and incorporating AMR reduction benefits in health technology assessment and economic modeling.

While coverage with some licensed vaccines such as influenza remains suboptimal even in developed countries such as the U.S. and Europe, it could be greatly improved by stronger recommendations and provider education in the form of continuing medical education programs for impact on AMR reduction. Advocacy for the safe and effective use of vaccines directed at medical professionals and the general public is provided by academic and public health institutions and is complemented by organizations such as Vaccines Europe, an EU-wide vaccine industry stakeholder group of major innovative research and development based vaccine companies (Jansen et al. 2018) and European "civil society organisations," advocating for vaccination by working with national policymakers, vaccine experts, and the general public to communicate the benefits of vaccination (Esposito et al. 2014; Laurent-Ledru et al. 2011). For example, Vaccines Europe provides information to the public regarding vaccine innovation and manufacturing processes and highlights evidence for vaccine safety and efficacy.

New vaccine candidates addressing important bacterial and viral pathogens for which vaccines currently do not exist are under development, as well as vaccines against parasitic infections such as malaria which often predispose children in endemic areas to invasive bacterial coinfections requiring antibiotic treatment (Were et al. 2011). Vaccines to prevent *C. difficile* or *S. aureus* infection, pneumococcal conjugate vaccines with extended serotype coverage, and vaccines to prevent infections with Gram negative bacteria and *M. tuberculosis* hold a profound promise not only to address these life threatening diseases, but also to help further curb antibiotic use and thereby prevent AMR. Incentives that could be provided to enable industry to develop new vaccines that are of public interest but may not be commercially viable would be similar to those used for the development of new antibiotics and include priority review vouchers, transferable regulatory data and marketing exclusivity, and research and development tax credits. In parallel, sustained investments in developing the human talent pool, which has undergone a significant reduction due to dramatic consolidation within the vaccine industry over the last decade, would provide an experienced workforce to innovate across vaccine research and development (Cawein et al. 2017).

Though this chapter is focused on human vaccines, of considerable importance will also be an emphasis on the development of veterinary vaccines to reduce the inappropriate widespread prophylactic use of antibiotics in animal and fish husbandry intended for human consumption. This is captured in the One Health Initiative, that is a collaborative interdisciplinary concept being supported by the CDC (https://www.cdc.gov/onehealth/index.html; http://www.onehealthinitiative.com/about.php) and the U.S. Department of Agriculture (https://www.usda.gov/topics/animals/one-health). For example, vaccination of farmed poultry against *Salmonella* is required in Europe but not mandated in the U.S. (Desin et al. 2013; Erickson and Reader's Digest 2018; USDA APHIS 2014). Broad use of *Salmonella* vaccines in farm animals would not only reduce cases of foodborne *Salmonella* infections, but also likely decrease the rise of multi drug resistant *Salmonella* strains.

Vaccines represent an important component of our armamentarium in the battle against resistant pathogens and are integral in the strategy to address this dire global threat. While much has been accomplished with respect to the development of vaccines and immunization strategies to address important public health challenges, there remain a large number of important human pathogens for which there is no available vaccine or for which current vaccines are suboptimal. Vaccination strategies and AMR considerations are intertwined in importance and, taken together, will drive development decisions and priorities in the decades to come.

Acknowledgements The authors thank the following Pfizer colleagues: Natasha Kushnir, PhD for scientific writing, Robert Donald, PhD and Kirstin Heinrich, MPH for critical review of the manuscript, and Dawn De Thomas for graphics preparation.

Disclosures All authors were employees of Pfizer at time of writing. The chapter preparation was funded by Pfizer.

References

Aanensen DM, Feil EJ, Holden MT, Dordel J, Yeats CA, Fedosejev A, Goater R, Castillo-Ramirez S, Corander J, Colijn C, Chlebowicz MA, Schouls L, Heck M, Pluister G, Ruimy R, Kahlmeter G, Ahman J, Matuschek E, Friedrich AW, Parkhill J, Bentley SD, Spratt BG, Grundmann H, European S.R.L. Working Group (2016) Whole-genome sequencing for routine pathogen surveillance in public health: a population snapshot of invasive staphylococcus aureus in Europe. MBio 7(3). https://doi.org/10.1128/mBio.00444-16

Adam HJ, Richardson SE, Jamieson FB, Rawte P, Low DE, Fisman DN (2010) Changing epidemiology of invasive Haemophilus influenzae in Ontario, Canada: evidence for herd effects and strain replacement due to Hib vaccination. Vaccine 28(24):4073–4078. https://doi.org/10.1016/j.vaccine.2010.03.075

Adler A, Miller-Roll T, Bradenstein R, Block C, Mendelson B, Parizade M, Paitan Y, Schwartz D, Peled N, Carmeli Y, Schwaber MJ (2015) A national survey of the molecular epidemiology of

Clostridium difficile in Israel: the dissemination of the ribotype 027 strain with reduced susceptibility to vancomycin and metronidazole. Diagn Microbiol Infect Dis 83(1):21–24. https://doi.org/10.1016/j.diagmicrobio.2015.05.015

Aguilo N, Gonzalo-Asensio J, Alvarez-Arguedas S, Marinova D, Gomez AB, Uranga S, Spallek R, Singh M, Audran R, Spertini F, Martin C (2017) Reactogenicity to major tuberculosis antigens absent in BCG is linked to improved protection against Mycobacterium tuberculosis. Nat Commun 8:16085. https://doi.org/10.1038/ncomms16085

Ahmed H, Davies F, Francis N, Farewell D, Butler C, Paranjothy S (2017) Long-term antibiotics for prevention of recurrent urinary tract infection in older adults: systematic review and meta-analysis of randomised trials. BMJ Open 7(5):e015233. https://doi.org/10.1136/bmjopen-2016-015233

Alderson MR (2016) Status of research and development of pediatric vaccines for Streptococcus pneumoniae. Vaccine 34(26):2959–2961. https://doi.org/10.1016/j.vaccine.2016.03.107

Ali A, An SJ, Cui C, Haque A, Carbis R (2014) Synthesis and immunogenicity evaluation of Salmonella enterica serovar Paratyphi A O-specific polysaccharide conjugated to diphtheria toxoid. Hum Vaccin Immunother 10(6):1494–1498. https://doi.org/10.4161/hv.28130

Alving CR (2002) Design and selection of vaccine adjuvants: animal models and human trials. Vaccine 20(Suppl 3):S56–S64. https://doi.org/10.1016/s0264-410x(02)00174-3

American Academy of Pediatrics Committee on Infectious Diseases; American Academy of Pediatrics Bronchiolitis Guidelines Committee (2014) Updated guidance for palivizumab prophylaxis among infants and young children at increased risk of hospitalization for respiratory syncytial virus infection. Pediatrics 134(2):415–420. https://doi.org/10.1542/peds.2014-1665

Andersen P, Scriba TJ (2019) Moving tuberculosis vaccines from theory to practice. Nat Rev Immunol 19(9):550–562. https://doi.org/10.1038/s41577-019-0174-z

Andrews JR, Qamar FN, Charles RC, Ryan ET (2018) Extensively drug-resistant typhoid – are conjugate vaccines arriving just in time? N Engl J Med 379(16):1493–1495. https://doi.org/10.1056/NEJMp1803926

Angulo FJ, Swerdlow DL (1995) Bacterial enteric infections in persons infected with human immunodeficiency virus. Clin Infect Dis 21(Suppl 1):S84–S93. https://doi.org/10.1093/clinids/21.supplement_1.s84

Anonymous (2018) Addressing barriers to optimal community-based vaccination. AJMC Persp:9–12

Antrobus RD, Berthoud TK, Mullarkey CE, Hoschler K, Coughlan L, Zambon M, Hill AV, Gilbert SC (2014) Coadministration of seasonal influenza vaccine and MVA-NP+M1 simultaneously achieves potent humoral and cell-mediated responses. Mol Ther 22(1):233–238. https://doi.org/10.1038/mt.2013.162

Arbeit RD, Karakawa WW, Vann WF, Robbins JB (1984) Predominance of two newly described capsular polysaccharide types among clinical isolates of Staphylococcus aureus. Diagn Microbiol Infect Dis 2(2):85–91. https://doi.org/10.1016/0732-8893(84)90002-6

Aslam S, Hamill RJ, Musher DM (2005) Treatment of Clostridium difficile-associated disease: old therapies and new strategies. Lancet Infect Dis 5(9):549–557. https://doi.org/10.1016/S1473-3099(05)70215-2

Bahl K, Senn JJ, Yuzhakov O, Bulychev A, Brito LA, Hassett KJ, Laska ME, Smith M, Almarsson O, Thompson J, Ribeiro AM, Watson M, Zaks T, Ciaramella G (2017) Preclinical and clinical demonstration of immunogenicity by mRNA vaccines against H10N8 and H7N9 influenza viruses. Mol Ther 25(6):1316–1327. https://doi.org/10.1016/j.ymthe.2017.03.035

Baker S, The HC (2018) Recent insights into Shigella. Curr Opin Infect Dis 31(5):449–454. https://doi.org/10.1097/QCO.0000000000000475

Baker CJ, Rench MA, Fernandez M, Paoletti LC, Kasper DL, Edwards MS (2003) Safety and immunogenicity of a bivalent group B streptococcal conjugate vaccine for serotypes II and III. J Infect Dis 188(1):66–73. https://doi.org/10.1086/375536

Baker CJ, Carey VJ, Rench MA, Edwards MS, Hillier SL, Kasper DL, Platt R (2014) Maternal antibody at delivery protects neonates from early onset group B streptococcal disease. J Infect Dis 209(5):781–788. https://doi.org/10.1093/infdis/jit549

Baliban SM, Allen JC, Curtis B, Amin MN, Lees A, Rao RN, Naidu G, Venkatesan R, Rao DY, Mohan VK, Ella KM, Levine MM, Simon R (2018) Immunogenicity and induction of functional antibodies in rabbits immunized with a trivalent typhoid-invasive nontyphoidal Salmonella Glycoconjugate formulation. Molecules 23(7). https://doi.org/10.3390/molecules23071749

Balsells E, Guillot L, Nair H, Kyaw MH (2017) Serotype distribution of Streptococcus pneumoniae causing invasive disease in children in the post-PCV era: a systematic review and meta-analysis. PLoS One 12(5):e0177113. https://doi.org/10.1371/journal.pone.0177113

Barel LA, Mulard LA (2019) Classical and novel strategies to develop a Shigella glycoconjugate vaccine: from concept to efficacy in human. Hum Vaccin Immunother 15(6):1338–1356. https://doi.org/10.1080/21645515.2019.1606972

Bartlett JG, Gerding DN (2008) Clinical recognition and diagnosis of Clostridium difficile infection. Clin Infect Dis 46(Suppl 1):S12–S18. https://doi.org/10.1086/521863

Bauer MP, Notermans DW, van Benthem BH, Brazier JS, Wilcox MH, Rupnik M, Monnet DL, van Dissel JT, Kuijper EJ, Group ES (2011) Clostridium difficile infection in Europe: a hospital-based survey. Lancet 377(9759):63–73. https://doi.org/10.1016/S0140-6736(10)61266-4

Beadling C, Slifka MK (2004) How do viral infections predispose patients to bacterial infections? Curr Opin Infect Dis 17(3):185–191

Beeler JA, van Wyke Coelingh K (1989) Neutralization epitopes of the F glycoprotein of respiratory syncytial virus: effect of mutation upon fusion function. J Virol 63(7):2941–2950

Beran J, Lickliter JD, Schwarz TF, Johnson C, Chu L, Domachowske JB, Van Damme P, Withanage K, Fissette LA, David MP, Maleux K, Schmidt AC, Picciolato M, Dieussaert I (2018) Safety and immunogenicity of 3 formulations of an investigational respiratory syncytial virus vaccine in nonpregnant women: results from 2 phase 2 trials. J Infect Dis 217(10):1616–1625. https://doi.org/10.1093/infdis/jiy065

Betsch C, Brewer NT, Brocard P, Davies P, Gaissmaier W, Haase N, Leask J, Renkewitz F, Renner B, Reyna VF, Rossmann C, Sachse K, Schachinger A, Siegrist M, Stryk M (2012) Opportunities and challenges of Web 2.0 for vaccination decisions. Vaccine 30(25):3727–3733. https://doi.org/10.1016/j.vaccine.2012.02.025

Bhatti MW (2019) Pakistan approaches Indian firm to buy vaccine against XDR typhoid, https://www.thenews.com.pk/print/431240-pakistan-approaches-indian-firm-to-buy-vaccine-against-xdr-typhoid. Accessed 29 Sept 2019

Block SL, Heikkinen T, Toback SL, Zheng W, Ambrose CS (2011) The efficacy of live attenuated influenza vaccine against influenza-associated acute otitis media in children. Pediatr Infect Dis J 30(3):203–207. https://doi.org/10.1097/INF.0b013e3181faac7c

Boston Consulting Group (2019) Vaccines to tackle drug resistant infections. An evaluation of R&D opportunities, https://vaccinesforamr.org/wp-content/uploads/2018/09/Vaccines_for_AMR.pdf. Accessed 8 Aug 2019

Bratzler DW, Dellinger EP, Olsen KM, Perl TM, Auwaerter PG, Bolon MK, Fish DN, Napolitano LM, Sawyer RG, Slain D, Steinberg JP, Weinstein RA, American Society of Health-System P, Infectious Diseases Society of A, Surgical Infection S, Society for Healthcare Epidemiology of A (2013) Clinical practice guidelines for antimicrobial prophylaxis in surgery. Surg Infect (Larchmt) 14(1):73–156. https://doi.org/10.1089/sur.2013.9999

Braye K, Ferguson J, Davis D, Catling C, Monk A, Foureur M (2018) Effectiveness of intrapartum antibiotic prophylaxis for early-onset group B Streptococcal infection: an integrative review. Women Birth 31(4):244–253. https://doi.org/10.1016/j.wombi.2017.10.012

Breiman RF, Butler JC, Tenover FC, Elliott JA, Facklam RR (1994) Emergence of drug-resistant pneumococcal infections in the United States. JAMA 271(23):1831–1835

Broniatowski DA, Jamison AM, Qi S, AlKulaib L, Chen T, Benton A, Quinn SC, Dredze M (2018) Weaponized health communication: twitter bots and Russian trolls amplify the vaccine debate. Am J Public Health 108(10):1378–1384. https://doi.org/10.2105/AJPH.2018.304567

Burack JH, Hahn JA, Saint-Maurice D, Jacobson MA (1994) Microbiology of community-acquired bacterial pneumonia in persons with and at risk for human immunodeficiency virus type 1 infection. Implications for rational empiric antibiotic therapy. Arch Intern Med 154(22):2589–2596

Butler JC, Hofmann J, Cetron MS, Elliott JA, Facklam RR, Breiman RF (1996) The continued emergence of drug-resistant Streptococcus pneumoniae in the United States: an update from the centers for disease control and prevention's pneumococcal sentinel surveillance system. J Infect Dis 174(5):986–993. https://doi.org/10.1093/infdis/174.5.986

Buurman ET, Timofeyeva Y, Gu J, Kim JH, Kodali S, Liu Y, Mininni T, Moghazeh S, Pavliakova D, Singer C, Singh S, Handke LD, Lotvin J, Prasad AK, Scully IL, Donald RGK, Jansen KU, Anderson AS (2019) A novel hexavalent capsular polysaccharide conjugate vaccine (GBS6) for the prevention of neonatal group B streptococcal infections by maternal immunization. J Infect Dis 220(1):105–115. https://doi.org/10.1093/infdis/jiz062

Campos PE, Suarez PG, Sanchez J, Zavala D, Arevalo J, Ticona E, Nolan CM, Hooton TM, Holmes KK (2003) Multidrug-resistant Mycobacterium tuberculosis in HIV-infected persons, Peru. Emerg Infect Dis 9(12):1571–1578. https://doi.org/10.3201/eid0912.020731

CARB-X (2017–2018) Progress against superbugs. Annual report 2017–2018, https://carb-x.org/wp-content/uploads/2018/09/CARB-X_AR-2017-18.pdf. Accessed 23 Sept 2019

Carmona Martinez A, Prymula R, Miranda Valdivieso M, Otero Reigada MDC, Merino Arribas JM, Brzostek J, Szenborn L, Ruzkova R, Horn MR, Jackowska T, Centeno-Malfaz F, Traskine M, Dobbelaere K, Borys D (2019) Immunogenicity and safety of 11- and 12-valent pneumococcal non-typeable Haemophilus influenzae protein D-conjugate vaccines (11vPHiD-CV, 12vPHiD-CV) in infants: results from a phase II, randomised, multicentre study. Vaccine 37(1):176–186. https://doi.org/10.1016/j.vaccine.2018.07.023

Caroom C, Tullar JM, Benton EG Jr, Jones JR, Chaput CD (2013) Intrawound vancomycin powder reduces surgical site infections in posterior cervical fusion. Spine (Phila Pa 1976) 38(14):1183–1187. https://doi.org/10.1097/BRS.0b013e31828fcfb5

Cawein A, Emini E, Watson M, Dailey J, Donnelly J, Tresnan D, Evans T, Plotkin S, Gruber W (2017) Human capital gaps in vaccine development: an issue for global vaccine development and global health. Ann N Y Acad Sci 1395(1):3–11. https://doi.org/10.1111/nyas.13316

Centers for Disease Control (1981) Pneumocystis pneumonia–Los Angeles. MMWR Morb Mortal Wkly Rep 30(21):250–252

Centers for Disease Control and Prevention (1999) Control of infectious diseases. MMWR Morb Mortal Wkly Rep 48(29):621–629

Centers for Disease Control and Prevention (2013a) Antibiotic resistance threats in the United States, 2013, https://www.cdc.gov/drugresistance/pdf/ar-threats-2013-508.pdf. Accessed 11 Jun 2019

Centers for Disease Control and Prevention (2013b) Ensuring the safety of vaccines in the United States, https://www.cdc.gov/vaccines/hcp/patient-ed/conversations/downloads/vacsafe-ensuring-bw-office.pdf. Accessed 30 Oct 2019

Centers for Disease Control and Prevention (2015) National action plan for combating antibiotic-resistant bacteria, https://www.cdc.gov/drugresistance/pdf/national_action_plan_for_combating_antibotic-resistant_bacteria.pdf. Accessed 15 Jun 2019

Centers for Disease Control and Prevention (2016) ABCs report: Haemophilus influenzae, 2014, https://www.cdc.gov/abcs/reports-findings/survreports/hib14.html. Accessed 3 Aug 2019

Centers for Disease Control and Prevention (2017) Health, United States, 2017, https://www.cdc.gov/nchs/data/hus/hus17.pdf. Accessed 17 Sept 2019

Centers for Disease Control and Prevention (2019) Antibiotic resistance threats in the United States, 2019, https://www.cdc.gov/drugresistance/pdf/threats-report/2019-ar-threats-report-508.pdf. Accessed 15 Nov 2019

Centers for Disease Control and Prevention (CDC) (2002) Progress toward elimination of Haemophilus influenzae type b invasive disease among infants and children–United States, 1998–2000. MMWR Morb Mortal Wkly Rep 51(11):234–237

Chatham House (2017) The value of vaccines in the avoidance of antimicrobial resistance. Centre on Global Health Security, The Royal Institute of International Affairs. Meeting Summary, https://www.chathamhouse.org/sites/default/files/events/2017-03-30-amr-vaccines-meeting-summary.pdf. Accessed 12 Jul 2019

Chen W (2015) Current advances and challenges in the development of Acinetobacter vaccines. Hum Vaccin Immunother 11(10):2495–2500. https://doi.org/10.1080/21645515.2015.1052354

Chu CY, Liu BK, Watson D, Szu SS, Bryla D, Shiloach J, Schneerson R, Robbins JB (1991) Preparation, characterization, and immunogenicity of conjugates composed of the O-specific polysaccharide of Shigella dysenteriae type 1 (Shiga's bacillus) bound to tetanus toxoid. Infect Immun 59(12):4450–4458

Clift C, Salisbury DM (2017) Enhancing the role of vaccines in combatting antimicrobial resistance. Vaccine 35(48 Pt B):6591–6593. https://doi.org/10.1016/j.vaccine.2017.09.053

Cochi SL, Broome CV, Hightower AW (1985) Immunization of US children with Hemophilus influenzae type b polysaccharide vaccine. A cost-effectiveness model of strategy assessment. JAMA 253(4):521–529

Cohen D, Ashkenazi S, Green MS, Gdalevich M, Robin G, Slepon R, Yavzori M, Orr N, Block C, Ashkenazi I, Shemer J, Taylor DN, Hale TL, Sadoff JC, Pavliakova D, Schneerson R, Robbins JB (1997) Double-blind vaccine-controlled randomised efficacy trial of an investigational Shigella sonnei conjugate vaccine in young adults. Lancet 349(9046):155–159. https://doi.org/10.1016/S0140-6736(96)06255-1

Cohen SH, Gerding DN, Johnson S, Kelly CP, Loo VG, LC MD, Pepin J, Wilcox MH, Society for Healthcare Epidemiology of A, Infectious Diseases Society of A (2010) Clinical practice guidelines for Clostridium difficile infection in adults: 2010 update by the society for healthcare epidemiology of America (SHEA) and the infectious diseases society of America (IDSA). Infect Control Hosp Epidemiol 31(5):431–455. https://doi.org/10.1086/651706

Cohen R, Cohen JF, Chalumeau M, Levy C (2017) Impact of pneumococcal conjugate vaccines for children in high- and non-high-income countries. Expert Rev Vaccines 16(6):625–640. https://doi.org/10.1080/14760584.2017.1320221

Crank MC, Ruckwardt TJ, Chen M, Morabito KM, Phung E, Costner PJ, Holman LA, Hickman SP, Berkowitz NM, Gordon IJ, Yamshchikov GV, Gaudinski MR, Kumar A, Chang LA, Moin SM, Hill JP, DiPiazza AT, Schwartz RM, Kueltzo L, Cooper JW, Chen P, Stein JA, Carlton K, Gall JG, Nason MC, Kwong PD, Chen GL, Mascola JR, McLellan JS, Ledgerwood JE, Graham BS, Team VRCS (2019) A proof of concept for structure-based vaccine design targeting RSV in humans. Science 365(6452):505–509. https://doi.org/10.1126/science.aav9033

Cross A, Artenstein A, Que J, Fredeking T, Furer E, Sadoff JC, Cryz SJ Jr (1994) Safety and immunogenicity of a polyvalent Escherichia coli vaccine in human volunteers. J Infect Dis 170(4):834–840. https://doi.org/10.1093/infdis/170.4.834

Crump JA, Luby SP, Mintz ED (2004) The global burden of typhoid fever. Bull World Health Organ 82(5):346–353

Cryz SJ Jr, Mortimer P, Cross AS, Furer E, Germanier R (1986) Safety and immunogenicity of a polyvalent Klebsiella capsular polysaccharide vaccine in humans. Vaccine 4(1):15–20. https://doi.org/10.1016/0264-410x(86)90092-7

Cryz SJ Jr, Furer E, Cross AS, Wegmann A, Germanier R, Sadoff JC (1987) Safety and immunogenicity of a Pseudomonas aeruginosa O-polysaccharide toxin A conjugate vaccine in humans. J Clin Invest 80(1):51–56. https://doi.org/10.1172/JCI113062

Cryz SJ Jr, Lang A, Rudeberg A, Wedgwood J, Que JU, Furer E, Schaad U (1997) Immunization of cystic fibrosis patients with a Pseudomonas aeruginosa O-polysaccharide-toxin A conjugate vaccine. Behring Inst Mitt (98):345–349

Cunha CB, Cunha BA (2006) Impact of plague on human history. Infect Dis Clin North Am 20(2):253–272. https://doi.org/10.1016/j.idc.2006.03.001

Dayan GH, Mohamed N, Scully IL, Cooper D, Begier E, Eiden J, Jansen KU, Gurtman A, Anderson AS (2016) Staphylococcus aureus: the current state of disease, pathophysiology and strategies for prevention. Expert Rev Vaccines 15(11):1373–1392. https://doi.org/10.1080/14760584.2016.1179583

Dbaibo G, Amanullah A, Claeys C, Izu A, Jain VK, Kosalaraksa P, Rivera L, Soni J, Yanni E, Zaman K, Acosta B, Ariza M, Arroba Basanta ML, Bavdekar A, Carmona A, Cousin L, Danier J, Diaz A, Diez-Domingo J, Dinleyici EC, Faust SN, Garcia-Sicilia J, Gomez-Go GD, Gonzales MLA, Hacimustafaoglu M, Hughes SM, Jackowska T, Kant S, Lucero M, Mares Bermudez J, Martinon-Torres F, Montellano M, Prymula R, Puthanakit T, Ruzkova R, Sadowska-Krawczenko I, Szymanski H, Ulied A, Woo W, Schuind A, Innis BL, Flu VECSG (2020) Quadrivalent influenza Vaccine Prevents Illness and Reduces Healthcare Utilization Across Diverse Geographic Regions During Five Influenza Seasons: A Randomized Clinical Trial. Pediatr Infect Dis J 39(1):e1–e10. https://doi.org/10.1097/INF.0000000000002504

Desin TS, Koster W, Potter AA (2013) Salmonella vaccines in poultry: past, present and future. Expert Rev Vaccines 12(1):87–96. https://doi.org/10.1586/erv.12.138

DeStefano F, Verstraeten T, Chen RT (2002) Hepatitis B vaccine and risk of multiple sclerosis. Expert Rev Vaccines 1(4):461–466. https://doi.org/10.1586/14760584.1.4.461

Di Renzo GC, Melin P, Berardi A, Blennow M, Carbonell-Estrany X, Donzelli GP, Hakansson S, Hod M, Hughes R, Kurtzer M, Poyart C, Shinwell E, Stray-Pedersen B, Wielgos M, El Helali N (2015) Intrapartum GBS screening and antibiotic prophylaxis: a European consensus conference. J Matern Fetal Neonatal Med 28(7):766–782. https://doi.org/10.3109/14767058.2014.934804

Donskey CJ (2017) Clostridium difficile in older adults. Infect Dis Clin North Am 31(4):743–756. https://doi.org/10.1016/j.idc.2017.07.003

Donta ST, Peduzzi P, Cross AS, Sadoff J, Haakenson C, Cryz SJ Jr, Kauffman C, Bradley S, Gafford G, Elliston D, Beam TR Jr, John JF Jr, Ribner B, Cantey R, Welsh CH, Ellison RT 3rd, Young EJ, Hamill RJ, Leaf H, Schein RM, Mulligan M, Johnson C, Abrutyn E, Griffiss JM, Slagle D et al (1996) Immunoprophylaxis against klebsiella and pseudomonas aeruginosa infections. The Federal Hyperimmune Immunoglobulin Trial Study Group. J Infect Dis 174(3):537–543. https://doi.org/10.1093/infdis/174.3.537

Doring G, Pfeiffer C, Weber U, Mohr-Pennert A, Dorner F (1995) Parenteral application of a Pseudomonas aeruginosa flagella vaccine elicits specific anti-flagella antibodies in the airways of healthy individuals. Am J Respir Crit Care Med 151(4):983–985. https://doi.org/10.1164/ajrccm/151.4.983

Doring G, Meisner C, Stern M, Flagella Vaccine Trial Study G (2007) A double-blind randomized placebo-controlled phase III study of a Pseudomonas aeruginosa flagella vaccine in cystic fibrosis patients. Proc Natl Acad Sci U S A 104(26):11020–11025. https://doi.org/10.1073/pnas.0702403104

Edelman R, Taylor DN, Wasserman SS, McClain JB, Cross AS, Sadoff JC, Que JU, Cryz SJ (1994) Phase 1 trial of a 24-valent Klebsiella capsular polysaccharide vaccine and an eight-valent Pseudomonas O-polysaccharide conjugate vaccine administered simultaneously. Vaccine 12(14):1288–1294. https://doi.org/10.1016/s0264-410x(94)80054-4

Elbahesh H, Saletti G, Gerlach T, Rimmelzwaan GF (2019) Broadly protective influenza vaccines: design and production platforms. Curr Opin Virol 34:1–9. https://doi.org/10.1016/j.coviro.2018.11.005

Endimiani A, Blackford M, Dasenbrook EC, Reed MD, Bajaksouszian S, Hujer AM, Rudin SD, Hujer KM, Perreten V, Rice LB, Jacobs MR, Konstan MW, Bonomo RA (2011) Emergence of linezolid-resistant Staphylococcus aureus after prolonged treatment of cystic fibrosis patients in Cleveland, Ohio. Antimicrob Agents Chemother 55(4):1684–1692. https://doi.org/10.1128/AAC.01308-10

Epstein SL (2018) Universal influenza vaccines: progress in achieving broad cross-protection in vivo. Am J Epidemiol 187(12):2603–2614. https://doi.org/10.1093/aje/kwy145

Erickson A, Reader's Digest (2018) Why Europeans don't refrigerate their eggs. Business Insider. https://www.businessinsider.com/why-europeans-dont-refrigerate-their-eggs-2018-4?r=DE&IR=T

Esposito S, Principi N, Cornaglia G, Group EVS (2014) Barriers to the vaccination of children and adolescents and possible solutions. Clin Microbiol Infect 20(Suppl 5):25–31. https://doi.org/10.1111/1469-0691.12447

Estrada LD, Schultz-Cherry S (2019) Development of a Universal influenza vaccine. J Immunol 202(2):392–398. https://doi.org/10.4049/jimmunol.1801054

European Medicines Agency; European Centre for Disease Prevention and Control (2009) Joint technical report: the bacterial challenge: time to react, https://www.ecdc.europa.eu/sites/default/files/media/en/publications/Publications/0909_TER_The_Bacterial_Challenge_Time_to_React.pdf. Accessed 27 Aug 2019

Falsey AR, Hennessey PA, Formica MA, Cox C, Walsh EE (2005) Respiratory syncytial virus infection in elderly and high-risk adults. N Engl J Med 352(17):1749–1759. https://doi.org/10.1056/NEJMoa043951

Falsey AR, Walsh EE, Capellan J, Gravenstein S, Zambon M, Yau E, Gorse GJ, Edelman R, Hayden FG, McElhaney JE, Neuzil KM, Nichol KL, Simoes EA, Wright PF, Sales VM (2008) Comparison of the safety and immunogenicity of 2 respiratory syncytial virus (rsv) vaccines–nonadjuvanted vaccine or vaccine adjuvanted with alum–given concomitantly with influenza vaccine to high-risk elderly individuals. J Infect Dis 198(9):1317–1326. https://doi.org/10.1086/592168

Fattom A, Matalon A, Buerkert J, Taylor K, Damaso S, Boutriau D (2015) Efficacy profile of a bivalent Staphylococcus aureus glycoconjugated vaccine in adults on hemodialysis: phase III randomized study. Hum Vaccin Immunother 11(3):632–641. https://doi.org/10.4161/hv.34414

Feasey NA, Dougan G, Kingsley RA, Heyderman RS, Gordon MA (2012) Invasive non-typhoidal salmonella disease: an emerging and neglected tropical disease in Africa. Lancet 379(9835):2489–2499. https://doi.org/10.1016/S0140-6736(11)61752-2

Feasey NA, Hadfield J, Keddy KH, Dallman TJ, Jacobs J, Deng X, Wigley P, Barquist L, Langridge GC, Feltwell T, Harris SR, Mather AE, Fookes M, Aslett M, Msefula C, Kariuki S, Maclennan CA, Onsare RS, Weill FX, Le Hello S, Smith AM, McClelland M, Desai P, Parry CM, Cheesbrough J, French N, Campos J, Chabalgoity JA, Betancor L, Hopkins KL, Nair S, Humphrey TJ, Lunguya O, Cogan TA, Tapia MD, Sow SO, Tennant SM, Bornstein K, Levine MM, Lacharme-Lora L, Everett DB, Kingsley RA, Parkhill J, Heyderman RS, Dougan G, Gordon MA, Thomson NR (2016) Distinct Salmonella Enteritidis lineages associated with enterocolitis in high-income settings and invasive disease in low-income settings. Nat Genet 48(10):1211–1217. https://doi.org/10.1038/ng.3644

Feldman C, Anderson R (2016) Epidemiology, virulence factors and management of the pneumococcus. F1000Res 5:2320. https://doi.org/10.12688/f1000research.9283.1

Feldman RA, Fuhr R, Smolenov I, Mick Ribeiro A, Panther L, Watson M, Senn JJ, Smith M, Almarsson PHS, Laska ME, Thompson J, Zaks T, Ciaramella G (2019) mRNA vaccines against H10N8 and H7N9 influenza viruses of pandemic potential are immunogenic and well tolerated in healthy adults in phase 1 randomized clinical trials. Vaccine 37(25):3326–3334. https://doi.org/10.1016/j.vaccine.2019.04.074

Fireman B, Black SB, Shinefield HR, Lee J, Lewis E, Ray P (2003) Impact of the pneumococcal conjugate vaccine on otitis media. Pediatr Infect Dis J 22(1):10–16. https://doi.org/10.1097/00006454-200301000-00006

Fleming-Dutra KE, Hersh AL, Shapiro DJ, Bartoces M, Enns EA, File TM Jr, Finkelstein JA, Gerber JS, Hyun DY, Linder JA, Lynfield R, Margolis DJ, May LS, Merenstein D, Metlay JP, Newland JG, Piccirillo JF, Roberts RM, Sanchez GV, Suda KJ, Thomas A, Woo TM, Zetts RM, Hicks LA (2016) Prevalence of inappropriate antibiotic prescriptions among US ambulatory care visits, 2010–2011. JAMA 315(17):1864–1873. https://doi.org/10.1001/jama.2016.4151

Forthal DN (2014) Functions of antibodies. Microbiol Spectr 2(4):1–17

Freeman J, Vernon J, Morris K, Nicholson S, Todhunter S, Longshaw C, Wilcox MH, Pan-European Longitudinal Surveillance of Antibiotic Resistance among Prevalent Clostridium difficile Ribotypes' Study G (2015) Pan-European longitudinal surveillance of antibiotic resistance among prevalent Clostridium difficile ribotypes. Clin Microbiol Infect 21(3):248 e9-248 e16 doi:https://doi.org/10.1016/j.cmi.2014.09.017

Frenck RW Jr, Creech CB, Sheldon EA, Seiden DJ, Kankam MK, Baber J, Zito E, Hubler R, Eiden J, Severs JM, Sebastian S, Nanra J, Jansen KU, Gruber WC, Anderson AS, Girgenti D (2017) Safety, tolerability, and immunogenicity of a 4-antigen Staphylococcus aureus vaccine (SA4Ag): results from a first-in-human randomised, placebo-controlled phase 1/2 study. Vaccine 35(2):375–384. https://doi.org/10.1016/j.vaccine.2016.11.010

Frenck RW Jr, Ervin J, Chu L, Abbanat D, Spiessens B, Go O, Haazen W, van den Dobbelsteen G, Poolman J, Thoelen S, Ibarra de Palacios P (2019) Safety and immunogenicity of a vaccine for extra-intestinal pathogenic Escherichia coli (ESTELLA): a phase 2 randomised controlled trial. Lancet Infect Dis 19(6):631–640. https://doi.org/10.1016/S1473-3099(18)30803-X

G7 Summit (2015) Leaders' declaration. Schloss Elmau, Germany, 7–8 June 2015, https://sustainabledevelopment.un.org/content/documents/7320LEADERS%20STATEMENT_FINAL_CLEAN.pdf. Accessed 23 Aug 2019

Gagneux-Brunon A, Lucht F, Launay O, Berthelot P, Botelho-Nevers E (2018) Vaccines for healthcare-associated infections: present, future, and expectations. Expert Rev Vaccines 17(5):421–433. https://doi.org/10.1080/14760584.2018.1470507

Garcon N, Di Pasquale A (2017) From discovery to licensure, the Adjuvant System story. Hum Vaccin Immunother 13(1):19–33. https://doi.org/10.1080/21645515.2016.1225635

GAVI. The Vaccine Alliance (2017) Monitoring & evaluation framework. Gavi strategy 2016–2020, https://www.gavi.org/about/strategy/phase-iv-2016-20/. Accessed 14 Sept 2019

Gaviola ML, McMillian WD, Ames SE, Endicott JA, Alston WK (2016) A retrospective study on the protective effects of topical vancomycin in patients undergoing multilevel spinal fusion. Pharmacotherapy 36(1):19–25. https://doi.org/10.1002/phar.1678

Gaynes R, Edwards JR, National Nosocomial Infections Surveillance S (2005) Overview of nosocomial infections caused by gram-negative bacilli. Clin Infect Dis 41(6):848–854. https://doi.org/10.1086/432803

GBD (2017) Typhoid and Paratyphoid Collaborators (2019) The global burden of typhoid and paratyphoid fevers: a systematic analysis for the Global Burden of Disease Study 2017. Lancet Infect Dis 19(4):369–381. https://doi.org/10.1016/S1473-3099(18)30685-6

Gefenaite G, Bijlsma MJ, Bos HJ, Hak E (2014) Did introduction of pneumococcal vaccines in the Netherlands decrease the need for respiratory antibiotics in children? Analysis of 2002 to 2013 data. Euro Surveill 19(44). https://doi.org/10.2807/1560-7917.es2014.19.44.20948

Gellatly SL, Hancock RE (2013) Pseudomonas aeruginosa: new insights into pathogenesis and host defenses. Pathog Dis 67(3):159–173. https://doi.org/10.1111/2049-632X.12033

Gerding DN (2004) Clindamycin, cephalosporins, fluoroquinolones, and Clostridium difficile-associated diarrhea: this is an antimicrobial resistance problem. Clin Infect Dis 38(5):646–648. https://doi.org/10.1086/382084

Gerding DN, Muto CA, Owens RC Jr (2008) Measures to control and prevent Clostridium difficile infection. Clin Infect Dis 46(Suppl 1):S43–S49. https://doi.org/10.1086/521861

Giannasca PJ, Zhang ZX, Lei WD, Boden JA, Giel MA, Monath TP, Thomas WD Jr (1999) Serum antitoxin antibodies mediate systemic and mucosal protection from Clostridium difficile disease in hamsters. Infect Immun 67(2):527–538

Giaquinto C, Dominiak-Felden G, Van Damme P, Myint TT, Maldonado YA, Spoulou V, Mast TC, Staat MA (2011) Summary of effectiveness and impact of rotavirus vaccination with the oral pentavalent rotavirus vaccine: a systematic review of the experience in industrialized countries. Hum Vaccin 7(7):734–748. https://doi.org/10.4161/hv.7.7.15511

Giufre M, Cardines R, Caporali MG, Accogli M, D'Ancona F, Cerquetti M (2011) Ten years of Hib vaccination in Italy: prevalence of non-encapsulated Haemophilus influenzae among invasive isolates and the possible impact on antibiotic resistance. Vaccine 29(22):3857–3862. https://doi.org/10.1016/j.vaccine.2011.03.059

Glanz JM, Newcomer SR, Daley MF, DeStefano F, Groom HC, Jackson ML, Lewin BJ, McCarthy NL, McClure DL, Narwaney KJ, Nordin JD, Zerbo O (2018) Association between estimated cumulative vaccine antigen exposure through the first 23 months of life and non-vaccine-targeted infections from 24 through 47 months of age. JAMA 319(9):906–913. https://doi.org/10.1001/jama.2018.0708

Glezen WP, Taber LH, Frank AL, Kasel JA (1986) Risk of primary infection and reinfection with respiratory syncytial virus. Am J Dis Child 140(6):543–546. https://doi.org/10.1001/archpedi.1986.02140200053026

Graham BS, Ambrosino DM (2015) History of passive antibody administration for prevention and treatment of infectious diseases. Curr Opin HIV AIDS 10(3):129–134. https://doi.org/10.1097/COH.0000000000000154

Greenwood B (2014) The contribution of vaccination to global health: past, present and future. Philos Trans R Soc Lond B Biol Sci 369(1645):20130433. https://doi.org/10.1098/rstb.2013.0433

Guerrant RL, Hughes JM, Lima NL, Crane J (1990) Diarrhea in developed and developing countries: magnitude, special settings, and etiologies. Rev Infect Dis 12(Suppl 1):S41–S50. https://doi.org/10.1093/clinids/12.supplement_1.s41

Haines CF, Moore RD, Bartlett JG, Sears CL, Cosgrove SE, Carroll K, Gebo KA (2013) Clostridium difficile in a HIV-infected cohort: incidence, risk factors, and clinical outcomes. AIDS 27(17):2799–2807. https://doi.org/10.1097/01.aids.0000432450.37863.e9

Hament JM, Kimpen JL, Fleer A, Wolfs TF (1999) Respiratory viral infection predisposing for bacterial disease: a concise review. FEMS Immunol Med Microbiol 26(3-4):189–195. https://doi.org/10.1111/j.1574-695X.1999.tb01389.x

Hampton LM, Farley MM, Schaffner W, Thomas A, Reingold A, Harrison LH, Lynfield R, Bennett NM, Petit S, Gershman K, Baumbach J, Beall B, Jorgensen J, Glennen A, Zell ER, Moore M (2012) Prevention of antibiotic-nonsusceptible Streptococcus pneumoniae with conjugate vaccines. J Infect Dis 205(3):401–411. https://doi.org/10.1093/infdis/jir755

Hardelid P, Ghebremichael-Weldeselassie Y, Whitaker H, Rait G, Gilbert R, Petersen I (2018) Effectiveness of live attenuated influenza vaccine in preventing amoxicillin prescribing in preschool children: a self-controlled case series study. J Antimicrob Chemother 73(3):779–786. https://doi.org/10.1093/jac/dkx463

Hargreaves RM, Slack MP, Howard AJ, Anderson E, Ramsay ME (1996) Changing patterns of invasive Haemophilus influenzae disease in England and Wales after introduction of the Hib vaccination programme. BMJ 312(7024):160–161. https://doi.org/10.1136/bmj.312.7024.160

Hasegawa K, Yamamoto K, Chiba N, Kobayashi R, Nagai K, Jacobs MR, Appelbaum PC, Sunakawa K, Ubukata K (2003) Diversity of ampicillin-resistance genes in Haemophilus influenzae in Japan and the United States. Microb Drug Resist 9(1):39–46. https://doi.org/10.1089/107662903764736337

Hatz CF, Bally B, Rohrer S, Steffen R, Kramme S, Siegrist CA, Wacker M, Alaimo C, Fonck VG (2015) Safety and immunogenicity of a candidate bioconjugate vaccine against Shigella dysenteriae type 1 administered to healthy adults: a single blind, partially randomized Phase I study. Vaccine 33(36):4594–4601. https://doi.org/10.1016/j.vaccine.2015.06.102

Haynes BF, Gilbert PB, McElrath MJ, Zolla-Pazner S, Tomaras GD, Alam SM, Evans DT, Montefiori DC, Karnasuta C, Sutthent R, Liao HX, DeVico AL, Lewis GK, Williams C, Pinter A, Fong Y, Janes H, DeCamp A, Huang Y, Rao M, Billings E, Karasavvas N, Robb ML, Ngauy V, de Souza MS, Paris R, Ferrari G, Bailer RT, Soderberg KA, Andrews C, Berman PW, Frahm N, De Rosa SC, Alpert MD, Yates NL, Shen X, Koup RA, Pitisuttithum P, Kaewkungwal J, Nitayaphan S, Rerks-Ngarm S, Michael NL, Kim JH (2012) Immune-correlates analysis of an HIV-1 vaccine efficacy trial. N Engl J Med 366(14):1275–1286. https://doi.org/10.1056/NEJMoa1113425

He M, Miyajima F, Roberts P, Ellison L, Pickard DJ, Martin MJ, Connor TR, Harris SR, Fairley D, Bamford KB, D'Arc S, Brazier J, Brown D, Coia JE, Douce G, Gerding D, Kim HJ, Koh TH, Kato H, Senoh M, Louie T, Michell S, Butt E, Peacock SJ, Brown NM, Riley T, Songer G, Wilcox M, Pirmohamed M, Kuijper E, Hawkey P, Wren BW, Dougan G, Parkhill J, Lawley TD

(2013) Emergence and global spread of epidemic healthcare-associated Clostridium difficile. Nat Genet 45(1):109–113. https://doi.org/10.1038/ng.2478

Hegerle N, Guiso N (2014) Bordetella pertussis and pertactin-deficient clinical isolates: lessons for pertussis vaccines. Expert Rev Vaccines 13(9):1135–1146. https://doi.org/10.1586/14760584.2014.932254

Hegerle N, Choi M, Sinclair J, Amin MN, Ollivault-Shiflett M, Curtis B, Laufer RS, Shridhar S, Brammer J, Toapanta FR, Holder IA, Pasetti MF, Lees A, Tennant SM, Cross AS, Simon R (2018) Development of a broad spectrum glycoconjugate vaccine to prevent wound and disseminated infections with Klebsiella pneumoniae and Pseudomonas aeruginosa. PLoS One 13(9):e0203143. https://doi.org/10.1371/journal.pone.0203143

Heikkinen T, Block SL, Toback SL, Wu X, Ambrose CS (2013) Effectiveness of intranasal live attenuated influenza vaccine against all-cause acute otitis media in children. Pediatr Infect Dis J 32(6):669–674. https://doi.org/10.1097/INF.0b013e3182840fe7

Heilmann KP, Rice CL, Miller AL, Miller NJ, Beekmann SE, Pfaller MA, Richter SS, Doern GV (2005) Decreasing prevalence of beta-lactamase production among respiratory tract isolates of Haemophilus influenzae in the United States. Antimicrob Agents Chemother 49(6):2561–2564. https://doi.org/10.1128/AAC.49.6.2561-2564.2005

Hidron AI, Kempker R, Moanna A, Rimland D (2010) Methicillin-resistant Staphylococcus aureus in HIV-infected patients. Infect Drug Resist 3:73–86

Hillier SL, Ferrieri P, Edwards MS, Ewell M, Ferris D, Fine P, Carey V, Meyn L, Hoagland D, Kasper DL, Paoletti LC, Hill H, Baker CJ (2019) A phase 2, randomized, control trial of Group B Streptococcus (GBS) type III capsular polysaccharide-tetanus toxoid (GBS III-TT) vaccine to prevent vaginal colonization with GBS III. Clin Infect Dis 68(12):2079–2086. https://doi.org/10.1093/cid/ciy838

Hindle Z, Chatfield SN, Phillimore J, Bentley M, Johnson J, Cosgrove CA, Ghaem-Maghami M, Sexton A, Khan M, Brennan FR, Everest P, Wu T, Pickard D, Holden DW, Dougan G, Griffin GE, House D, Santangelo JD, Khan SA, Shea JE, Feldman RG, Lewis DJ (2002) Characterization of Salmonella enterica derivatives harboring defined aroC and Salmonella pathogenicity island 2 type III secretion system (ssaV) mutations by immunization of healthy volunteers. Infect Immun 70(7):3457–3467. https://doi.org/10.1128/iai.70.7.3457-3467.2002

Hiramatsu K, Aritaka N, Hanaki H, Kawasaki S, Hosoda Y, Hori S, Fukuchi Y, Kobayashi I (1997a) Dissemination in Japanese hospitals of strains of Staphylococcus aureus heterogeneously resistant to vancomycin. Lancet 350(9092):1670–1673. https://doi.org/10.1016/S0140-6736(97)07324-8

Hiramatsu K, Hanaki H, Ino T, Yabuta K, Oguri T, Tenover FC (1997b) Methicillin-resistant Staphylococcus aureus clinical strain with reduced vancomycin susceptibility. J Antimicrob Chemother 40(1):135–136. https://doi.org/10.1093/jac/40.1.135

Hirschtick RE, Glassroth J, Jordan MC, Wilcosky TC, Wallace JM, Kvale PA, Markowitz N, Rosen MJ, Mangura BT, Hopewell PC (1995) Bacterial pneumonia in persons infected with the human immunodeficiency virus. Pulmonary Complications of HIV Infection Study Group. N Engl J Med 333(13):845–851. https://doi.org/10.1056/NEJM199509283331305

HIV.gov (2020) Guidelines for the prevention and treatment of opportunistic infections in adults and adolescents with HIV. https://clinicalinfo.hiv.gov/en/guidelines/adult-and-adolescent-opportunistic-infection/whats-new-guidelines. Accessed 20 Sept 2020

Hoban D, Felmingham D (2002) The PROTEKT surveillance study: antimicrobial susceptibility of Haemophilus influenzae and Moraxella catarrhalis from community-acquired respiratory tract infections. J Antimicrob Chemother 50(Suppl S1):49–59. https://doi.org/10.1093/jac/dkf810

Holden MT, Hsu LY, Kurt K, Weinert LA, Mather AE, Harris SR, Strommenger B, Layer F, Witte W, de Lencastre H, Skov R, Westh H, Zemlickova H, Coombs G, Kearns AM, Hill RL, Edgeworth J, Gould I, Gant V, Cooke J, Edwards GF, McAdam PR, Templeton KE, McCann A, Zhou Z, Castillo-Ramirez S, Feil EJ, Hudson LO, Enright MC, Balloux F, Aanensen DM, Spratt BG, Fitzgerald JR, Parkhill J, Achtman M, Bentley SD, Nubel U (2013) A genomic portrait of the emergence, evolution, and global spread of a methicillin-resistant Staphylococcus aureus pandemic. Genome Res 23(4):653–664. https://doi.org/10.1101/gr.147710.112

Hsu DC, O'Connell RJ (2017) Progress in HIV vaccine development. Hum Vaccin Immunother 13(5):1018–1030. https://doi.org/10.1080/21645515.2016.1276138

Huang DB, Mohanty A, DuPont HL, Okhuysen PC, Chiang T (2006) A review of an emerging enteric pathogen: enteroaggregative Escherichia coli. J Med Microbiol 55(Pt 10):1303–1311. https://doi.org/10.1099/jmm.0.46674-0

Huttner A, Hatz C, van den Dobbelsteen G, Abbanat D, Hornacek A, Frolich R, Dreyer AM, Martin P, Davies T, Fae K, van den Nieuwenhof I, Thoelen S, de Valliere S, Kuhn A, Bernasconi E, Viereck V, Kavvadias T, Kling K, Ryu G, Hulder T, Groger S, Scheiner D, Alaimo C, Harbarth S, Poolman J, Fonck VG (2017) Safety, immunogenicity, and preliminary clinical efficacy of a vaccine against extraintestinal pathogenic Escherichia coli in women with a history of recurrent urinary tract infection: a randomised, single-blind, placebo-controlled phase 1b trial. Lancet Infect Dis 17(5):528–537. https://doi.org/10.1016/S1473-3099(17)30108-1

Immunization Action Coalition (2019) Haemophilus influenzae type b (Hib): questions and answers, https://www.immunize.org/catg.d/p4206.pdf. Accessed 19 Sept 2019

Ingels H, Rasmussen J, Andersen PH, Harboe ZB, Glismann S, Konradsen H, Hoffmann S, Valentiner-Branth P, Lambertsen L, Danish Pneumococcal Surveillance Collaboration G (2012) Impact of pneumococcal vaccination in Denmark during the first 3 years after PCV introduction in the childhood immunization programme. Vaccine 30(26):3944–3950. https://doi.org/10.1016/j.vaccine.2012.03.060

Institute of Medicine (US) Vaccine Safety Committee (1994) Adverse events associated with childhood vaccines: evidence bearing on causality. National Academies Press (US) The National Academies Collection: Reports funded by National Institutes of Health, Washington, DC. https://doi.org/10.17226/2138

Iuliano AD, Roguski KM, Chang HH, Muscatello DJ, Palekar R, Tempia S, Cohen C, Gran JM, Schanzer D, Cowling BJ, Wu P, Kyncl J, Ang LW, Park M, Redlberger-Fritz M, Yu H, Espenhain L, Krishnan A, Emukule G, van Asten L, Pereira da Silva S, Aungkulanon S, Buchholz U, Widdowson MA, Bresee JS, Global Seasonal Influenza-associated Mortality Collaborator N (2018) Estimates of global seasonal influenza-associated respiratory mortality: a modelling study. Lancet 391(10127):1285–1300. https://doi.org/10.1016/S0140-6736(17)33293-2

Jacobs MR (2003) Worldwide trends in antimicrobial resistance among common respiratory tract pathogens in children. Pediatr Infect Dis J 22(8 Suppl):S109–S119. https://doi.org/10.1097/00006454-200308001-00002

Jacobs MR, Felmingham D, Appelbaum PC, Gruneberg RN, Alexander Project G (2003) The Alexander Project 1998–2000: susceptibility of pathogens isolated from community-acquired respiratory tract infection to commonly used antimicrobial agents. J Antimicrob Chemother 52(2):229–246. https://doi.org/10.1093/jac/dkg321

Jansen KU, Anderson AS (2018) The role of vaccines in fighting antimicrobial resistance (AMR). Hum Vaccin Immunother 14(9):2142–2149. https://doi.org/10.1080/21645515.2018.1476814

Jansen KU, Knirsch C, Anderson AS (2018) The role of vaccines in preventing bacterial antimicrobial resistance. Nat Med 24(1):10–19. https://doi.org/10.1038/nm.4465

Jares Baglivo S, Polack FP (2019) The long road to protect infants against severe RSV lower respiratory tract illness. F1000Res 8. https://doi.org/10.12688/f1000research.18749.1

Johanesen PA, Mackin KE, Hutton ML, Awad MM, Larcombe S, Amy JM, Lyras D (2015) Disruption of the gut microbiome: clostridium difficile infection and the threat of antibiotic resistance. Genes (Basel) 6(4):1347–1360. https://doi.org/10.3390/genes6041347

Johnson S, Oliver C, Prince GA, Hemming VG, Pfarr DS, Wang SC, Dormitzer M, O'Grady J, Koenig S, Tamura JK, Woods R, Bansal G, Couchenour D, Tsao E, Hall WC, Young JF (1997) Development of a humanized monoclonal antibody (MEDI-493) with potent in vitro and in vivo activity against respiratory syncytial virus. J Infect Dis 176(5):1215–1224. https://doi.org/10.1086/514115

Jones RN (2010) Microbial etiologies of hospital-acquired bacterial pneumonia and ventilator-associated bacterial pneumonia. Clin Infect Dis 51(Suppl 1):S81–S87. https://doi.org/10.1086/653053

Joseph C, Togawa Y, Shindo N (2013) Bacterial and viral infections associated with influenza. Influenza Other Respir Viruses 7(Suppl 2):105–113. https://doi.org/10.1111/irv.12089

Kamtchoua T, Bologa M, Hopfer R, Neveu D, Hu B, Sheng X, Corde N, Pouzet C, Zimmermann G, Gurunathan S (2013) Safety and immunogenicity of the pneumococcal pneumolysin derivative PlyD1 in a single-antigen protein vaccine candidate in adults. Vaccine 31(2):327–333. https://doi.org/10.1016/j.vaccine.2012.11.005

Kash JC, Taubenberger JK (2015) The role of viral, host, and secondary bacterial factors in influenza pathogenesis. Am J Pathol 185(6):1528–1536. https://doi.org/10.1016/j.ajpath.2014.08.030

Kelly CP, Pothoulakis C, LaMont JT (1994) Clostridium difficile colitis. N Engl J Med 330(4):257–262. https://doi.org/10.1056/NEJM199401273300406

Kennedy DA, Read AF (2017) Why does drug resistance readily evolve but vaccine resistance does not? Proc Biol Sci 284(1851). https://doi.org/10.1098/rspb.2016.2562

Khoshnood S, Heidary M, Haeili M, Drancourt M, Darban-Sarokhalil D, Nasiri MJ, Lohrasbi V (2018) Novel vaccine candidates against Mycobacterium tuberculosis. Int J Biol Macromol 120(Pt A):180–188. https://doi.org/10.1016/j.ijbiomac.2018.08.037

Kim H, Webster RG, Webby RJ (2018) Influenza virus: dealing with a drifting and shifting pathogen. Viral Immunol 31(2):174–183. https://doi.org/10.1089/vim.2017.0141

Kingsley RA, Msefula CL, Thomson NR, Kariuki S, Holt KE, Gordon MA, Harris D, Clarke L, Whitehead S, Sangal V, Marsh K, Achtman M, Molyneux ME, Cormican M, Parkhill J, MacLennan CA, Heyderman RS, Dougan G (2009) Epidemic multiple drug resistant Salmonella Typhimurium causing invasive disease in sub-Saharan Africa have a distinct genotype. Genome Res 19(12):2279–2287. https://doi.org/10.1101/gr.091017.109

Klein KC, Diehl EB (2004) Relationship between MMR vaccine and autism. Ann Pharmacother 38(7-8):1297–1300. https://doi.org/10.1345/aph.1D293

Klemm EJ, Shakoor S, Page AJ, Qamar FN, Judge K, Saeed DK, Wong VK, Dallman TJ, Nair S, Baker S, Shaheen G, Qureshi S, Yousafzai MT, Saleem MK, Hasan Z, Dougan G, Hasan R (2018) Emergence of an extensively drug-resistant salmonella enterica serovar typhi clone harboring a promiscuous plasmid encoding resistance to fluoroquinolones and third-generation cephalosporins. MBio 9(1). https://doi.org/10.1128/mBio.00105-18

Koch A, Cox H, Mizrahi V (2018) Drug-resistant tuberculosis: challenges and opportunities for diagnosis and treatment. Curr Opin Pharmacol 42:7–15. https://doi.org/10.1016/j.coph.2018.05.013

Kohanski MA, Dwyer DJ, Collins JJ (2010) How antibiotics kill bacteria: from targets to networks. Nat Rev Microbiol 8(6):423–435. https://doi.org/10.1038/nrmicro2333

Kotloff KL, Simon JK, Pasetti MF, Sztein MB, Wooden SL, Livio S, Nataro JP, Blackwelder WC, Barry EM, Picking W, Levine MM (2007) Safety and immunogenicity of CVD 1208S, a live, oral DeltaguaBA Deltasen Deltaset Shigella flexneri 2a vaccine grown on animal-free media. Hum Vaccin 3(6):268–275. https://doi.org/10.4161/hv.4746

Kotloff KL, Nataro JP, Blackwelder WC, Nasrin D, Farag TH, Panchalingam S, Wu Y, Sow SO, Sur D, Breiman RF, Faruque AS, Zaidi AK, Saha D, Alonso PL, Tamboura B, Sanogo D, Onwuchekwa U, Manna B, Ramamurthy T, Kanungo S, Ochieng JB, Omore R, Oundo JO, Hossain A, Das SK, Ahmed S, Qureshi S, Quadri F, Adegbola RA, Antonio M, Hossain MJ, Akinsola A, Mandomando I, Nhampossa T, Acacio S, Biswas K, O'Reilly CE, Mintz ED, Berkeley LY, Muhsen K, Sommerfelt H, Robins-Browne RM, Levine MM (2013) Burden and aetiology of diarrhoeal disease in infants and young children in developing countries (the Global Enteric Multicenter Study, GEMS): a prospective, case-control study. Lancet 382(9888):209–222. https://doi.org/10.1016/S0140-6736(13)60844-2

KPMG LLP (2014) The global economic impact of anti-microbial resistance, https://home.kpmg/content/dam/kpmg/pdf/2014/12/amr-report-final.pdf. Accessed 28 Aug 2019

Kubler-Kielb J, Vinogradov E, Mocca C, Pozsgay V, Coxon B, Robbins JB, Schneerson R (2010) Immunochemical studies of Shigella flexneri 2a and 6, and Shigella dysenteriae type 1 O-specific polysaccharide-core fragments and their protein conjugates as vaccine candidates. Carbohydr Res 345(11):1600–1608. https://doi.org/10.1016/j.carres.2010.05.006
Kuehne SA, Cartman ST, Heap JT, Kelly ML, Cockayne A, Minton NP (2010) The role of toxin A and toxin B in Clostridium difficile infection. Nature 467(7316):711–713. https://doi.org/10.1038/nature09397
Kwong JC, Maaten S, Upshur RE, Patrick DM, Marra F (2009) The effect of universal influenza immunization on antibiotic prescriptions: an ecological study. Clin Infect Dis 49(5):750–756. https://doi.org/10.1086/605087
Kyaw MH, Lynfield R, Schaffner W, Craig AS, Hadler J, Reingold A, Thomas AR, Harrison LH, Bennett NM, Farley MM, Facklam RR, Jorgensen JH, Besser J, Zell ER, Schuchat A, Whitney CG, Active Bacterial Core Surveillance of the Emerging Infections Program N (2006) Effect of introduction of the pneumococcal conjugate vaccine on drug-resistant Streptococcus pneumoniae. N Engl J Med 354(14):1455–1463. https://doi.org/10.1056/NEJMoa051642
Kyne L, Kelly CP (1998) Prospects for a vaccine for Clostridium difficile. BioDrugs 10(3):173–181. https://doi.org/10.2165/00063030-199810030-00001
Kyne L, Warny M, Qamar A, Kelly CP (2001) Association between antibody response to toxin A and protection against recurrent Clostridium difficile diarrhoea. Lancet 357(9251):189–193. https://doi.org/10.1016/S0140-6736(00)03592-3
Lai CC, Lin SH, Liao CH, Sheng WH, Hsueh PR (2014) Decline in the incidence of invasive pneumococcal disease at a medical center in Taiwan, 2000–2012. BMC Infect Dis 14:76. https://doi.org/10.1186/1471-2334-14-76
Langermann S, Mollby R, Burlein JE, Palaszynski SR, Auguste CG, DeFusco A, Strouse R, Schenerman MA, Hultgren SJ, Pinkner JS, Winberg J, Guldevall L, Soderhall M, Ishikawa K, Normark S, Koenig S (2000) Vaccination with FimH adhesin protects cynomolgus monkeys from colonization and infection by uropathogenic Escherichia coli. J Infect Dis 181(2):774–778. https://doi.org/10.1086/315258
Laurent-Ledru V, Thomson A, Monsonego J (2011) Civil society: a critical new advocate for vaccination in Europe. Vaccine 29(4):624–628. https://doi.org/10.1016/j.vaccine.2010.11.004
Laxminarayan R, Matsoso P, Pant S, Brower C, Rottingen JA, Klugman K, Davies S (2016) Access to effective antimicrobials: a worldwide challenge. Lancet 387(10014):168–175. https://doi.org/10.1016/S0140-6736(15)00474-2
Leffler DA, Lamont JT (2015) Clostridium difficile infection. N Engl J Med 372(16):1539–1548. https://doi.org/10.1056/NEJMra1403772
Leroux-Roels G, Maes C, Willekens J, De Boever F, de Rooij R, Martell L, Bedell L, Wittke F, Slobod K, Dull P (2016) A randomized, observer-blind Phase Ib study to identify formulations and vaccine schedules of a trivalent Group B Streptococcus vaccine for use in non-pregnant and pregnant women. Vaccine 34(15):1786–1791. https://doi.org/10.1016/j.vaccine.2016.02.044
Leroux-Roels G, Bebia Z, Maes C, Aerssens A, De Boever F, Grassano L, Buffi G, Margarit I, Karsten A, Cho S, Slobod K, Corsaro B, Henry O (2019) Safety and immunogenicity of a second dose of an investigational maternal trivalent Group B streptococcus vaccine in non-pregnant women 4-6 years after a first dose: results from a phase 2 trial. Clin Infect Dis. https://doi.org/10.1093/cid/ciz737
Lessa FC, Mu Y, Bamberg WM, Beldavs ZG, Dumyati GK, Dunn JR, Farley MM, Holzbauer SM, Meek JI, Phipps EC, Wilson LE, Winston LG, Cohen JA, Limbago BM, Fridkin SK, Gerding DN, McDonald LC (2015) Burden of Clostridium difficile infection in the United States. N Engl J Med 372(9):825–834. https://doi.org/10.1056/NEJMoa1408913
Levine MM, Simon R (2018) The gathering storm: is untreatable typhoid fever on the way? MBio 9(2). https://doi.org/10.1128/mBio.00482-18
Levy SB, Marshall B (2004) Antibacterial resistance worldwide: causes, challenges and responses. Nat Med 10(12 Suppl):S122–S129. https://doi.org/10.1038/nm1145

Linhares AC, Velazquez FR, Perez-Schael I, Saez-Llorens X, Abate H, Espinoza F, Lopez P, Macias-Parra M, Ortega-Barria E, Rivera-Medina DM, Rivera L, Pavia-Ruz N, Nunez E, Damaso S, Ruiz-Palacios GM, De Vos B, O'Ryan M, Gillard P, Bouckenooghe A, Human Rotavirus Vaccine Study G (2008) Efficacy and safety of an oral live attenuated human rotavirus vaccine against rotavirus gastroenteritis during the first 2 years of life in Latin American infants: a randomised, double-blind, placebo-controlled phase III study. Lancet 371(9619):1181–1189. https://doi.org/10.1016/S0140-6736(08)60524-3

Louie TJ, Miller MA, Mullane KM, Weiss K, Lentnek A, Golan Y, Gorbach S, Sears P, Shue YK, Group OPTCS (2011) Fidaxomicin versus vancomycin for Clostridium difficile infection. N Engl J Med 364(5):422–431. https://doi.org/10.1056/NEJMoa0910812

Lowy I, Molrine DC, Leav BA, Blair BM, Baxter R, Gerding DN, Nichol G, Thomas WD Jr, Leney M, Sloan S, Hay CA, Ambrosino DM (2010) Treatment with monoclonal antibodies against Clostridium difficile toxins. N Engl J Med 362(3):197–205. https://doi.org/10.1056/NEJMoa0907635

Lu B, Li D, Cui Y, Sui W, Huang L, Lu X (2014) Epidemiology of Group B streptococcus isolated from pregnant women in Beijing, China. Clin Microbiol Infect 20(6):O370–O373. https://doi.org/10.1111/1469-0691.12416

Madhi SA, Klugman KP, Vaccine Trialist G (2004) A role for Streptococcus pneumoniae in virus-associated pneumonia. Nat Med 10(8):811–813. https://doi.org/10.1038/nm1077

Madhi SA, Cunliffe NA, Steele D, Witte D, Kirsten M, Louw C, Ngwira B, Victor JC, Gillard PH, Cheuvart BB, Han HH, Neuzil KM (2010) Effect of human rotavirus vaccine on severe diarrhea in African infants. N Engl J Med 362(4):289–298. https://doi.org/10.1056/NEJMoa0904797

Magill SS, Edwards JR, Bamberg W, Beldavs ZG, Dumyati G, Kainer MA, Lynfield R, Maloney M, McAllister-Hollod L, Nadle J, Ray SM, Thompson DL, Wilson LE, Fridkin SK, Emerging Infections Program Healthcare-Associated I, Antimicrobial Use Prevalence Survey T (2014) Multistate point-prevalence survey of health care-associated infections. N Engl J Med 370(13):1198–1208. https://doi.org/10.1056/NEJMoa1306801

Mancini F, Monaci E, Lofano G, Torre A, Bacconi M, Tavarini S, Sammicheli C, Arcidiacono L, Galletti B, Laera D, Pallaoro M, Tuscano G, Fontana MR, Bensi G, Grandi G, Rossi-Paccani S, Nuti S, Rappuoli R, De Gregorio E, Bagnoli F, Soldaini E, Bertholet S (2016) One dose of Staphylococcus aureus 4C-staph vaccine formulated with a novel TLR7-dependent adjuvant rapidly protects mice through antibodies, effector CD4+ T cells, and IL-17A. PLoS One 11(1):e0147767. https://doi.org/10.1371/journal.pone.0147767

Mani S, Wierzba T, Walker RI (2016) Status of vaccine research and development for Shigella. Vaccine 34(26):2887–2894. https://doi.org/10.1016/j.vaccine.2016.02.075

Marchisio P, Esposito S, Bianchini S, Dusi E, Fusi M, Nazzari E, Picchi R, Galeone C, Principi N (2009) Efficacy of injectable trivalent virosomal-adjuvanted inactivated influenza vaccine in preventing acute otitis media in children with recurrent complicated or noncomplicated acute otitis media. Pediatr Infect Dis J 28(10):855–859. https://doi.org/10.1097/INF.0b013e3181a487b4

Marks F, von Kalckreuth V, Aaby P, Adu-Sarkodie Y, El Tayeb MA, Ali M, Aseffa A, Baker S, Biggs HM, Bjerregaard-Andersen M, Breiman RF, Campbell JI, Cosmas L, Crump JA, Espinoza LM, Deerin JF, Dekker DM, Fields BS, Gasmelseed N, Hertz JT, Van Minh HN, Im J, Jaeger A, Jeon HJ, Kabore LP, Keddy KH, Konings F, Krumkamp R, Ley B, Lofberg SV, May J, Meyer CG, Mintz ED, Montgomery JM, Niang AA, Nichols C, Olack B, Pak GD, Panzner U, Park JK, Park SE, Rabezanahary H, Rakotozandrindrainy R, Raminosoa TM, Razafindrabe TJ, Sampo E, Schutt-Gerowitt H, Sow AG, Sarpong N, Seo HJ, Sooka A, Soura AB, Tall A, Teferi M, Thriemer K, Warren MR, Yeshitela B, Clemens JD, Wierzba TF (2017) Incidence of invasive salmonella disease in sub-Saharan Africa: a multicentre population-based surveillance study. Lancet Glob Health 5(3):e310–e323. https://doi.org/10.1016/S2214-109X(17)30022-0

Marty FM, Yeh WW, Wennersten CB, Venkataraman L, Albano E, Alyea EP, Gold HS, Baden LR, Pillai SK (2006) Emergence of a clinical daptomycin-resistant Staphylococcus aureus isolate during treatment of methicillin-resistant Staphylococcus aureus bacteremia and osteomyelitis. J Clin Microbiol 44(2):595–597. https://doi.org/10.1128/JCM.44.2.595-597.2006

Matias G, Taylor R, Haguinet F, Schuck-Paim C, Lustig R, Shinde V (2014) Estimates of mortality attributable to influenza and RSV in the United States during 1997–2009 by influenza type or subtype, age, cause of death, and risk status. Influenza Other Respir Viruses 8(5):507–515. https://doi.org/10.1111/irv.12258

McDonald LC, Gerding DN, Johnson S, Bakken JS, Carroll KC, Coffin SE, Dubberke ER, Garey KW, Gould CV, Kelly C, Loo V, Shaklee Sammons J, Sandora TJ, Wilcox MH (2018) Clinical practice guidelines for clostridium difficile infection in adults and children: 2017 update by the Infectious Diseases Society of America (IDSA) and Society for Healthcare Epidemiology of America (SHEA). Clin Infect Dis 66(7):987–994. https://doi.org/10.1093/cid/ciy149

McFarland LV (1995) Epidemiology of infectious and iatrogenic nosocomial diarrhea in a cohort of general medicine patients. Am J Infect Control 23(5):295–305. https://doi.org/10.1016/0196-6553(95)90060-8

McGann P, Snesrud E, Maybank R, Corey B, Ong AC, Clifford R, Hinkle M, Whitman T, Lesho E, Schaecher KE (2016) Escherichia coli Harboring mcr-1 and blaCTX-M on a novel IncF plasmid: first report of mcr-1 in the United States. Antimicrob Agents Chemother 60(7):4420–4421. https://doi.org/10.1128/AAC.01103-16

McKenzie R, Walker RI, Nabors GS, Van De Verg LL, Carpenter C, Gomes G, Forbes E, Tian JH, Yang HH, Pace JL, Jackson WJ, Bourgeois AL (2006) Safety and immunogenicity of an oral, inactivated, whole-cell vaccine for Shigella sonnei: preclinical studies and a Phase I trial. Vaccine 24(18):3735–3745. https://doi.org/10.1016/j.vaccine.2005.07.014

McLellan JS, Chen M, Leung S, Graepel KW, Du X, Yang Y, Zhou T, Baxa U, Yasuda E, Beaumont T, Kumar A, Modjarrad K, Zheng Z, Zhao M, Xia N, Kwong PD, Graham BS (2013) Structure of RSV fusion glycoprotein trimer bound to a prefusion-specific neutralizing antibody. Science 340(6136):1113–1117. https://doi.org/10.1126/science.1234914

McNeely TB, Shah NA, Fridman A, Joshi A, Hartzel JS, Keshari RS, Lupu F, DiNubile MJ (2014) Mortality among recipients of the Merck V710 Staphylococcus aureus vaccine after postoperative S. aureus infections: an analysis of possible contributing host factors. Hum Vaccin Immunother 10(12):3513–3516. https://doi.org/10.4161/hv.34407

Merck (2016) Zinplava. Prescribing information, https://www.merck.com/product/usa/pi_circulars/z/zinplava/zinplava_pi.pdf. Accessed 28 Sept 2019

Mertz D, Kim TH, Johnstone J, Lam PP, Science M, Kuster SP, Fadel SA, Tran D, Fernandez E, Bhatnagar N, Loeb M (2013) Populations at risk for severe or complicated influenza illness: systematic review and meta-analysis. BMJ 347:f5061. https://doi.org/10.1136/bmj.f5061

Meynet E, Laurin D, Lenormand JL, Camara B, Toussaint B, Le Gouellec A (2018) Killed but metabolically active Pseudomonas aeruginosa-based vaccine induces protective humoral- and cell-mediated immunity against Pseudomonas aeruginosa pulmonary infections. Vaccine 36(14):1893–1900. https://doi.org/10.1016/j.vaccine.2018.02.040

Micoli F, Rondini S, Gavini M, Lanzilao L, Medaglini D, Saul A, Martin LB (2012) O:2-CRM(197) conjugates against Salmonella Paratyphi A. PLoS One 7(11):e47039. https://doi.org/10.1371/journal.pone.0047039

Miriagou V, Tassios PT, Legakis NJ, Tzouvelekis LS (2004) Expanded-spectrum cephalosporin resistance in non-typhoid Salmonella. Int J Antimicrob Agents 23(6):547–555. https://doi.org/10.1016/j.ijantimicag.2004.03.006

Moffitt K, Malley R (2016) Rationale and prospects for novel pneumococcal vaccines. Hum Vaccin Immunother 12(2):383–392. https://doi.org/10.1080/21645515.2015.1087625

Mogasale V, Maskery B, Ochiai RL, Lee JS, Mogasale VV, Ramani E, Kim YE, Park JK, Wierzba TF (2014) Burden of typhoid fever in low-income and middle-income countries: a systematic, literature-based update with risk-factor adjustment. Lancet Glob Health 2(10):e570–e580. https://doi.org/10.1016/S2214-109X(14)70301-8

Mok W (2018) Vaccine investment strategy: short list. Gavi, The Vaccine Alliance. Board Meeting. Geneva, Switzerland, 6–7 June 2018, https://www.gavi.org/about/governance/gavi-board/minutes/2018/6-june/. Accessed 7 Oct 2019.

Morris DE, Cleary DW, Clarke SC (2017) Secondary bacterial infections associated with influenza pandemics. Front Microbiol 8:1041. https://doi.org/10.3389/fmicb.2017.01041
Morrissey I, Maher K, Williams L, Shackcloth J, Felmingham D, Reynolds R, Surveillance BWPoR (2008) Non-susceptibility trends among Haemophilus influenzae and Moraxella catarrhalis from community-acquired respiratory tract infections in the UK and Ireland, 1999–2007. J Antimicrob Chemother 62(Suppl 2):97–103. https://doi.org/10.1093/jac/dkn356
Moura I, Spigaglia P, Barbanti F, Mastrantonio P (2013) Analysis of metronidazole susceptibility in different Clostridium difficile PCR ribotypes. J Antimicrob Chemother 68(2):362–365. https://doi.org/10.1093/jac/dks420
Mousa JJ, Kose N, Matta P, Gilchuk P, Crowe JE Jr (2017) A novel pre-fusion conformation-specific neutralizing epitope on the respiratory syncytial virus fusion protein. Nat Microbiol 2:16271. https://doi.org/10.1038/nmicrobiol.2016.271
Mukesi M, Iweriebor BC, Obi LC, Nwodo UU, Moyo SR, Okoh AI (2019) Prevalence and capsular type distribution of Streptococcus agalactiae isolated from pregnant women in Namibia and South Africa. BMC Infect Dis 19(1):179. https://doi.org/10.1186/s12879-019-3809-6
N'Cho HS, Masunda KPE, Mukeredzi I, Manangazira P, Govore E, Duri C, Aubert RD, Martin H, Gonese E, Vere M, Tippett Barr BA, Balachandra S, Strysko J, Davis WW, Appiah GD, Mintz E (2019) Notes from the field: typhoid fever outbreak – Harare, Zimbabwe, October 2017–February 2018. MMWR Morb Mortal Wkly Rep 68(2):44–45. https://doi.org/10.15585/mmwr.mm6802a5
Nair H, Nokes DJ, Gessner BD, Dherani M, Madhi SA, Singleton RJ, O'Brien KL, Roca A, Wright PF, Bruce N, Chandran A, Theodoratou E, Sutanto A, Sedyaningsih ER, Ngama M, Munywoki PK, Kartasasmita C, Simoes EA, Rudan I, Weber MW, Campbell H (2010) Global burden of acute lower respiratory infections due to respiratory syncytial virus in young children: a systematic review and meta-analysis. Lancet 375(9725):1545–1555. https://doi.org/10.1016/S0140-6736(10)60206-1
National Institute of Allergy and Infectious Diseases (NIAID) (2016) Large-scale HIV vaccine trial to launch in South Africa. NIH-Funded Study Will Test Safety, Efficacy of Vaccine Regimen, https://www.niaid.nih.gov/news-events/large-scale-hiv-vaccine-trial-launch-south-africa. Accessed 11 Jul 2019
National Vaccine Advisory Committee (2016) A call for greater consideration for the role of vaccines in National strategies to combat antibiotic-resistant bacteria: recommendations from the National Vaccine Advisory Committee, https://www.hhs.gov/sites/default/files/nvpo/nvac/reports/nvac-antibioticresistance.pdf. Accessed 14 Sept 2019
Nelson MR, Shanson DC, Hawkins DA, Gazzard BG (1992) Salmonella, Campylobacter and Shigella in HIV-seropositive patients. AIDS 6(12):1495–1498. https://doi.org/10.1097/00002030-199212000-00012
Nemes E, Geldenhuys H, Rozot V, Rutkowski KT, Ratangee F, Bilek N, Mabwe S, Makhethe L, Erasmus M, Toefy A, Mulenga H, Hanekom WA, Self SG, Bekker LG, Ryall R, Gurunathan S, DiazGranados CA, Andersen P, Kromann I, Evans T, Ellis RD, Landry B, Hokey DA, Hopkins R, Ginsberg AM, Scriba TJ, Hatherill M, Team CS (2018) Prevention of M. tuberculosis infection with H4:IC31 Vaccine or BCG revaccination. N Engl J Med 379(2):138–149. https://doi.org/10.1056/NEJMoa1714021
Nesta B, Pizza M (2018) Vaccines against Escherichia coli. Curr Top Microbiol Immunol 416:213–242. https://doi.org/10.1007/82_2018_111
Neu HC (1992) The crisis in antibiotic resistance. Science 257(5073):1064–1073. https://doi.org/10.1126/science.257.5073.1064
Ngwuta JO, Chen M, Modjarrad K, Joyce MG, Kanekiyo M, Kumar A, Yassine HM, Moin SM, Killikelly AM, Chuang GY, Druz A, Georgiev IS, Rundlet EJ, Sastry M, Stewart-Jones GB, Yang Y, Zhang B, Nason MC, Capella C, Peeples ME, Ledgerwood JE, McLellan JS, Kwong PD, Graham BS (2015) Prefusion F-specific antibodies determine the magnitude of RSV neutralizing activity in human sera. Sci Transl Med 7(309):309ra162. https://doi.org/10.1126/scitranslmed.aac4241

Nordmann P, Naas T, Poirel L (2011) Global spread of Carbapenemase-producing Enterobacteriaceae. Emerg Infect Dis 17(10):1791–1798. https://doi.org/10.3201/eid1710.110655

Novavax (2019a) Novavax announces presentation of phase 3 data from RSV maternal immunization program at 37th annual meeting of the European Society for Pediatric Infectious Diseases, https://www.globenewswire.com/news-release/2019/05/01/1813825/0/en/Novavax-Announces-Presentation-of-Phase-3-Data-from-RSV-Maternal-Immunization-Program-at-37th-Annual-Meeting-of-the-European-Society-for-Pediatric-Infectious-Diseases.html. Accessed 6 Oct 2019

Novavax (2019b) Novavax announces topline results from phase 3 prepareTM trial of ResVax™ for prevention of RSV disease in infants via maternal immunization, http://ir.novavax.com/news-releases/news-release-details/novavax-announces-topline-results-phase-3-preparetm-trial. Accessed 11 Oct 2019

Nyirenda TS, Gilchrist JJ, Feasey NA, Glennie SJ, Bar-Zeev N, Gordon MA, MacLennan CA, Mandala WL, Heyderman RS (2014) Sequential acquisition of T cells and antibodies to nontyphoidal Salmonella in Malawian children. J Infect Dis 210(1):56–64. https://doi.org/10.1093/infdis/jiu045

O'Neill J (2014) Antimicrobial resistance: tackling a crisis for the health and wealth of nations. https://amr-review.org/sites/default/files/AMR%20Review%20Paper%20-%20Tackling%20a%20crisis%20for%20the%20health%20and%20wealth%20of%20nations_1.pdf. Accessed 20 Sept 2020

O'Neill J (2016a) Tackling drug-resistant infections globally: final report and recommendations. https://dlcs.io/file/wellcome/5/b28644797_160525_Final%20paper_with%20cover.pdf. Accessed 20 Sept 2020

O'Neill J (2016b) Vaccines and alternative appoaches: reducing our dependence on antimicrobials. The Review on Antimicrobial Resistance. https://amr-review.org/sites/default/files/Vaccines%20and%20alternatives_v4_LR.pdf. Accessed 20 Sept 2020

Obiero CW, Ndiaye AGW, Scire AS, Kaunyangi BM, Marchetti E, Gone AM, Schutte LD, Riccucci D, Auerbach J, Saul A, Martin LB, Bejon P, Njuguna P, Podda A (2017) A phase 2a randomized study to evaluate the safety and immunogenicity of the 1790GAHB generalized modules for membrane antigen vaccine against Shigella sonnei administered intramuscularly to adults from a Shigellosis-endemic country. Front Immunol 8:1884. https://doi.org/10.3389/fimmu.2017.01884

Octavia S, Sintchenko V, Gilbert GL, Lawrence A, Keil AD, Hogg G, Lan R (2012) Newly emerging clones of Bordetella pertussis carrying prn2 and ptxP3 alleles implicated in Australian pertussis epidemic in 2008–2010. J Infect Dis 205(8):1220–1224. https://doi.org/10.1093/infdis/jis178

Olaru ID, Mtapuri-Zinyowera S, Feasey N, Ferrand RA, Kranzer K (2019) Typhoid Vi-conjugate vaccine for outbreak control in Zimbabwe. Lancet Infect Dis 19(9):930. https://doi.org/10.1016/S1473-3099(19)30425-6

Orr N, Katz DE, Atsmon J, Radu P, Yavzori M, Halperin T, Sela T, Kayouf R, Klein Z, Ambar R, Cohen D, Wolf MK, Venkatesan MM, Hale TL (2005) Community-based safety, immunogenicity, and transmissibility study of the Shigella sonnei WRSS1 vaccine in Israeli volunteers. Infect Immun 73(12):8027–8032. https://doi.org/10.1128/IAI.73.12.8027-8032.2005

Ozgur SK, Beyazova U, Kemaloglu YK, Maral I, Sahin F, Camurdan AD, Kizil Y, Dinc E, Tuzun H (2006) Effectiveness of inactivated influenza vaccine for prevention of otitis media in children. Pediatr Infect Dis J 25(5):401–404. https://doi.org/10.1097/01.inf.0000217370.83948.51

Parry CM, Ribeiro I, Walia K, Rupali P, Baker S, Basnyat B (2019) Multidrug resistant enteric fever in South Asia: unmet medical needs and opportunities. BMJ 364:k5322. https://doi.org/10.1136/bmj.k5322

Patel MM, Steele D, Gentsch JR, Wecker J, Glass RI, Parashar UD (2011) Real-world impact of rotavirus vaccination. Pediatr Infect Dis J 30(1 Suppl):S1–S5. https://doi.org/10.1097/INF.0b013e3181fefa1f

PATH (2019) RSV Vaccine and mAb Snapshot. https://path.azureedge.net/media/documents/RSV-snapshot-2019_08_28_High_Resolution_PDF.pdf. Accessed 17 Oct 2019

Peltola H, Rod TO, Jonsdottir K, Bottiger M, Coolidge JA (1990) Life-threatening Haemophilus influenzae infections in Scandinavia: a five-country analysis of the incidence and the main clinical and bacteriologic characteristics. Rev Infect Dis 12(4):708–715. https://doi.org/10.1093/clinids/12.4.708

Peltola H, Aavitsland P, Hansen KG, Jonsdottir KE, Nokleby H, Romanus V (1999) Perspective: a five-country analysis of the impact of four different Haemophilus influenzae type b conjugates and vaccination strategies in Scandinavia. J Infect Dis 179(1):223–229. https://doi.org/10.1086/314535

Peng Z, Jin D, Kim HB, Stratton CW, Wu B, Tang YW, Sun X (2017) Update on antimicrobial resistance in Clostridium difficile: resistance mechanisms and antimicrobial susceptibility testing. J Clin Microbiol 55(7):1998–2008. https://doi.org/10.1128/JCM.02250-16

Penn-Nicholson A, Tameris M, Smit E, Day TA, Musvosvi M, Jayashankar L, Vergara J, Mabwe S, Bilek N, Geldenhuys H, Luabeya AK, Ellis R, Ginsberg AM, Hanekom WA, Reed SG, Coler RN, Scriba TJ, Hatherill M, team T-s (2018) Safety and immunogenicity of the novel tuberculosis vaccine ID93 + GLA-SE in BCG-vaccinated healthy adults in South Africa: a randomised, double-blind, placebo-controlled phase 1 trial. Lancet Respir Med 6(4):287–298. https://doi.org/10.1016/S2213-2600(18)30077-8

Pepin J, Valiquette L, Cossette B (2005) Mortality attributable to nosocomial Clostridium difficile-associated disease during an epidemic caused by a hypervirulent strain in Quebec. CMAJ 173(9):1037–1042. https://doi.org/10.1503/cmaj.050978

Perry J, Waglechner N, Wright G (2016) The prehistory of antibiotic resistance. Cold Spring Harb Perspect Med 6(6). https://doi.org/10.1101/cshperspect.a025197

Pfizer (2018) Independent data monitoring committee recommends discontinuation of the phase 2b STRIVE clinical trial of Staphylococcus aureus vaccine following planned interim analysis. https://www.pfizer.com/news/press-release/press-release-detail/independent_data_monitoring_committee_recommends_discontinuation_of_the_phase_2b_strive_clinical_trial_of_staphylococcus_aureus_vaccine_following_planned_interim_analysis. Accessed 21 Aug 2019

Pilishvili T, Lexau C, Farley MM, Hadler J, Harrison LH, Bennett NM, Reingold A, Thomas A, Schaffner W, Craig AS, Smith PJ, Beall BW, Whitney CG, Moore MR, Active Bacterial Core Surveillance/Emerging Infections Program N (2010) Sustained reductions in invasive pneumococcal disease in the era of conjugate vaccine. J Infect Dis 201(1):32–41. https://doi.org/10.1086/648593

Plotkin S (2014) History of vaccination. Proc Natl Acad Sci U S A 111(34):12283–12287. https://doi.org/10.1073/pnas.1400472111

Polage CR, Gyorke CE, Kennedy MA, Leslie JL, Chin DL, Wang S, Nguyen HH, Huang B, Tang YW, Lee LW, Kim K, Taylor S, Romano PS, Panacek EA, Goodell PB, Solnick JV, Cohen SH (2015) Overdiagnosis of Clostridium difficile infection in the molecular test era. JAMA Intern Med 175(11):1792–1801. https://doi.org/10.1001/jamainternmed.2015.4114

Pollard SL, Malpica-Llanos T, Friberg IK, Fischer-Walker C, Ashraf S, Walker N (2015) Estimating the herd immunity effect of rotavirus vaccine. Vaccine 33(32):3795–3800. https://doi.org/10.1016/j.vaccine.2015.06.064

Polsky B, Gold JW, Whimbey E, Dryjanski J, Brown AE, Schiffman G, Armstrong D (1986) Bacterial pneumonia in patients with the acquired immunodeficiency syndrome. Ann Intern Med 104(1):38–41. https://doi.org/10.7326/0003-4819-104-1-38

Poolman JT, Wacker M (2016) Extraintestinal pathogenic Escherichia coli, a common human pathogen: challenges for vaccine development and progress in the field. J Infect Dis 213(1):6–13. https://doi.org/10.1093/infdis/jiv429

Pozsgay V, Glaudemans CP, Robbins JB, Schneerson R (1993) Synthesis of a tetrasaccharide donor corresponding to the O-specific polysaccharide of Shigella dysenteriae type 1. Carbohydr Res 244(2):259–273. https://doi.org/10.1016/0008-6215(83)85006-x

Prasso JE, Deng JC (2017) Postviral complications: bacterial pneumonia. Clin Chest Med 38(1):127–138. https://doi.org/10.1016/j.ccm.2016.11.006

Pray L (2008) Antibiotic R&D: resolving the paradox between unmet medical need and commercial incentive. Cambridge Healthtech Institute, Needham, MA

Prymula R, Szenborn L, Silfverdal SA, Wysocki J, Albrecht P, Traskine M, Gardev A, Song Y, Borys D (2017) Safety, reactogenicity and immunogenicity of two investigational pneumococcal protein-based vaccines: results from a randomized phase II study in infants. Vaccine 35(35 Pt B):4603–4611. https://doi.org/10.1016/j.vaccine.2017.07.008

Qamar FN, Yousafzai MT, Khalid M, Kazi AM, Lohana H, Karim S, Khan A, Hotwani A, Qureshi S, Kabir F, Aziz F, Memon NM, Domki MH, Hasan R (2018) Outbreak investigation of ceftriaxone-resistant Salmonella enterica serotype Typhi and its risk factors among the general population in Hyderabad, Pakistan: a matched case-control study. Lancet Infect Dis 18(12):1368–1376. https://doi.org/10.1016/S1473-3099(18)30483-3

Raviglione M, Marais B, Floyd K, Lonnroth K, Getahun H, Migliori GB, Harries AD, Nunn P, Lienhardt C, Graham S, Chakaya J, Weyer K, Cole S, Kaufmann SH, Zumla A (2012) Scaling up interventions to achieve global tuberculosis control: progress and new developments. Lancet 379(9829):1902–1913. https://doi.org/10.1016/S0140-6736(12)60727-2

Rello J, Krenn CG, Locker G, Pilger E, Madl C, Balica L, Dugernier T, Laterre PF, Spapen H, Depuydt P, Vincent JL, Bogar L, Szabo Z, Volgyes B, Manez R, Cakar N, Ramazanoglu A, Topeli A, Mastruzzo MA, Jasovich A, Remolif CG, Del Carmen SL, Andresen Hernandez MA, Ruiz Balart C, Kremer I, Molnar Z, von Sonnenburg F, Lyons A, Joannidis M, Burgmann H, Welte T, Klingler A, Hochreiter R, Westritschnig K (2017) A randomized placebo-controlled phase II study of a Pseudomonas vaccine in ventilated ICU patients. Crit Care 21(1):22. https://doi.org/10.1186/s13054-017-1601-9

Rerks-Ngarm S, Pitisuttithum P, Nitayaphan S, Kaewkungwal J, Chiu J, Paris R, Premsri N, Namwat C, de Souza M, Adams E, Benenson M, Gurunathan S, Tartaglia J, McNeil JG, Francis DP, Stablein D, Birx DL, Chunsuttiwat S, Khamboonruang C, Thongcharoen P, Robb ML, Michael NL, Kunasol P, Kim JH, Investigators M-T (2009) Vaccination with ALVAC and AIDSVAX to prevent HIV-1 infection in Thailand. N Engl J Med 361(23):2209–2220. https://doi.org/10.1056/NEJMoa0908492

Review on Antimicrobial Resistance (2016) Declaration by the pharmaceutical, biotechnology and diagnostics industries on combating antimicrobial resistance. https://amr-review.org/sites/default/files/Declaration_of_Support_for_Combating_AMR_Jan_2016.pdf. Accessed 16 Jun 2019

Rey-Jurado E, Kalergis AM (2017) Immunological features of respiratory syncytial virus-caused pneumonia-implications for vaccine design. Int J Mol Sci 18(3). https://doi.org/10.3390/ijms18030556

Riddle MS, Kaminski RW, Williams C, Porter C, Baqar S, Kordis A, Gilliland T, Lapa J, Coughlin M, Soltis C, Jones E, Saunders J, Keiser PB, Ranallo RT, Gormley R, Nelson M, Turbyfill KR, Tribble D, Oaks EV (2011) Safety and immunogenicity of an intranasal Shigella flexneri 2a Invaplex 50 vaccine. Vaccine 29(40):7009–7019. https://doi.org/10.1016/j.vaccine.2011.07.033

Riddle MS, Kaminski RW, Di Paolo C, Porter CK, Gutierrez RL, Clarkson KA, Weerts HE, Duplessis C, Castellano A, Alaimo C, Paolino K, Gormley R, Gambillara Fonck V (2016) Safety and immunogenicity of a candidate bioconjugate vaccine against Shigella flexneri 2a administered to healthy adults: a single-blind, randomized phase I study. Clin Vaccine Immunol 23(12):908–917. https://doi.org/10.1128/CVI.00224-16

Robbins JB, Schneerson R (1990) Polysaccharide-protein conjugates: a new generation of vaccines. J Infect Dis 161(5):821–832. https://doi.org/10.1093/infdis/161.5.821

Robbins JB, Chu C, Watson DC, Szu SC, Daniels EM, Lowe CU, Schneerson R (1991) O-specific side-chain toxin-protein conjugates as parenteral vaccines for the prevention of shigellosis and related diseases. Rev Infect Dis 13(Suppl 4):S362–S365. https://doi.org/10.1093/clinids/13.supplement_4.s362

Robbins JB, Kubler-Kielb J, Vinogradov E, Mocca C, Pozsgay V, Shiloach J, Schneerson R (2009) Synthesis, characterization, and immunogenicity in mice of Shigella sonnei O-specific oligosaccharide-core-protein conjugates. Proc Natl Acad Sci U S A 106(19):7974–7978. https://doi.org/10.1073/pnas.0900891106

Rose F, Roovers S, Fano M, Harloff-Helleberg S, Kirkensgaard JJK, Hejnaes K, Fischer P, Foged C (2018) Temperature-induced self-assembly of the Group B Streptococcus (GBS) fusion antigen GBS-NN. Mol Pharm 15(7):2584–2593. https://doi.org/10.1021/acs.molpharmaceut.8b00101

Rudnick W, Liu Z, Shigayeva A, Low DE, Green K, Plevneshi A, Devlin R, Downey J, Katz K, Kitai I, Krajden S, Ostrowska K, Richardson D, Richardson S, Sarabia A, Silverman M, Simor AE, Tyrrell G, McGeer A, Toronto Invasive Bacterial Diseases N (2013) Pneumococcal vaccination programs and the burden of invasive pneumococcal disease in Ontario, Canada, 1995–2011. Vaccine 31(49):5863–5871. https://doi.org/10.1016/j.vaccine.2013.09.049

Russo TA, Johnson JR (2003) Medical and economic impact of extraintestinal infections due to Escherichia coli: focus on an increasingly important endemic problem. Microbes Infect 5(5):449–456

Safarchi A, Octavia S, Luu LD, Tay CY, Sintchenko V, Wood N, Marshall H, McIntyre P, Lan R (2015) Pertactin negative Bordetella pertussis demonstrates higher fitness under vaccine selection pressure in a mixed infection model. Vaccine 33(46):6277–6281. https://doi.org/10.1016/j.vaccine.2015.09.064

Saha S, Kapoor S, Tariq R, Schuetz AN, Tosh PK, Pardi DS, Khanna S (2019) Increasing antibiotic resistance in Clostridioides difficile: a systematic review and meta-analysis. Anaerobe 58:35–46. https://doi.org/10.1016/j.anaerobe.2019.102072

Sahastrabuddhe S, Saluja T (2019) Overview of the typhoid conjugate vaccine pipeline: current status and future plans. Clin Infect Dis 68(Supplement_1):S22–S26. https://doi.org/10.1093/cid/ciy884

Sanchez TH, Brooks JT, Sullivan PS, Juhasz M, Mintz E, Dworkin MS, Jones JL, Adult/Adolescent Spectrum of HIVDSG (2005) Bacterial diarrhea in persons with HIV infection, United States, 1992–2002. Clin Infect Dis 41(11):1621–1627. https://doi.org/10.1086/498027

Sanofi (2017) Sanofi ends development of Clostridium difficile vaccine. https://www.sanofi.com/-/media/Project/One-Sanofi-Web/Websites/Global/Sanofi-COM/Home/media-room/press-releases/2017/2017-12-01-22-00-00-1216392-en.pdf. Accessed 1 Jul 2019

Sastry M, Zhang B, Chen M, Joyce MG, Kong WP, Chuang GY, Ko K, Kumar A, Silacci C, Thom M, Salazar AM, Corti D, Lanzavecchia A, Taylor G, Mascola JR, Graham BS, Kwong PD (2017) Adjuvants and the vaccine response to the DS-Cav1-stabilized fusion glycoprotein of respiratory syncytial virus. PLoS One 12(10):e0186854. https://doi.org/10.1371/journal.pone.0186854

Schmidt CS, White CJ, Ibrahim AS, Filler SG, Fu Y, Yeaman MR, Edwards JE Jr, Hennessey JP Jr (2012) NDV-3, a recombinant alum-adjuvanted vaccine for Candida and Staphylococcus aureus, is safe and immunogenic in healthy adults. Vaccine 30(52):7594–7600. https://doi.org/10.1016/j.vaccine.2012.10.038

Schmoele-Thoma B, Falsey AR, Walsh EE, Swanson K, Zareba A, Cooper D, Gruber W, Jansen KU, Radley D, Scott D, Dormitzer P (2019) Phase 1/2, first-in-human study of the safety, tolerability, and immunogenicity of a RSV prefusion F-based subunit vaccine candidate. IDWeek Washington, DC 2-6 Oct 2019 PO2755

Schrag S, Gorwitz R, Fultz-Butts K, Schuchat A (2002) Prevention of perinatal group B streptococcal disease. Revised guidelines from CDC. MMWR Recomm Rep 51(RR-11):1–22

Scorza FB, Pardi N (2018) New kids on the block: RNA-based influenza virus vaccines. Vaccines (Basel) 6(2). https://doi.org/10.3390/vaccines6020020

Sharma SK, Katoch K, Sarin R, Balambal R, Kumar Jain N, Patel N, Murthy KJR, Singla N, Saha PK, Khanna A, Singh U, Kumar S, Sengupta A, Banavaliker JN, Chauhan DS, Sachan S, Wasim M, Tripathi S, Dutt N, Jain N, Joshi N, Penmesta SRR, Gaddam S, Gupta S, Khamar B, Dey B, Mitra DK, Arora SK, Bhaskar S, Rani R (2017) Efficacy and safety of mycobacterium indicus pranii as an adjunct therapy in category II pulmonary tuberculosis in a randomized trial. Sci Rep 7(1):3354. https://doi.org/10.1038/s41598-017-03514-1

Shen AK, Cooke MT (2019) Infectious disease vaccines. Nat Rev Drug Discov 18(3):169–170. https://doi.org/10.1038/d41573-018-00011-6

Sheppard DC, Yeaman MR, Welch WH, Phan QT, Fu Y, Ibrahim AS, Filler SG, Zhang M, Waring AJ, Edwards JE Jr (2004) Functional and structural diversity in the Als protein family of Candida albicans. J Biol Chem 279(29):30480–30489. https://doi.org/10.1074/jbc.M401929200

Shokeir AA, Hussein MI (1999) The urology of pharaonic Egypt. BJU Int 84(7):755–761. https://doi.org/10.1046/j.1464-410x.1999.00313.x

Simioni J, Hutton EK, Gunn E, Holloway AC, Stearns JC, McDonald H, Mousseau A, Schertzer JD, Ratcliffe EM, Thabane L, Surette MG, Morrison KM (2016) A comparison of intestinal microbiota in a population of low-risk infants exposed and not exposed to intrapartum antibiotics: The Baby & Microbiota of the Intestine cohort study protocol. BMC Pediatr 16(1):183. https://doi.org/10.1186/s12887-016-0724-5

Simoes EA, Tan DH, Ohlsson A, Sales V, Wang EE (2001) Respiratory syncytial virus vaccine: a systematic overview with emphasis on respiratory syncytial virus subunit vaccines. Vaccine 20(5-6):954–960. https://doi.org/10.1016/s0264-410x(01)00388-7

Simor AE (2010) Diagnosis, management, and prevention of Clostridium difficile infection in long-term care facilities: a review. J Am Geriatr Soc 58(8):1556–1564. https://doi.org/10.1111/j.1532-5415.2010.02958.x

Smith MJ, Woods CR (2010) On-time vaccine receipt in the first year does not adversely affect neuropsychological outcomes. Pediatrics 125(6):1134–1141. https://doi.org/10.1542/peds.2009-2489

Spigaglia P (2016) Recent advances in the understanding of antibiotic resistance in Clostridium difficile infection. Ther Adv Infect Dis 3(1):23–42. https://doi.org/10.1177/2049936115622891

Spigaglia P, Barbanti F, Mastrantonio P, European Study Group on Clostridium d (2011) Multidrug resistance in European Clostridium difficile clinical isolates. J Antimicrob Chemother 66(10):2227–2234. https://doi.org/10.1093/jac/dkr292

Steele AD, Hay Burgess DC, Diaz Z, Carey ME, Zaidi AK (2016) Challenges and opportunities for typhoid fever control: a call for coordinated action. Clin Infect Dis 62(Suppl 1):S4–S8. https://doi.org/10.1093/cid/civ976

Steinhoff M, Goldblatt D (2003) Conjugate Hib vaccines. Lancet 361(9355):360–361. https://doi.org/10.1016/S0140-6736(03)12441-5

Tack DM, Marder EP, Griffin PM, Cieslak PR, Dunn J, Hurd S, Scallan E, Lathrop S, Muse A, Ryan P, Smith K, Tobin-D'Angelo M, Vugia DJ, Holt KG, Wolpert BJ, Tauxe R, Geissler AL (2019) Preliminary Incidence and Trends of Infections with Pathogens Transmitted Commonly Through Food – Foodborne Diseases Active Surveillance Network, 10 U.S. Sites, 2015-2018. MMWR Morb Mortal Wkly Rep 68(16):369–373. https://doi.org/10.15585/mmwr.mm6816a2

Tagliabue A, Rappuoli R (2018) Changing priorities in vaccinology: antibiotic resistance moving to the top. Front Immunol 9:1068. https://doi.org/10.3389/fimmu.2018.01068

Tameris MD, Hatherill M, Landry BS, Scriba TJ, Snowden MA, Lockhart S, Shea JE, McClain JB, Hussey GD, Hanekom WA, Mahomed H, McShane H, Team MATS (2013) Safety and efficacy of MVA85A, a new tuberculosis vaccine, in infants previously vaccinated with BCG: a randomised, placebo-controlled phase 2b trial. Lancet 381(9871):1021–1028. https://doi.org/10.1016/S0140-6736(13)60177-4

Taylor J, Hafner M, Yerushalmi E, Smith R, Bellasio J, Vardavas R, Bienkowska-Gibbs T, Rubin J (2014a) Estimating the economic costs of antimicrobial resistance: model and results. SantaMonica, CA: RAND Corporation https://www.rand.org/content/dam/rand/pubs/research_reports/RR900/RR911/RAND_RR911.pdf. Accessed 28 Jun 2019

Taylor LE, Swerdfeger AL, Eslick GD (2014b) Vaccines are not associated with autism: an evidence-based meta-analysis of case-control and cohort studies. Vaccine 32(29):3623–3629. https://doi.org/10.1016/j.vaccine.2014.04.085

Tenover FC, Tickler IA, Persing DH (2012) Antimicrobial-resistant strains of Clostridium difficile from North America. Antimicrob Agents Chemother 56(6):2929–2932. https://doi.org/10.1128/AAC.00220-12

The IMpact-RSV Study Group (1998) Palivizumab, a humanized respiratory syncytial virus monoclonal antibody, reduces hospitalization from respiratory syncytial virus infection in high-risk infants. Pediatrics 102(3 Pt 1):531–537

The Lancet (2017) National progress on antimicrobial resistance. Lancet 389(10084):2082. https://doi.org/10.1016/S0140-6736(17)31433-2

The Organisation for Economic Co-operation and Development (OECD) (2019) Antimicrobial resistance: tackling the burden in the European Union. https://www.oecd.org/health/health-systems/AMR-Tackling-the-Burden-in-the-EU-OECD-ECDC-Briefing-Note-2019.pdf. Accessed 08 Jan 2020

The White House (2014) Executive order – combating antibiotic-resistant bacteria. https://obamawhitehouse.archives.gov/the-press-office/2014/09/18/executive-order-combating-antibiotic-resistant-bacteria. Accessed 16 Sept 2019

The White House (2015) National action plan for combating antibiotic-resistant bacteria. https://obamawhitehouse.archives.gov/sites/default/files/docs/national_action_plan_for_combating_antibotic-resistant_bacteria.pdf. Accessed 16 Sept 2019

Thornsberry C, Kirven LA (1974) Antimicrobial susceptibility of Haemophilus influenzae. Antimicrob Agents Chemother 6(5):620–624. https://doi.org/10.1128/aac.6.5.620

Thornton J (2019) Polio returns to the Philippines. Lancet 394(10205):1217. https://doi.org/10.1016/S0140-6736(19)32263-9

Tian JH, Fuhrmann SR, Kluepfel-Stahl S, Carman RJ, Ellingsworth L, Flyer DC (2012) A novel fusion protein containing the receptor binding domains of C. difficile toxin A and toxin B elicits protective immunity against lethal toxin and spore challenge in preclinical efficacy models. Vaccine 30(28):4249–4258. https://doi.org/10.1016/j.vaccine.2012.04.045

Tomczyk S, Lynfield R, Schaffner W, Reingold A, Miller L, Petit S, Holtzman C, Zansky SM, Thomas A, Baumbach J, Harrison LH, Farley MM, Beall B, McGee L, Gierke R, Pondo T, Kim L (2016) Prevention of antibiotic-nonsusceptible invasive pneumococcal disease with the 13-valent pneumococcal conjugate vaccine. Clin Infect Dis 62(9):1119–1125. https://doi.org/10.1093/cid/ciw067

Tomeny TS, Vargo CJ, El-Toukhy S (2017) Geographic and demographic correlates of autism-related anti-vaccine beliefs on Twitter, 2009-15. Soc Sci Med 191:168–175. https://doi.org/10.1016/j.socscimed.2017.08.041

Tong SY, Davis JS, Eichenberger E, Holland TL, Fowler VG Jr (2015) Staphylococcus aureus infections: epidemiology, pathophysiology, clinical manifestations, and management. Clin Microbiol Rev 28(3):603–661. https://doi.org/10.1128/CMR.00134-14

Tribble D, Kaminski R, Cantrell J, Nelson M, Porter C, Baqar S, Williams C, Arora R, Saunders J, Ananthakrishnan M, Sanders J, Zaucha G, Turbyfill R, Oaks E (2010) Safety and immunogenicity of a Shigella flexneri 2a Invaplex 50 intranasal vaccine in adult volunteers. Vaccine 28(37):6076–6085. https://doi.org/10.1016/j.vaccine.2010.06.086

Tristram S, Jacobs MR, Appelbaum PC (2007) Antimicrobial resistance in Haemophilus influenzae. Clin Microbiol Rev 20(2):368–389. https://doi.org/10.1128/CMR.00040-06

Trovato M, D'Apice L, Prisco A, De Berardinis P (2018) HIV vaccination: a roadmap among advancements and concerns. Int J Mol Sci 19(4). https://doi.org/10.3390/ijms19041241

Tsaban G, Ben-Shimol S (2017) Indirect (herd) protection, following pneumococcal conjugated vaccines introduction: a systematic review of the literature. Vaccine 35(22):2882–2891. https://doi.org/10.1016/j.vaccine.2017.04.032

USDA APHIS (2014) Salmonella enteritidis on table-egg farms in the United States. https://www.aphisusda.gov/animal_health/nahms/poultry/downloads/layers2013/Layers2013_is_SEpdf. Accessed 8 Sept 2019

Valneva (2016) Valneva's pseudomonas aeruginosa candidate (VLA43) did not confirm positive vaccine effect in phase II/III trial. https://valneva.com/wp-content/uploads/2019/06/2016_06_02_Valneva_Pseudomonas_PR_EN.pdf. Accessed 23 Aug 2019

Van Boeckel TP, Gandra S, Ashok A, Caudron Q, Grenfell BT, Levin SA, Laxminarayan R (2014) Global antibiotic consumption 2000 to 2010: an analysis of national pharmaceutical sales data. Lancet Infect Dis 14(8):742–750. https://doi.org/10.1016/S1473-3099(14)70780-7

van den Dobbelsteen G, Fae KC, Serroyen J, van den Nieuwenhof IM, Braun M, Haeuptle MA, Sirena D, Schneider J, Alaimo C, Lipowsky G, Gambillara-Fonck V, Wacker M, Poolman JT (2016) Immunogenicity and safety of a tetravalent E. coli O-antigen bioconjugate vaccine in animal models. Vaccine 34(35):4152–4160. https://doi.org/10.1016/j.vaccine.2016.06.067

Van Der Meeren O, Hatherill M, Nduba V, Wilkinson RJ, Muyoyeta M, Van Brakel E, Ayles HM, Henostroza G, Thienemann F, Scriba TJ, Diacon A, Blatner GL, Demoitie MA, Tameris M, Malahleha M, Innes JC, Hellstrom E, Martinson N, Singh T, Akite EJ, Khatoon Azam A, Bollaerts A, Ginsberg AM, Evans TG, Gillard P, Tait DR (2018) Phase 2b controlled trial of M72/AS01E vaccine to prevent tuberculosis. N Engl J Med 379(17):1621–1634. https://doi.org/10.1056/NEJMoa1803484

Ventola CL (2016a) Immunization in the United States: recommendations, barriers, and measures to improve compliance: Part 1: Childhood vaccinations. P T 41(7):426–436

Ventola CL (2016b) Immunization in the United States: recommendations, barriers, and measures to improve compliance: Part 2: Adult vaccinations. P T 41(8):492–506

Vesikari T, Karvonen A, Prymula R, Schuster V, Tejedor JC, Cohen R, Meurice F, Han HH, Damaso S, Bouckenooghe A (2007) Efficacy of human rotavirus vaccine against rotavirus gastroenteritis during the first 2 years of life in European infants: randomised, double-blind controlled study. Lancet 370(9601):1757–1763. https://doi.org/10.1016/S0140-6736(07)61744-9

Vidunas E, Mathews A, Weaver M, Cai P, Koh EH, Patel-Brown S, Yuan H, Zheng ZR, Carriere M, Johnson JE, Lotvin J, Moran J (2016) Production and characterization of chemically inactivated genetically engineered clostridium difficile toxoids. J Pharm Sci 105(7):2032–2041. https://doi.org/10.1016/j.xphs.2016.04.017

Vignesh R, Shankar EM, Murugavel KG, Kumarasamy N, Sekar R, Irene P, Solomon S, Balakrishnan P (2008) Urinary infections due to multi-drug-resistant Escherichia coli among persons with HIV disease at a tertiary AIDS care centre in South India. Nephron Clin Pract 110(1):c55–c57. https://doi.org/10.1159/000151533

von Gottberg A, de Gouveia L, Tempia S, Quan V, Meiring S, von Mollendorf C, Madhi SA, Zell ER, Verani JR, O'Brien KL, Whitney CG, Klugman KP, Cohen C, Investigators G-S (2014) Effects of vaccination on invasive pneumococcal disease in South Africa. N Engl J Med 371(20):1889–1899. https://doi.org/10.1056/NEJMoa1401914

von Gottberg A, de Gouviea L, Tempia S, Quan V, Meiring S, von Mollendorf C, Madhi SA, Klugman KP, Whitney CG, Cohen C (2016) Ongoing pneumococcal disease declines and an indirect effect of vaccination, South Africa, 2005–2015. 10th International Symposium on Pneumococci and Pneumococal Disease (ISPPD) Glasgow, Scotland 28 Jul 2016 PO01b 156

von Reyn CF, Mtei L, Arbeit RD, Waddell R, Cole B, Mackenzie T, Matee M, Bakari M, Tvaroha S, Adams LV, Horsburgh CR, Pallangyo K, DarDar Study G (2010) Prevention of tuberculosis in Bacille Calmette-Guerin-primed, HIV-infected adults boosted with an inactivated whole-cell mycobacterial vaccine. AIDS 24(5):675–685. https://doi.org/10.1097/QAD.0b013e3283350f1b

Voth DE, Ballard JD (2005) Clostridium difficile toxins: mechanism of action and role in disease. Clin Microbiol Rev 18(2):247–263. https://doi.org/10.1128/CMR.18.2.247-263.2005

Wahid R, Kotloff KL, Levine MM, Sztein MB (2019) Cell mediated immune responses elicited in volunteers following immunization with candidate live oral Salmonella enterica serovar Paratyphi A attenuated vaccine strain CVD 1902. Clin Immunol 201:61–69. https://doi.org/10.1016/j.clim.2019.03.003

Walker NF, Meintjes G, Wilkinson RJ (2013) HIV-1 and the immune response to TB. Future Virol 8(1):57–80. https://doi.org/10.2217/fvl.12.123

Walsh C (2000) Molecular mechanisms that confer antibacterial drug resistance. Nature 406(6797):775–781. https://doi.org/10.1038/35021219

Walsh TR, Weeks J, Livermore DM, Toleman MA (2011) Dissemination of NDM-1 positive bacteria in the New Delhi environment and its implications for human health: an environmental point prevalence study. Lancet Infect Dis 11(5):355–362. https://doi.org/10.1016/S1473-3099(11)70059-7

Ward JI, Lum MK, Hall DB, Silimperi DR, Bender TR (1986) Invasive Haemophilus influenzae type b disease in Alaska: background epidemiology for a vaccine efficacy trial. J Infect Dis 153(1):17–26. https://doi.org/10.1093/infdis/153.1.17

Weinberger DM, Malley R, Lipsitch M (2011) Serotype replacement in disease after pneumococcal vaccination. Lancet 378(9807):1962–1973. https://doi.org/10.1016/S0140-6736(10)62225-8

Were T, Davenport GC, Hittner JB, Ouma C, Vulule JM, Ong'echa JM, Perkins DJ (2011) Bacteremia in Kenyan children presenting with malaria. J Clin Microbiol 49(2):671–676. https://doi.org/10.1128/JCM.01864-10

Widmer K, Zhu Y, Williams JV, Griffin MR, Edwards KM, Talbot HK (2012) Rates of hospitalizations for respiratory syncytial virus, human metapneumovirus, and influenza virus in older adults. J Infect Dis 206(1):56–62. https://doi.org/10.1093/infdis/jis309

Wiegand PN, Nathwani D, Wilcox MH, Stephens J, Shelbaya A, Haider S (2012) Clinical and economic burden of Clostridium difficile infection in Europe: a systematic review of healthcare-facility-acquired infection. J Hosp Infect 81(1):1–14. https://doi.org/10.1016/j.jhin.2012.02.004

Wilcox MH, Gerding DN, Poxton IR, Kelly C, Nathan R, Birch T, Cornely OA, Rahav G, Bouza E, Lee C, Jenkin G, Jensen W, Kim YS, Yoshida J, Gabryelski L, Pedley A, Eves K, Tipping R, Guris D, Kartsonis N, Dorr MB, Modify I, Investigators MI (2017) Bezlotoxumab for Prevention of Recurrent Clostridium difficile Infection. N Engl J Med 376(4):305–317. https://doi.org/10.1056/NEJMoa1602615

World Health Organization (2014a) Global tuberculosis report. https://www.who.int/tb/publications/global_report/gtbr14_executive_summary.pdf. Accessed 9 Jul 2019

World Health Organization (2014b) Status of vaccine research and development for Paratyphoid fever prepared for WHO PD-VAC. https://www.who.int/immunization/research/meetings_workshops/Paratyphoid_VaccineRD_Sept2014.pdf. Accessed 14 Sept 2019

World Health Organization (2015) Global action plan on antimicrobial resistance. https://apps.who.int/iris/bitstream/handle/10665/193736/9789241509763_eng.pdf. Accessed 11 Jul 2019

World Health Organization (2017a) Global priority list of antibiotic-resistant bacteria to guide research, discovery, and development of new antibiotics. http://www.who.int/medicines/publications/WHO-PPL-Short_Summary_25Feb-ET_NM_WHO.pdf. Accessed 20 Jun 2019

World Health Organization (2017b) Guidelines for the prevention and control of carbapenem-resistant Enterobacteriaceae, Acinetobacter baumannii and Pseudomonas aeruginosa in health care facilities. https://apps.who.int/iris/bitstream/handle/10665/259462/9789241550178-eng.pdf. Accessed 23 Aug 2019

World Health Organization (2018) Global tuberculosis report. https://www.who.int/tb/publications/global_report/tb18_ExecSum_web_4Oct18.pdf. Accessed 13 Jul 2019

World Health Organization (2019a) Global observatory on health R&D. https://www.who.int/research-observatory/monitoring/processes/health_products/en/. Accessed 22 Jun 2019

World Health Organization (2019b) Global vaccine safety blueprint 2.0 background research. https://www.who.int/vaccine_safety/publications/2019_Landscape_Analysispdf. Accessed 30 Oct 2019

Yong D, Toleman MA, Giske CG, Cho HS, Sundman K, Lee K, Walsh TR (2009) Characterization of a new metallo-beta-lactamase gene, bla(NDM-1), and a novel erythromycin esterase gene carried on a unique genetic structure in Klebsiella pneumoniae sequence type 14 from India. Antimicrob Agents Chemother 53(12):5046–5054. https://doi.org/10.1128/AAC.00774-09

Zaman K, Dang DA, Victor JC, Shin S, Yunus M, Dallas MJ, Podder G, Vu DT, Le TP, Luby SP, Le HT, Coia ML, Lewis K, Rivers SB, Sack DA, Schodel F, Steele AD, Neuzil KM, Ciarlet M (2010) Efficacy of pentavalent rotavirus vaccine against severe rotavirus gastroenteritis in

infants in developing countries in Asia: a randomised, double-blind, placebo-controlled trial. Lancet 376(9741):615–623. https://doi.org/10.1016/S0140-6736(10)60755-6
Zambon MC (2001) The pathogenesis of influenza in humans. Rev Med Virol 11(4):227–241
Zhang F, Lu YJ, Malley R (2013) Multiple antigen-presenting system (MAPS) to induce comprehensive B- and T-cell immunity. Proc Natl Acad Sci U S A 110(33):13564–13569. https://doi.org/10.1073/pnas.1307228110
Zhang X, Yang F, Zou J, Wu W, Jing H, Gou Q, Li H, Gu J, Zou Q, Zhang J (2018) Immunization with Pseudomonas aeruginosa outer membrane vesicles stimulates protective immunity in mice. Vaccine 36(8):1047–1054. https://doi.org/10.1016/j.vaccine.2018.01.034
Zhou F, Shefer A, Kong Y, Nuorti JP (2008) Trends in acute otitis media-related health care utilization by privately insured young children in the United States, 1997–2004. Pediatrics 121(2):253–260. https://doi.org/10.1542/peds.2007-0619
Zhou H, Thompson WW, Viboud CG, Ringholz CM, Cheng PY, Steiner C, Abedi GR, Anderson LJ, Brammer L, Shay DK (2012) Hospitalizations associated with influenza and respiratory syncytial virus in the United States, 1993–2008. Clin Infect Dis 54(10):1427–1436. https://doi.org/10.1093/cid/cis211

Index

H. Panwar et al. (eds.), *Sustainable Agriculture Reviews 49*, Sustainable Agriculture Reviews 49, https://doi.org/10.1007/978-3-030-58259-3

The manufacturer's authorised representative in the EU is Springer Nature Customer Service Centre GmbH, Europaplatz 3, 69115 Heidelberg, Germany. If you have any concerns regarding our products, please contact ProductSafety@springernature.com

Printed and bound by CPI Group (UK) Ltd, Croydon, CR0 4YY
30/09/2026
02225501-0011